Informatics and Nursing

Opportunities and Challenges

Fifth Edition

Informatics and Nursing
Opportunities and Challenges

Fifth Edition

Jeanne Sewell, MSN, RN-BC
Associate Professor, School of Nursing
College of Health Sciences
Georgia College & State University
Milledgeville, Georgia

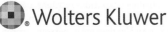 Wolters Kluwer

Philadelphia • Baltimore • New York • London
Buenos Aires • Hong Kong • Sydney • Tokyo

Acquisitions Editor: Christina C. Burns
Product Manager: Meredith Brittain
Editorial Assistant: Cassie Berube
Production Project Manager: Cynthia Rudy
Design Coordinator: Holly McLaughlin
Illustration Coordinator: Jennifer Clements
Manufacturing Coordinator: Karin Duffield
Prepress Vendor: SPi Global

5th edition

9 8 7 6 5 4 3 2 1

Printed in China

Library of Congress Cataloging-in-Publication Data
Sewell, Jeanne P., author.
  Informatics and nursing : opportunities and challenges / Jeanne Sewell. —
Fifth edition.
       p. ; cm.
  Includes bibliographical references.
  ISBN 978-1-4511-9320-6
  I. Title.
  [DNLM: 1. Nursing Informatics. 2. Computers. 3. Internet. 4. Medical Records Systems, Computerized. WY 26.5]
  RT50.5
  610.73—dc23
                                                                              2015013707

LWW.com

About the Author

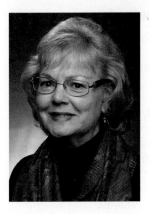

Jeanne Sewell, an associate professor of nursing at Georgia College & State University in Milledgeville, Georgia, is board certified as an informatics nurse specialist. Her credentials include a postgraduate certificate in nursing informatics from Duke University, a Master of Science in Nursing at the University of Maryland at Baltimore, a Bachelor of Science in Nursing at Georgia Regents University–Medical College of Georgia, and a nursing diploma from Georgia Baptist School of Nursing, now Georgia Baptist College of Nursing at Mercer University.

Jeanne's expertise is nursing informatics, nursing education, and the scholarship of teaching and learning. She has received several teaching awards, including the Georgia College & State University 2015 Scholarship of Teaching and Learning Award. She teaches traditional face-to-face classes, as well as blended and online classes, across the nursing curriculum in the following programs: baccalaureate in nursing, RN-BSN, master of science in nursing, and doctor of nursing practice. She has served as a consultant in nursing education and as a speaker at statewide, national, and international conferences.

Jeanne has clinical nursing experience in a variety of settings, including nursing administration, outpatient care, critical care, medical-surgical care, and pediatric nursing. Her interest in nursing informatics began in the early 1980s as she was completing graduate studies, when different clinical information systems began integration.

Contributors

Contributors to the Fifth Edition

Omega Finney, MSN, RN-BC
Informaticist
Piedmont Healthcare
Atlanta, Georgia

Karen Frith, PhD, RN, NEA-BC
Professor and Associate Dean, Undergraduate
Programs
College of Nursing, The University of Alabama in
Huntsville
Huntsville, Alabama

Linda Q. Thede, PhD, RN-BC
Professor Emerita of Nursing
Kent State University
Kent, Ohio

Contributors to the Fourth Edition

Deborah Ariosto, PhD, MSN, RN
Director, Patient Care Informatics
Vanderbilt University Medical Center
Nashville, Tennessee

Pamela J. Correll, RN, MS
Nursing Informatics Consultant
Maine Center for Disease Control and Prevention
Public Health Nursing Program
Bangor, Maine

Karen Frith, PhD, RN, NEA-BC
Professor and Associate Dean, Undergraduate
Programs
College of Nursing, The University of Alabama in
Huntsville
Huntsville, Alabama

Judy Hornbeck, MHSA, BSN, RN
Highland, Illinois

Reviewers

Kerry Allen, MSN
Associate Professor
Southern Adventist University
Collegedale, Tennessee

Kim Amer, PhD, RN
Associate Professor
DePaul University
Chicago, Illinois

Mary Boylston, MSN, EdD
Professor
Eastern University
St. Davids, Pennsylvania

Elizabeth Carlson, PhD
Associate Professor and Systems Leadership DNP
Program Director
Rush University, College of Nursing
Chicago, Illinois

Laura Clayton, PhD, RN, CNE
Assistant Professor of Nursing Education
Shepherd University
Shepherdstown, West Virginia

Prudence Dalrymple, PhD, MS in Informatics
Research and Teaching Professor
Drexel University
Philadelphia, Pennsylvania

Jeff Dowdy, MLIS
Graduate Librarian
Ina Dillard Russell Library, Georgia College &
State University
Milledgeville, Georgia

Tresa Dusaj, PhD(c)
Assistant Professor
Monmouth University
West Long Branch, New Jersey

**Robert Elshaw, MSN, RN-BC, ANCC Board
Certified Informatics Nurse**
Adjunct Faculty
Ursuline College
Pepper Pike, Ohio

Willy Fahlman, BScN, MEd, EdD
Sociology Faculty
Athabasca University
Athabasca, Alberta

Mary Fairbanks, MS, DNP, RN, PHN
Associate Professor
Bemidji State University
Bemidji, Minnesota

Matthew Gaines, AAS
Technical Support Tech
Division on Information Technology, Georgia
College & State University
Milledgeville, Georgia

Debbie Greene, PhD, RN, CNE
Associate Professor and Assistant Director for
Undergraduate Nursing Programs
School of Nursing, Georgia College & State
University
Milledgeville, Georgia

Janis Hayden, EdD, MSN, RN
Professor
St. Francis Medical Center, College of Nursing
Peoria, Illinois

Arlene Holowaychuk, RN, MSN, CNE
Assistant Professor, Preceptor Coordinator
Bon Secours Memorial College of Nursing
Richmond, Virginia

Michelle Hornack, MSN, BSN
Assistant Professor of Nursing
Graceland University
Independence, Missouri

Janice Jones, PhD, RN, CNS
Clinical Professor
University at Buffalo
Buffalo, New York

Rebecca Koeniger-Donahue, PhD, APRN
Professor of Practice
Simmons College
Boston, Massachusetts

Elizabeth Kostas-Polston, PhD, APRN, WHNP-BC, FAANP
Assistant Professor
University of South Florida
Tampa, Florida

Anne Krouse, PhD
Professor
Widener University
Chester, Pennsylvania

Katherine Leigh, DNP, RN
Assistant Professor
Troy University
Dothan, Alabama

Barry Lung, MSN, RN-BC
Informaticist
Byron, Georgia

Rosemary Macy, PhD, RN, CNE, CHSE
Associate Professor
Boise State University
Boise, Idaho

Patricia Martin, MSN
Associate Professor
West Kentucky Community and Technical College
Paducah, Kentucky

Priscilla Okunji, RN-BC, PhD
Nursing Faculty
Howard University
Washington, District of Columbia

Jill Pence, MSN, BSN, RN, CNE
Assistant Professor
Samford University
Birmingham, Alabama

Rorey Pritchard, EdS, MSN, RN-BC, CNOR, CNE
Clinical Assistant Professor
University of Wisconsin, Eau Claire
Eau Claire, Wisconsin

Leandro Resurreccion, BSZ, BSN, MSN, EdD
Professor of Nursing
Oakton Community College
Des Plaines, Illinois

Luis M. Cabret Rios, RN, MSN, APRN, FNP-BC, DNP(s)
Nursing Instructor
Turabo University
Gurabo, Puerto Rico

Nicole Robert, MSN, RN
Faculty Mentor
Thomas Edison State College
Zachary, Louisiana

Lisa Shaffer, MS, MBA
Adjunct Instructor
Galen College of Nursing
Cincinnati, Ohio

Bonnie Stegman, PhD, MSN, RN
Assistant Professor of Nursing and Coordinator
of the BSN Online Completion Program
Maryville University, St. Louis
St. Louis, Missouri

Sharon Stoten, DNP
Assistant Professor
Indiana University East, School of Nursing
Richmond, Indiana

Debra Sullivan, PhD, MSN
Assistant Professor
Middle Tennessee State University
Murfreesboro, Tennessee

Jeanne Tucker, PhD, MSN, RN, HSAD, CHES
Assistant Professor of Nursing
Patty Hanks Shelton School of Nursing
Abilene, Texas

Laureen Turner, MSN, DNP
Instructor
University of San Francisco
San Francisco, California

Denyce Watties-Daniels, MSN
Assistant Professor
Coppin State University
Baltimore, Maryland

Bonnie K. Webster, MS, RN, BC
Assistant Professor
University of Texas, Medical Branch in Galveston,
School of Nursing
Galveston, Texas

Kathleen Williams, MSN, RN-BC (Informatics)
Assistant Professor
Charleston Southern University
North Charleston, South Carolina

Ronda Yoder, PhD, ARNP
Nursing Faculty
Pensacola Christian College
Pensacola, Florida

Preface

Advancements in computer technology and the Internet have made the use of informatics pervasive in our society worldwide. Simply stated, informatics is the use of computers to discover, manipulate, and understand information. Informatics is required to achieve the nursing transformation mentioned by the 2010 Institute of Medicine (IOM) report, *The Future of Nursing*, which includes enabling nurses to be full partners in redesigning healthcare in the United States and to engage in effective workforce planning and policymaking (Committee on the Robert Wood Johnson Foundation Initiative on the Future of Nursing at the Institute of Medicine, Robert Wood Johnson Foundation, & IOM, 2011).

The first edition of this textbook, *Computers in Nursing*, which was published in 1999, was one of the first textbooks to address core informatics competencies for all nurses. Each edition, including this fifth edition, was designed to capture the innovative advancements in nursing informatics core competencies and applications and to teach students how informatics should be integrated into practice. This edition focuses on the best of the fourth edition, such as office computing software, interoperability, consumer informatics, telehealth, and clinical information systems, plus new topics that have entered the field since the last edition, such as social media use guidelines, software and hardware developments, and updates on meaningful use. Each chapter now includes a Quality and Safety Education for Nurses (QSEN) scenario designed to stimulate critical thinking. The book's companion webpage at http://thepoint.lww.com/sewell5e includes many resources for students—for example, a sample database and spreadsheets, as well information on APA templates and e-mail signatures—along with a wealth of resources

for instructors (see the "Additional Resources" section later in this preface for more information). The goal was to make it all interesting—and yes, thought-provoking—to you, the reader. For example, QSEN scenarios, as well as application and competencies critical thinking exercises, align with each chapter's objectives. In the decade and a half since the first edition published, nursing and the entire healthcare arena have come to recognize the importance of informatics.

The major accrediting organizations for nursing, American Association of Colleges of Nursing (AACN) and the National League for Nursing (NLN), have identified informatics as an essential competency for all nurses, ranging from the beginning practitioner to the doctor of nursing practice (DNP), doctor of philosophy (PhD), and doctor of nursing science (DNSc) (AACN, 1996, 2006, 2008, 2010, 2011; NLN, 2008, 2015). A call for nursing education to adopt informatics competencies for all levels of education came from the TIGER Initiative, aimed at using informatics for improving practice with evidence-based information (The TIGER Initiative Foundation, 2014).

Evidence-based decision making using informatics tools should be implemented in healthcare redesign as well as in improvements in data collection and information infrastructure. The textbook includes information on how to discover scholarly journal articles and websites with healthcare information for evidence-based decision making. The learner is introduced to Medline/PubMed, from the U.S. National Library of Medicine, a free library available to users worldwide. Clearly, there is agreement that informatics is an essential tool to address the need to provide evidence-based care with improved outcomes for individuals and populations.

AUDIENCE

The information in this textbook is what every nurse should know. Besides providing information for anyone who is just beginning to learn about nursing informatics, the book is designed for use either as a text for a course in nursing informatics or with a curriculum in which informatics is a vertical strand. Here is a unit-by-unit breakdown of how the material could be used:

- Unit I, Informatics Basics, and Unit II, Computer Applications for Your Professional Career, provide background information that would be useful in undergraduate and graduate introductory courses, or as an introduction to computers and information management.
- Unit III, Information Competency, would be useful at any point in a curriculum.
- Unit IV, The Evolving Healthcare Paradigm, and Unit V, Healthcare Informatics, provide information that would be useful at more advanced levels.
- Unit VI, Computer Uses in Healthcare Beyond Clinical Informatics, can be used as a whole or its individual chapters matched with a course.

International Council of Nurses, the Healthcare Information and Management Systems Society (HIMSS) TIGER Initiative, and two United States nursing accrediting bodies provide direction for incorporating nursing informatics as a core competency into all levels of education programs.

ORGANIZATION AND STRUCTURE

In this fifth edition, the six units were redesigned to improve the organization and flow of the content.

Unit I, Informatics Basics, introduces readers to new guidelines for use of electronic communication with social and professional networking. Chapter 1 (Introduction to Nursing Informatics: Managing Healthcare Information) provides an overview of nursing informatics, including the differences between computers and informatics, the rationale for having basic informatics skills, and the need to be computer fluent and information literate. Chapters 2 (Essential Computer and Software Concepts) and 3 (Basic Computer Networking Concepts) cover essential computer and software concepts, as well as information related to how computers network and communicate. Nurses often use computers without knowing the terminology and the possibilities and limitations of information technology. Chapter 4 (Social and Professional Networking) examines guidelines for use of social and professional networking media. Ethical and legal implications for use of social networking sites are discussed.

Unit II, Computer Applications for Your Professional Career, provides information on the recent versions of office software, including Google Drive, Apache OpenOffice.org, and Microsoft Office. The chapters include additional information to assist the growing number of Mac users. Chapter 5 (Authoring Scholarly Word Documents) demonstrates how to use word processing software to format papers using American Psychological Association writing style. It also addresses the differences between writing a paper for a class assignment and writing for publication. Chapter 6 (Authoring Scholarly Slide Presentations) emphasizes best practices for presentation design. Chapter 7 (Mastering Spreadsheet Software to Assess Quality Outcomes Using Numbers) addresses best practices for designing worksheets and charts. Chapter 8 (Databases: Creating Information from Data) provides an explanation of how databases work, including a short tutorial to assist students in designing a simple database that addresses a nursing care issue. The database concepts discussed are relative to any database, such as the digital library or Internet search engines.

Unit III, Information Competency, includes updated information on this topic. Chapter 9 (Information Literacy: A Road to Evidence-Based Practice) includes information on use of the PICO (patient/problem—intervention—comparison—outcome) research approach, and it includes how to evaluate health information found on the Internet and how to analyze scholarly articles. Chapter 10 (Finding Knowledge in the Digital Library Haystack) reviews how to search digital libraries and use filters from PubMed, the free National Library of Medicine digital library. Chapter 11 (Mobile Computing) covers the latest mobile computing devices and resources.

In Unit IV, The Evolving Healthcare Paradigm, Chapters 12 (Informatics Benefits for the

Consumer) and 13 (The Empowered Consumer) address information for empowering healthcare consumers, the importance of personal health records, and challenges consumers face accessing and understanding health information. Chapters 14 (Interoperability at the National and the International Levels) and 15 (Nursing Documentation in the Age of the Electronic Health Record) discuss standards and terminology necessary for interoperability and data abstraction from electronic records using standardized terminology for documenting the electronic health record.

Unit V, Healthcare Informatics, focuses on use of informatics in the healthcare setting. Chapter 16 (Nursing Informatics: Theoretical Basis, Education Program, and Profession) explores informatics as a nursing specialty, including information on the theory base for nursing informatics, educational programs, and professional organizations. Chapter 17 (Electronic Healthcare Information Systems, Electronic Health Records, and Meaningful Use) reviews the progress toward implementation of the electronic health record (EHR), as well as "meaningful use" and the implications for improving healthcare delivery. Chapter 18 (Design Considerations for Healthcare Information Systems) provides an overview of healthcare information systems, systems selection, and the systems life cycle, a process used to plan and implement a computer system. Chapter 19 (Quality Measures and Specialized Electronic Healthcare Information Systems) reviews information on specialized electronic healthcare information systems and quality measures to improve care outcomes. Chapter 20 (Electronic Healthcare System Issues) covers issues associated with the use of information systems. When documentation moved from paper to electronic systems, new problems emerged that nurses need to understand in order to mitigate. Finally, Chapter 21 (Evolving Trends in Telehealth) addresses exciting new developments in telehealth, which allows supplementation of face-to-face care with technology that supports care delivery in the patient's home, emergency departments, and intensive care units.

Unit VI, Computer Uses in Healthcare Beyond Clinical Informatics, includes the use of informatics in other nursing settings. Chapter 22 (Educational Informatics: e-Learning) describes the use of informatics in nursing education. Chapter 23 (Informatics in Management and Quality Improvement) covers management information technology tools. Chapter 24 (Informatics and Research) discusses the use of informatics for nursing research. Chapter 25 (Legal and Ethical Issues) addresses the legal and ethical challenges that informatics introduces, encompassing data breaches and copyright issues.

Information on the newest computer and software features is included in the textbook appendix. This overview may serve as a course lesson, depending on the computer knowledge of the students. Key terms in each of the book's chapters are defined in the glossary. Because nursing students often identify information technology terminology as new and challenging, the glossary terms provide learning support.

In summary, the topics in this textbook address informatics competencies and applications needed by all nurses, now and in the near future. Nurses with communication skills enhanced with the use of technology, computer fluency, information literacy skills, and knowledge of informatics terminology and clinical information systems can assist in shaping nursing practice to improve patient outcomes and to contribute to the scholarship of nursing.

ADDITIONAL RESOURCES

Informatics and Nursing includes additional resources for both instructors and students that are available on the book's companion website at http://thepoint.lww.com/sewell5e.

Instructors

Approved adopting instructors will be given access to the following additional resources:

- **Ebook:** Allows access to the book's full text and images online.
- **PowerPoint Slides:** Provide an easy way for you to integrate the textbook with your students' classroom experience through either slide shows or handouts.

- **Case Studies:** Bring the content to life through real-world situations with these scenarios, which can be used as class activities or group assignments.
- **Test Generator:** Lets you put together exclusive new tests from a bank to help you assess your students' understanding of the material. These questions are formatted to match the NCLEX (National Council Licensure Examination), so that your students can have practice with the question types covered in this important examination.
- **Suggested answers to the QSEN scenarios found in the book.**
- **QSEN Map:** Shows how the book content integrates QSEN competencies.
- **BSN Essentials Competencies Map:** Shows how the book content integrates American Association of Colleges of Nursing (AACN) Essentials of Baccalaureate Education for Professional Nursing Practice competencies.
- **TIGER Competencies Map:** Shows how the book content integrates Technology Informatics Guiding Educational Reform (TIGER) competencies.
- **Image Bank:** Contains all the illustrations and tables from the book in formats suitable for printing and incorporating into PowerPoint presentations and Internet sites.
- **Strategies for Effective Teaching:** Offer creative approaches for engaging students.
- **Learning Management System Cartridges.**

Students

Students who have purchased *Informatics and Nursing*, fifth edition, have access to the following additional resources:

- **Journal Articles:** One article per chapter offers access to current research available in Wolters Kluwer journals.
- **Weblinks:** These URLs point readers to helpful online resources for each chapter.
- **Acronyms:** This list of abbreviations and their spell outs demystifies the alphabet soup of the informatics field.

- **Additional Information and Examples:** Users can download digital versions of examples used for the office software chapters, among others, from thePoint.
- Plus a **Spanish-English Audio Glossary, Nursing Professional Roles and Responsibilities**, and **Learning Objectives**.

See the inside front cover of this text for more details, including the passcode you will need to gain access to the website.

REFERENCES

American Association of Colleges of Nursing. (1996). The essentials of master's education for advanced practice nursing. Retrieved from http://www.aacn.nche.edu/education-resources/MasEssentials96.pdf

American Association of Colleges of Nursing. (2006). The essentials of doctoral education for advanced nursing practice. Retrieved from http://www.aacn.nche.edu/publications/position/DNP Essentials.pdf

American Association of Colleges of Nursing. (2008). The essentials of baccalaureate education for professional nursing practice. Retrieved from http://www.aacn.nche.edu/education-resources/BaccEssentials08.pdf

American Association of Colleges of Nursing. (2010). The research-focused doctoral program in nursing: Pathways to excellence. Retrieved from http://www.aacn.nche.edu/education-resources/PhDPosition.pdf

American Association of Colleges of Nursing. (2011). The essentials of master's education in nursing. Retrieved from http://www.aacn.nche.edu/education-resources/Masters Essentials11.pdf

Committee on the Robert Wood Johnson Foundation Initiative on the Future of Nursing at the Institute of Medicine, Robert Wood Johnson Foundation, & Institute of Medicine. (2011). *The future of nursing: Leading change, advancing health.* Washington, DC: National Academies Press.

National League for Nursing. (2008). *Preparing the next generation of nurses to practice in a technology-rich environment: An informatics agenda.* New York: NLN Press.

National League for Nursing. (2015). A vision for the changing faculty role: Preparing students for the technological world of health care. Retrieved from http://www.nln.org/docs/default-source/about/nln-vision-series-%28position-statements%29/a-vision-for-the-changing-faculty-role-preparing-students-for-the-technological-world-of-health-care.pdf?sfvrsn=0

Technology Informatics Guiding Education Reform. (2014). *The TIGER initiative.* Retrieved from http://www.thetiger-initiative.org/

Acknowledgments

Several colleagues contributed to this fifth textbook edition. Jeff Dowdy shared his librarian expertise for Chapter 10 edits on digital libraries. Linda Thede, who has expertise with nursing taxonomy, wrote the revisions for Chapter 15 on nursing documentation. Barry Lung, a nursing informatics expert and a recently retired informatics consultant, provided his expertise for Chapters 18, 19, and 20 edits on clinical information systems. Omega Finney, who is certified as an informatics nurse specialist and works as an informatics nurse specialist at Piedmont Healthcare, provided the updates for Chapter 16 on nursing informatics. She also wrote the section in that chapter titled A Day in the Life of an Informatics Nurse Specialist. Omega is a recipient of an Informatics Nurse of the Year award at Piedmont Healthcare. Karen Frith, who is board certified as an advanced nurse executive, wrote and updated Chapters 23 and 24 on research and administrative tools. Matthew Gaines, an information technology specialist, provided his technical support expertise for the updated appendix on hardware and software. In addition, the feedback from peer reviewers, faculty, and students who have used the textbook helped to guide the changes and updates. Numerous others assisted in editing and rewriting, including Meredith Brittain, a Supervisory Product Development Editor at Wolters Kluwer.

I appreciate the opportunity to have coauthored the third and fourth editions of the textbook with Linda Thede. Thanks also go to my husband, faculty colleagues, and friends for their support while preparing this edition. Finally, I extend a special thanks to my mother, Daisy Penny, for fostering my love of nursing and nursing informatics.

Contents

6. Authoring Scholarly Slide Presentations 82

7. Mastering Spreadsheet Software to Assess Quality Outcomes Using Numbers 99

Informatics Basics

Informatics is too often viewed solely as one of its components instead of as a whole. Its primary goal is information management, but knowledge of each of these divisions is a necessary part of informatics. This opening unit introduces these components and then focuses on the tool of informatics: the computer.

Chapter 1 presents a brief overview of informatics (what it is, the factors that are making it increasingly important in healthcare) and takes a look at its components (information management, computer competency, and information literacy). Chapter 2 addresses essential computer and software concepts, including technical terminology that you may not be aware of even if you grew up using computers. Basic computer networking concepts are the focus of Chapter 3, whereas the last chapter in this unit, Chapter 4, addresses social and professional networking.

CHAPTER 1

Introduction to Nursing Informatics: Managing Healthcare Information

OBJECTIVES

After studying this chapter, you will be able to:

1. Distinguish between the computer and informatics.

2. Define nursing informatics.

3. Describe some of the forces inside and outside healthcare that are driving a move toward a greater use of informatics.

4. Explain the need for all nurses to have basic skills in informatics.

5. Interpret the need for nurses to be computer fluent and information literate in today's healthcare environment.

KEY TERMS

Aggregated data

Computer fluency

Computer literacy

Data

Deidentified data

Electronic health record (EHR)

Electronic Numerical Integrator and Computer (ENIAC)

Evidence-based care

Genomics

Healthcare informatics

Health information technology (HIT)

Informatics

Information literacy

Information technology

Interoperable

Listserv

Nursing informatics

Office of the National Coordinator for Health Information Technology (ONC)

Protocols

Quality and Safety Education for Nurses (QSEN)

Secondary data

Technology Informatics Guiding Educational Reform (TIGER)

In attempting to arrive at the truth, I have applied everywhere for information, but in scarcely an instance have I been able to obtain hospital records fit for any purposes of comparison. If they could be obtained, they would enable us to decide many other questions besides the ones alluded to. They would show subscribers how their money was being spent, what amount of good was really being done with it, or whether the money was not doing mischief rather than good ... (Nightingale, 1863, p. 176).

INFORMATICS INTRODUCTION

What is informatics? Isn't it just about computers? Taking care of patients is nursing's primary concern, not thinking about computers! It is common for some nurses to have these thoughts. Transitions are always difficult, and a transition to using more technology in managing information is no exception. The use of **information technology** (IT) in healthcare is **informatics**, and its focus is information management, not computers. The quality of future patient care and nursing practice is dependent upon nurses effectively using informatics.

Information management is an integral part of nursing. Think about your practice for a minute. What besides your nursing education and experience do you depend upon when providing care for patients? You need to know the patient's history, medical conditions, medications, laboratory results, and more. Could you care for a patient without this information? How this information is organized and presented affects the care that you can provide, as well as the time you spend finding it.

The old way is to record and keep the information for a patient's current admission in a paper chart. Today, with several specialties, consults, medications, laboratory reports, and procedures, the paper chart is inadequate. A well-designed information system, developed with you and for you, can facilitate finding and using information that you need for patient care. Informatics skills enable you to participate in and benefit from this process. Informatics does not perform miracles; it requires an investment by you, the clinician, to assist those who design information systems so the systems are helpful and do not impede your workflow.

If healthcare is to improve, it is imperative that there be a workforce that can innovate and implement **health information technology (HIT)** (American Health Information Management Association & American Medical Informatics Association, 2006, p. 3). There are two roles in informatics: the informatics nurse specialist and the clinician who must use HIT. This means that in essence every nurse has a role in informatics. Information, the subject of informatics, is the structure on which healthcare is built. Except for purely technical procedures (of which there are few, if any), a healthcare professional's work revolves around information. Is the laboratory report available? When is Mrs. X for surgery scheduled? What are the contraindications for the prescribed drug? What is Mr. Y's history? What orders did the physician leave for Ms. Z? Where is the latest x-ray report?

An important part of healthcare information is nursing documentation. When information systems designed for nursing exist, the documentation can expand our knowledge of what constitutes quality healthcare. Have you ever wondered if the patient for whom you provided care had an outcome similar to others with the same condition? From nursing documentation, are you easily able to see the relationship between nursing diagnoses, interventions, and outcomes for your patients? Without knowledge of these chain events, you have only your intuition and old knowledge to use when making decisions about the best interventions in patient care. Observations tend to be self-selective; however, there is better information on which to base patient care. Informatics can furnish the information needed to see these relationships and to provide care based on actual patient **data**, which are facts stored in the computer.

If Florence Nightingale were with us today, she would be a champion of the push toward more use of healthcare IT. Information in a paper chart essentially disappears into a black hole after discharging a patient. Because we cannot easily access it, we cannot learn from it and use it in future patient care. This realization is international. Many countries, especially those with a national health service, have long realized the need to be able to use information buried in charts. Tommy Thompson, the former United States Secretary of Health and Human Services, is quoted as saying "the most remarkable feature of this 21st century medicine is that we hold it together with 19th century paperwork" (Committee on Government Reform, 2004).

The introduction of bills in the U.S. Congress backed up Thompson's statement. The President's Information Technology Advisory Committee (PITAC) created support for greater use of informatics. PITAC responsibilities transferred to the President's Council of Advisors on Science and Technology in the Office of Science and Technology Policy in 2005 (Office of Science and Technology Policy, 2013).

In 2004, President Bush called for adoption of **interoperable electronic health records (EHRs)** for most Americans by 2014. He also established the position of National Coordinator for Health Information Technology. The **Office of the National Coordinator for Health Information Technology (ONC)** released the first Federal Health HIT strategic plan for 2008–2012, which focused on two goals—patient-focused healthcare and population health. The common themes for the goals included privacy and security, interoperability, adoption, and collaborative governance. The 2011–2015 strategic plan was released with a mission to improve health and healthcare for all Americans through information and technology. The strategic plan expanded on the initial plan with five goals that affect nurses and healthcare (Box 1-1).

BOX 1-1   2011–2015 Strategic Plan Goals

1. Achieve adoption and information exchange through meaningful use of health IT.
   a. Accelerate adoption of electronic medical records.
   b. Facilitate information exchange to support meaningful use of electronic health records.
   c. Support health IT adoption and information exchange for public health and populations with unique needs.
2. Improve care, improve population health, and reduce healthcare costs through the use of health IT.
   a. Support more sophisticated uses of EHRs and other health IT to improve health system performance.
   b. Better manage care, efficiency, and population health through EHR-generated reporting measures.
   c. Demonstrate health IT–enabled reform of payment structures, clinical practices, and population health management.
   d. Support new approaches to the use of health IT in research, public and population health, and national health security.
3. Inspire confidence and trust in health IT.
   a. Protect confidentiality, integrity, and availability of health information.
   b. Inform individuals of their rights and increase the transparency regarding the uses of protected health information.
   c. Improve safety and effectiveness of health IT.
4. Empower individuals with health IT to improve their health and the healthcare system.
   a. Engage individuals with health IT.
   b. Accelerate individual and caregiver access to their electronic health information in a format they can use and reuse.
   c. Integrate patient-generated health information and consumer health IT with clinical applications to support patient-centered care.
5. Achieve rapid learning technological advancement.
   a. Lead the creation of a learning health system to support quality, research, and public and population health.
   b. Broaden the capacity of health IT through innovation and research.

Adapted from HealthIT.gov (2011).

To fulfill these goals, information, which is the structure on which healthcare is built, can no longer be managed with paper. If we are to provide **evidence-based care**, we must make the mountains of data hidden in medical records reveal their secrets. Bakken (2001) proposed the need for five components to provide evidence-based care:

1. Standardization of terminologies and structures used in documentation.
2. The use of digital information.
3. Standards to permit healthcare data exchange between heterogeneous entities.
4. The ability to capture data relevant to the actual care provided.
5. Competency among practitioners to use these data.

All of these components are parts of informatics.

The Affordable Care Act (ACA), signed into law in 2010, made improvements in healthcare coverage, lowered costs, and increased access to care (HHS.gov/HealthCare, 2014). To be able to assess ACA compliance and care outcomes, all nurses must have data analysis skills, and there is an increased need for informatics nurse specialists.

The complexity of today's healthcare milieu, added to the explosion of knowledge, makes it impossible for any clinician to remember everything needed to provide high-quality patient care. Additionally, healthcare consumers today want their healthcare providers to integrate all known relevant scientific knowledge when providing care. We have passed the time when the unaided human mind can perform this feat. The changes in practice that are needed as new knowledge becomes available require modern information management tools as well as a commitment by healthcare professionals to evidence-based practice.

INFORMATICS DISCIPLINE

Informatics is about managing information. The tendency to relate it to computers comes from the fact that the ability to manage large amounts of information was born with the computer and progressed as computers became more powerful and commonplace. However, human ingenuity is the crux of informatics. The term "informatics" originated from the Russian term "informatika"

(Sackett & Erdley, 2002). A Russian publication, Oznovy Informatiki (Foundations of Informatics), published in 1968, is credited with the origins of the general discipline of informatics (Bansal, 2002, p. 10). At that time, the term related to the context of computers. The term "medical informatics" was the first term to identify informatics in healthcare. It meant information technologies concerned with patient care and the medical decision-making process. Another definition stated that medical informatics is complex data processing by the computer to create new information.

As with many healthcare enterprises, there was debate about whether "medical" referred only to informatics focusing on physician concerns or whether it refers to all healthcare disciplines. We now recognize that other disciplines, such as nursing, are a part of healthcare and have a body of knowledge separate from medicine. For this reason, we more commonly use the term **healthcare informatics**. In essence, informatics is the management of information, by using cognitive skills and the computer.

Healthcare Informatics

Healthcare informatics focuses on managing information in all healthcare disciplines. It is an umbrella term that describes the capture, retrieval, storage, presenting, sharing, and use of biomedical information, data, and knowledge for providing care, problem solving, and decision making (Shortliffe & Blois, 2001). The purpose is to improve the use of healthcare data, information, and knowledge in supporting patient care, research, and education (Delaney, 2001). The focus is on the subject, information, rather than the tool, the computer. This is analogous to using another data acquisition tool, the stethoscope, to gather information about heart and lung sounds (Figure 1-1). This distinction is not always obvious because mastery of computer skills is necessary to manage the information. We use the computer to acquire, organize, manipulate, and present the information. The computer will not produce anything of value without human direction. That includes human input for how, when, and where the data are acquired, treated, interpreted, manipulated, and presented. Informatics provides that human direction.

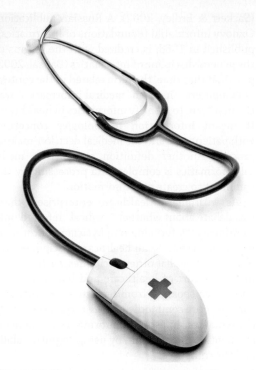

Figure 1-1. The computer as a data acquisition tool. (shutterstock.com/JIL Photo.)

Nursing Informatics

Healthcare has many disciplines; thus, it is not surprising that healthcare informatics has many specialties, of which nursing is one. The American Nurses Association (ANA) recognized **nursing informatics** as a subspecialty of nursing in 1992. The first administration of the informatics certification examination was fall of 1995 (Newbold, 1996). Managing information pertaining to nursing is the focus of nursing informatics. Specialists in this area study how we acquire, manipulate, store, present, and use nursing information. Informatics nurse specialists work with clinical nurses to identify nursing needs for information and support. These specialists work with system developers to design systems that work to complement the practice needs of nurses.

Informatics nurse specialists bring to system development and implementation a viewpoint that supports the needs of the clinical end user. The objective is an information system that is not only user friendly for data input but also presents the clinical nurse with needed information in a manner that is timely and useful. This is not to say that nursing informatics stands alone; it is an integral part of the interdisciplinary field of healthcare informatics, hence related to and responsible to all the healthcare disciplines. (The nursing informatics subspecialty will be explored in more detail in Chapter 16.)

Definitions of Nursing Informatics

The term *nursing informatics* was probably first used and defined by Scholes and Barber in 1980 in their address that year to the MEDINFO conference in Tokyo. There is still no definitive agreement on exactly what this term means. As Simpson (1998) once said, defining nursing informatics is difficult because it is a moving target. The original definition said that nursing informatics was the use of computer technology in all nursing endeavors: nursing services, education, and research (Scholes & Barber, 1980). Hannah et al. (1994) wrote another early definition that followed the broad definition by Scholes and Barber. Hannah et al. (1994) defined nursing informatics as any use of information technologies in carrying out nursing functions. Like the definition by Scholes and Barber, the one by Hannah et al. focused on the technology. The interpretations of those definitions meant any use of the computer, from word processing to the creation of artificial intelligence for nurses, as long as the computer use involved the practice of professional nursing.

The shift from a technology orientation in definitions to one that is more information oriented started in the mid-1980s with Schwirian (Staggers & Thompson, 2002). Schwirian (1986) created a model for use as a framework for nursing informatics investigators. The model consisted of four elements arranged in a pyramid with a triangular base. The top of the pyramid was the desired goal of nursing informatics activity and the base was composed of three elements: (1) users (nurses and students), (2) raw material or nursing information, and (3) the technology, which is computer hardware and software. They all interact in nursing informatics activity to achieve a goal. The intention of the model was as a stimulus for research.

The first widely circulated definition that moved from technology to concepts was from Graves and Corcoran (Staggers & Thompson, 2002). They defined nursing informatics as "a combination of computer science, information science and nursing science designed to assist in the management and processing of nursing data, information and knowledge to support the practice of nursing and the delivery of nursing care" (Graves & Cocoran, 1989, p. 227). This definition secured the position of nursing informatics within the practice of nursing and placed the emphasis on data, information, and knowledge (Staggers & Thompson, 2002). Many consider it the seminal definition of nursing informatics.

Turley (1996), after analyzing previous definitions, added another discipline, cognitive science, to the base for nursing informatics. Cognitive science emphasizes the human factor in informatics. Its focus is the nature of knowledge, its components, development, and use. Goossen (1996), thinking along the same lines, used the definition by Graves and Corcoran as a basis and expanded the meaning of nursing informatics to include the thinking that is done by nurses to make knowledge-based decisions and inferences for patient care. By using this interpretation, he felt that nursing informatics should focus on analyzing and modeling the cognitive processing for all areas of nursing practice. Goossen also stated that nursing informatics should look at the effects of computerized systems on nursing care delivery.

In 1992, the first ANA definition added the role of the informatics nurse specialist to the definition by Graves and Corcoran. The 2014 ANA definition of the specialty of nursing informatics (NI) has expanded from the original 2001 definition. Originally, it stated that this specialty combines nursing, information, and computer sciences for the purpose of managing and communicating data, information, and knowledge to support nurses and healthcare providers in decision making (American Nurses Association, 2001). An update in 2008 included the term wisdom to the data, information, and knowledge continuum (American Nurses Association, 2008). The 2015 definition states that "NI supports consumers, patients, the interprofessional healthcare team, and other stakeholders in their decision making in all roles and settings to achieve desired outcomes. This support is accomplished through the use of information structures, information processes, and information technology" (American Nurses Association, 2015, p. 12). ANA states that the goal of NI is to optimize information management and communication to improve the health of individuals, families, populations, and communities.

Staggers and Thompson (2002), who believe that the evolution of definitions will continue, pointed out that in all of the current definitions, the role of the patient is underemphasized. Some early definitions included the patient, but as a passive recipient of care. With the advent of the Internet, more and more patients are taking an active role in their healthcare. This factor not only changes the dynamics of healthcare but also permits a definition of nursing informatics that recognizes that patients as well as healthcare professionals are consumers of healthcare information. For example, patients may participate in keeping their medical records current. Staggers and Thompson (2002) also pointed out that we overlooked the role of the nurse as an integrator of information. They recommended including it in future definitions.

Despite these definitions, the focus of much of today's practice informatics is still on capturing data at the point of care and presenting it in a manner that facilitates the care of an individual patient. Although this is a vital first step, we must give thought to **secondary data** analysis, or analysis of data for purposes other than the purpose of the original collection. You can make decisions based on actual patient care data by using **aggregated data**, or the same piece(s) of data. For example, you can analyze outcomes of a given intervention for many patients. Understanding how informatics can serve you as an individual nurse, as well as the profession, puts you in a position to work with informatics nurse specialists to retrieve data needed to improve patient care.

QSEN Scenario

After sharing that you are learning about informatics with a nursing colleague, the colleague asks you what informatics has to do with the quality and safety of nursing practice. How would you respond?

FORCES DRIVING MORE USE OF INFORMATICS IN HEALTHCARE

The ultimate goal of healthcare informatics is a lifetime EHR with decision support systems. These records will include standardized data, permit consumers to access their records, and provide for secondary use of healthcare data. Ultimately, when emergency medical services and primary care facilities have access to and can contribute to the EHR, there are immense possibilities to provide seamless care and communication with patients. Forces driving more use of informatics in healthcare include national initiatives, nursing, healthcare consumer empowerment, patient safety, and costs.

National Forces

Federal efforts behind a move to EHRs include the creation of the Office of the National Coordinator for Health Information Technology (ONC). Several seminal reports aimed at improving healthcare, all of which foresee a large role for IT, were published by the Institute of Medicine (IOM), which is an independent body that acts as an adviser to the U.S. government to improve healthcare. Their report *Health Professions Education: A Bridge to Quality* (Greiner & Knebel, 2003) includes informatics as a core competency required of all healthcare professionals. In the report *Crossing the Quality Chasm: A New Health System for the 21st Century* (Committee on Quality of Health Care in America & Institute of Medicine, 2001), HIT is seen as an important force in improving healthcare. Some of the HIT themes in this report are a national information infrastructure, computerized clinical data, use of the Internet, clinical decision support, and evidence-based practice integration. (See Chapter 14 for more information on U.S. government efforts.)

The pervasive use of technology in healthcare is another driving force. Technologies to manage care, such as electronic health records, smart beds, computerized intravenous pumps, and telehealth, are examples of technology that although it assists nurses to improve patient care outcomes (Needleman, 2013), needs to be understood and managed. Other forces such as the changing healthcare environment and increasing patient acuity are affecting the move toward informatics.

Nursing Forces

Nursing also recognized the need for informatics. In 1962, before conceptualization of the term informatics, Dr. Harriet Werley understood the value of nursing data and insisted that the ANA make research about nursing information a priority. Nurses wrote many articles about informatics in the intervening years. In 1982, Gary Hales at the University of Texas, Austin, started the journal *Computers in Nursing* as a mimeograph sheet. Although today it is a full-fledged journal in its fourth decade, in 1982 few nurses realized the value of and need for informatics.

The Robert Wood Johnson Foundation (2010) study revealed that nurses believe technology can improve workflow, communication, and documentation; however, many technologies are still not "user-friendly." Although technology has the potential to improve nursing, there is still work that must be done. The bedside clinician has an integral role in that work. The clinical nurse with essential nursing competencies can and must assist in designing user-friendly technologies that improve care delivery and care outcomes.

Nursing Organizations

In 1993, the National Center for Nursing Research released the report *Nursing Informatics: Enhancing Patient Care* (Pillar & Golumbic, 1993), which set the following six program goals for nursing informatics research:

1. Establish a nursing language (useful in computerized documentation).
2. Develop methods to build clinical information databases.
3. Determine how nurses give patient care using data, information, and knowledge.
4. Develop and test patient care decision support systems.
5. Develop workstations that provide nurses with needed information.
6. Develop appropriate methods to evaluate nursing information systems.

The above are still pertinent, although today number three would include wisdom.

In 1997, the Division of Nursing of the Health Resources and Services Administration convened the National Advisory Council on Nurse Education and Practice. The council produced the *National Informatics Agenda for Education and Practice*, which made the following five recommendations (National Advisory Council on Nurse Education and Practice, 1997, p. 8):

1. Educate nursing students and practicing nurses in core informatics content.
2. Prepare nurses with specialized skills in informatics.
3. Enhance nursing practice and education through informatics projects.
4. Prepare nursing faculty in informatics.
5. Increase collaborative efforts in nursing informatics.

The National League for Nursing (NLN) (2008) published a position paper outlining recommendations for preparing nurses to work in an environment that uses technology. The paper outlined recommendations for nursing faculty, deans/directors/chairs, and the NLN. Examples of recommendations included the need for faculty to achieve informatics competencies and incorporate informatics into the nursing curriculum.

The American Association of Colleges of Nursing's (AACN's) Essentials for baccalaureate, master's, and doctoral education lists of core competencies include many recommendations in the area of information and healthcare technologies. Examples include the use of information and communication technologies, the use of ethics in the application of technology, and the enhancement of one's knowledge using information technologies (AACN, 2006, 2008, 2011).

The ANA has been another force moving nursing toward the effective use of informatics. In 1992, they published two documents, Standards of Practice for Nursing Informatics and The Scope of Practice for Nursing Informatics. In 2008, *Nursing Informatics: Scope & Standards of Practice* combined the two publications into one document. The publication of the most recent edition was 2014.

The American Organization of Nurse Executives (AONE) (2012) issued a position paper on the Nursing Informatics (NI) Executive Leader. The paper identifies that nursing leaders are key to influencing healthcare reform in all settings where they bridge the new practice delivery models with the right technology. AONE recognizes the importance of clinical data captured with the EHR in decision making. AONE recommends master's and doctoral education for the NI Executive Leader.

The **Technology Informatics Guiding Educational Reform (TIGER)** Initiative originated after several years of planning, with a 2-day invitation-only conference starting October 30, 2006. TIGER's objective is to make nursing informatics competencies part of every nurse's skillset, with the aim of making informatics the stethoscope of the 21st century (Technology Guiding Educational Reform, 2007). TIGER is working to ensure that nursing can be fully engaged in the digital era of healthcare by ensuring that all nurses are educated in using informatics, empowering them to deliver safer, high-quality, evidence-based care.

Patient Safety

Patient safety is a primary concern and the one that drives many informatics initiatives. At least 10 patient safety databases use aggregated healthcare data to identify safety issues. Aggregated data are data from more than one source and grouped for comparison. Most, such as the National Healthcare Safety Network (NHSN) from the Centers for Disease Control and Prevention (CDC) and the National Database of Nursing Quality Indicators from ANA, are voluntary. Two safety databases, the vaccine adverse event report system from the CDC and the U.S. Food and Drug Administration (FDA), are mandatory.

The **Quality and Safety Education for Nurses (QSEN)** Institute is an initiative initially funded by the Robert Wood Johnson Foundation. The Case Western Reserve University now hosts the QSEN Institute (QSEN Institute, 2014). QSEN Institute initiatives unfolded with four phases. Phase I addressed IOM's five competencies—patient-centered care, teamwork and collaboration, evidence-based practice, quality improvement, and informatics—plus safety, for six goals. Phase II integrated the competencies in pilot nursing programs. Phase III continued to promote the implementation and evaluation of knowledge, skills, and attitudes associated with the six competencies. Phase IV addressed the recommendation of the 2010 Institute of Medicine report *The Future of Nursing: Campaign for Action*, by funding initiatives supporting academic progression in nursing.

The QSEN Institute competencies developed in Phase II are online at http://qsen.org/competencies/ for prelicensure and graduate education. Many nursing programs use the competencies in the design of curricula. The categories for the competencies are as follows:

- Patient-centered care
- Teamwork and collaboration
- Evidence-based practice
- Quality improvement
- Safety
- Informatics.

Some other informatics implementations that focus on safety include barcode medication administration (BCMA) and computerized provider order entry (CPOE). A well-designed CPOE system cannot only prevent transcription errors but, when combined with a patient's record, can also flag any condition that might present a hazard or would need additional assessment. Clinical decision support systems that provide clinicians with suggested care information or remind busy clinicians of items easy to forget or overlook are also being pushed to improve patient safety. (CPOE will be further discussed in Chapters 17, 18 and 19.)

Costs

Healthcare costs are also driving the move to using informatics. One example is the Leapfrog Group (http://leapfroggroup.org/). Upset by the rising cost of healthcare, in 1998, a group of chief executives of leading corporations in the United States discussed how they could have an influence on its quality and affordability (Leapfrog Group, 2014a). The executives were spending billions of dollars on healthcare for their employees, but they lacked a way of assessing its quality or comparing healthcare providers. The Business Roundtable provided the initial funding, and this group took the name "Leapfrog Group" in November 2000. The 1999 IOM report, *To Err Is Human*, which reported up to 98,000 preventable hospital deaths and recommended that large employers use their purchasing power to improve the quality and safety of healthcare, gave further impetus to the move.

Today, the Robert Wood Johnson Foundation, Leapfrog members, and others also support the Leapfrog Group. Their mission is to support healthcare decisions by those who use and pay for healthcare and promote high-value healthcare using incentives and awards (Leapfrog Group, 2014b). Efforts toward the mission are met by collecting data voluntarily submitted by hospitals and posting this information on The Hospital Safety Score Web site (http://www.leapfroggroup.org/cp). Consumers can use this Web site to check the outcomes of hospitals in their areas for selected procedures.

Members of the Leapfrog Group also educate their employees about patient safety and the importance of comparing healthcare providers. They offer financial incentives to their covered employees for selecting care from hospitals that meet their standards. Healthcare providers without information systems will have a difficult time providing the information that healthcare buyers demand and could see a loss of patients.

As healthcare informatics moves to solve these problems, the need for interdisciplinary, enterprise-wide, information management becomes clearer. The advances of HIT coupled with the evolution of the EHR create a steady progression to this end. Integration of HIT, however, is not without its perils. Any discipline that is not ready for this integration may find itself lost in the process. For nursing to be a part of healthcare informatics, all nurses must become familiar with the value of nursing data, how to capture date, the terminology needed to capture it, and methods for analyzing and manipulating it. True integration of data from all healthcare disciplines will improve patient care and the patient experience, as well as enabling economic gains.

THE INFORMATION MANAGEMENT TOOL: COMPUTERS

In 1850, the collection of all the medical knowledge known to the Western world would fit into two large volumes, making it possible for one person to read and assimilate the entire information. The situation today is dramatically different. The number of journals available in healthcare and the research that fills them is increasing many times over. Even in the early 1990s, if physicians read two journal articles a day, by the end of a year, they would be 800 years behind in their reading (McDonald, 1994). In the early 2000s, there was an expectation that the healthcare clinician might know something about 10,000 different diseases and syndromes, 3,000 medications, 1,100 laboratory tests, and the information in the more than 400,000 articles added to the biomedical information each year (Davenport & Glaser, 2002). The number of journals, books, blogs, and news articles is growing exponentially on a daily basis. Additionally, current knowledge is constantly changing: one can expect much of one's knowledge to be obsolete in 5 years or less.

In healthcare, the increase in knowledge has led to the development of many specialties, such as respiratory therapy, neonatology, and gerontology, and subspecialties within each of these. The proliferation of the specialties spawned the development of many miraculous treatments. However, the number of specialties can fractionalize healthcare, resulting in difficulty gaining an overview of the entire patient. Additionally, the pressure of accomplishing the tasks necessary for a patient's physical recovery usually leaves little time for perusing a patient's record and putting together the bits and pieces so carefully charted by each discipline. Even if time is available, there is simply so much data, in so many places, that it is difficult to merge the data with the knowledge that a healthcare provider has learned, as well as with new knowledge to provide the best patient care. We are drowning in data but lack the time and skills to transform it to useful information or knowledge.

The historical development of the computer as a tool to manage information is evident. The first information management task "computerized" was numeric manipulation. Although not technically a computer by today's terminology, the first successful computerization tool was the abacus, which was developed about 3000 BC. Although even when one developed skill and speed, the operator of the abacus still had to manipulate data mentally (Dilson, 1968). All the abacus did was store the results step-by-step. Slide rules came next in 1622 (The Oughtred Society, 2011), but like the abacus, they required a great deal of skill on the part of the operator. The first machine to add and subtract by itself was Blaise Pascal's "arithmetic machine," built between 1642 and 1644 AD (Freiberger & Swaine, 2013). The first "computer" to be a commercial success was Jacquard's weaving machine built in 1803 ("Jacquard, Joseph Marie (1752–1834)," 2011). Its efficiency so frightened workers at the mill where it was built that they rioted, broke apart the machine, and sold the parts. Despite this setback, the machine proved a success because it introduced a cost-effective way of producing goods.

Early computers designed by Charles Babbage in the mid-19th century, although never built, laid the foundation for modern computers (Barile, 2007). The first successful use of an automatic calculating machine was the 1900 census. Herman Hollerith (who later started IBM) used the Jacquard Loom concept of punch cards to create a machine that enabled the 1900 census takers to compile the results in 1 year instead of the 10 required for the 1890 census (Bellis, 2013). The first computer by today's perception was the **Electronic Numerical Integrator and Computer (ENIAC)** built by people at the Moore School of Engineering at the University of Pennsylvania in partnership with the U.S. government. When completed in 1946, it consisted of 18,000 vacuum tubes, 70,000 resistors, and 5 million soldered joints. It consumed enough energy to dim the lights in an entire section of Philadelphia (Moye, 1996). The progress in hardware since then is phenomenal; today's smartphones have more processing power than ENIAC did!

COMPUTERS AND HEALTHCARE

The use of computers in healthcare originated in the late 1950s and early1960s as a way to manage financial information. The development of a few computerized patient care applications in the late 1960s followed. Some of these hospital information systems included patient diagnoses and other patient information as well as care plans based on physician and nursing orders. Because they lacked processing power, most of these systems were unable to deliver the needs of users and never became widely used.

Early Healthcare Informatics Systems

One interesting early use of the computer in patient care was the Problem-Oriented Medical Information System (PROMIS) begun by Dr. Lawrence Weed in 1968 at the University Medical Center in Burlington, Vermont (McNeill, 1979). The importance of this system is that it was the first attempt to provide a total, integrated system that covered all aspects of healthcare including patient treatment. It was patient oriented and used the problem-oriented medical record (POMR) as its framework. The unit featured an interactive touch screen and had a reputation for fast responsiveness (Schultz, 1988). At its height, it consisted of more than 60,000 frames of knowledge.

The design of PROMIS was to overcome four problems that are still with us today: lack of care coordination, reliance on memory, lack of recorded logic of delivered care, and lack of an effective feedback loop (Jacobs, 2009). The system provided a wide array of information to all healthcare providers. All disciplines recorded their observations and plans and related them to a specific problem. This broke down barriers between disciplines, making it possible to see the relationship between conditions, treatments, costs, and outcomes. Unfortunately, this system never was widely accepted. To embrace it meant a change in the structure of healthcare, something that did not begin until the 1990s, when managed care in all its variations reinvigorated a push toward more patient-centered information systems, a push that continues today.

In 1967, the development of another early system, the Help Evaluation through Logical Processing (HELP) system, was developed by the Informatics Department at the University of Utah School of Medicine. The first implementation was in a heart catheterization laboratory and a post–open-heart intensive care unit (ICU). It is today hospital-wide and operational in many hospitals in the Intermountain Healthcare system (Gardner et al., 1999; OpenClinical, 2013). HELP is not only a hospital information system but it also integrates a sophisticated clinical decision support system that provides information to clinical areas. HELP was the first hospital information system that collected data for clinical decision making and integrated it with a medical knowledge base. Clinicians accepted the system. HELP demonstrated that a clinical support system is feasible and can reduce healthcare costs without sacrificing quality.

Progression of Information Systems

As the science of informatics has progressed, changes in information systems occurred. Originally, computerized clinical information systems were process oriented. That is, implementation was to computerize a specific process, for example, billing, order entry, or laboratory reports. This led to the creation of different software systems for different departments, which unfortunately could not share data, creating a need for clinicians to enter data more than once. An attempt to share data by integrating data from disparate systems is a difficult and sometimes impossible task. Lack of the use of standard terminology and **protocols** (a system of rules) complicates the transfer of data between different systems. Even when possible, the results are often disappointing and can leave negative impressions of computerization in users' minds.

Newer systems, however, are organized by data. Data-designed systems use the same piece of data many times, thus requiring entry of data only once. The basis of primary design is how data are gathered, stored, and used in an entire institution rather than on a specific process such as pharmacy or laboratory. For example, when a healthcare provider places a medication order, the system has access to all the information about a patient including his or her diagnosis, age, weight, allergies, and eventually **genomics**, as well as the medications that he or she is currently taking. The system can also match the order and patient information against knowledge such as what drugs are incompatible with the prescribed drug, the dosage of the drug, and the appropriateness of the drug for this patient. If there are difficulties, the system can deliver warnings at the initial order time of the medication instead of requiring clinician intervention either in the pharmacy or at the time of administration. A data-driven system allows the dietician planning the patient's diet and the nurse providing patient care and doing discharge planning, access to the same information. This integration enables a more complete picture of a patient than one that would be available when separate systems handle dietetics and nursing.

Evidence-based practice will result not only from research and practice guidelines but also from unidentifiable (data minus any patient identification) **aggregated data** from actual patients. It will also be possible to see how patients with a given genomics react to a drug, thus helping the clinician in prescribing drugs. These same aggregated data will help clinicians make decisions by providing information about treatments that are most effective for given conditions, replacing the current system which is too often based on "what we have always done" rather than empirical information. These systems will use computers that are powerful enough to process data so that the creation of information is "on the fly," or immediately when requested. Systems that incorporate these features will require a new way of thinking. Instead of having all one's knowledge in memory, one must be comfortable both with needing to access information, knowing how and where to find it, and with changing one's practice to accommodate new knowledge.

Computerization will affect healthcare professionals in other ways. Some jobs will change focus. As nurses, we may find that our job as a patient care coordinator has shifted from transcribing and checking orders to accessing this information on the computer. To preserve our ability to provide full care for our patients, and as an information integrator for other disciplines, we will need to make our information needs known to those who design the systems. To accomplish this, we all need to be aware of the value of both our data and our experience. We need to be able to identify the data we need to perform our job, as well as to appreciate the value of the data that others add to the healthcare system.

BENEFITS OF INFORMATICS

The information systems described earlier will bring many benefits to healthcare. These benefits will result in the ability to improve patient care outcomes by creating and using aggregated data, preventing errors, easing working conditions, and providing better healthcare records.

Benefits for Healthcare in General

One of the primary benefits of informatics is that previously buried data in inaccessible records become usable. Informatics is not only about collecting data but also about making it useful. The capture of data electronically in a structured manner allows for retrieval and use of data in different ways, both to assimilate information easily about one patient and as aggregated data. (Aggregated data will be further discussed in Chapter 8.)

Table 1-1 shows some aggregated data for postsurgical infections sorted by physician and then by the organism. Because infections for some patients are caused by two different pathogens, as presented in Table 1-1, you see two entries for some patients; however, this is all produced from only one entry of the data. With just a few clicks of a mouse, the system can organize these same data by unit to show the number of infections on each unit. This is possible because data that are structured, as in Table 1-1 and standardized, can be presented in many different views.

When examining aggregated data, patterns emerge that might otherwise take several weeks or months to become evident or might never become evident. When patterns, such as the prevalence of infections for Dr. Smith emerge (see Table 1-1), it is possible to investigate what this physician's patients have in common. However, one must use caution. The aggregated data in Table 1-1 are insufficient to draw conclusions; the data serve only as an indication of a problem and provide clues for where to start investigating. Aggregated data are a type of information or even knowledge, but wisdom in this case says that these data are not sufficient for drawing hard conclusions. Any shared data, outside of an agency or with those

TABLE 1-1   Aggregated Data

First Name	Last Name	Unit	Surgery	Physician	Pathogen
Charles	Babbage	3 West	Cholecystectomy	Black	*E. coli*
Jack	Of All Trades	4 West	Appendectomy	Black	*Strep*
George	Washington	4 West	Tonsillectomy	Black	*Strep*
John	Wayne	2 East	Herniorrhaphy	Greene	*E. coli*
Gloria	Swanson	2 East	Cholecystectomy	Greene	*E. coli*
Gloria	Swanson	2 East	Cholecystectomy	Greene	*Strep*
Susan	Anthony	3 West	Tubal ligation	Jones	*Strep*
Alexander	Hamilton	2 East	Cholecystectomy	Smith	*E. coli*
Florence	Dayingale	4 West	Hysterectomy	Smith	*E. coli*
Abigail	Adams	2 East	Herniorrhaphy	Smith	*Staph*
Johnny	Appleseed	3 West	Open reduction, left femur	Smith	*Staph*
Davey	Jones	3 West	Transurethral resection	Smith	*Staph*
Alexander	Hamilton	2 East	Cholecystectomy	Smith	*Strep*
Florence	Dayingale	4 West	Hysterectomy	Smith	*Strep*

Note: Fictitious patient names are used here to help in understanding the concept; real secondary data should be unidentifiable.

E. coli, Escherichia coli; Staph, Staphylococcus; Strep, Streptococcus.

who do not need to have personal information about a patient, must be **deidentified**, that is, there should be no way to identify the patient from the data.

Informatics through information systems can improve communication between all healthcare providers, which will improve patient care and reduce stress. Additional benefits for healthcare include making the storage and retrieval of healthcare records much easier, quicker retrieval of test results, printouts or screens of needed information organized to meet the needs of the user, and fewer lost charges because of easier methods of recording charges. Another benefit will come from saving time and money by computerizing administrative tasks such as staffing and scheduling.

Benefits for the Nursing Profession

Each healthcare discipline will benefit from its investment in informatics. In nursing, informatics will not only enhance practice but also add to the development of nursing science.

Informatics will improve documentation and, when properly implemented, not increase the time spent in documentation. Nurses spend more than 15% to 25% of their time documenting patient care (Gugerty et al., 2007; Yee et al., 2012). Entering vital signs both in nursing notes and on a flow sheet wastes time and invites errors. In a well-designed clinical documentation system, data entered once, retrieved, and presented in many different forms should meet the needs of users.

Paper documentation methods create other problems such as inconsistency and irregularity in charting as well as the lack of data for evaluation and research as mentioned above. An electronic clinical information system can remind users of the need to provide data in areas one is apt to forget and can provide a list of terms that can be "clicked" to enter data. There is a vast improvement in the ability to use patient data for both quality control and research when documentation is complete and electronic.

Despite Florence Nightingale's emphasis on data, for much of nursing's history, nursing data have not been valued. Florence Nightingale used data to create the predecessor of the pie graph to demonstrate that the real enemy in the Crimean War was not the Russians but poor sanitation. This communication of information in a way that was comprehended easily caused the British to understand the value of sanitation in military hospitals.

They are either buried in paper patient records that make retrieving it economically infeasible or, worse, discarded when a patient is discharged, hence unavailable for building nursing science. With the advent of electronic clinical documentation, nursing data can be a part of the EHR and be available to researchers for building evidence-based nursing knowledge. It will also allow the inclusion of nursing information in overall healthcare evidence-based care. The Maryland report on the use of technology to address the nursing shortage demonstrated that informatics could be used to improve staff morale and the efficiency of patient care (Gugerty et al., 2007). For example, paper request forms can be eliminated, easy communication of work announcements can be more easily communicated, the time for in-services can be reduced, and empty shifts can be filled by using Internet software.

In understanding the role and value that informatics adds to nursing, it is necessary to recognize that the profession is cognitive, rather than one confined to tasks. Providing data to support this is a joint function of nursing informatics and clinicians. Identifying and determining how to facilitate data collection is an informatics skill that all nurses need.

SKILLS NEEDED BY ALL NURSES

The need to manage complex amounts of data in patient care demands that all nurses, regardless of specialty area, have informatics skills (Gaumer et al., 2007; Nelson, 2007). Informatics skills for all nurses require basic computer skills as one component (American Nurses Association, 2008). Another skill needed for proficiency in informatics is **information literacy**. The ANA, NLN, AONE, and AACN have identified both computer and information literacy skills as necessary for evidence-based practice.

Computer Fluency

The information age described the 20th century. The present century will be the information-processing age, that is the use of data and information to create more information and knowledge. The broad use of the term "**computer literacy**" means the ability to perform various tasks with a computer. Given the rapid changes in technology and in nursing, perhaps thinking in terms of **computer fluency** rather than literacy provides a better perspective on computer use. This term implies that you have an adequate foundation in computer concepts to enable you to learn new computer skills and programs independently (Committee on Information Technology Literacy, 2013). Thus, an individual needs a lifelong commitment to acquiring new skills for being more effective in work and personal life. Computer literacy is a temporary state, whereas computer fluency is dynamic and involves being able to increase one's ability to effectively use a computer when needed.

A perusal of archives in a **Listserv** (an e-mail discussion list that has participants who discuss various aspects of a topic) in informatics reveals periodic requests for instruments to measure the computer competency of staff. Unfortunately, there is little agreement on specific competencies needed, let alone an instrument to measure this, but there is consensus that it involves knowledge, attitude, and competencies in the use of computers, computer technology, and hardware and software. Nurses must be able to visualize the overall benefits to nursing practice and patient care outcomes. More than a decade and a half ago, Simpson (1998) pointed out the need for nurses to master computers to avoid extinction. A computer is a mind tool that frees us from the mental drudgery of data processing, just as the bulldozer frees us from the drudgery of digging and moving dirt. Similar to the bulldozer, however, we must use the computer intelligently or damage can result.

Given the forces moving healthcare toward more use of informatics, it is important for nurses to learn the skills associated with using a computer for managing information. Additionally, knowing how to use graphical interfaces and application programs such as word processing, spreadsheets, databases, and presentation programs is as an important an element in a professional career as is mastering technology skills. Just as anatomy and physiology provide a background for learning about disease processes and treatments, computer fluency skills are necessary to appreciate more complex informatics concepts (McNeil & Odom, 2000) and for learning clinical applications (Nagelkerk et al., 1998).

Ronald and Skiba (1987) were the first to look at computer competencies required for nurses. In the late-1990s and early part of this century, this issue was revisited, but the focus became the use of computer skills as part of informatics skills (McCannon & O'Neal, 2003; McNeil et al., 2003; Utley-Smith, 2004). Staggers et al. (2001, 2002) defined four levels of informatics competencies for practicing nurses. The first two pertain to all nurses, and the last two pertain to informatics nurse specialists:

1. The beginning nurse should possess basic information management and computer technology skills. Accomplishments should include the ability to access data, use a computer for communication, use basic desktop software, and use decision support systems.
2. Experienced nurses should be highly skilled in using information management and computer technology to support their major area of practice. Additional skills for the experienced nurse include being able to make judgments on the basis of trends and patterns within data elements and to collaborate with informatics nurse specialists to suggest improvements in nursing systems.
3. The informatics nurse specialist should be able to meet the information needs of practicing nurses by integrating and applying information, computer, and nursing sciences.
4. The informatics innovator will conduct informatics research and generate informatics theory.

A matrix with a listing of the informatics competencies by nursing informatics functional areas is included in the Nursing Informatics: Scope & Standards of Practice (American Nurses Association, 2014).

Information Literacy

Information literacy, or the ability to know when one needs information, and how to locate, evaluate, and effectively use it (National Forum on Information Literacy, 2011), is an informatics skill. Although it involves computer skills, similar to informatics, it requires critical thinking and problem solving. Information literacy is part of the foundation for evidence-based practice and provides nurses with the ability to be intelligent information creators and consumers in today's electronic environment.

Computer fluency that enables nurses to be both information literate and informatics capable in their practice is an expectation of any educated nurse. In Figure 1-2, you can see that the skill of computer literacy is needed to develop computer fluency. Nurse clinicians need both those skills as well as information literacy and a basic knowledge of nursing informatics. The informatics nurse specialist needs all those skills, knowledge of the

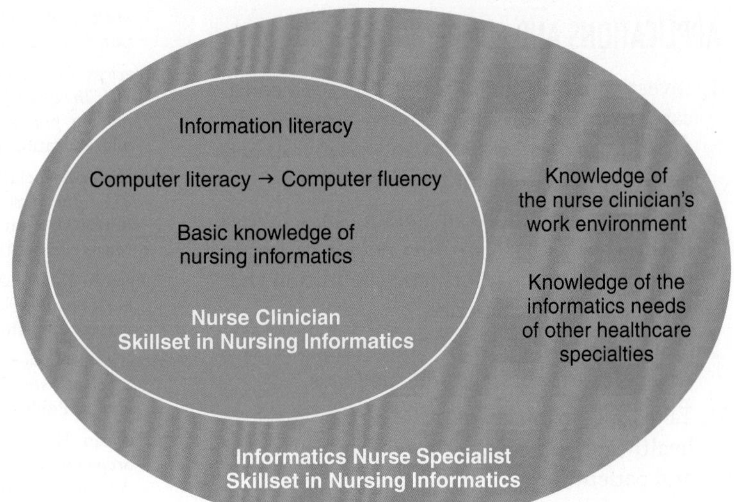

Information literacy

Computer literacy → Computer fluency

Basic knowledge of
nursing informatics

**Nurse Clinician
Skillset in Nursing Informatics**

Knowledge of
the nurse clinician's
work environment

Knowledge of the
informatics needs
of other healthcare
specialties

**Informatics Nurse Specialist
Skillset in Nursing Informatics**

Figure 1-2. Skillset in nursing informatics.

nurse clinician's work environment, and knowledge of the informatics needs of other healthcare specialties.

Unit II, addressing basic computer skills, emphasizes concepts that promote the ability to learn new applications. These chapters provide information underlying the use of informatics in professional life. The chapters in Unit III build upon these principles to allow the reader to start to gain new informatics skills, including the ability to find and evaluate information from electronic sources. The chapters in Units IV, V, and VI allow the reader to develop skills necessary to work with informatics nurse specialists in providing effective information systems and the use of nursing data.

SUMMARY

The changes of healthcare in transition affect nursing. Part of these changes involves informatics. Whether the change will be positive or negative for patient care and nursing depends on nurses. For the change to be positive, nurses need to develop skills in information management, known in healthcare as informatics. To gain these skills, a background in both computer and information literacy skills is necessary.

The expansion of knowledge logarithmically limits the human minds ability to manage data and information. The use of technology tools to aid the human mind has become mandatory. Healthcare has been behind most industries in using technology to manage its data. However, government- and private-level forces are working to change this. With these pressures, healthcare informatics is rapidly expanding. Nursing is one of many subspecialties in healthcare informatics. Embracing informatics will allow nurses to assess and evaluate practice just as a stethoscope allows the evaluation and assessment of a patient.

The use of computers in healthcare started in the 1960s, mostly in financial areas, but with the advance in computing power and the demand for clinical data, as nurses we are using computers more and more in clinical areas. With this growth has come a change in focus for information systems from providing solutions for just one process to an enterprise-wide patient-centered system that focuses on data. This new focus provides the functionality that allows the use of one piece of data in multiple ways. To understand and work with clinical systems, as well as to fulfill other professional responsibilities, nurses need to be computer fluent, information literate, and informatics knowledgeable.

APPLICATIONS AND COMPETENCIES

1. Investigate one of the forces outside health-care that are driving a move toward the greater use of informatics and briefly discuss some pros and cons for this force.

2. Using the definitions of nursing informatics in this chapter or from other resources, create your own nursing informatics definition that applies to clinical practice.

3. Support the statement: "The computer is a tool of informatics, but not the focus."

4. Take one instance of informatics used in healthcare and analyze its effect on nurses and patient care.

5. Using Table 1-1, analyze what other data would be needed to draw conclusions from infection control data.

6. List reasons why every nurse needs to have informatics skills.

7. Do a library search for an article on nursing information literacy or nursing informatics competencies. Compose talking points for the article, as well as citing the source of the article.

8. Analyze all the information beyond your immediate knowledge that you need and use in caring for one of your patients on just one shift. Where does this information originate? When do you need it for care? How do you obtain it? How do you use it?

9. Write one or two paragraphs on how you now think a practicing nurse can use computer fluency and information literacy to advance in a career. Save this and at the end of this book, compare it with how you then see these two skills affecting a nursing career.

REFERENCES

American Health Information Management Association, & American Medical Informatics Association. (2006). *Building the workforce for health information transformation*. Retrieved from http://www.amia.org/sites/amia.org/files/Workforce_2006.pdf

American Association of Colleges of Nursing. (2006, October). *The essentials of doctoral education for advanced nursing practice*. Retrieved from http://www.aacn.nche.edu/DNP/pdf/Essentials.pdf

American Association of Colleges of Nursing. (2008, October 20). *The essentials of baccalaureate education for professional nursing practice*. Retrieved from http://www.aacn.nche.edu/education/pdf/baccessentials08.pdf

American Association of Colleges of Nursing. (2011, March 21). *The essentials of master's education in nursing*. Retrieved from http://www.aacn.nche.edu/Education/pdf/Master'sEssentials11.pdf

American Nurses Association. (2001). *Scope and standards of nursing informatics practice*. Washington, DC: American Nurses Publishing.

American Nurses Association. (2008). *Nursing informatics: Scope and standards of practice*. Washington, DC: American Nurses Publishing.

American Nurses Association. (2015). *Nursing informatics: Scope and standards of practice* (2nd ed.). Washington, DC: American Nurses Publishing.

American Organization of Nurse Executives. (2012). *Position paper: Nursing Informatics Executive Leader*. Retrieved from http://www.aone.org/resources/leadership%20tools/PDFs/AONE_Technology_Committee_CNIO_Position_Paper.pdf

Barile, M. (2007). *Babbage, Charles (1791-1871)*. Retrieved from http://scienceworld.wolfram.com/biography/Babbage.html

Bakken, S. (2001). An informatics infrastructure is essential for evidence-based practice. *Journal of the American Medical Informatics Association, 8*(3), 199–201.

Bansal, M. (2002). *Medical informatics: A primer*. Cincinnati, OH: McGraw-Hill.

Bellis, M. (2013). *Herman Hollerith—Punch cards*. Retrieved from http://inventors.about.com/library/inventors/blhollerith.htm

Committee on Government Reform. (2004, July 14). *Health informatics: What is the prescription for success in intergovernmental information sharing and emergency response?* Retrieved from http://www.gpo.gov/fdsys/pkg/CHRG-108hhrg98120/html/CHRG-108hhrg98120.htm

Committee on Quality of Health Care in America, & Institute of Medicine. (2001). *Crossing the quality chasm: A new health system for the 21st century*. Retrieved from http://books.nap.edu/catalog.php?record_id=10027#toc

Davenport, T. H., & Glaser, J. (2002). Just-in-time delivery comes to knowledge management. *Harvard Business Review, 80*(7), 107–111. Retrieved from http://hbswk.hbs.edu/archive/3049.html

Delaney, C. (2001). Health informatics and oncology nursing. *Seminars in Oncology Nursing, 17*(1), 2–6.

Dilson, J. (1968). *The abacus: A pocket computer*. New York, NY: St. Martin's Press.

Freiberger, P. A., & Swaine, M. R. (2013). *Arithmetic machine—Encyclopedia Britannica*. Retrieved from http://www.britannica.com/EBchecked/topic/725527/Pascaline

Gardner, R. M., Pryor, T. A., & Warner, H. R. (1999). The HELP hospital information system: Update 1998. *International Journal of Medical Informatics, 54*(3), 169–182. doi: S1386505699000131.

Gaumer, G. L., Koeniger-Donohue, R., Friel, C., et al. (2007). Use of information technology by advanced practice nurses. *CIN: Computers Informatics Nursing, 25*(6), 344–352. doi: 10.1097/01.NCN.0000299656.59519.06.

Goossen, W. T. (1996). Nursing information management and processing: A framework and definition for systems analysis, design and evaluation. *International Journal of Biomedical Computing, 40*(3), 187–195.

Graves, J. R., & Cocoran, S. (1989). The study of nursing informatics. *Image: Journal of Nursing Scholarship, 21,* 227–231.

Greiner, A. C., & Knebel, E. (Eds.). (2003). *Health professions education: A bridge to quality.* Washington, DC: National Academy Press.

Gugerty, B., Maranda, M. J., Beachley, M., et al. (2007, May). *Challenges and opportunities in documentation of the nursing care of patients.* Retrieved from http://www.mbon.org/commission2/documenation_challenges.pdf

Hannah, K. J., Ball, M. J., & Edwards, M. J. A. (1994). *Introduction to nursing informatics.* New York, NY: Springer-Verlag.

HealthIT.gov. (2011, September 12). *Federal health information technology plan: 2011-2015.* Retrieved from http://www.healthit.gov/policy-researchers-implementers/health-it-strategic-planning

HHS.gov/HealthCare. (2014, June 24). *About the law.* Retrieved from http://www.hhs.gov/healthcare/rights/

Jacobs, L. (2009). Interview with Lawrence Weed, MD- The father of the problem-oriented medical record looks ahead. *Permanente Journal, 13*(3), 84–89.

Jacquard, Joseph Marie (1752–1834). (2011). *The Hutchinson biography database.* 1.

Leapfrog Group. (2014a). *About Leapfrog.* Retrieved from http://www.leapfroggroup.org/about_leapfrog

Leapfrog Group. (2014b). *The Leapfrog Group fact sheet.* Retrieved from http://www.leapfroggroup.org/about_us/leapfrog-factsheet

McCannon, M., & O'Neal, P. V. (2003). Results of a national survey indicating information technology skills needed by nurses at time of entry into the work force. *Journal of Nursing Education, 42*(8), 327–340.

McDonald, M. D. (1994). Telecognition for improving health. *Healthcare Forum Journal, 37*(2), 18–21.

McNeil, B. J., & Odom, S. K. (2000). Nursing informatics education in the United States: Proposed undergraduate curriculum. *Health Informatics Journal, 6*(1), 32–38.

McNeil, B. J., Elfrink, V. L., Bickford, C. J., et al. (2003). Nursing information technology knowledge, skills, and preparation of student nurses, nursing faculty, and clinicians: A U.S. survey. *Journal Nursing Education, 42*(8), 341–349.

McNeill, D. G. (1979). Developing the complete computer-based information system. *Journal of Nursing Administration, 9*(11), 34–46.

Moye, W. T. (1996, January), *ENIAC: The army-sponsored revolution.* Retrieved from http://ftp.arl.army.mil/mike/comphist/96summary/

Nagelkerk, J., Ritolo, P. M., & Vandort, P. J. (1998). Nursing informatics: The trend of the future. *Journal of Continuing Education in Nursing, 29*(1), 17–21.

National Advisory Council on Nurse Education and Practice. (1997, December). *A national informatics agenda for nursing education and practice.* Retrieved from http://eric.ed.gov/?id=ED449700

National Forum on Information Literacy. (2011). *National forum on information literacy: 21st century skills.* Retrieved from http://infolit.org/

National League for Nursing. (2008). *Position statement: Preparing the next generation of nurses to practice in a technology-rich environment: An informatics agenda.* Retrieved from http://www.nln.org/aboutnln/PositionStatements/informatics_052808.pdf

National Research Council (U.S.) Committee on Information Technology Literacy. (1999). *Being fluent with information technology.* Washington, DC: National Academy Press. Retrieved from http://www.nap.edu/catalog.php?record_id=6482

Needleman, J. (2013). Increasing acuity, increasing technology, and the changing demands on nurses. *Nursing Economics, 31*(4), 200–202. Retrieved from http://www.nursingeconomics.net/

Nelson, R. (2007). U.S. hospitals need staffing makeover. *American Journal of Nursing, 107*(12), 19. doi: 10.1097/01.NAJ.0000301004.88450.83.

Newbold, S. K. (1996). The informatics nurse and the certification process. *Computers in Nursing, 14*(2), 84–85, 88.

Nightingale, F. (1863). *Notes on hospitals* (3rd ed.). London, England: Longman, Green, Longman, Roberts, & Green.

Office of Science and Technology Policy. (2013, September 29). *Science, technology and innovation.* Retrieved from http://www.whitehouse.gov/administration/eop/ostp

OpenClinical. (2013, July 9). *HELP OpenClinical AI systems in clinical practice.* Retrieved from http://www.openclinical.org/aisp_help.html

Pillar, B., & Golumbic, N. (1993). *Nursing informatics: Enhancing patient care.* Bethesda, MD: National Center for Nursing Research, U.S. Department of Health and Human Services.

QSEN Institute. (2014). *QSEN—Quality & safety education for nurses.* Retrieved from http://qsen.org/

Robert Wood Johnson Foundation. (2010, August 5). *Improving the nurse work environment on medical-surgical units through technology.* Retrieved from http://www.rwjf.org/en/research-publications/find-rwjf-research/2010/08/improving-the-nurse-work-environment-on-medical-surgical-units-t.html

Ronald, J., & Skiba, D. (1987). *Guidelines for basic computer education in nursing.* New York, NY: National League for Nursing.

Sackett, K. M., & Erdley, W. S. (2002). The history of health care informatics. In S. Englebardt & R. Nelson (Eds.), *Healthcare informatics from an interdisciplinary approach* (pp. 453–477). St. Louis, MO: Mosby.

Scholes, M., & Barber, B. (1980). Towards nursing informatics. In D. A. D. Lindberg & S. Kaihara (Eds.), *MEDINFO: 1980* (pp. 7–73). Amsterdam, the Netherlands: North Holland.

Schultz, J. R. (1988). A history of the PROMIS technology: An effective human interface. In A. Goldberg (Ed.),

A history of personal workstations (pp. 1–46). Reading, MA: Addison-Wesley.

Schwirian, P. (1986). The NI pyramid—A model for research in nursing informatics. *CIN: Computers in Nursing, 4*(3), 134–136.

Shortliffe, E. H., & Blois, M. S. (2001). The computer meets medicine: Emergence of a discipline. In E. H. Shortliffe & L. E. Perrault (Eds.), *Medical informatics: Computer applications in healthcare* (pp. 3–40). New York, NY: Springer-Verlag.

Simpson, R. (1998). The technologic imperative: A new agenda for nursing education and practice, part 1. *Nursing Management, 29*(9), 22–24.

Staggers, N., Gassert, C. A., & Curran, C. (2001). Informatics competencies for nurses at four levels of practice. *Journal of Nursing Education, 40*(7), 303–316.

Staggers, N., Gassert, C. A., & Curran, C. (2002). *Results of a Delphi study to determine informatics competencies for nurses at four levels of practice.* Retrieved from http://www.nursing-informatics.com/niassess/NIcompetencies_Staggers.pdf

Staggers, N., & Thompson, C. B. (2002). The evolution of definitions for nursing informatics: A critical analysis and revised definition. *Journal of the American Medical Association, 9*(3), 255–261.

Technology Guiding Educational Reform. (2007). *The TIGER initiative: Evidence and informatics transforming nursing: 3-year action steps toward a 10-year vision.* Retrieved from http://www.thetigerinitiative.org/docs/TIGERInitiativeSummaryReport_001.pdf

The Oughtred Society. (2013, December 14). *Slide rule history.* Retrieved from http://www.oughtred.org/history.shtml

Turley, J. (1996). Toward a model for nursing informatics. *Image: Journal of Nursing Scholarship, 28*(4), 309–313.

Utley-Smith, Q. (2004). 5 competencies needed by new baccalaureate graduates. *Nursing Education Perspectives, 25*(4), 166–170.

Yee, T., Needleman, J., Pearson, M., et al. (2012). The influence of integrated electronic medical records and computerized nursing notes on nurses' time spent in documentation. *Computers, Informatics, Nursing: CIN, 30*(6), 287–292. doi: 10.1097/NXN.0b013e31824af835

2

Essential Computer and Software Concepts

OBJECTIVES

After studying this chapter, you will be able to:

1. Discuss the differences in operating systems.
2. Discuss the pros and cons of cloud computing.
3. Differentiate between the various types of software copyright.
4. Demonstrate competencies using universal text editing features.
5. Explain efficient methods for managing digital files.

KEY TERMS

Applications (Apps)	Freeware	Proprietary
Apple iCloud	Google Drive	Public-domain software
Backup	Graphical user interface (GUI)	Save As
Clipboard		Shareware
Cloud computing	Hibernate	Sleep mode
Crash	OneDrive	Software piracy
Encryption	Open source	Speech recognition
Export	Operating system	Synchronize (sync)

The need to manage complex amounts of data in patient care demands that all nurses, regardless of specialty area, have informatics skills (Gaumer et al., 2007). This requires understanding some basic computer concepts. In this chapter, you will learn about some of the essential computer and software concepts that provide computers with the ability to make our life easier. Essential computer concepts refer to the type of computer device concepts refer to the type of computer device and the associated operating system software. The concepts also refer to how to access software features, where software is stored on the device, and how to remotely access files. Other essentials include understanding the types of software copyright and implications of copyright piracy issues. It is also important to know how to maximize the use of hardware and software by using universal editing features and efficiently managing digital files.

Application programs are the various types of software, such as office software and web browsers. Because access to the Internet from different devices using Wi-Fi is almost ubiquitous in many parts of the world, cloud computing is emerging as a standard.

OPERATING SYSTEMS

The computer, despite all its parts, will do nothing but act as an expensive paperweight unless told what to do. As you know, all computers require an operating system and application programs to work. The **operating system** functions as the traffic controller or the brains of the computer. The operating system is the most important program on your computer. It coordinates input from the keyboard with output on the screen, responds to mouse and touch pad clicks, heeds commands to save a file, retrieves files, and transmits commands to printers and other peripheral devices (Webopedia, 2013). The operating system provides access to applications, such as office software and e-mail.

Computer **applications (apps)** work with a specific operating system (OS). Thus, the operating system that you select determines which apps you can run. Today, there are four main OSs for personal computers: Microsoft Windows OS, Mac OSX, Linux, and Google Chrome OS. Microsoft Windows OS has the majority of the market share, followed by the Mac OSX and Linux (Net Applications.com, 2013). Microsoft released the first version of Windows OS in 1985. Bill Gates and Paul Allen started Microsoft with the vision that personal computing was a "path to the future" (Microsoft, 2013a). Apple Computer released the first version of an OS for the Mac in 1984 (Sanford, 2015). Linux was released as a free and open-source OS in 1991 (Linux.org, 2013). Linux, an unsupported OS, is more popular with "tech gurus" and used on less than 5% of personal computers. However, because of its stability and affordability, users utilize Linux for web servers. Google released the Chrome OS in 2012 as the operating system for Chromebook laptops (Chromium Projects, 2013; Google, 2011, May 11). Chrome OS, which is an open-source project, represents a paradigm shift. The Chrome OS is a combination of web browser and operating system.

Prior to the point and click **graphical user interface** (**GUI**—pronounced "gooey") that we use today, computers used the DOS (disk operating system). DOS was text based and required the user to remember a set of commands, such as Delete, Run, Copy, and Rename. The computer screens were black and generally only displayed text and numbers. Unlike GUI, DOS allowed for only one program at a time to run, there was no sharing of information between programs, and there was no point and click for entering commands.

Vannevar Bush is responsible for developing the concept of a graphical interface in 1945, almost 40 years prior to use by Apple and Windows OSs (Mesa, 1998). Bush's research team at the Department of Defense called the Advanced Research Project Agency (ARPA) also developed the mouse that allowed for pointing and clicking. Douglas C. Engelbart and his research team continued to develop the GUI concept. When Engelbart's project lost funding, most of his research team went to work for Palo Alto Research Center (PARC), a Xerox company. Xerox is the company responsible for developing the first personal computer in 1973. However, Xerox never marketed the early product that used a GUI, named Xerox Alto, because it cost $40,000.

Apple Computer released the first Macintosh with an OS that used a GUI and a mouse in January of 1984 for $2,495 (Oldcomputers.net, 2013). In November 1985, Microsoft shipped Windows 1, which had an OS that used a GUI and a mouse (Microsoft, 2013a). The introduction of a GUI with the ability to use a mouse to point and click revolutionized computing, as we know it today.

CLOUD COMPUTING

Cloud computing refers to the ability to access software and file storage on remote computers using the Internet. Many of the cloud computing office applications and file storage resources provide the ability to share files and folders with others. Examples of cloud computing software include office applications such as word processing and spreadsheets, note-taking, and picture and

TABLE 2-1	Cloud Computing Resource Examples		
Cloud Computing Application	**URL**	**Includes Office Applications**	**Includes File Storage**
Microsoft OneDrive	https://onedrive.live.com/	X	X
Google Drive	https://drive.google.com	X	X
Zoho	http://www.zoho.com/	X	X
Apple iCloud	http://icloud.com	X	X ,
Dropbox	https://www.dropbox.com/		X
Box	http://www.box.net/		X
IDrive	http://www.idrive.com/		X
ADrive	http://www.adrive.com/		X

For additional information on how cloud computing storage works, go to http://communication.howstuffworks.com/cloud-storage.htm

video sharing apps. Many of the cloud computing resources provide 2 to 200 GB of free file storage (Table 2-1).

Cloud Office Apps

Microsoft created an office application for which the software is completely online. Subscribers can access the Microsoft Office programs and the files that they create from devices connected to the Internet such as a tablet or a smartphone. Known as Microsoft Office 365, it is available for Windows and Mac computers and includes Word, PowerPoint, Excel, and Outlook. The Windows version also includes OneNote, Publisher, and Access (Microsoft, 2013b). Users can purchase the cloud software by the month or year. The subscription license allows for use on up to five devices. Users always have the latest editions of the office apps. Microsoft Office 365 also provides off-site file storage capabilities using **OneDrive** (formally named SkyDrive).

Another app that enables cloud sharing of files is OneDrive. It is downloadable for personal computers, tablets, and smartphones. It is available to Mac and Windows users who have Microsoft Office installed on their computer.

OneDrive allows the user to choose files to **sync (synchronize)** between a computer device and the OneDrive cloud.

Another cloud sharing app is **Google Drive**. It includes a word processor, presentation program, spreadsheet, a drawing program, and a way to create forms. Files created using Google drive programs can be shared and edited with others. Additionally, files such as photos may be placed on the Google Drive folder on your computer for storage or sharing. Users can create files and save them to Google Drive even when off-line. When the user is online, these files will be synced with all devices to which the user has given permission that have the app installed.

Apple iCloud began to include the office apps, Pages, Numbers, and Keynote (a presentation program) as of 2013. The iCloud office apps allow for file sharing using the iCloud e-mail address. Users also can turn on and sync mail, contacts, find my iPhone, notes, reminders, and calendar. Like OneDrive and Google Drive, iCloud syncs the files with all devices. However, iCloud differs from the other cloud office solutions as it is accessed using a web browser, but it is not a downloadable app.

Sharing Files in the Cloud

The ability to create and edit files using cloud computing apps is a great feature as is the ability to share and edit files simultaneously with other users. Common cloud computing sharing features include the ability to determine if:

- A file is publicly visible on the web where anyone can search and view.
- A file is visible to anyone who has the link without a sign in.
- A file is private and a sign in is necessary to access the file.
- Shared users can have the ability to view the file.
- Shared users have the ability to edit the file.
- Shared users have the ability to make comments on the file.

File sharing is often used by a group of students working on a course project, committee members who need to share minutes and meeting documents, users who need others to sign up for participation, and users disseminating online surveys. The sharing access is dependent upon the need of the file owner who, with a click of the mouse, can change the status of sharing.

Advantages and Limitations of Using the Cloud

There are many advantages of using cloud applications and files. Advantages include:

- **Backup of important documents**. **Backup** is a term that means a duplicate copy of a file. Because disasters and accidents occur, it is best to back up files and have the backup located in a geographically different location than where the original document is stored. This is particularly important for papers that you do not wish to recreate.
- **Share and edit**. As noted earlier, the ability to share and edit files with others. The ability to access and edit files from any device connected to the Internet that has the appropriate software.

Likewise, there are limitations of using cloud computing. For example:

- **No control over the cloud site**. Since the user is not the owner of the site, there is no control on the availability. The site could be unavailable due to maintenance or your connection to the Internet could be down.

- **Target for cyber criminals**. Popular cloud computing sites are targets for cyber criminals.
- **Concerns about safety of the information**. Safety of the information in the files on the cloud computing site. Generally, files with patient or student information should not be located on a cloud computing web site without encrypting the files. Some cloud computing sites offer site encryption, but for a fee. Users cannot view encrypted data without a secret code. (More information about encryption is located in the "Disk and Data Encryption" section later in this chapter.)

Users must determine their personal comfort zone for using cloud computing. Reputable cloud computing sites take special precautions for keeping their associated resources safe. Be sure to take time to review the information on cloud resources privacy before making a decision about using it.

> ### QSEN Scenario
> You work at a clinic that provides free healthcare services and computers for patients to use. One of the patients asks for recommendations for storing health information on a computer. How would you respond?

SOFTWARE PROGRAM COPYRIGHT

Many commercial vendors believe that the users are not buying software, but instead buying a license to use it. Software licenses indicate the terms of use for the software. Software vendors may specify the number of computers or devices for software installation. There are other types of software licenses besides those of the commercial software, such as open source, shareware, freeware, public domain, and commercial. It is important to know, understand, and abide by the software copyright policies for programs you use.

Open Source

Open-source software has copyright protection, but the software source code is available to anyone who wants it. The idea behind this is that by making source code available, many programmers, who are not concerned with financial gain, will make improvements to the code and produce a more useful, bug-free product (Beal, 2013). The basis of this concept is using peer review to find and eliminate bugs, a process that is unfortunately absent in proprietary programs. Open source grew in the technological community as a response to proprietary software owned by corporations. Google, for example, has many open-source software projects for developers (Google Developers, 2013).

Shareware

Some software is distributed as **shareware**. You can often find software of this type on the Internet. The developers of shareware encourage users to give copies to friends and colleagues to try out. They request that anyone who uses the program after a trial period pay them a fee. Registration information is included in the program. Continuing to use shareware without paying the registration fee is software piracy. In many cases, users cannot access the program after a given period. There is a terms of use statement when the program is installed. Shareware has copyright protection.

Freeware

Freeware is an application the programmer has decided to make freely available to anyone who wishes to use it. Usually, it is closed source with some restricted usage rights. Although you may use freeware without paying, the author usually maintains the copyright. Unless the program is open source, a user cannot do anything with the program other than what the author specifies. Some freeware programs available on the Internet are in the public domain and for which the author states that they can be used any way the user desires, including making changes. When users accept software through any channel but a reputable reseller, they should be certain that they know whether the software is proprietary, shareware, freeware, or in the public domain. Unless using a very well-known vendor, you should use a virus checker to verify that the file does not have a virus before installing it. Freeware has copyright protection.

Public-Domain Software

Public-domain software is software with no copyright restrictions. Because there is no ownership, you can use the software without restrictions. Most of us are not familiar with public-domain software.

An example is the GNU operating system used with Linux (Free Software Foundation, 2011). Another example is the source code used for the Veteran's Administration electronic health record (EHR), VistA. The source code is public domain under US copyright law (17 U.S.C. § 105) and is licensed as open source under WorldVistA (HRSA, 2013).

Commercial Software

Commercial software is **proprietary**. Commercial software has copyright protection and you must purchase it. The terms of use display when you install the software. Users must accept the terms of use in order to install the software.

Today, installation of most proprietary software such as Microsoft Office Suite requires the user to register the software—a process that generally requires an Internet (online) connection. During installation, one must enter a number or code, such as the serial number, product key, or some other designation. The location of the information is on the installation disks or the envelope in which the software disk came. Once this code is entered the program checks to see if the program was previously registered before allowing installation.

Some products that allow trial periods will give the user a chance to register either after a given number of days or when it is installed after purchasing it. Product numbers may be matched to a number in the computer BIOS, an acronym for basic input output system (Fisher, 2013). A chip on the computer motherboard stores the software. Should the hard disk **crash** (become unresponsive), the user can reinstall the software on a new disk on that computer if the user still has the registration information. Keep the numbers for all commercial software in several safe places!

Software Piracy

Today, given the ease with which the legitimacy of programs can be verified, pirated software is more of a problem than illegal installations of legitimate software. Most problems are from countries outside the Western world. According to the 2011 Business Software Report, the value of software theft in 2011 was 63.4 billion dollars (Business Software Alliance, 2013). Globally, the piracy rate was 42% although the piracy rate in the United States was 19%. In 1992, Congress passed the

Software Copyright Protection Bill, which raised **software piracy** from a misdemeanor to a felony (Nicoll, 1994). Penalties for piracy can be up to $100,000 for statutory damages and fines of up to $250,000. Penalties might also include a jail term for up to 5 years for people involved with the crime.

Healthcare is not immune from prosecution. A hospital in Illinois received a $161,000 fine after engaging in unauthorized software duplication (Chicago hospital caught pirating, 1997). Organizations without an enforced software oversight policy are possible candidates for investigation.

Spending less for software is always tempting, but beware of pirated copies. Besides opening the owners up to lawsuits, jail terms, and economic losses, pirated software can carry viruses that can harm the computer. The Business Software Alliance is so serious about pirated software that it provides an online method of reporting software piracy at https://reporting.bsa.org/usa/home.aspx.

MANAGING DIGITAL FILES

Although many of us have used computers for the majority of our lives, we may not be aware of efficient ways to manage digital files. Working with computers entails lifelong learning. The best way to learn is to self-assess your skills, set goals, and practice the new techniques. Examples include learning how to organize files on a hard drive (Figure 2-1) (see this book's companion web site at thepoint. lww.com/sewell5e for help with this), keyboard shortcuts, managing file extensions, using the clipboard, using encryption software, and putting the computer on standby or suspend mode.

Keyboard Shortcuts

There are universal keyboard shortcuts for Windows and Mac software programs that do not require the use of menus or the mouse. The Ctrl (control) key for Windows is the same as the Command key on the Mac. There are keyboard shortcuts for web browsers and for office software applications (Table 2-2). A comprehensive listing of keyboard shortcuts is online:

- Windows—http://windows.microsoft.com/en-us/windows/keyboard-shortcuts
- Mac—http://support.apple.com/kb/ht1343

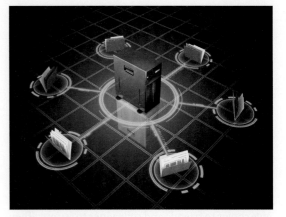

Figure 2-1. File folders on a hard drive (shutterstock. com/Andrea Danti).

Managing File Extensions

File extensions, or the three or four letters after the period in a file name, differ between applications. The file extension instructs the computer which program to use to open the file. It is an automatic extension assigned to the file name when saving the file. To learn which file extensions belong to which programs, see http://www.webopedia.com/quick_ref/fileextensions.asp. Commercial office software, such as Microsoft Office and Apple iWork, include file extension translators and sometimes allow you to open files created with other similar software. You can open files created with Apache OpenOffice Writer in Word 2013, but in Word 2010, you will encounter a message that says that Word cannot open the file because of a problem with the contents. Answer yes and it will ask you if you wish to recover the data; saying yes opens the file. You can download documents created with Google Docs in a Word format. If a word processing document allows you to save a file as an .rtf (rich text format), most other word processors can open it.

Saving a File as a Different Type

To save a file in a different format in many software programs, use "**Save As**" from the File menu. Then when the save screen appears, near the bottom of the screen, click on the triangle at the end of the "Save As Type" box and select the type of file you need from the drop-down box (Figure 2-2).

TABLE 2-2 Universal Keyboard Shortcuts		
Windows	**Mac**	**Action**
Ctrl + A	Command + A	Select all items
Ctrl + C	Command + C	Copy selected items to clipboard
Ctrl + X (or Shift + Insert)	Command + X	Cut selected items
Ctrl + V	Command + V	Paste selected items
Windows logo key + S	Command + Shift + 4	Clip a part of a window
Windows + N	Command + N	Open a new web browser window
Windows + N	Command + N	Open a new web browser tab
Ctrl + Z	Command + Z	Undo
Ctrl + Y	Command + Y	Redo
Ctrl + S	Command + S	Save

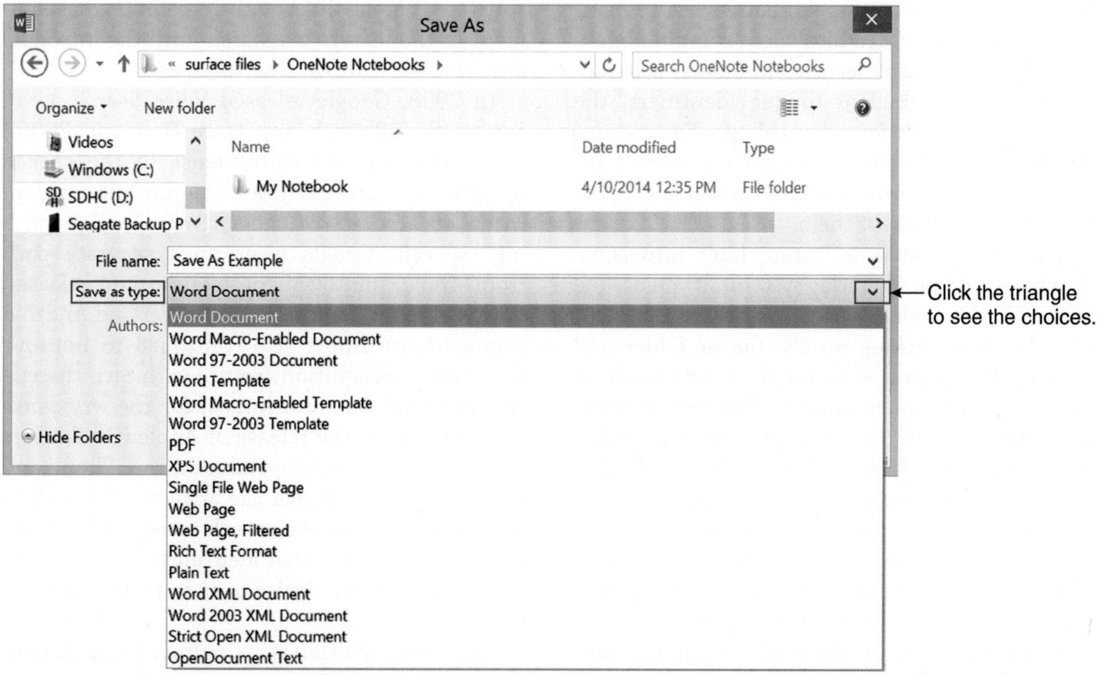

Figure 2-2. How to save as a different file format. (Used with permission from Microsoft.)

For the Apple iWork Pages, choose **Export** from the File menu. Another work around for sharing word processing files is to save the file in a universal format, rich text format (rtf).

The Clipboard

The **clipboard** is where cut or copied items are stored. It is a universal feature for Windows and Mac computers. For Microsoft Windows programs, it functions as a scrapbook layering each change the user makes for Microsoft Software. You can see what is on the clipboard in a Microsoft product by clicking on the Home tab and the arrow in the lower right corner of the clipboard group. (Free clipboard viewers are available for download for use with non-Microsoft software.) Mac computers store only the last change. In a Mac, the clipboard empties anytime you close a file or turn off the computer. In Windows programs, all items stay on the clipboard until you either clear it manually, exit ALL Microsoft products, or turn off the computer. After closing all Microsoft products, the last item placed on the clipboard will remain.

Disk and Data Encryption

Because computers are tools that we use to manage private and secure files such as online banking, files with social security numbers, program passwords, and student unique identifiers, the data are vulnerable for cyber thieves. You can use **encryption** software to encrypt an entire hard drive or encrypt selected files. To access encrypted files, you must decrypt them.

File encryption is a feature built into some Windows and Mac operating systems. If you use the professional version of Windows, you can encrypt files, by right-clicking on the file or folder and clicking Properties → General → Advanced → and clicking on the checkbox for Encrypt contents to secure data. On the Mac, open the Disk Utility and select File → New → Disk Image from Folder. Select the folder that you want to encrypt and then select the type of encryption from the drop-down menu. You will have a choice of the recommended 128-bit AES encryption or 256-bit encryption, which is slower, but more secure.

If your version of Windows is not the professional version or you wish more encryption options, you can also use free encryption software available as a download from the Internet such as TrueCrypt or Axcrypt. You can also search the Internet for reviews of encryption software or go to http://dottech.org/15996/need-to-encrypt-your-files-let-axcrypt-or-truecrypt-do-the-job-for-you/.

The good and the bad about file encryption is that it works. Thieves will not be able to steal private data. However, if you forget the password used to encrypt the file, you will not be able to view the file contents.

OTHER COMPUTER FEATURES

Features added since the first personal computers appeared in the late 1970s and early 1980s make them easier to use.

Speech Recognition

Speech recognition, or the ability to translate the spoken work into text, has been available for decades, but slow computer processors hindered its development. The other problems that prevented popular use included the time necessary to train the program and the expensiveness of the software (Pinola, 2011). Advances in the development of the feature stagnated until the introduction of the feature on smartphones.

In 2008, Google released Voice Search as an app in the iPhone's app store (Ionescu, 2008). The popularity and convenience of the speech recognition feature triggered significant developments in accuracy of the software "understanding" speech. Google went on a separate path from Apple, improved the feature, and released Voice Search to the Chrome Browser and Android smartphones. Apple also continued to improve the speech recognition feature with Siri, the virtual personal assistant known for the wry sense of humor. With the release of Apple iOS 7, users can change Siri's voice gender on the iPhone and iPad. Google and Apple use analytics from all of their users to improve speech recognition. Apple is using geolocation that identifies the geographical location of the device user to make improvements (Campbell, 2013).

Speech recognition is an improved feature with the most recent Windows and Apple computers.

On Windows computers, you must activate the speech recognition through the Control Panel → Speech Recognition menu. Microsoft prompts users to use a headset with a microphone and to complete a tutorial. On the Mac, the feature is located in the Apple Preferences System menu.

Additionally, there are commercially available programs that allow one to dictate to the computer. One of the most popular for general work is Dragon Speaking Naturally by Nuance Corporation. Nuance Corporation also has a version for medical dictation. Although, some training is helpful, the program will learn with use. Not only is this program capable of translating spoken word to text, but it will read the text back.

Sleep Mode

If you want to access your computer files quickly after taking a break from working without turning off the computer, you can use the **sleep mode**. On many devices automatic activation of sleep mode occurs after a given period of inactivity. Sleep mode is available on all computers, including tablets and smartphones. The sleep mode saves energy, but the computer is not off. Be aware that if you do not save the active files before using the sleep mode and the battery drains, you will lose your most recent changes.

Some Windows operating systems and Android phones provide an option to **hibernate**. Hibernate is a deeper sleep than sleep mode. In the hibernate mode, all of the active files in memory are saved safely to the computer hard drive. From either sleep or hibernate mode, moving the mouse will awaken the computer to the state in which you left it, but when the computer is in hibernate mode, it will require a little longer to awaken.

Handling Minor Problems

As robust as today's computers are, they sometimes get themselves tangled up and, through no fault of the user, refuse to respond to commands. This is most apt to happen to an individual program, not the entire computer. If you are working in a computer laboratory, or on an agency computer, if this happens, leave the computer alone and notify the laboratory or network manager. If, however, you are home, you can do some things.

If you receive a message saying, "This program is not responding" with a request to shut it down, you have no choice except to say yes. The computer may or may not shut down. If it does not, this is the time to use what is affectionately referred to as the "three-finger salute," because it requires three fingers to execute. To carry it out, you press down and hold the Ctrl, Alt, and Delete keys until you get a menu on which one of the choices is to open the task manager (Microsoft Operating Systems). From there, you can locate the offending program and click the End Task button (Figure 2-3). You may then get still another window telling you that the program is not responding and asking you if you want to end it. You may need to tell it yes more than once! However, eventually it will close the program. After letting it rest for a few minutes, you can then restart that program if you wish. On the Mac, click on the Apple icon, and then Force Quit from the menu to close a nonresponding program.

The biggest drawback is that when a program crashes, you will lose whatever you have not saved, which is a reason to save continually as you work! However, most of today's programs will do a backup save every 10 or 15 minutes, a time that you can set in the preferences. After a program crash, when you reopen the program, a message appears stating that program did not close properly last time and presents a listing of files that were open and not saved. The best approach is to look at each file and select the latest version.

On rare occasions, the above approach does not work, and the computer seems bent on doing its own thing with absolutely no regard for what you want. No matter what you do, you cannot seem to get its attention. Programmers of operating systems, knowing that despite all their efforts this can occasionally happen, have provided an out. To turn off a nonresponding computer, press the power button (yes, the power button on the CPU) and hold it down until the computer turns off! If you are using a laptop or other mobile device, you may need to remove the battery for a minute to cut off its power. Afterward, you can restart the computer, and it will probably be back to normal! Beyond this, see your computer guru!

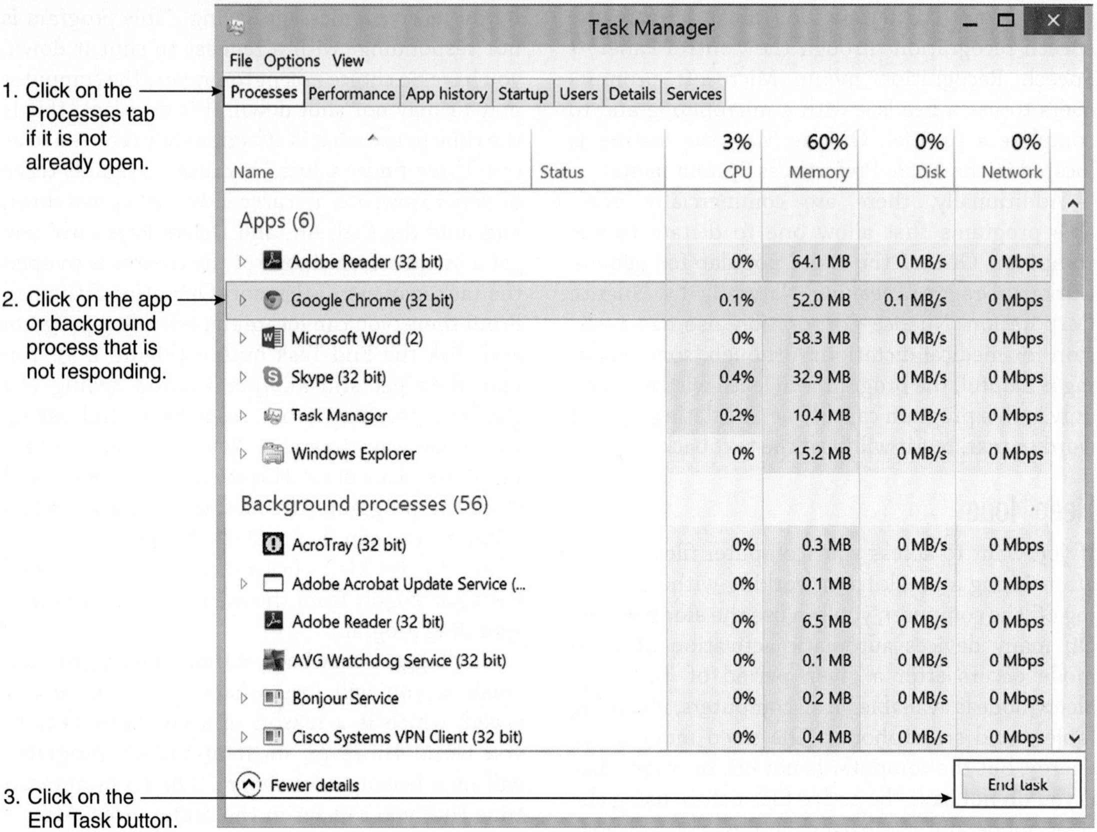

Figure 2-3. Closing a nonresponsive program. (Used with permission from Microsoft.)

SUMMARY

Many different types of software are useful in managing information. There are two main classifications of software: operating systems and application software. An operating system determines what application software you can use.

Cloud computing is pervasive in the use of computers with Internet access. Cloud computing encompasses use of remote servers and software, file storage resources, and the ability to work synchronously and asynchronously using shared files and folders with others. However, there are pros and cons to its use.

Knowledge of software program copyright is required to avoid software piracy. All but public-domain software used is proprietary and copyrighted. Using a copyrighted program without following the rules for use is software piracy.

Using computers and managing files efficiently may require you to learn new processes.

Cyber criminals are in constant search of private and unsecured files and computer hard drive data. Users should master the use of encryption software to secure data. Finally, users should use energy-saving sleep modes to save energy, battery life, and computer files.

APPLICATIONS AND COMPETENCIES

1. Identify the current operating system on the computer you are using.

2. Are you using cloud computing on a desktop/laptop, phone, or tablet? If so, which cloud computing software are you using? Do an Internet search to identify cloud computing resources that may help you or others. Summarize your findings.

3. Conduct an Internet search for examples of software piracy. Write up the talking points of the findings.

4. A friend gives you a CD-ROM with a program on it for you to install. What things should you consider before doing so?

5. You wish to install a program that you have at home on another computer. What things should you consider?

6. Explore keyboard shortcuts for the computer(s) you use. Identify at least two new shortcuts for you to use. Discuss the advantages for use.

7. Select and use encryption software to encrypt a sample file, decrypt the file, and shred and delete the file. What precautions must users take when using encryption software? What are the advantages? Summarize your findings.

8. Are you using computer speech recognition? Explain the advantages and disadvantages for use.

REFERENCES

Beal, V. (2013, September 4). *What is open source software?* Retrieved from http://www.webopedia.com/DidYouKnow/Computer_Science/2005/open_source.asp

Business Software Alliance. (2013). *2011 piracy study*. Retrieved from http://globalstudy.bsa.org/2011/

Campbell, M. (2013, September 12). Apple looks to geolocation for enhanced speech recognition. *Apple Insider*. Retrieved from http://appleinsider.com/articles/13/09/12/apple-looks-to-geolocation-for-enhanced-speech-recognition

Chicago hospital caught pirating. (1997, January). *Healthcare Informatics*, 20.

Chromium Projects. (2013). *Chromium OS*. Retrieved from http://www.chromium.org/chromium-os

Fisher, T. (2013). *BIOS (basic input output system)*. Retrieved from http://pcsupport.about.com/od/termsb/p/bios.htm

Free Software Foundation. (2011). *About GNU operating system*. Retrieved from http://www.gnu.org/gnu/about-gnu.html

Gaumer, G. L., Koeniger-Donohue, R., Friel, C., et al (2007). Use of information technology by advanced practice nurses. *CIN: Computers, Informatics, Nursing*, 25(6), 344–352. Retrieved from http://journals.lww.com/cinjournal/pages/default.aspx

Google. (2011, May 11). *A new kind of computer: Chromebook*. Retrieved from http://googleblog.blogspot.com/2011/05/new-kind-of-computer-chromebook.html?utm_source=feedburner&utm_medium=feed&utm_campaign=Feed%3A+blogspot%2FMKuf+%28Official+Google+Blog%29&utm_content=Google+Reader

Google Developers. (2013, February 22). *Open source programs office*. Retrieved from https://developers.google.com/open-source/

Health Resources and Services Administration (HRSA). (2013). *What is public domain software?* Retrieved from http://www.hrsa.gov/healthit/toolbox/HealthITAdoptiontoolbox/OpenSource/pubdomainsoftware.html

Ionescu, D. (2008, November 14). iPhone gets Google search by voice. *PC World*. Retrieved from http://www.techhive.com/article/153871/search.html

Linux.org. (2013). *What is Linux*. Retrieved from http://www.linux.org/threads/what-is-linux.4076/

Mesa, A. (1998). *A history of graphical user interface*. Retrieved from http://applemuseum.bott.org/sections/gui.html

Microsoft. (2013a). *A history of Windows highlights from the first 25 years*. Retrieved from http://windows.microsoft.com/en-in/windows/history

Microsoft. (2013b). *Office*. Retrieved from http://office.microsoft.com/en-us/

Net Applications.com. (2013). *Desktop operating system market share*. Retrieved from http://www.netmarketshare.com/operating-system-market-share.aspx?qprid=8&qpcustomd=0

Nicoll, L. H. (1994). Modern day pirates: Software users and abusers. *Journal of Nursing Administration*, 24(1), 18–20. Retrieved from http://journals.lww.com/jonajournal/pages/default.aspx

Oldcomputers.net. (2013). *Macintosh computer*. Retrieved from http://oldcomputers.net/macintosh.html

Pinola, M. (2011, November 2). *Speech recognition through the decades: How we ended up with Siri*. PC World. Retrieved from http://www.techhive.com/article/243060/speech_recognition_through_the_decades_how_we_ended_up_with_siri.html?page=2

Sanford, G. (2015). *Apple-history*. Retrieved from http://apple-history.com/

Webopedia. (2013). *Operating system*. Retrieved from http://www.webopedia.com/TERM/o/operating_system.html

CHAPTER 3

Basic Computer Networking Concepts

OBJECTIVES

After studying this chapter, you will be able to:

1. Discuss the overall technology of computer networking.
2. Provide examples for use of intranet, extranet, and virtual private networks.
3. Analyze the different methods of connecting to the Internet.
4. Discuss the different types of malware.
5. Describe effective methods to protect against malware.

KEY TERMS

Advanced encryption standard (AES)

Adware

Bandwidth

Botnet

Broadband

Campus area network (CAN)

Computer virus

Distributed denial of service (DDoS)

Digital subscriber line (DSL)

Dynamic IP address

E-mail virus

Extranet

Firewall

Hardwire

Hoax

Internet protocol (IP)

Internet service provider (ISP)

Intranet

IP address

Local area network (LAN)

Keylogger

Malware

Metropolitan area network (MAN)

Modem

Network

Network authentication

Nodes

Pharming

Phishing

Plain old telephone service (POTS)

Protocols

Router

Social engineering

Spyware

Static IP address

Transmission control protocol (TCP)

Trojan horse

Universal resource locator (URL)

Virtual private network (VPN)

Warez

Web browser (browser)

Wide area network (WAN)

Wi-Fi protected access (WPA)

Wi-Fi protected access 2 (WPA2)

Wired equivalent privacy (WEP)

Wireless (Wi-Fi)

Worm

Urban legend

A nurse encounters a patient with an unfamiliar disease. From an e-mail message, the nurse learns that a document on a computer in another country has information about caring for patients with this disease. Within 60 seconds of logging on to the Internet, the nurse prints out the document. This ability to exchange information on a global scale is changing the world. Healthcare professionals do not have to wait for information to become available in a journal in the country in which they live. Nurses and other healthcare professionals can and do use computers to **network** with colleagues all over the world. Network refers to the connection of two or more computers, which allows the computers to communicate.

Healthcare depends on communication: communication between the nurse and the patient, communication between healthcare professionals, communication about organizational issues, and communication with the public. As you can see, computer networking augments the methods used today to communicate in healthcare. Since the first computers talked to each other in the late 1960s, networking has progressed to the point where not only computers in an organization are connected to each other but also institutions are connected to a worldwide network known as the Internet.

This chapter discusses information on networking, from both a historical and working perspective. It introduces terminology pertinent to networking that you can use when talking about a problem with an information technology specialist or participating on a committee related to networking technology. Finally, there is comprehensive information about online security, security threats, and methods to protect you and your computer from security threats.

A HISTORICAL PERSPECTIVE OF THE INTERNET

The development of the Internet was one of the positive legacies of the Cold War. It served as a means of communication that would survive a nuclear war and provide the most economical use from then scarce, large computer resources. The journey from ARPANET (Advanced Research Projects Agency NETwork), which was established in 1969 to connect four nodes—the University of California, Los Angeles; Stanford Research Institute; the University of California, Santa Barbara; and the University of Utah (Howe, 2012, September 13)—to today's Internet, has been amazing. It is "one of the most successful examples of the benefits of sustained investment and commitment to research and development of information infrastructure" (Internet Society, 2013a, para 1).

In August 1962, J.C.R. Licklider of MIT wrote the first recorded description of networking in a series of memos. The concepts expressed were similar to those used in today's Internet. His vision was a "globally interconnected set of computers through which everyone could quickly access data and programs from any site" (Internet Society, 2013a, para 5). The underlying technical feature of the Internet is open architecture networking (Internet Society, 2013a). That is, the choice of how connected networks were set up, or their network architecture, was immaterial as long as they could work with other networks. Computer communication required a way of packaging the data and the development of **protocols** for data transfer.

The U.S. Defense Advanced Research Projects Agency (DARPA) began researching computer communication technologies in 1973. Examples of protocols DARPA researchers created are **TCP (transmission control protocol)** and **IP (Internet protocol)**. In 1986, the National Science Foundation developed a major backbone Internet communication service using NSFNET (Internet Society, 2013b). Today, there are thousands of backbones across the world, which allows instantaneous computer communication.

The government, industry, and academia have been, and continue to be, partners in evolving and implementing the Internet. The free and open access to basic documents, especially protocol specifications, was key to the rapid growth of the Internet. The development of faster **bandwidth** speeds was another key factor.

NETWORK CONNECTIONS ESSENTIALS

The Internet is, as its last three letters indicate, a network. Granted, it is a worldwide, amorphous network of interconnected computers, but it still is a network. Nothing in the world before has become so quickly assimilated into daily use as the Internet. In the early 1990s, the Internet was relatively unknown by all but a few academics. By the summer of 1993, the popular culture took note of this phenomenon, as evidenced by a cartoon in the New Yorker showing two dogs at a computer, with one remarking to the other, "On the Internet no one knows you are a dog" (Aikat, 1997, August 27). Since then, the Internet changed how and with whom we communicate. The Internet crosses national boundaries disregarding long-established international protocols. Laws designed for national entities are inadequate with the pervasive Internet (Figure 3-1).

A network (Figure 3-2) can range in size from a connection between a smartphone and a personal computer (PC) to the worldwide, multiuser computer connection—the Internet. The network name relates to the variation in network size and the number and location of connected computers.

- LAN or **local area network** is a network confined to a small area such as a building or groups of buildings (Webopedia, 2013a).
- WAN or **wide area network** is a network that encompasses a large geographical area. A

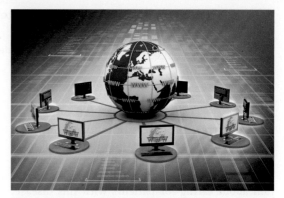

Figure 3-1. The global Internet (shutterstock.com/ramcreations).

WAN might be two or more LANs (Webopedia, 2013b).
- CAN or **campus area network** is a network that encompasses a defined geographic area, such as a college campus (Webopedia, 2013c).
- MAN or **metropolitan area network** is a network that encompasses a city or town (Webopedia, 2013d).

Construction of the Internet (architecture) varies, often depending on the purpose of the network. Client–server and peer-to-peer are examples of Internet architecture types.

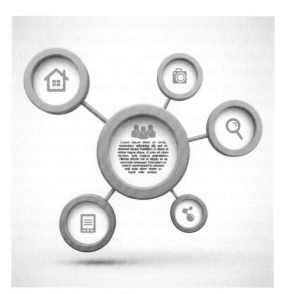

Figure 3-2. Network (shutterstock.com/3d_kot).

- In client–server architecture, clients or workstation computers rely on the server to run a program or access data. The server is often located in a remote setting (Webopedia, 2013e).
- With peer-to-peer (P2P) architecture, each computer operates as a standalone, but can exchange files with other computers on that network (Webopedia, 2013f).

In healthcare, we use the client–server architecture to use the electronic medical record, often with a thin client. A thin client might have only a keyboard and monitor, but not have a hard drive, instead depending upon the server to process data.

Types of Networks

There are three main types of networks for Internet use: **intranet**, **extranet**, and **virtual private network (VPN)**. The intranet is a private network within an organization, which allows users of an organization to share information. It may include features similar to the Internet, such as e-mail, mailing lists, and user groups. An extranet is an extension of an intranet with added security features. It provides accessibility to the intranet to a specific group of outsiders, often business partners. Access requires a valid username and password.

A VPN allows an organization to communicate confidentially (Beal, 2015, February 16). The VPN transmits a file using an encrypted tunnel blocking view of the file by others. The VPN is an intranet with an extra layer of security that operates as an extranet. A VPN provides access to patient data to authorized users who are not physically present in the healthcare setting such as allowing a physician or nurse practitioner at home to see a patient's electronic health record (EHR). They can also be used for patient portals or places where patients can renew prescriptions, make appointments, and send messages.

Network Connections

Networks connect physically with a variety of materials, such as twisted-wire cables, phone lines, fiber-optic lines, or radio waves. Computers wired together are **hardwired**. When you see the term "hard" with another item, this means that the item is permanent or that it physically exists.

Most healthcare agency networks, even those that use **wireless**, are to some extent hardwired.

Wireless (Wi-Fi) transmissions are limited in distance, so they do not compete with other radio traffic. During the wireless system installation, **nodes**, or wireless devices that pick up signals sent by a user and transmit them to the central server or rebroadcast them to another node, are placed at strategic locations throughout the institution. They also transmit signals back to the user's computer. A node consists of a tiny router with a few wireless cards and antennas. Determination of node placements occurs after a thorough assessment of the building or premises. Successful wireless communication depends on an adequate number of nodes and their placement. The distance of a device from the node will affect both the speed of transmission and whether one can use the network. The number of users per node also affects the speed of transmission.

Wireless transmission is less secure than hardwired transmission because the signal is available for use by anyone in range (Joan, 2011). Wi-Fi security measures include **wired equivalent privacy (WEP)**, **Wi-Fi protected access (WPA)**, and **Wi-Fi protected access 2 (WPA2)**. WPA2 is better security than WPA because it uses an **advanced encryption standard (AES)**.

Connection to a Wi-Fi network requires the use of a modem and router (Figure 3-3). The **modem** connects with the **Internet service provider**

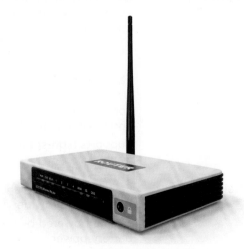

Figure 3-3. Cable modem and wireless router (shutterstock.com/Maxx-Studio).

(ISP) and the **router** connects multiple computers to the same network (PC.net, 2013). The router has one or two antennas, which may be internal, to transmit the Wi-Fi signal. Sometimes, the one device contains the router and modem. In home networks, **digital subscriber line (DSL)** and television (TV) cable often connect the router to the Internet. In some rural areas, Internet users may connect using a dial-up modem through a regular telephone line. This type of connection is a **POTS (plain old telephone service)**. Another type of connection, especially in less developed countries, is through a satellite.

Network authentication is a standard for home and work computer networks. In the home setting, the authentication code is often located on the router. If it is not, it is imperative that the network owners know the authentication code. All users must enter the authentication code to access a secure Wi-Fi network. Without the code, no new devices such as a smartphone or tablet computer can connect to the network.

Network Connection Speed

Today, most Internet connections use **broadband**. This term applies to many different types of network connections and refers to the bandwidth, or how much data the connection can transmit at the same time. The size of the broadband connection determines the speed of the network connection. The greater the bandwidth, the greater the simultaneous information transmission, just as a six-lane highway will permit more cars to travel at the same time. POTS (plain old telephone service) transmits only a single frequency at one time; hence, a broadband connection offers more speed. There are different broadband connections available for using the Internet, such as DSL, cable, satellite, and fiber-optic cable (Table 3-1).

TABLE 3-1 Pros and Cons of Broadband Connection Types		
Connection Type	**Pros**	**Cons**
Fiber-optic cable	Supports high-speed data transfer Excellent signal reliability	More fragile than wire More expensive than DSL
Digital subscriber lines (DSLs)	Faster than dial-up Uses a regular phone line (can use the phone and Internet connection at the same time) Easy to install	Available only where there is phone service Connection speed slowed by longer distances from the provider
Television cable	Faster than dial-up and DSL Uses a television cable connection (can use Internet and television at the same time) Supports high-speed data transfer	Available only where there is cable television service
Satellite	Faster than dial-up and DSL Available worldwide Can be powered by generator or battery power	Affected by weather (heavy cloud cover and storms) More expensive than DSL and cable Requires use of a satellite dish

IP Addresses

To make it possible for each computer on the Internet to be electronically located, each has an **IP address**, even the one you use to connect to the Internet at home. There are four sets of numbers separated by periods or dots in an IP address (similar to Figure 3-4). Each set of numbers can range from 0 to 255. Because numbers are difficult for most people to remember, and because they may change, each computer also has an assigned name (ICANN, 2013). The Internet **domain name system** translates the computer name into its IP address each time when sending a message. Therefore, when there is a requirement for an IP numerical address change, only the domain name system updates.

IP addresses can be static or dynamic. A **static IP address** is the same each time the computer connects to the Internet. A **dynamic IP address** changes each time a user connects to the Internet. To facilitate each online computer having its own IP address, each ISP has a given number of IP addresses, which they then assign to online computers, in either a static or a dynamic format.

Domain Name System

In 1998, the Internet Corporation for Assigned Names and Numbers (ICANN) was established to keep the Internet "secure, stable and interoperable" (ICANN, 2013). ICANN is a nonprofit organization for the world. It works with individual government advisory organizations to determine the domain names. To obtain a domain name, users register the domain name with ICANN. The domain name suffix or ending provides information about the web page sponsor.

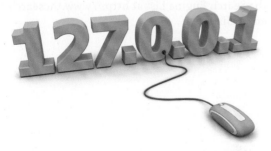

Figure 3-4. IP address (shutterstock.com/Matthias Pahl).

The term top-level domain (TLD) describes the domain suffix name. Originally, there were five domain suffixes. Today, there are over 250. The domain name is read from the right to the left. The far right is the TLD. The specific descriptors are located to the left of the TLD. The IP address is invisible. One should pay attention to the TLD in a web address because people intent on deceiving others will take the name of the computer address of a respected organization and obtain an Internet address with that name but with a different TLD. In the address bar of a **web browser**, enter the same web address, except use a different TLD to determine if others have used it.

THE WORLD WIDE WEB

The World Wide Web is a network within the Internet that allows hypertext documents to be accessed using software known as a web browser. The web is "governed" and maintained by the World Wide Web Consortium (W3C). This organization "tries to enforce compatibility and agreement among industry members in the adoption of new standards defined by the W3C. Different vendors offer incompatible versions of HTML (hypertext markup language), causing inconsistency on the display of Web pages. The consortium tries to get all those vendors to implement a set of core principles and components, which are chosen by the consortium" (Wikipedia, 2013a).

Web Browsers

A web browser, or just browser, is a tool enabling users to retrieve and display files from the Internet. Web browsers use the client–server model of networking to retrieve a web document. The browser on the client computer requests a file from the server using a transmission protocol known as hypertext transfer protocol (HTTP). The server has special server software for using the protocol to receive the message, find the file, and send it back to the requesting computer.

It is important to understand that there are many web browsers (Table 3-2), not just the desktop icon, that came with the computer. It is a good idea to have more than one to use because

TABLE 3-2 **Examples of Popular Web Browsers**

Web Browser Name	Web Address
Chrome	https://www.google.com/intl/en/chrome/browser/
Firefox	http://www.mozilla.org/en-US/firefox/new/
Internet Explorer	http://windows.microsoft.com/en-us/internet-explorer/download-ie
Opera	http://www.opera.com/
Safari	http://www.apple.com/safari/

pages that will not display correctly with one web browser may work correctly with another one. The search feature varies with web browsers. For example, Chrome and Safari integrated the search feature with the web address bar for instead of a separate search window.

Troubleshooting an URL

All web documents have an URL (pronounced "Earl"), which stands for **universal resource locator**. The URL usually begins with http or https. A final "s" in a website's URL beginning letters (https://) indicates the website is secure. URLs always contain descriptors, a domain name (a unique name that identifies a website), and may include a folder name, a file name, or both. In Figure 3-5, starting at the end of the URL, the file name is "index.html" and the folder names are "evidence-based-reports" and "findings" and "research"; "evidence-based-reports" is located in the "findings" folder, and the "findings" folder is located in the "research" folder. If the URL ends with a forward slash (/), it designates a folder, and if it ends with a dot (.) and other letters, it is a file. The top-level domain name is ".gov" and the descriptors are www.ahrq. If you use an URL that does not open a page, try modifying the URL by deleting first the file name and then the folder(s) until you return to the domain or computer website address. Along the way, you may receive an error message that you do not have access to this file or folder; if that happens, just keep deleting between forward slashes. Often, the website organization and the address of the page for which you are searching changed. Once at the website address, you may be able to search for the file. If neither of these tricks works, use a search engine to see if the page still exists.

Choosing a Search Engine

Web browsers allow you to choose a search engine. The choice you make depends on the purpose of the search. There are almost 300 different search engines, but you should consider narrowing your choice to only two or three. For a comprehensive listing of search engines, go to the Search Engine List at http://www.thesearch-enginelist.com/.

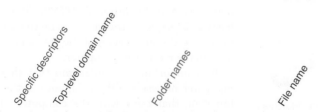

http://www.ahrq.gov/research/findings/evidence-based-reports/index.html

Figure 3-5. Anatomy of an URL.

TABLE 3-3   Web Browser Terminology

Term	Definition
Active server page (ASP)	Allows access to databases to present real-time data based upon the user's request (Web Wiz, 2013)
Active X controls	Small programs used to allow animation or to install Microsoft security updates. Installation might be necessary to use a website. Users must identify legitimacy before using (Microsoft Safety & Security Center, 2013).
Bookmarks/ Favorites	Allows the user to save links to favorite websites from a menu. Can save links to a web browser or to a personal cloud bookmarking site
Java	A programming language that some websites use to display data (Java, 2013). Is compiled before it can be run (Burns, 2013)
JavaScript	A scripting language (differs from Java) used to make web pages interactive. Often used for online polling and quizzes (Chapman, 2013). Must be placed inside an HTML (web) document (Burns, 2013)
Plug-ins/Add-ons	A helper program for a web browser that increases the functionality of the browser. Examples include Adobe Acrobat Reader and Shockwave.
Streaming	Allows delivery of audio and/or video to the user before downloading the entire file
Web cookies	Allows a website to save a message to the user's computer from a web server. Examples include remembering a log-in and password for a website or form auto completion (Beal, 2013a).

The way you change search engines to use is browser specific. The procedure often changes with new editions of web browser. An easy way to identify the changing procedure is to enter terms with the name of the web browser and "change search engine" into a search engine. Sometimes, selecting a choice for a search engine is from the web address bar or search engine window. Other times, the feature is in the configuration menu for the web browser.

Web Browser Terminology

Terminology used for web browsers causes confusion; however, there is terminology that is essential to know. Table 3-3 provides a list of some of the more common terms used in connection with the web and their definitions.

ONLINE SECURITY

One does not have to be web familiar to have heard about web security problems. A perceptive user can prevent most security issues. Before becoming overly paranoid about security breaches, know that most of the problems occur if one is lax about Internet security. Anyone connecting to the Internet with any type of broadband connection needs to protect their computer systems against invaders or viruses. POTS users, although less vulnerable, also need to take precautions.

Computer Malware

Computer malware refers to all forms of computer software designed by criminals, specifically to damage or disrupt a computer system, often for a profit. Several types of such programs exist, all of which operate differently, but they all change a computer to suit the aims of the perpetuator. The criminals use two techniques for the malware attacks, **social engineering** and drive-by-download (Krishna et al., 2013).

Social engineering tricks the victims into downloading and installing malware. For example, you may receive an e-mail message asking you to view a video or an "alert" that your video software is out of date with instructions to click to update. Of course, the false "video update" click installs the malware. Drive-by-download occurs when the web page design includes the malware. Opening the web page triggers the download and installation of the malware. It is possible for malware to hide in advertisements of reputable websites such as *Los Angeles Times* and *US News* (Infosecurity Magazine, 2013, October 11; Mimosao, 2013, September 6). Of course, attacked websites take immediate action to address the problem as soon as they identify the threats. Unfortunately, the problem is like Whack-a-Mole where after correcting one problem, another one appears.

Although all computer users are vulnerable to a malware infection, there are preventative measures that we can employ. Like healthcare diseases, it is important to understand the problems and vulnerabilities. The language of the "dark world" sounds like child play, but make no mistake, it is a serious lucrative business for cyber criminals.

Botnet

Botnet (also known as a zombie army) is a growing malware threat (Figure 3-6). It is a group of computers connected to the Internet that, unbeknownst to their owners, have software installed on their computers to forward items such as spam or viruses to other Internet computers (Rouse, 2012). The botnet owner is termed a "herder," the infected computer is a "drone" or "zombie," and computer resources used to trap malware are termed "honeypots" (Shadowserver, 2005a,

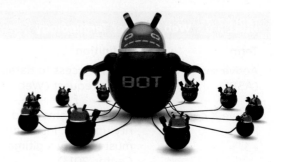

Figure 3-6. Botnet herder (shutterstock.com/Gunnar Assmy).

2005b). Botnets may lurk on popular websites such as social networking, financial institutions, online advertisements, online auction sites, and online stores (Arbor Networks, 2013).

Use of botnets is for click fraud, **distributed denial of service (DDoS)**, **keylogger**, **warez**, and spam. Click fraud occurs when directing a zombie computer to send fake clicks to an advertising affiliate network in order to abscond with an award from visiting the site. DDoS occurs when the herder directs all the computers in its botnet to send requests to the same site at the same time. This overwhelms the site and prevents legitimate access to the website for a long time. The cyber crooks have even demanded ransom money to release the hijacked website. Botnets might use malicious keylogger software to trace and steal passwords and bank account numbers. They can also steal, store, or gain access to illegal and pirated software known as **warez**.

Phishing and Pharming

Phishing and **pharming** are older forms of web scams, and both try to get an individual to reveal personal information such as a bank account number or a social security number. Phishing and pharming are easy to detect. In phishing, the victim received an e-mail message with a web address hyperlink in it, with instructions to go to this website to confirm an account or perform some other task that will involve revealing personal information. Although the hyperlink text in the message looks authentic, clicking it will take a user to a website that is not the one seen in the URL in the message, although it may be a mirror image of the real one.

Subject: adp_subj

ADP **Pressing Communication**

Note No.: 98489

http://randallpetersonhomes.com/
wp-content/plugins/zabicyenusa/
chkpayroladp.html

Valued ADP Partne
Your Refused Yes **Click to follow link** ⟩rd(s) have been delivered to the web site:
Enter Into website here
Please review the following information:
lease note that your bank account will be debited within 1 banking day for the sum shown on the Summary(s).
ease DO NOT reply to this message. auomatic informational system can't accept incoming email.
Please Contact your ADP Benefits Authority.
This message was sent to valid clients in your system that approach ADP Netsecure.
As general, thank you for being with ADP as your business companion!
Ref: 98489

Figure 3-7. E-mail scam.

You can check the true owner of a site by going to the site http://whois.com and entering a web address into the space at the top left. To copy the URL easily, tap Ctrl (Command) + L, which will place your insertion point on the address bar and select the entire address. To copy the URL, tap Ctrl (Command) + C. You can then paste it into the whois website by putting your insertion point into the window and tapping Ctrl (Command) + V.

You can protect against this type of fraud by placing the mouse pointer over the hyperlinked web address to see the real address of the link (Figure 3-7). Notice that some letters are missing from the left side of the e-mail. Often, the persons committing the fraud do not know English, so they do not recognize the errors caused by cut-and-paste (H. Patrick, personal communication, July 24, 2014). Broken English and copy/paste errors should make e-mail receivers alerted to phishing, scamming, virus, or other fraud schemes. However, the perpetrators committing e-mail fraud are getting more sophisticated every day. The e-mail example in Figure 3-7 is classified as spoofing because the sender was

disguised as ADP (Automatic Data Processing), a company that provides payroll services.

Pharming, on the other hand, results when an attacker infiltrates a domain name server and changes the routing for addresses. Thus, when users of that domain name server enter an URL for a pharmed site, they are "pharmed" to the evil site. It results from inadequate security for the domain name server. Protection against this type of attack rests with those who maintain the DNS servers.

> **QSEN Scenario**
>
> You are teaching a group of patients about how to avoid phishing and pharming types of e-mails. What information will you share?

Computer Viruses

A type of malware that you hear about most often is a **computer virus**. A computer virus is a small software program. The design of the program is to execute and replicate itself without your knowledge.

Before the widespread use of the Internet, a disk inserted into the computer's drive usually introduced them. Today, computer viruses usually arrive from the Internet, with an e-mail attachment, a greeting card, or an audio or video file. They can corrupt or delete data on your computer or use your e-mail program to send themselves to everyone in your address book or even erase your hard drive.

Like the human variety, computer viruses cause varying degrees of harm. Some can damage hardware, but others only cause annoying effects. Although a virus may exist on a computer, it cannot infect the computer until you run the program with the attached virus. After their initial introduction, sharing infected files and sending e-mails with infected attachments spread the viruses without the knowledge of the user.

E-mail Virus

E-mail messages may have an **e-mail virus**. A file created by a legitimate program, such as a word processor or a spreadsheet, might hide the virus. To prevent this type of virus, most antivirus programs thoroughly vet each e-mail message.

Worm

A **worm** is a small piece of malware that uses security holes and computer networks to replicate itself. It is not completely a virus in that it does not require a human to run a program to become active; rather, it is a subclass of virus because it replicates itself. To accomplish replication, the worm scans the network for another machine with the same security hole and, using this, copies itself to the new machine, which in turn repeats this action creating an ever-growing mass of infection. Unlike a plain virus, worms do not need to attach themselves to an existing program. They always cause harm to a network, even if only by consuming bandwidth. Some worms include a "payload," or code that is designed to do more than just spread the worm. A payload may delete files on the host computer or encrypt files. The perpetuator then demands a ransom to unencrypt the file. Payloads can also create a "backdoor," or way into a theoretically secure system that bypasses security and is undetected (Wikipedia, 2013b).

Trojan Horse

A **Trojan horse** is not technically a virus because it does not replicate itself. Like the historical Trojan horse, it masquerades as something it is

not. For example, a Trojan horse may appear to be a program that performs a useful action or is fun, such as a game, but in reality, when the program runs, it places malicious software on your computer or create a backdoor. Trojan horses do not infect other files or self-replicate.

A keylogger Trojan is malicious software that monitors keystrokes, placing them in a file and sending it to the remote attacker (Landesman, 2013). Some keyloggers record all keystrokes; others are sophisticated enough to log keys only when you open a specific site such as a bank account. Parents who monitor their children's online activities also use this type of software. Some sites prevent keylogging by having a user use the mouse to point to a visual cue instead of using the keyboard.

Adware and Spyware

Adware and **spyware** are neither a virus nor spam. Most adware is legitimate, but some software that functions as adware is actually spyware, which at the very least is a nuisance, or it may actually invade your privacy by tracking your Internet travels or installing malicious code (Beal, 2013b, May 5).

Adware

Adware is software that is often a legitimate revenue source for companies that offer free software. Software programs, games, or utilities, designed and distributed as freeware, often provide their software in a sponsored mode (Beal, 2013b). In this mode, depending on the vendor, most or all of the features are enabled, but pop-up advertisements appear when you use the program. Paying to register the software will remove the advertisements. This software is not malicious, but just randomly displays paid advertisements when the program is used. It does not track your habits or provide personal information to a third party but is a legitimate source of income to those who provide free software.

Spyware

Spyware, in contrast to adware, tracks your web surfing to tailor advertisements for you. Some adware unfortunately is spywares (Beal, 2013b). This has given legitimate adware a bad name. Spyware is similar to a Trojan horse because it masquerades as what it is not. Downloading and installing peer-to-peer file-swapping products, such as those allowing users to swap music files, are a common way to infect computers. Although spyware appears to operate like legitimate adware, it is usually a separate program that can monitor keystrokes, including passwords and credit card numbers, and transmit this information to a third party. It can also scan your hard drive, read cookies, and change default home pages on web browsers. Sometimes, a licensing agreement, which few of us read before clicking "Accept," informs users of the spyware installation with the program, although this information is usually in obtuse, hard-to-read legalese or misleading double-edged statements.

Protection Against Malware

Whether malware is a type of virus, spyware, or Trojan horse is not important. What is important is to protect the computer against malware, or if a computer is infected, an alert allows for prompt removal. The first line of protection is to be careful of sites whose reputations are unknown. Downloading a file that you find in an open web search is always problematic. If you really must download the file, scan the file with your antivirus program before installing or executing it. In fact, this is a good standard procedure with any downloaded file, no matter what the source.

Take the following steps as protection against malware (Umstead, 2013, February 25):

- Avoid password reuse.
- Use strong passwords.
- Use antivirus software and keep it updated.
- Avoid getting too personal with the public on social networking sites (e.g., do not share the following: your phone number, physical address, inappropriate or provocative photos, use of alcohol or drugs, or messages attacking others).
- Do not open e-mail from strangers.
- Do not open e-mail attachments you were not expecting to receive.
- Always keep your antimalware software updated.
- Always download the latest operating system and software updates. Many of the updates fix security holes.
- Avoid believing you are invulnerable to malware—robot computers attack randomly.

Firewalls

A **firewall** for computers is like a firewall in a building; it acts to block destructive forces. Computer firewalls work closely with a router program to filter the traffic both coming into and, for many firewalls, going out of a network or a private computer. The difficulty comes with deciding what to accept, that is, what level of security to set. For networks such as those in healthcare agencies, the network administrator sets the limits.

For a private computer, the best method is to accept the defaults. Windows software includes a firewall. Reputable antivirus software will manage the Windows firewall and alert you of a security risk if the firewall is off. Given that new methods of attack as well as new viruses come on the scene almost daily, make sure that the firewall is on. In addition to the Windows firewall, most wireless routers for home use include a built-in hardware firewall.

If in a Windows computer, you install antimalware software that includes a firewall, be sure to turn off the Windows firewall. The reason is that having both operating can cause conflicts because both firewalls are doing the same task, which creates performance issues. Additionally, you would have to configure both firewalls identically to make it work at all.

Antivirus Software

Antivirus software protects against more malware than just viruses, although it is still referred to with this term. Depending on the version you install, this software often provides SOME protection against e-mail and Internet malware. Even if you have antivirus software on your computer, the first step toward protecting one's data is to keep a backup of important files stored in another geographical location. There are many different vendors of antivirus software, including free versions, some of which are of high quality (Rubenking, 2013).

Details may differ between vendors, but antivirus software operates by scanning files or your computer's memory or both, looking for patterns based on the signatures or definitions of known viruses that may indicate an infection. Continually update your antivirus software, because malware authors are continually creating new ways to attack computers. In fact, once installed on your computer, most antivirus software immediately goes to the Internet and downloads updates. Most antivirus software allows you to make continual updating automatic, for example, every Tuesday at noon. If the computer is not online at that time, or if you do not set automatic updates, you need to access the software and manually update it, preferably daily.

Antivirus software performs three types of scans. One is a custom scan for which you designate the folder or file that you wished scanned. The second is a quick scan in which the software finds any malware currently active on your computer. A deep or full scan detects anything that missed by the quick scan, but which rarely is. A custom scan, such as you would do for anything downloaded from the Internet, generally takes only a few minutes. A quick scan can take 15 to 30 minutes or less while a deep or full scan, depending on the number of files on your computer, can take two to four hours. This process uses much of the computer's processing ability and usually slows down any work that you may wish to do. Therefore, you may want to set the scan for times when the computer is on but not in use.

Once you install and update antivirus software, run a deep or full scan of the entire computer. Afterward, depending on the software and your choice, you may be able to configure the software to scan specific files or folders at intervals that you set automatically (McDowell & Householder, 2013). Scanning any e-mail attachments of web downloads is an excellent way to protect your system from malware.

The response when an antivirus program finds a virus varies with the software. Some software packages present you with a dialog box asking you if you would like the virus removed, and others will remove the virus without asking you. For many, you can set a preference.

Today, most antivirus software detects and removes both viruses and spyware as well as provides firewall-type protection. However, consider downloading a separate antimalware application in addition to the antivirus software (Henry, 2013, August 21). You can have both antimalware and antivirus on your computer; however, never have more than one in "active protection mode" or running any other protection at the same time. Use the second antimalware software to scan at a different time than the antivirus software. Occasionally, one product will detect something that the other one missed. Once installed, antivirus software operates in the background and checks all the incoming and outgoing data for malicious operations. However, you still need to keep your operating system and all software updated as well as have the latest version of both the antivirus program and virus definitions.

Hoaxes

The world has never known a shortage of practical jokers or those who enjoy sending sensational news to friends. Unfortunately, an e-mail **hoax** lends itself beautifully to these misguided individuals.

Virus Hoaxes

E-mails that warn of viruses are hoaxes 99% of the time. Although, with few exceptions, these hoaxes are not harmful, they are a waste of time and clutter up the Internet and internal networks with useless messages. Hoaxes sound very credible, frequently citing sources such as an official from Microsoft or Symantec. The message contains the information that this virus will destroy a hard drive or perform other dire computer damage. They always tell the recipient to forward this message to anyone she or he knows. Despite containing the statement "This is not a hoax," such messages are usually a hoax. Discard these messages and do not forward them. When there is a real virus, you are most likely to hear about it in the regular mass media, especially if the virus is new and your antivirus program does not have any protection against it. If you believe that there might be a kernel of truth in the warning, before passing it on, check it with a site such as Hoax-Slayer at http://hoax-slayer.com/. You can find good tips on spotting an e-mail hoax at http://urbanlegends.about.com/cs/nethoaxes/ht/emailhoax.htm.

Urban Legends

Urban legends often are stories thought to be factual by those who pass them on. They may be cautionary or moralistic tales passed on by those who believe them. They may or may not be true, but are generally sensationalist, distorted, or exaggerated. You might find an urban legend in a news story, but today, most urban legends arrive via e-mail. The sender alleges that the incident happened to someone they or their friends know.

Before passing on such information, check with a site that reports on urban legends, such as Snopes (http://www.snopes.com/). The e-mail may even state that Snopes reported the story is true. Check yourself; this is generally a false statement and a case of attempted social engineering.

Damaging Hoaxes

Damaging hoaxes are a malicious practical joke spread by e-mail. A user receives a message saying that if a file named "such and such" is on the recipient's computer, the recipient should delete it immediately, because it is a logical virus that will execute in so many days and damage the computer, files, and so on. Included are elaborate instructions for how to determine whether the file is on the computer and equally elaborate instructions for deleting it. Believing the malicious hoax, a user finds the file and deletes it. Unfortunately, often, the file is part of the operating system or other application program on the computer. Deleting the file causes a problem when the system or application program needs that file. Repairing the damage is often a lengthy chore.

If a recipient has any doubt that a message such as the one discussed in the previous paragraph is a malicious practical joke, after finding the file, he or she should maximize the *Find Screen* and look at the creation of the file date (use the details view). The recipient will probably find that the file creation date shows that the duration mentioned in the warning has exceeded long ago, and hence, the file is not malicious. If the file is part of the operating system, the date will be the installation date of the operating system or the last update date. As a rule of thumb, except for deleting files that were user created with an application program, proceed very cautiously in deleting any file. Know exactly what the file that is to be deleted does, and be 100% certain that it is not an important file. A good way to discover what a file does is to enter the name into a web search tool.

Characteristics of E-mail Hoaxes

E-mail warnings should arouse suspicions if any of the following characteristics are present (McDowell & Householder, 2011):

- The message says that tragic consequences will occur if you do not perform a given action.
- The message states you will receive money or a gift certificate for performing an action.

- Instructions or attachments claim to protect you from a virus that is undetectable by antivirus software.
- The message says that it is not a hoax.
- The logic is contradictory.
- There are multiple spelling or grammatical errors.
- You are asked to forward the message.
- The message has already been forwarded multiple times, which is evidenced by a trail of e-mail headers in the body of the message.

Security Pitfalls

Believing that antivirus software and firewalls once installed are 100% effective is a guaranteed step toward problems. Although combining these technologies with good security habits reduces risks, frequent software updates further mitigate risks (McDowell, 2013). If you do not protect your computer, believing that there is nothing important on it, it becomes a fertile field for use by attackers who, unbeknownst to you, plant software to make your computer part of a botnet owner's herd. Some operating systems will not install a program without informing you, but it is only a matter of time until attackers learn to bypass this. Slowing down of your computer may be a sign that there are other processes or programs running in the background without your permission, usually to yours or the Internet's detriment. Ignoring patches for either the operating system or the software is big risk situation.

SUMMARY

The time since the first two computers "talked" to each other to today's Internet has been short, but it has been a long journey. Never before in history have the methods of communication been as rapidly changed. The worldwide reach of the Internet and its features, such as e-mail, provide the tools that are creating a truly international community.

Ways of connecting to the Internet have speeded up connections from the original 300 baud (slow enough to read the text as it was sent to your computer) to 56 kilobytes per second for POTS and up to 1,000 megabits per second for fiber, with the potential to keep increasing.

Building on the use of protocols that created the Internet, the World Wide Web has introduced a new level of knowledge dissemination. From the original, HTML language has come variations such as Java and ASP (active server pages), which have added new features to the web.

Organizations, understanding the benefits of Internet connections, have created network connections such as LANs and WANs. Unfortunately, people intent on doing damage to others have also been active in creating botnets, viruses, Trojan horses, and other methods of spying on web users or producing damages. Fortunately, methods of protecting against these threats have kept up, and with common sense, it is possible to protect oneself against damages. Computer networking is here to stay and will continue to expand the ways that it can be used, limited not by technology but by imagination and the willingness to adopt new methods.

APPLICATIONS AND COMPETENCIES

1. Classify the networking architecture used in a hospital nursing unit setting. Consider the equipment used to chart patient data, control intravenous infusions, access medications, and control blood sugars.

2. Analyze the methods you use to connect to the Internet for work and personal use. What are the differences and similarities?

3. Compare two different web browsers. Identify how you change the preferences, for example, the search engine or the ability to sync.

4. Do an Internet search that extends your understanding of intranets, extranets, and VPNs. Summarize your finding along with examples for their use.

5. Contrast three types of malware. Discuss how the malware might infect a computer.

6. You receive a lengthy e-mail, the idea of which is that child's nursery rhyme "Sing a Song of Sixpence" is a coded message to recruit pirates. The e-mail states that it has been checked with Snopes and it is true. Check it with an urban legend checker. What did you find?

REFERENCES

Aikat, D. (1997, August 27). *On the Internet no one knows you are a dog*. Retrieved from http://www.unc.edu/depts/jomc/academics/dri/idog.html

Arbor Networks. (2013, October 15). *Atlas summary reports: Global botnets*. Retrieved from http://atlas.arbor.net/summary/botnets

Beal, V. (2013a). *What are cookies and what do cookies do?* Retrieved from http://www..com/DidYouKnow/Internet/2007/all_about_cookies.asp

Beal, V. (2015, February 16). *Virtual private network (VPN) study guide*. Retrieved from http://www.webopedia.com/DidYouKnow/Internet/virtual_private_network_VPN.asp

Beal, V. (2013b). *The difference between adware & spyware*. Retrieved from http://www.webopedia.com/DidYouKnow/Internet/2004/spyware.asp

Burns, J. (2013). *Java vs. JavaScript: Similarities and differences*. Retrieved from http://www.htmlgoodies.com/beyond/javascript/article.php/3470971/Java-vs-JavaScript.htm

Chapman, S. (2013). *What is JavaScript?* Retrieved from http://www.java.com/en/download/faq/whatis_java.xml

Howe, W. (2012, September 13). *A brief history of the Internet*. Retrieved from http://www.walthowe.com/navnet/history.html

Henry, A. (2013, August 13). *The difference between antivirus and anti-malware (and which to use)*. Retrieved from http://lifehacker.com/the-difference-between-antivirus-and-anti-malware-and-1176942277

Infosecurity Magazine. (2013, October 11). *"Bad"-Bing: Search site ads are serving up malware*. Retrieved from http://threatpost.com/malware-campaign-leverages-ad-networks-sends-victims-to-blackhole

International Corporation for Assigned Names and Numbers (ICANN). (2013). *What does ICANN do?* Retrieved from http://www.icann.org/en/participate/what-icann-do.html

Internet Society. (2013a). *A brief history of the Internet*. Retrieved from http://www.internetsociety.org/internet/what-internet/history-internet/brief-history-internet

Internet Society. (2013b). *A brief history of the Internet & related networks*. Retrieved from http://www.internet-society.org/internet/what-internet/history-internet/brief-history-internet-related-networks

Java. (2013). *What is Java technology and why do I need it?* Retrieved from http://www.java.com/en/download/faq/whatis_java.xml

Joan, B. (2011, July 27). *Difference between WPA and WPA2*. Retrieved from http://www.differencebetween.net/technology/difference-between-wpa-and-wpa2/

Krishna, J., Venkatasubramanian, K., West, A. G., et al. (2013). Analyzing and defending against web-based malware. *ACM Computing Surveys, 45*(4), 49:1–49:35.

Landesman, M. (2013). *What is a keylogger trojan?* Retrieved from http://antivirus.about.com/od/whatisavirus/a/keylogger.htm

McDowell, M. (2013, February 16). *Security top (ST06-002) debunking some common myths*. Retrieved from https://www.us-cert.gov/ncas/tips/ST06-002

McDowell, M., & Householder, A. (2013, February 8). *Security tip (ST04-005) understanding anti-virus software.* Retrieved from http://www.us-cert.gov/ncas/tips/ST04-005

McDowell, M., & Householder, A. (2011, March 11). *Security tip (ST04-009) identifying hoaxes and urban legends.* Retrieved from http://www.us-cert.gov/ncas/tips/ST04-009

Microsoft Safety & Security Center. (2013). *Protect yourself when you use Active X controls.* Retrieved from http://www.microsoft.com/security/pc-security/activex.aspx

Mimosao, M. (2013, September 6). *Malware campaign leverages ad networks, sends victims to blackhole.* Retrieved from http://threatpost.com/malware-campaign-leverages-ad-networks-sends-victims-to-blackhole

PC.net. (2013). *What is the difference between a router and a modem?* Retrieved from http://pc.net/helpcenter/answers/difference_between_router_and_modem

Rouse, M. (2012). *Botnet (zombie army).* Retrieved from http://searchsecurity.techtarget.com/definition/botnet

Rubenking, N. J. (2013, May 8). *The best free antivirus for 2013.* Retrieved from http://www.pcmag.com/article2/0,2817,2388652,00.asp

Shadowserver. (2005a). *Botnets.* Retrieved from http://www.shadowserver.org/wiki/pmwiki.php/Information/Botnets

Shadowserver. (2005b). *Honeypots.* Retrieved from http://www.shadowserver.org/wiki/pmwiki.php/Information/Honeypots

Umstead, M. (2013, February 25). *Eight ways to avoid malware attacks.* Retrieved from http://limerick.patch.com/groups/marc-umsteads-blog/p/bp--eight-ways-to-avoid-malware-attacks

Webopedia. (2013a). *Local-area network.* Retrieved from http://www.webopedia.com/TERM/L/local_area_network_LAN.html

Webopedia. (2013b). *Wide-area network.* Retrieved from http://www.webopedia.com/TERM/W/wide_area_network_WAN.html

Webopedia. (2013c). *CAN.* Retrieved from http://www.webopedia.com/TERM/C/CAN.html

Webopedia. (2013d). *MAN.* Retrieved from http://www.webopedia.com/TERM/M/MAN.html

Webopedia. (2013e). *Client/server architecture.* Retrieved from http://www.webopedia.com/TERM/C/client_server_architecture.html

Webopedia. (2013f). *Peer-to-peer architecture.* Retrieved from http://www.webopedia.com/TERM/P/peer_to_peer_architecture.html

Web Wiz. (2013). *What are active server pages (Classic ASP).* Retrieved from http://www.webwiz.co.uk/kb/asp-tutorials/what-is-asp.htm

Wikipedia. (2013a). *World Wide Web Consortium.* Retrieved from http://en.wikipedia.org/wiki/World_Wide_Web_Consortium

Wikipedia. (2013b). *Computer worm.* Retrieved from http://en.wikipedia.org/wiki/Computer_worm

CHAPTER 4

Social and Professional Networking

OBJECTIVES

After studying this chapter, you will be able to:

1. Explain how collective intelligence has implications for improving nursing practice.
2. Compare and contrast three social media apps pertinent to professional networking.
3. Discuss how to use social media safely.
4. Examine the ethical and legal implications for breaches of health information privacy by health professionals.
5. Compare and contrast the guidelines for use of social media for the National Council of State Boards of Nursing (NCSBN) and the American Nurses Association (ANA).
6. Relate the differences between three collaborative sharing software applications.
7. Discuss professional nursing use of e-mail in the workplace and home.

KEY TERMS

Blog

Chat

Cloud computing

Collective intelligence

E-mail

Facebook

FaceTime

FaceTime Audio

Folksonomy

Hacked

Hashtag

Internet radio

Internet telephone

LinkedIn

Listserv

Microblogging

Out-of-office reply

Photo sharing

Plaxo

Podcasting

Podcatching

Professional networking

Real simple syndication (RSS)

ResearchGate

Rich Site Summary (RSS)

Skype

Social bookmarking

Social media

Social networking

Text speak

Tumblr

Twitter

Two-factor authentication

Universal resource locator (URL)

Video sharing

Vimeo

Voice over the Internet Protocol (VoIP)

Web 2.0

Web conferencing

Webcast

Webinar

Wiki

Wikipedia

YouTube

Christina is a nurse in the quality improvement department of a rural county hospital. Kerrie is a nurse in a critical care step-down unit. Both Christina and Kerrie (not their real names) are working on nursing degrees and have become dependent on electronic communication, but both have had to devise a "workaround" to get access to the Internet. Christina has access to **e-mail** and the Internet from her hospital but not at home. In the evenings and on weekends, she takes her laptop and textbooks and drives to the local library or sandwich shop to check e-mail and complete online course assignments. Kerrie does not have e-mail or Internet access at work, so to stay in touch with her instructors and fellow students, she checks e-mail using her smartphone during breaks.

As with the example of two nurses, online communication is so important to daily life that when it is not easily available, people go out of their way to become connected. Free Wi-Fi (wireless fidelity) connections to the Internet have become a selling point for coffee shops and hotels. (The Wi-Fi Alliance is a trade group that owns Wi-Fi, which is the trademark to Wi-Fi.) The Internet has given us inexpensive asynchronous discussions, synchronous instant communication, e-mail, electronic mailing lists, and the library known as the World Wide Web (WWW). Creative users, not content to have the WWW as just a repository of information, have given us social networking tools, interactive websites, instant news, and personal opinions not regulated by traditional media.

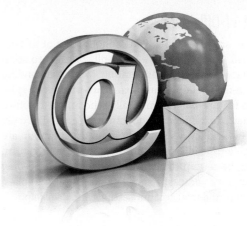

Figure 4-1. E-mail (shutterstock.com/amaster-photographer).

E-MAIL

As you know, an e-mail client is software used to access e-mail from an e-mail server so the user can view and read it. An e-mail server is simply a computer anywhere in the world that uses server software to receive and make e-mail available for those who have an account on that server (Figure 4-1). Users have a variety of choices for e-mail accounts including work and school and website services, such as Google Gmail and Yahoo! Mail. You can access e-mail from any computer, smartphone, or tablet using the Internet or cellular services.

E-mail users should consider having several e-mail accounts, each with a different purpose. For example, use one e-mail account for official communication with coworkers and colleagues. Students should use an account dedicated to official school communication with other students and faculty. Use a third e-mail account, with free online e-mail software or a home ISP (Internet service provider), for personal communication. In addition, consider using a fourth e-mail account for online shopping to trap potential resulting spam. If you have more than one e-mail address, you may want to configure your e-mail client to download all e-mail to single e-mail app. For example, today's smartphones and tablets allow you to configure the settings to access all of your e-mail accounts with a single e-mail app.

E-mail Signature

E-mail written by professionals should include a signature with the sender's name, title, company name, and geographical location. A signature is similar to the return address on a postal letter; however, avoid including personal information such as street addresses and home phone numbers. Most signatures are of one to five lines; personalized signatures might include a favorite quotation. Use the e-mail Help menu for instructions on how to create a signature. More information on e-mail signatures is available on this book's companion website at thepoint.lww.com/sewell5e.

Out-of-Office Replies

There are times when you cannot access or answer e-mail. However, your e-mail will continue to accumulate. To show consideration for those sending you e-mail, set up an automatic **out-of-office reply**. This feature will automatically send an out-of-office e-mail to each person who sent you e-mail. The reply should include a short note indicating that you are unable to read e-mail and the date of your return. Also, be certain to change the setting to send only once to an address. To activate out-of-office replies, go to your e-mail account settings and use Help.

Managing E-mail

You can save yourself time by taking a few minutes to organize and manage e-mail (Table 4-1). All e-mail clients have Help menus to guide you through the organization process. Use e-mail alerts to assist in prioritizing the e-mail. Alerts include flags, stars, and font colors. Use e-mail filters to file incoming e-mail into designated folders automatically. You can also use filters to send personal alerts from specified senders.

Spam

Spam is the electronic version of junk postal mail, except that it shifts the costs of advertising to the receiver; it exists because it is a cheap way to advertise. It also fills the Internet with unwanted messages. Spam is not only a nuisance; it is potentially harmful. As annoying as spam can be, it is important to recognize it to proactively limit or eliminate it. A first clue that an e-mail is junk is the sender's e-mail address. If you do not know the sender, the e-mail is probably junk. Learn how to

TABLE 4-1	Managing E-mail: Tools May Vary According to the E-mail Agent	
Tools	Function	How to Use
Folders and labels	Provide a way to categorize e-mail	Drag and drop e-mail into the folders or create a filter to move the e-mail to the folder automatically. Examples of categories are committees, school, and work.
		If using a filter to move e-mail into a folder, consider providing yourself an alert that the e-mail has arrived.
Flags or stars	Used to give a visual alert for importance and/or follow-up	After you have read the e-mail, you can click a flag or star to indicate importance and follow-up.
Colors	Provide a visual cue to help organize e-mail	Create rules to use color to categorize e-mail.
Sound	Provides an auditory alert for the arrival of e-mail	Use sound alerts to check e-mail as it arrives into the mailbox.
Filters	Provide rules to the software to perform actions on e-mail	Use filters to delete spam that escapes your Internet mail provider's spam filter. Use filters to apply rules to perform an action on e-mail automatically with identified senders, receivers, subject, and/or message words.

develop e-mail filters and rules to control spam. Some ISPs will automatically designate messages that they believe are dangerous as junk or spam. It is a good idea to check this folder because they are not always accurate.

E-mail clients all have an option for marking e-mail as spam. Once you designate a message as spam or junk, all messages from that address will go to the junk or spam folder. E-mail users must be knowledgeable about spamming practices and malware, such as phishing and pharming.

You should never open a known spam message or any attachment that you do not expect or know what it is! Keep in mind that many of these messages look official and you may not realize that it is spam. If you think that a message might be genuine, for example, it is from a vendor with whom you have business, call the telephone number that you have previously saved to check the legitimacy of the message. Never click on any URL in a suspicious e-mail. Also, know that an ISP never sends e-mails to notify you of anything! They use regular mail. A little paranoia with e-mail is a good thing. Finally, users should never purchase a product or service advertised from unsolicited e-mail.

Spam generated by robot computers may constantly change the e-mail address of the fake sender. You can create rules that identify conditions for managing the spam. For example, the first condition might be "look for specified words in the subject or message." The second condition is what to do next, such as filing the e-mail in the spam or in the delete folder.

E-mail Etiquette

E-mail etiquette is essential for professional communication. The rules for creating e-mail are important. First, always include a short pertinent subject line. When replying to e-mail, make sure to include appropriate information from the prior message. In general, e-mail should be short and to the point, but not too short. The recipient may misinterpret a message that is too short as being abrupt or curt.

Users may use acronyms and emoticons in informal e-mail, but they are not appropriate for professional communication. Acronyms use the first letter of words or word parts to communicate a meaning (Table 4-2). Emoticons (emotional icons), sometimes called smileys, are created using the keyboard (Table 4-3) or e-mail graphics. Use the appropriate font, case, and colors when writing e-mail. According to e-mail etiquette, use of all uppercase (all caps) indicates the user is shouting. Use font colors thoughtfully. Depending on the content of the e-mail message, the recipient might interpret a red-colored font as swearing. See Box 4-1 for e-mail recommendations.

TABLE 4-2 Common E-mail Acronyms

Acronym	Meaning
BTW	By the way
FAQ	Frequently asked questions
f2f	Face-to-face
FWIW	For what it is worth
<g>	Grin
IMO or IMHO	In my opinion or in my humble opinion
OTOH	On the other hand

TABLE 4-3 Common E-mail Emoticons

Emoticon	Meaning
☺ or :)	Smiley
☹ or :(	Frown
:O	Shock or disappointment
;)	Wink
> :(or > :O	Upset or angry

BOX 4-1 E-mail Recommendations

Managing Accounts
- Be familiar with your employer's policy on the use of official e-mail.
- Use employer e-mail only for official business.
- Use several e-mail accounts—one for official e-mail, one for school e-mail, and the others for personal activities.

Sending E-mail
- Always check your e-mail for spelling, grammar, and punctuation before sending.
- Include a signature with contact information (title, organization, address).
- Be aware that all e-mails, even if deleted, are potentially discoverable.

- Be sure that your e-mail does not violate common decency laws.
- Never open attachments that you do not expect to receive.
- Never send confidential information in e-mail.
- Use e-mail appropriately—never use it to avoid face-to-face communication.

Managing E-mail
- Create e-mail filters and rules to avoid spam and other unwanted e-mails.
- Never respond to spam.
- Organize your e-mail by using folders and alerts.
- Try to respond to e-mail within 24 hours.

WEB 2.0

Social media tools allow us to communicate with colleagues worldwide and to stay abreast of standards of care and practice. History has taught us through recent devastating disasters that electronic networking provides a means for organizing and delivering healthcare; providing volunteer assistance, pharmaceuticals, and medical supplies; and providing care to those in need. Nurses trapped within disasters were able to connect to the Internet and chronicle events by using messaging, e-mail, and blogs.

O'Reilly and others coined the term **Web 2.0** to describe what online companies/services that survived the dot.com bubble burst in 2000 had in common (O'Reilly & Battelle, 2009). Web 2.0 emerged as a social technology that provides a rich medium to nurses and other healthcare professionals for interactive networking. A professional networking website is like a visit to your colleague's office or home where you can see personal pictures and other decor that reflect his or her ideas and personality. Before the concept of Web 2.0 existed, we used the web to read; now, we use it to read, interact, and write. Information sharing can be images, video, data, or text. The provider determines the format and users create and share information.

SOCIAL AND PROFESSIONAL NETWORKING

Social media allows people to share their stories, pictures, videos, and thoughts with others online using the Internet (Figure 4-2). **Professional networking** is a subset of social media, where interactions focus on business themes. Social media has four main classifications: networking sites, blogging, microblogging, and content sharing.

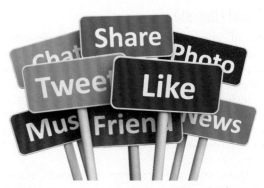

Figure 4-2. Social media (shutterstock.com/Oleksiy Mark).

Networking Sites

Social networking sites such as Facebook, LinkedIn, Plaxo, and ResearchGate serve to connect millions of users worldwide. All allow for professional networking and are available as separate apps for smartphones and tablets. Each site is slightly different, but all meet the needs of people who have a particular interest who want to connect and share content.

Academia and corporate businesses initially shunned use of social networking. Today, many colleges, universities, and hospitals have a presence on Facebook and embrace the use of the social media to connect with groups of users on a more personal level and a sense of community. Examples of use at colleges and universities include connecting with enrolled students and alumni. Box 4-2 includes a sample of nursing professional associations with a social networking presence.

Social networking services have a short history beginning with Friendster in 2002 (Buckley, 2010). In 2009, Friendster ceased to exist (McMillan, 2013, February 27). It is now a gaming site. It was followed by MySpace (https://myspace.com/), which began in 2003 and was the most popular until 2008 when Facebook took over. Facebook began in February 2004 when Mark Zuckerberg and three of his college friends decided to connect with other students by using a website from a Harvard University dorm (Zeeva, 2013). One month later, the social networking site was in use by students at Columbia, Yale, and Stanford universities. Nine years later, the site had more than 1.15 billion active users (Facebook, 2014a). In 2013, 819 million users accessed the site from mobile devices monthly. According to Facebook, 8% of the users lived outside the United States and Canada.

Facebook (http://www.facebook.com/) provides the ability for users to create personal pages and groups and includes e-mail messaging and chat features. Groups target smaller audiences, such as organizations or businesses. Groups can be open, where all can view postings, or closed. A closed group is private and requires an invitation to participate or view postings. A chat bar at the bottom of the browser shows online Facebook member friends' names. Facebook will deliver chat messages instantly to an online Facebook friend. Chat messages are private and can include one or more friends and use text, photos, or video. To learn more about Facebook, go to https://www.facebook.com/help/.

LinkedIn (https://www.linkedin.com) is a professional networking site. Like Facebook, the users can choose individuals and groups with whom they want to connect. LinkedIn provides a way to connect with other business professionals, share information, or look for new career opportunities. LinkedIn is unique in that users can build professional profiles, post resumes, and search for jobs. To learn more about LinkedIn, go to http://help.linkedin.com/.

Plaxo (http://www.plaxo.com/) is a social networking online address book. Plaxo is a cloud computing address book. Plaxo app syncs the cloud address book with other devices, such as smartphones and tablets. Birthday alerts of contacts and a variety of ecards (electronic greeting cards) provide a social aspect for the app. Some of the greeting cards are free and others required a small fee. To learn more about Plaxo, go to http://help.plaxo.com.

ResearchGate (http://www.researchgate.net/) is a professional networking site for researchers and scientists. It allows members to share research, post published papers, and collaborate with others. Similar to LinkedIn, members can build a profile that includes education, work experience, and

---

BOX 4-2 Examples of Professional Associations Using Social Networking Sites

Look for the following groups in Facebook, LinkedIn, and Twitter:

- American Nurses Association
- AACN (American Association of Critical-Care Nurses)
- PubMed
- HIMSS (Healthcare Information and Management Systems Society)
- MERLOT (Multimedia Educational Resources for Learning and Online Teaching)

current position. Members can also use the site to post and find jobs. ResearchGate also allows members to post peer-reviewed work and supplementary resources, such as data sets. Member can also post papers that have not been peer-reviewed to obtain feedback from others. To learn more about ResearchGate, go to https://help.researchgate.net/ResearchGate_FAQs.

Nurses, professional nursing organizations, libraries, and corporations are avid users of Facebook, LinkedIn, and Plaxo. ResearchGate allows users to share professional scholarship and search for jobs. The trend of connecting with people where they tend to gather electronically will continue.

QSEN Scenario

You are a member of a professional practice committee. One of the items under discussion is the development of a policy for nurses' uses of social networking websites. What resources might you recommend to use as references for the policy?

Blogs

A **blog** is an online weblog or discussion about thoughts or topics of interest (Figure 4-3). Although blogs can be collaborative, more often, one person, known as a blogger, starts them.

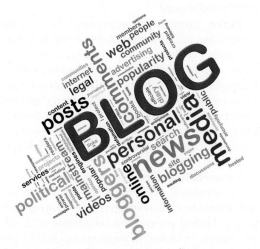

Figure 4-3. Blog (shutterstock.com/Ribah).

Reader comments generally revolve around the blogger's posts. Blog posts appear in reverse chronological order. Good bloggers update their blog regularly. Google Blog Search (http://www.google.com/blogsearch), Technorati (http://technorati.com/), and BlogSearchEnging.org (http://www.blogsearchengine.org/) are search engines specifically for blogs.

There are many different ways to use blogs in education and healthcare. Because blogs are websites, nursing educators can easily incorporate their use into online course content. Nursing students might use family blogs that share experiences about care for a loved one with medical problems as case studies. Patient-centered blogs provide insight into those affected by the illnesses.

Blogs may share information about a particular health topic. One example is scoliosis blogs (http://www.scoliosisblogs.com/), a website with choices of many blogs about scoliosis. Health blogs have varying authors, including healthcare professionals, patients, and others who are interested in certain topics, read widely on the subjects, and want to share their knowledge. One such case is Dave deBronkart, a cancer survivor and advocate for participatory medicine and patient engagement, who has a blog titled e-Patient Dave (http://www.epatientdave.com/). Nurses in both hospital and education settings use blogs to share learning. For example, the nurses at Saint Joseph Hospital (Orange, California) created a nursing research blog (http://evidencebasednursing.blogspot.com/search/label/ResearchatSt.JosephHospital0Orange) where they communicate the research activities of their staff as well as the results of group discussions about research articles.

A blog is easy to create using free tools such as Google's Blogger (http://www.blogger.com/start), WordPress (http://wordpress.com/), LiveJournal (http://www.livejournal.com/), and Xanga (http://www.xanga.com/). Many blog creation tools allow readers to post comments to the postings. Blog quality and content vary, from personal musings to those that are more serious and informative. Like all web sources, blog readers should assess the validity and currency of the information. (Chapter 9 includes information on evaluating websites.) Blog readers need to understand the blog purpose and the blog authors' authority for writing the content (Billings, 2009). Other features that may be included with the blog design tools include design templates, **RSS (real simple syndication)** feeds, a language translator, and analytics.

RSS Feeds

You can subscribe to **RSS** feeds for websites such as news and blogs to notify you when there is new information on a website. RSS feed is an acronym for both **Real Simple Syndication and Rich Site Summary** feeds (your choice). The orange icon on a web page or in the location bar (see Figure 4-4) indicates the news feed capability. You can have RSS feeds of new items from websites including electronic library searches, news, and blogs sent to your e-mail account. The RSS icon became the industry standard denoting RSS feed availability in December 2005. By using the Help menu in your web browser or e-mail application, you can easily create an RSS feed for any site where you see the icon. For more information on RSS feeds, go to https://support.google.com/feedburner/answer/79408. You can also search YouTube for information about RSS feeds.

Microblogging

Text messaging, Twitter, and chat are very popular text-based communication tools worldwide. They are examples of microblogging applications. **Microblogging** refers to very brief web journaling. A microblog could be simply a sentence fragment.

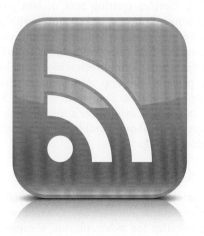

Figure 4-4. RSS feeds icon (shutterstock.com/vector illustration).

The immediacy of text-based communication resulted in the development of a new language system called "**text speak**" that uses letter, numbers, and symbols instead of spelling out words. For example, instead of "I have a question for you," the text-based representation would be "?4U." No standard invokes the meaning of words used in text messaging. However, in English, the alphabet letter, number, or symbol that invokes meaning of a word is commonly used. For example, the letter r is used for the word "are," the number 2 for the word "to," and number 4 is used instead of "for." Webopedia has an extensive listing of abbreviations used for quick messaging at http://www.Webopedia.com/quick_ref/textmessageabbreviations.asp. Abbreviated language works well for quick communication of information, but it is not appropriate for use in a professional setting, such as school or workplace communication.

The prevalent use of smartphones and tablets allows messaging to become the preferred method (over e-mail) for many communications. It is relatively unobtrusive and provides the ability for instant communication. Messaging is a feature in online services such as Google Chat, Yahoo! Messenger, and Skype. It is also a standard feature for social and professional networking sites. Smartphones use multimedia messaging (multimedia message service [MMS]) features, which allow for the use of photos and videos in messaging.

Messaging use continues to be a controversial topic. In school classrooms, students message each other in class similar to the days some of us passed paper notes. Teachers voice concern that the students are inattentive to classroom lessons. Instant messaging raises many questions. Should there be laws against drivers who text while operating vehicles? It is against the law in some states and still under debate in others (Governors Highway Safety Association, 2014, January).

Twitter

Twitter (http://twitter.com/) is a mini-blogging platform. You, or anyone, can send messages of 140 characters or less, known as "tweets," to family, friends, or the general web community. Twitter also allows users to post photos and short videos. Twitter requires users to register and create a log-in and password, but the service is free. The difference

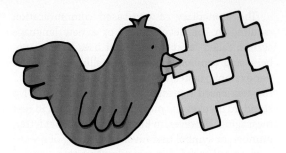

Figure 4-5. Twitter (shutterstock.com/Diego Schtutman).

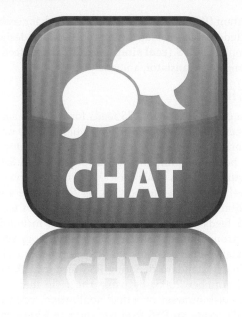

Figure 4-6. Chat (shutterstock.com/faysal).

between Twitter and messaging is that tweets are shared with collective others. It allows you to connect with others who share your interests or might be interested in what you have to say. Subscribing to another user's content is called "following." When subscribing to someone, you are the person's "follower."

Users can tweet, retweet (share the tweet with others), or reply to a Tweeter. A tweet can be text or include images, or video clips. The @ sign is a connector symbol for the Tweeter's name, for example, @jeannesewell. The # sign or **hashtag** identifies the keyword or topic of the Tweet, for example, #nursinginformatics (Figure 4-5).

Twitter allows us to keep up with breaking news from professional organizations such as the Future of Nursing, Interdisciplinary Nursing Quality Research Initiative, HealthIT, and the Centers for Disease Control and Prevention. Use the search window to enter the Tweeter name or a keyword. The tweets for the organizations or people you are following will show up on your Twitter home page. The tweets are a great way to keep up with your particular interests. Twitter users, when in natural disasters, sent tweets to inform the affected people about various situations. To learn more about how to use Twitter, go to https://support.twitter.com/.

Chat

Chat is interactive e-mail that has been around for a long time, but it has morphed into newer types. Both messaging and chat can involve two or more individuals. Chat and messaging are optional features available in course Learning Management Systems (LMSs). In this milieu, the computer screen shows a list of the participants as they enter the chat room. Some chat software allows users to use their real names or a "handle or alias." Chat users type their conversation and tap the Enter key to send the message. Others in the chat room respond with their replies (Figure 4-6).

Tumblr

Tumblr is part microblog and part social networking. Besides posting text, it lets you post and customize photos, links, quotes, videos, and e-mails from wherever you are. Tumblr prompts new users to find other microblogs to follow by using keywords. Tumblr microblogs can be public or private. The app also includes chat and messaging features. Similar to Twitter, Tumblr users can repost other user's microblog entries. To learn more about Tumblr, go to http://www.tumblr.com/help.

Content Sharing

Content sharing is a component of social media and professional networking. Content is shared using websites for video, photos, a combination of images/video, and online radio. New content sharing websites continue to emerge.

Video Sharing

Popular **video sharing** websites include **YouTube** (http://www.youtube.com/) and **Vimeo** (https://vimeo.com/). Both sites include the ability to search and find video as well as post user-generated video. User-generated video must adhere to the terms of the website and not violate copyrights. To upload video, you must register with the service and create a log-in and password. Instructions for user-generated YouTube videos are online at *Getting Started on YouTube* (https://support.google.com/youtube/answer/3309389). Instructions for user-generated Vimeo videos are online at *Create Something New* (http://vimeo.com/create).

Photo/Video Sharing

Photo sharing is a popular social media form. Examples of photo sharing websites include Flickr (http://www.flickr.com/), Picasa (http://picasa.google.com/), Instagram (http://instagram.com/), Pinterest (https://www.pinterest.com/), Snapfish (http://www.snapfish.com), and Shutterfly (http://www.shutterfly.com/). The sites provide the ability to share photos with others as well as the ability to upload files. As with other video sharing sites, users must register and create a log-in and password to share photos. Flickr, Picasa, Instagram, and Pinterest allow sharing of photos and videos. Snapfish and Shutterfly allow for sharing only photos, as well as commercial services for printing individual photos, photo books, cards, and calendars. Users must adhere to the website terms of use and copyright law.

Internet Radio

Internet radio is a social media form for streaming audio using the Internet. There are numerous Internet radio sites. Pandora (http://pandora.com/), Live365 (www.live365.com), and Last.fm (http://www.last.fm) allow users to select radio channels by selecting artists or themes. Some Internet radio sites are also music stores where users can purchase album tracks.

Pros and Cons for Using Social Media for Professional Networking

There are pros and cons for using social media for professional networking. The pros include the ability to communicate and collaborate with other nurses and healthcare professionals (Baker, 2013; Piscotty et al., 2013; Prinz, 2011, July). Healthcare organizations can market services to the public. The cons relate to legal and ethical issues including breaching the Health Insurance Portability and Accountability Act (HIPAA) of 1996 or not adhering to healthcare institution policies (Anderson & Puckrin, 2011; Breslin, 2009; McBride, 2009). Nurses and healthcare providers who indiscriminately share stories, photos, and video related to practice, face serious punishments.

Nurses and healthcare providers who indiscriminately share stories, photos, and video related to practice face serious punishments. Indiscriminate use of social media is not only unethical but may be illegal. Examples of penalties include dismissal from a nursing program, termination from work as a nurse, revoking of a nursing license by the state board of nursing, lawsuits, fines, jail, or imprisonment (Lazzarotti, 2011, May 8; "Nurses sacked after posting pictures of themselves online wearing incontinence pads and tweet patients' personal details, 2013", October 29; Tappendorf, 2013; Valinsky, 2013, March 1; Wilson, 2012, March 7).

The National Council of State Boards of Nursing (NCSBN) and the American Nurses Association (ANA) collaborated on a set of guidelines for social media. You can access the NCSBN guidelines and video, *Social Media Guidelines for Nurses*, from https://www.ncsbn.org/2930.htm. The social media guidelines are available as an Adobe Reader file and include:

- Confidentiality and privacy issues related to nurses' use
- Possible consequences for misuse
- Common myths and misunderstandings
- Tips to avoid problems
- Several scenarios of inappropriate uses reported to boards of nursing

Examples from the NCSBN guidelines of inappropriate use of social and electronic media include a nurse who took unauthorized photos of a client with his personal cell phone. The nurse received sanctions by the state board of nursing and was required to complete continuing education on ethics, professional boundaries, patient privacy, and confidentiality. In another case, a nursing student was expelled from the nursing program after taking a picture of a little boy recovering from cancer and posting it on Facebook. In both cases, there was no malice intended, but the actions were unethical and illegal.

The ANA (2011) developed a tool kit for social media online at http://www.nursingworld.org/FunctionalMenuCategories/AboutANA/Social-Media/Social-Networking-Principles-Toolkit. The tool kit includes a Webinar, fact sheet, tip card, poster, and social networking principles. The Webinar provides users with continuing education credit and is associated with a small fee. The *Principles for Social Networking and the Nurse* is a free Adobe Reader download for ANA members. It includes an overview of social networking in nursing, principles for use, and the foundation for social networking as it relates to the ANA codes of ethics, scope and standards of practice, and the social policy statement.

Safe Networking

Social and professional networking privacy policies remain in constant flux. It is important that users read the privacy policies before selecting a networking site. Social media sites allow users to choose privacy settings. Unless the user customizes the settings, the default setting is for information to be public. Facebook users, for example, can select who can view posts, block viewers from posts, review and edit photo tags, and manage connections (Facebook, 2014b).

Have you or a friend had their social media account hacked? **Hacked** refers to unauthorized use of the account. It can occur by a hacker exploiting a website security flaw or a network security breach. For example, in February 2013, Twitter alerted the public that hackers had illegal access to e-mail addresses, usernames, and passwords for 250,000 Twitter users (McHugh, 2013, February 1; Twitter Blogs, 2013, February 1). Twitter sent e-mail to users of the compromised accounts stating that Twitter had reset e-mail passwords. They asked users to create a new password and provided advice on how to create a strong password.

In October 2013, cyber thieves stole private information from 2.9 million Adobe customers, including names and information customer billing order information. Adobe sent an e-mail to customers alerting them of possible customer Adobe IDs and encrypted passwords compromise because of the security breach (LeClaire, 2013,

October 4). The e-mail stated that Adobe reset all passwords after the breach. A reset password link allowed customers to set a new password.

Many websites use a **two-factor authentication**, which requires personal information for account changes to prevent unauthorized users from hacking your account. Twitter began using two-factor authentication after the 2013 security breach. Cyber criminals have a variety of motives and some are malicious. For example, criminals may fraudulently assume your identity or use your account to send spam. The best way to protect your social media account is to change the settings to require two-factor authentication for any account changes. Requiring you to enter a code sent to your cell phone as a text message before making account changes is an excellent way to protect your account(s). In addition, Twitter, Facebook, Yahoo!, and other social media sites require two-factor authentication.

Think carefully before sharing your location away from home, such as when taking a trip. Many social media sites allow users to show their location using the smartphone or tablet GPS (global positioning system). If the location information is public, it alerts would-be robbers of theft opportunities. If you choose to share your location away from home, change the privacy settings of the posting to be visible to only your friends.

The National Consumers League (http://www.nclnet.org/technology/9-safe-computing/152-social-networking-security-and-safety-tips) provides the following security and safety tips:

- Keep financial and private information secure.
- Visualize social networking sites as cyberspace billboards.
- Verify information about friends met on the Internet, such as where employed. If you decide to meet with the person, be sure to use a public place.
- Be aware of "con artists" who are looking for victims.

COLLABORATIVE SHARING AND COLLECTIVE INTELLIGENCE

There are a number of web resources available to foster collaborative sharing in addition to websites designed specifically for social media and networking. Group discussion forums and wikis are forums that support collaboration as do e-mail lists (listservs). Group collaboration is possible using Internet telephone and teleconferencing with Webcasts and Webinar. Cloud office suite software provides ways that one or more users can create word processing, spreadsheets, and presentations synchronously or asynchronously. Video and audio podcasts provide a means for sharing ideas with other. Users might use **social bookmarking** to share favorite websites, tag them with keywords, and share the sites with other.

Collaborative sharing maximizes the **collective intelligence** or the intelligence that emerges from group collaboration (Johnson et al., 2010). Analysis of data, which collected over time, allows new patterns to emerge results in new knowledge. The notion of collective intelligence has implications for changes in the educational process and the nursing profession. Collective intelligence applications in nursing and nursing education provide opportunities for grassroots problem-solving and knowledge construction by nurses and students worldwide. Collective intelligence requires some type of regulation; it is often provided by users of the site. Examples include user recommendations on eBay or Amazon and reviews of various travel facilities.

Group Discussion Forums

There are group discussion forums for every topic imaginable. Finding the right one is easy. You can search the web by using the terms "online nursing communities," "nursing discussion lists," or "nursing listserv." If you are interested in a specialty forum, include the name of the specialty in the search.

Listservs

A **listserv** is an e-mail discussion list of a group of people with a common interest such as pediatric nursing. Those belonging to the list, called subscribers, receive all messages sent to the listserv mailing address. Users can reply to the original message or start a new thread with a new message. Subscriptions are managed from a different address or a website.

The archives of many e-mail lists as well as classroom chat rooms are organized by the subject line in the message. To preserve the thread, when sending a message to the group that pertains to the same subject, use the reply feature. If you will be starting a new topic, start a new message; do not use the reply feature.

Wikis

A **wiki** is an example of collaborative knowledge sharing (Figure 4-7). A "wiki" is a piece of server software that allows users to freely create and edit content on a web page using any web browser. The word "wiki" is Hawaiian for "quick" (Wikipedia Contributors, 2013a). The person who creates the wiki, the "owner," hosts a wiki site. The "owner" can then invite others into the site. Editing authority may be public, as in Wikipedia or by those invited to participate in the wiki.

Wikipedia (http://en.wikipedia.org/) is a popular, free, publically edited, online encyclopedia, which began in 2001. Within the first 9 months of development, users had contributed 10,000 articles (Wikipedia Contributors, 2013b); as of December 2013, there were more than 30 million articles. Users collaboratively create and improve Wikipedia articles. Tabs at the top of the article provide a means for collaborative discussion on the topic, editing the page, or viewing the history of changes (an audit trail). Changes can always be undone. Contributors should note that their computer Internet address will be publically available in the edit history.

To prevent vandalism of popular pages, some Wikipedia articles are "semi-protected," meaning that only registered users can make changes to

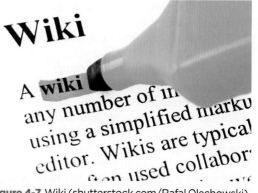

Figure 4-7. Wiki (shutterstock.com/Rafal Olechowski).

the articles. The strength of Wikipedia is that it provides information on an ever-expanding number of topics. Critics are quick to point out that the quality of articles is inconsistent. However, Wikipedia flags questionable articles or those that they believe are incomplete with information such as "This article may require cleanup to meet Wikipedia's quality standards. No cleanup reason has been specified. Please help improve this article if you can" or "citation needed." For technical information, Wikipedia is often one of the most up to date and the best sources of information.

The design of wiki websites allows for sharing and collaborative work on documents. Users can use wikis for research endeavors, committee work, clubs, classrooms, and knowledge management. Wikis can be private or public, for example, a wiki designed for committee work or nursing research would be private. The wiki administrator identifies the membership using e-mail addresses, and the wiki automatically e-mails members with information on how to register for the wiki website. Wiki websites for personal use often include a file manager, the ability to upload and download files, a text editor, and support for hyperlinks. Some wiki sites are available for private use without advertising; others charge a fee.

There are numerous free wiki sites available. When selecting a wiki site, consider the purpose of the site, restrictions for numbers of users, and file sizes. Also, consider having to pay special fees to make the site free of advertisements and private. Examples (in alphabetical order) include the following:

- DooWiki (http://www.doowikis.com/)
- Google sites (http://sites.google.com/)
- Wikidot (http://www.wikidot.com/)
- Wikispaces (http://www.wikispaces.com/)
- XWiki (http://www.xwiki.com)
- Zoho Wiki (http://wiki.zoho.com/)

The culture of the group is a factor that affects the effectiveness of collaboration. Users must be willing to share knowledge and exchange ideas. They must be open-minded and willing to seek new knowledge. Users must have the technical skills to upload and edit documents when using wikis as an updatable knowledge management repository.

Internet Telephone

Internet telephone or telephony refers to computer software and hardware that can perform functions usually associated with a telephone. **Voice over Internet Protocol (VoIP)** is the terminology for telephony products. VoIP provides a means to make a telephone call anywhere in the world with voice and video by using the Internet, thereby bypassing the phone company (Figure 4-8). Many educational institutions and businesses are switching from the conventional telephone to VoIP phones, which allow the user to use robust features similar to those on smartphones, such as conference and video calling.

The free versions of VoIP software apps provide phone communication from computer to computer. Skype (http://www.skype.com) is an example of VoIP software. **Skype** allows free Skype-to-Skype voice and video calls, instant messaging, and file sharing (Skype, 2013). For an Internet call, all you need is a microphone, speakers, and a sound card. If you have a video camera, you can have video calls. The connection, computer processor, and software determine the number of people and quality of the connection. For a small fee, you can choose to call telephone numbers on mobile phones and landlines, send text messages, and have group video calls with up to ten people. You can also download the software for your smartphone or even purchase a Skype phone that allows you to make phone calls using Wi-Fi.

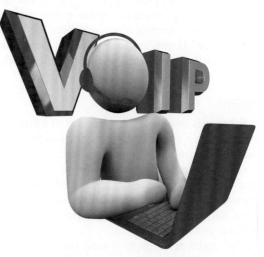

Figure 4-8. VoIP phone (shutterstock.com/iQoncept).

Vonage (http://www.vonage.com/) and Evaphone (http://evaphone.com/) are examples of two other VoIP products. In 2013, Apple introduced **FaceTime Audio** with iOS (operating system) 7 (Guarino, 2013, September 28). FaceTime Audio allows Apple iPhone and iPad users to call others with an iPhone or iPad over Wi-Fi. The **FaceTime** app allows for video calls over Wi-Fi. FaceTime Audio and FaceTime work internationally. Because FaceTime connects users with Wi-Fi, international calls are free.

Teleconferencing

Conference calls by using the telephone are a way of life for those belonging to committees whose members live in different geographical locations. You can add videos, such as slideshows and other visuals, to the meeting in **web conferencing**. Some web conferencing software features the ability of participants to mark up documents or images as well as "chat" by using a keyboard. Web conferencing is similar to an open telephone call, but with the added element of video. Most web conferencing software allow recording of the sessions and sharing the recording with others afterward. Participants can participate using a computer or a telephone connection.

Webcast

A **Webcast** is a one-way presentation, usually with video, to an audience who may be present either in a room or in a different geographical location. The Webcast host often provides methods for the distant audience to ask questions. Users can view the Webcast "live" or as a recording. The host can distribute the recording to others as a link on a web page or as an e-mail file attachment.

Webinar

A **Webinar**, on the other hand, is more like a live seminar. Users must log in to a website address. Although there is a speaker, the audience can ask questions during the presentation, and the speaker can ask for feedback. Webinar software is available for enterprise and individual use. Faculty who teach courses online may use Webinar software for office hours. Healthcare organizations use the software to conduct meetings, save employees inconvenience,

and travel costs. Professional organizations often offer free Webinars to their members.

Webinar software is available as a standalone or as embedded with an LMS. Webinar software usually provides a means for video, audio, and chat. Free trial versions of Webinar software are available for individual use. For more information, search the Internet by using the term "Webinar."

Cloud Office Suite Software

Web 2.0 **cloud computing** includes tools that allow groups of users to work together virtually. Many of the tools are free and very easy to use. The only requirement is the use of a computer with an Internet connection. Examples of online office suites that allow group collaboration are Google Drive (https://drive.google.com/), Microsoft OneDrive (https://onedrive.live.com), and Zoho Office (http://www.zoho.com). Cloud computing office suites include word processing, spreadsheet, and presentation software. The documents can be created off-site or online and then uploaded where they can be shared and edited by others. Editing can be synchronous or asynchronous. Additionally, users can download and save documents from the cloud.

Podcasts

Online **podcasts** allow anyone with the appropriate hardware and software to listen or view audio and video content on the web. Some developers publish podcasts as a theme series on a specific subject and make the podcasts available as RSS feeds. For example, Medscape and the ANA have educational podcasts available for nursing. You can listen to a podcast by using an MP3/video player such as those built into smartphones and tablets or software such as iTunes and Windows Media Player.

You can download free **podcatching** software from the Internet. Podcatching software "catches" podcasts. It is the name for software that allows users to aggregate podcast feeds and play podcasts on their computers, smartphones, and tablet devices. Examples include iTunes (http://www.apple.com/itunes/download/) and Juice (http://juicereceiver.sourceforge.net/). To subscribe to a podcast, open the command to subscribe in podcatching software and then copy and paste the URL for the podcast.

Nursing educators are taking advantage of podcasting by recording their lectures and then uploading them as a podcast to the iTunes store, iTunes U, or campus podcasting servers for use in the "flipped classroom" where learners view the lecture as a homework assignment and then practice learning in class with case studies and other problem-based learning approaches. Some publishers also offer free how-to videos such as the American Journal of Nursing videos at http://journals.lww.com/ajnonline/pages/collectiondetails.aspx?TopicalCollectionId=15. Students create podcasts using smartphones and computers with built-in cameras to display school learning projects.

Social Bookmarking

Bookmark is a term for identifying a favorite website. Social bookmarking allows you to save bookmarks to the cloud where they are available on all of your computers, smartphone, and tablets with an Internet connection. Diigo (https://www.diigo.com/), Delicious (http://delicious.com/), and Reddit (http://www.reddit.com/) are examples of social bookmarking sites where people share and tag their favorite websites. At these sites, you can add your favorite websites to tag keywords and see tags identified by others. Digg (http://digg.com/) is a social news site that allows contributors to add links to articles. Contributors can click a "thumbs up" icon if they "digg" the link, make comments, and share the link with others using Twitter or Facebook. Social bookmarking site tags use folksonomy taxonomies.

A folksonomies taxonomy is "... social tagging of diverse content such as documents, images, blog entries, links, and keywords" (Kaminski, 2009, p. 3). Folksonomies are a form of collective intelligence. The tags are word descriptors, often achieved by collaborative group consensus. "Tag clouds" refers to the collection of **folksonomy** tags. Their appearance varies on websites.

There are numerous tag cloud generators available for website authors. The generators provide options for either entering a **universal resource locator (URL)** of a website or entering specific tags and the associated links. Users may also have the option to choose colors, fonts, and styles of the tag clouds and then copy the code to use on their websites so that the tag cloud is visible to others. The variety of visual representations of tag clouds is a feature of folksonomies.

SUMMARY

E-mail is a predominant way of everyday communication for busy nurses. E-mail signatures and out-of-office replies facilitate professional communication. E-mail RSS feeds allow us to have a just-in-time news delivered to an e-mail or other preferred news reader(s). When healthcare professionals effectively use these new tools, they improve healthcare, both in the practice of the professional and for the patient.

The WWW provides many opportunities for professional networking. As the web matured, many new features were added, such as the interaction permitted by Web 2.0 for computer, smartphones, and tablet devices. Use of blogs and networking sites, such as Facebook, LinkedIn, Plaxo, and ResearchGate, provides opportunities to develop professional collaboration with other nurses. Microblogging sites, such as Twitter, chat, and Tumblr, provide means for instant communication. Social networking sites provide a way for groups to interact with public and private notes, photos, and other media. From the sharing of documents to discussion groups, these features make possible a collective intelligence as many people from all geographical areas and walks of life contribute their knowledge in such formats as wikis, cloud office suite applications, and social bookmarking. Grass Roots Media has become a possibility with media-sharing apps such as YouTube, Vimeo, and picture sharing, all of which can be useful in healthcare for providing both continuing education and patient education.

Unfortunately, the immediacy of communication has blurred the lines for social and professional responsibility to respect and advocate for patients. Incidents occurred where nurses and other healthcare providers breached the trust and confidentiality of patients with social media. As a result, the NCSBN and ANA created guidelines and principles for professional use of social media.

APPLICATIONS AND COMPETENCIES

1. Examine the technology use policies and procedures for your educational or healthcare provider workplace facility for:
   a. Setting up an e-mail account
   b. Use of the institution's e-mail server
   c. Maintaining privacy of e-mail
   d. Use of social networking sites
   e. Use of approved e-mail attachments
   f. E-mail communication with patients and families by healthcare providers

2. Identify at least two ways that collective intelligence has implications for improving nursing practice. Explain the benefits and compare your experiences with other student colleagues.

3. Compare and contrast three social media apps pertinent to professional networking.

4. Conduct a literature search in a digital library to find an article that extends your understanding about using social media safely.

5. Search the digital library and Internet for social media privacy breaches made by nurses and healthcare workers over the past 3 years. Discuss the ethical and legal implications for the practice breaches.

6. Compare and contrast the guidelines for use of social media for the National Council State Boards of Nursing (NCSBN) and the American Nurses Association (ANA). Describe the use of the guidelines in your school and workplace settings.

7. Explain the differences between three collaborative sharing software applications. Discuss the current use of collaborative sharing software applications in your school or workplace setting.

8. Find a site that interests you with an RSS feed. Create a news feed for the site. Discuss the reason you selected the website and the newsreader you used for the RSS feed.

REFERENCES

American Nurses Association. (2011, September). *Fact sheet—Navigating the world of social media*. Retrieved from http://www.nursingworld.org/FunctionalMenuCategories/AboutANA/Social-Media/Social-Networking-Principles-Toolkit/Fact-Sheet-Navigating-the-World-of-Social-Media.pdf

Anderson, J., & Puckrin, K. (2011). Social network use: A test of self-regulation. *Journal of Nursing Regulation*, 2(1), 36–41. Retrieved from http://jnr.metapress.com/

Baker, D. (2013). Social networking and professional boundaries. *AORN Journal*, 97(5), 501–506. doi: 10.1016/j.aorn.2013.03.001.

Billings, D. M. (2009). Wikis and blogs: Consider the possibilities for continuing nursing education. *Journal of Continuing Education in Nursing*, 40(12), 534–535. doi: 10.3928/00220124-20091119-10.

Breslin, T. (2009, September 15). *When social networking enters the workplace*. Retrieved from http://massnurses.org/news-and-events/p/openItem/3013

Buckley, N. (2010). *The origins of Friendster*. Retrieved from http://social-networking.limeWebs.com/friendster-history.htm

Facebook. (2014a). *Key facts—Facebook's latest news, announcements and media resources*. Retrieved from https://newsroom.fb.com/Key-Facts

Facebook. (2014b). *Facebook help center: Privacy*. Retrieved from https://www.facebook.com/help/445588775451827

Governors Highway Safety Association. (2014, January). *State distracted driving laws*. Retrieved from http://www.ghsa.org/html/stateinfo/laws/cellphone_laws.html

Guarino, S. (2013, September 28). *iOS 7 how-to: Make FaceTime Audio calls and check out how much data they use 9 to 5 Mac*. Retrieved from http://9to5mac.com/2013/09/28/ios-7-how-to-make-facetime-audio-calls-and-check-how-much-data-they-use/

Johnson, L., Levine, A., Smith, R., et al. (2010). *The 2010 horizon report*. Austin, TX: The New Media Consortium. Retrieved from http://www.nmc.org/pdf/2010-Horizon-Report.pdf

Kaminski, J. (2009). Folksonomies boost Web 2.0 functionality. *Online Journal of Nursing Informatics*, 13(2), 8. Retrieved from http://www.nursing-informatics.com/folksonomies.pdf

Lazzarotti, J. (2011, May 8). *Registered nurse fired for Facebook posting while treating patients*. Retrieved from http://www.workplaceprivacyreport.com/2011/05/articles/social-networking-1/resigtered-nurse-fired-for-facebook-posting-while-treating-patients/

LeClaire, J. (2013, October 4). Adobe resets passwords after massive data breach. *Top Tech News*. Retrieved from http://www.toptechnews.com/story.xhtml?story_title=Adobe_Resets_Passwords_after_Massive_Data_Breach&story_id=12000DGEZ4YO

McBride, D. (2009). Misuses of social networking may have ethical implications for nurses. *ONS Connect*, 24(7), 17. Retrieved from http://connect.ons.org/

McHugh, M. (2013, February 1). 250,000 user accounts attacked in Twitter security breach. *Digital Trends*. Retrieved from http://www.digitaltrends.com/social-media/twitter-security-breach/

McMillan, R. (2013, February 27). *The Friendster autopsy: How a social network dies*. Retrieved from http://www.wired.com/wiredenterprise/2013/02/friendster-autopsy/

Davie, E. (2013, October 29). Nurses sacked after posting pictures of themselves online wearing incontinence pads and tweet patients' personal details. *MailOnline*. Retrieved from http://www.dailymail.co.uk/news/article-2433011/Nurses-sacked-posting-pictures-online-wearing-incontinence-pads-tweet-patients-personal-details.html#ixzz2j8y6icwg

O'Reilly, T., & Battelle, J. (2009, October). *Web squared: Web 2.0 five years on. Web 2.0 summit*. Retrieved from http://www.Web2summit.com/Web2009/public/schedule/detail/10194

Piscotty, R., Voepel-Lewis, T., Lee, S. H., et al. (2013). To tweet or not to tweet? Nurses, social media, and patient care. *Nursing Management*, 44(5), 52–53. doi: 10.1097/01.NUMA.0000429012.15882.d9.

Prinz, A. (2011). Professional social networking for nurses. *American Nurse Today*, 6(7), 30–32. Retrieved from http://www.americannursetoday.com/article.aspx?id=8016

Skype. (2013). *What is Skype?* Retrieved from http://www.skype.com/en/what-is-skype/

Tappendorf, J. (2013, September 16). *Nurse fired for Facebook posts shared by coworker "friend"*. Retrieved from http://strategicallysocial.blogspot.com/2013/09/nurse-fired-for-facebook-posts-shared.html

Twitter Blogs. (2013, February 1). *Keeping our users secure*. Retrieved from https://blog.twitter.com/2013/keeping-our-users-secure

Valinsky, J. (2013, March 1). Swiss nurse in trouble over posting with a corps on Facebook. *The Daily Dot*. Retrieved from http://www.dailydot.com/news/swiss-nurse-facebook-corpse-bdsm/

Wikipedia Contributors. (2013a). *Wiki*. Retrieved from http://en.wikipedia.org/wiki/Wiki

Wikipedia Contributors. (2013b). *Wikipedia*. Retrieved from http://en.wikipedia.org/wiki/Wikipedia

Wilson, K. A. C. (2012, March 7). Gresham woman banned from social networking after posting nude photo of nursing home patient on Facebook. *OregonLive: The Oregonian*. Retrieved from http://www.oregonlive.com/gresham/index.ssf/2012/03/gresham_woman_banned_from_soci.html

Zeeva, D. (2013, February 21). The ultimate history of Facebook (infographic). *Socialmedia Today*. Retrieved from http://socialmediatoday.com/daniel-zeevi/1251026/ultimate-history-facebook-infographic

Computer Applications for Your Professional Career

Some of us grew up in the world of computers and look at the time before they existed as the dark ages. However, some feel uncomfortable in the world of computers. No matter where you are on the continuum, you need to master digital literacy skills to write, calculate numbers, analyze data, and create presentations in your professional and personal lives. All the chapters in this unit focus on improving productivity and allowing sharing of documents.

Chapter 5 addresses mastering word processing skills to write scholarly documents. The American Psychological Association 6th edition writing style, the one commonly used in nursing literature, is the example used to discuss word processing features applied in scholarly documents. The chapter also includes information on special considerations needed for academic papers and journal manuscripts. Other word processing features covered include mail merge, collaborating with others using cloud computing resources, and creating a table of contents.

Chapter 6, on presentations, addresses the pluses and minuses of using slide presentation software and offers help in making presentations truly informational. The chapter also includes the theoretical and pedagogical use of visuals in presentations.

Chapter 7 examines spreadsheet software to manage, analyze, and display numerical data. The chapter investigates the mathematical priority in formulas, tips for better spreadsheets, and the use of charts (graphs), as well as other spreadsheet features, such as protecting data. As in Chapters 6 and 7, best practices for design and resources for learning new skills are discussed.

Finally, Chapter 8 introduces databases, which are the key ingredient of all information systems. The chapter covers concepts common to all databases, including web-based databases, such as tables, queries, forms, and reports. The basic database concepts should help the reader understand databases that nurses commonly use, including the electronic medical record, the digital library, and online shopping.

CHAPTER 5

Authoring Scholarly Word Documents

OBJECTIVES

After studying the chapter, you will be able to:

1. Apply the use of new word processing skills.
2. Compare scholarly papers written for the academic setting with those written for peer-reviewed nursing journals.
3. Explain the differences between free and commercial word processors.
4. Design a word processing document using American Psychological Association (APA) sixth edition style.
5. Discuss the rationale for using paragraph headings.
6. Apply competencies formatting a table using APA style.

KEY TERMS

Abstract

Academic papers

APA (American Psychological Association) Sixth Style

Body of the paper

Default setting

Endnotes

Figures

Footnotes

Grammar check

Journal manuscripts

Keywords

Line spacing

Mail merge

Margins

Page break (hard page return or forced page break)

Page header

Page ruler

Paragraph heading

Plagiarism

References

Repeat header row

Scholarly writing

Self-plagiarism

Spelling check

Table of contents

Tables

Title page

Track changes

Writing bias

Writing is an essential communication tool for nurses. It is a learned skill and, like other nursing skills, takes practice. Yogi Berra, a famous baseball player, once said, "If you don't know where you are going, you'll end up someplace else" ("Things people said: Yogi Berra," 2014). Berra's quote applies to writing. Effective writing has a clear focus. This chapter focuses on writing and formatting scholarly documents using word processing software. It includes common word processing software features used to enhance written communication.

Scholarly nurse **writing** is a synthesis of information that contributes to the discipline of nursing. The basis for scholarly papers is the research findings, peer-reviewed literature written by other experts, and possibly case studies. Major papers take on an iterative process with a series of changes so that the information is clear, organized, succinct, and complete. There are differences between academic papers and journal manuscripts. The audience for **academic papers** is the instructor or professor. The audience for **journal manuscripts** is all of the journal readers.

Scholarly papers use a strict writing style format. A style is a way to format the paper, cite, and credit resources. It provides a familiar structure that assists the reader to understand the information in the text. There are many citation styles. Examples of other styles include AMA (American Medical Association), MLA (Modern Language Arts), and Chicago. The sixth edition of *Publication Manual of the American Psychological Association* (**APA**), a style for authoring scholarly papers in many nursing education programs, journals, and textbooks, is the citation style example for this chapter.

There are many resources for using APA style, but unfortunately, some provide erroneous instructions. It is best to use a primary source and obtain a copy of the APA *Publication Manual*. The sixth edition of the *APA Style Guide to Electronic References* provides additional guidelines for electronic sources (American Psychological Association, 2012). In addition to reference manuals, APA provides online tutorials, *Basics of APA Style* and *What's New in the Sixth Edition*, at http://www.apastyle.org/learn/tutorials/.

STEPS FOR WRITING A SCHOLARLY PAPER

This section describes how to prepare scholarly documents, with a focus on using a word processor as a writing tool.

Step 1: Researching the Paper Topic

Once you are clear about the audience for the paper, start a comprehensive literature review to narrow the paper topic. The paper topic should add to the body of knowledge for nursing. Consider using several approaches for selecting the paper topic. Conduct an initial broad literature search as well as articles published by the journal(s) that is/are under consideration. Search for peer-reviewed resources, which have references. Experts scrutinize peer-reviewed resources prior to publication to assure that the information is valid, applicable, pertinent, and current. When selecting a topic, look for gaps in literature information, as well as current topics without literature updates for 5 or more years.

For the initial search to identify a topic, explore a digital library, such as your academic library databases or PubMed (http://www.ncbi.nlm.nih.gov/pubmed), using the keywords for the paper topic. (See Chapter 10 for detailed information on using the digital library.) You may also find the website *Jane: Journal/author name estimator* at http://biosemantics.org/jane/ helpful (The Biosemantics Group, 2007). Jane is a database that allows users to locate journal articles written on the same topic. You can search Jane using keywords, a title, or an abstract.

Step 2: Choosing the Word Processing Tool

In order to work efficiently and focus on writing, use the word processor as a tool that works for you. Three popular word processing programs, Microsoft Word, Apache OpenOffice Writer, and Google Drive Docs, are used for examples of writing features. Microsoft Word and Apple Pages are commercial word processors. You can download OpenOffice, which is free, to a desktop or laptop computer from http://www.openoffice.org/download/. Google Docs is a free cloud computing word processor. You can download the Google Drive app to your desktop, laptop, smartphone, and tablet from https://tools.google.com/dlpage/drive. All three word processors work on Windows and Apple platforms.

Step 3: Writing the Paper

After identifying and researching the topic, outline the paper and begin to write. Do not worry about writing the perfect sentences at the first attempt. Simply write down all of your thoughts. You can begin writing in any section. You do not need to begin with the introduction. You can always go back and edit or reorganize the flow of the paper. Use the word processing software to format and edit the paper.

Outlining the paper helps you to visualize the organization. It also allows you to identify **paragraph headings**, which are topics and subtopics discussed in the paper. Ways to use a word processor to create an outline are:

- Use the paragraph style tool.
- Use the automatic numbering tool.
- Use the outline tool (Word).

The paragraph style tool has additional benefits in addition to creating an outline. For example, use paragraph styles to create paragraph headings to group and organize the information when writing the paper. Word uses paragraph headings created using the style tool to generate a table of contents. Selecting one of the multilevel automatic numbering tools is another outlining option. In Word, you can use the outline tool in the View ribbon menu. The chapter section "Automatics Bullets and Numbers" has additional discussion of the feature. See the "Paragraph Headings" later in this section for more information.

Changing the Word Processor Default Settings

When formatting a document that uses a citation style, change the default settings of the document to match the citation style first. **Default setting** refers to the software presets. Examples of setting changes needed for APA include line spacing, margins, default font, and paragraph headings.

Line Spacing

The default **line spacing** in word processors is to single space. Change the setting to double space for the entire document. The line spacing can be set as

the default line spacing with Word by clicking on the Paragraph menu > Double-line spacing > Set as Default. In Writer, click on Paragraph > More Options > Double spacing. In Docs, click on the Format menu > Line spacing > Double.

There should be no extra spacing between paragraphs. If you see extra spacing, open the Paragraph menu on the word processor and change the settings to zeros (0s) for before and after "spacing" for Word and Docs and before and after "paragraph" for Writer.

Margins

The **margins** should be at least 1-inch wide on all four sides of each page. The default font for most word processors is for 1-inch margins. Verify the margin settings. The feature is available from the Page Layout menu in Word, Page Properties menu in Writer, and File > Page Setup in Docs.

Default Font

Look at the word processor default font setting. The default font for Word is Calibri. Times New Roman is the default for Writer and Docs, so no change is necessary. To change the default font in Word, click on the Font menu. Change the font to Times New Roman, Regular, and Size 12. Click on the Default button. You have the option of changing the default font to only the current document, or all documents, based on the Normal template. To change the font in Docs, you must create a template with the font change.

Paragraph Headings

Paragraph headings name the sections of a paper. They assist the reader to understand what to anticipate in the section. Format the paragraph heading for each of the five APA heading styles (Table 5-1). To make the modification, type the paragraph heading using the APA font type, size, and style for each heading number. Use the mouse to highlight the paragraph heading in the document and then from the paragraph style tool, use the mouse to right-click the corresponding heading number and select "update to match" for Word, "update" for Writer, or "apply" for Docs. The process takes only a few minutes.

Page Header

A **page header** is a separate section located at the top of a page. APA sixth edition style requires the page header for the **title page** to differ from the rest on the document. On the title page, the

TABLE 5-1   APA Headings Compared with Outline Levels

Roman Numeral Outline Convention	Paragraph Style Heading Equivalent	APA Formatting
I, II, III, IV, etc.	H1	Title style, centered, and boldface
A, B, C, D, etc.	H2	Title style, flush left, and boldface
1, 2, 3, 4, etc.	H3	Sentence style, indented, and ends with a period
a), b), c), d), etc.	H4	Sentence style, indented, boldface, and italicized, and ends with a period
(1), (2), (3), (4), etc.	H5	Sentence style, indented, italicized, and ends with a period

Source: American Psychological Association (2011, p. 62).

header begins with the words "Running head:" (where only the "R" is capitalized) followed by an abbreviated title in ALL CAPITAL LETTERS that is 50 letters and spaces or less. The page header beginning on page 2 with the abstract omits the words Running head.

The page number must be on the same line as the page header title. Format the header so that the document title is flush left and the page number on the far right. The procedure differs slightly according to the type of word processor.

If you use Word, to create the page header, start with the title page. Insert the page number first and the running head with the abbreviated title second. Click Insert from the ribbon menu > Header & Footer Page Number > Simple Plain Number > Right. (IMPORTANT: Using the Header & Footer design tools, *place a check* in the checkbox for *Different First Page*.) After the number inserts, click flush left on the paragraph formatting menu. Type the words "Running head:" and then the abbreviated title for the paper in all capital letters. Use the Word Count tool in the Review > Proofing menu to verify that the abbreviated title is 50 words and spaces or less. Click on the space immediately to the right of the running head. Next, click the tab key twice to move the pager number back in place as flush right. Click the Esc key to close the edit page header window.

To insert the abbreviated title without "Running head:" on the abstract page, scroll down to page 2. Right-click on the page header to show the Header & Footer tools menu. *Unclick* the checkbox for *Different First Page*. Remove the words "Running head:" from the page header on page 2. Click the escape key to exit the page header menu. To understand more about the process, go to http://thepoint.lww.com/sewell5e.

If you use Writer, click on Page Options > Header tab from the Page Style Defaults menu > and place a check in the checkbox for *Header On*. Add the running head title. Click on the Insert menu > Insert Fields > Page Number to add the page number. Click to the left of the page number and click the tab key twice to move the page number to be flush right on the page. The procedure is similar using Docs. The word count tool is in the Tools menu for Writer and Docs. However, there is a caveat with creating the page header. Neither Writer nor Docs allows for using two different page headers. If Writer or Docs, you need to create two files—the title page would be a separate file from the text document. For more information on page styles and numbering with Writer, go to https://wiki.openoffice.org/wiki/Documentation/OOoAuthors_User_Manual/Writer_Guide/Page_numbering and with Docs, go to https://support.google.com/drive/answer/86629?hl=en.

THE APA PAPER FORMATTING REQUIREMENTS

The APA paper includes four main sections: title page, abstract, body of the paper, and reference list. You must insert a **page break** (also called **hard page return** or **forced page**), a word processing menu feature, to separate each of the sections. When using Word, Writer, and Docs, to insert a page break, tap the Ctrl (Command) key + Enter key. Do not use the Enter key to give the appearance of a page break.

Title Page

The **title page**, according to APA *Publication Manual*, has the running head, page number, author name, and institutional affiliation (2011, p. 23). The author note may be pertinent for journal publications, but it is optional. Teachers might modify the requirements for the title page to include a course number and date; however, that is a variance from APA style. A page break separates the title page from the abstract.

Abstract and Keywords

The **abstract** summarizes the information presented in the paper. The information should include a description of the findings. According to the APA *Publication Manual*, the abstract should reflect keywords and assist others to find the paper in an electronic database. Although the abstract is at the beginning of the paper, you do not need to write it first. You may want to outline what you intend to include in the paper and then finalize it after you finished writing the paper.

There are three main formatting features for the abstract. Use the word "Abstract" for the page title on the first line of the abstract and center it. Do not use a boldface font. The abstract title is in "title case" with the letter "A" capitalized and the rest of the word in lower case. The first paragraph of the abstract is not indented. Add keywords following the last paragraph of the abstract. **Keywords** are tags used to identify the topics discussed in the documents. They serve as search terms for the paper. The word *"Keywords:"* is in italics and indented using the tab key. According to APA *Publication Manual* (2011, p. 229), tabs should be set at ½ inch or five to seven spaces. The default tab length for most word processors is ½ inch.

Body of the Paper

The **body of the paper** begins with an introduction and ends with a conclusion or summary. Indent all paragraphs in the body of the paper. Use paragraph headings to assist the reader to visualize organization of the paper. When writing the paper, pay attention to paragraph length. If you have a paragraph that is shorter than three sentences or longer than half a page, consider revising it. Each sentence in a paragraph should relate to the topic sentence or theme of the paragraph.

Introduction

Begin the body of the paper on page three with the title of the paper, centered, and in title case. The title of the paper for the introduction should be the same as the title page. The introduction should state the purpose of the paper. It should be clear, concise, and provide a roadmap on how you develop the purpose for the paper.

Citing Sources

All scholarly papers require the author(s) to credit sources using citations used within the body of the paper. Each citation corresponds with a reference list entry. When using APA style, you display the citations between a set of parentheses. Other styles, like AMA (American Medical Association), use superscript numbers in the paper that corresponds with a reference list number. Chapter 6 in the APA *Publication Manual* includes all of the specifics necessary for crediting sources. If you are citing electronic resources, such as open access journals, databases, and social media, use the information in the APA style supplement, *APA Style Guide to Electronic References*, sixth edition. The supplement is available as an electronic book. For a quick reference, use the Purdue University Online Writing Lab website at https://owl.english.purdue.edu/owl/resource/560/01/.

Quotations

Use quotations sparingly, if at all. If using a quotation, cite it and include a page or paragraph number where the reader can locate the information. It is always best to paraphrase information, which means representing the ideas of other authors (may be one or more) in your own words. Paraphrasing often clarifies information (Norquist, 2014).

When using a quotation that is less than 40 words, include it in the paragraph enclosed with double quotation marks. For quotations 40 words or over, indent and use as a block of text with no quotation marks (American Psychological Association, 2011, p. 171). Insert the quotation citation after the period of the last sentence. Use the Increase Indent tool in Word, Writer, and Docs to create the block quote.

Plagiarism

Plagiarism is using another's work as your own. Two common types of plagiarism include:

- Copying the exact text written by others without citing the source
- Reordering the words of a source text without citing the source
- Self-plagiarism (see the section Special Considerations for Journal Manuscripts in this chapter)

To review a succinct source with examples of plagiarism, go to Types of Plagiarism at http://www.plagiarism.org/plagiarism-101/types-of-plagiarism/. An excellent tutorial on how to avoid plagiarism is VAIL (Virtual Academic Integrity Laboratory) at http://www-apps.umuc.edu/vailtutor/.

Mitigating Writing Bias

Chapter 3 of the APA *Publication Manual* includes useful information to mitigate bias in writing. **Writing bias** is distortion of information that others might interpret as prejudice. Examples where the writer might inadvertently introduce bias include terminology used for labels, gender, sexual orientation, racial and ethnic identity, disabilities, and age. Our cultural norms can introduce unintended wording that is offensive to others.

Using Acronyms

Acronyms are abbreviations made up of the parts of words or word phrases. Use stand-alone acronyms sparingly. With one exception, always write out the meaning of an acronym with the first use, followed by the acronym in parentheses. The exception is that if the *Merriam-Webster's Collegiate Dictionary fifth edition* displays it as a word (rather than an abbreviation), it is okay to use only the acronym without its spelled-out meaning. Examples in nursing include IQ, HIV, and AIDS (American Psychological Association, 2011, p. 107).

Tables and Figures

Use tables and figures when they are essential to convey information to the reader. Always refer to and explain information in tables and figures within the text (Webb, 2009). Check the author guidelines for any limitations on the number of tables and figures. The placement and formatting of the tables and figures differ with type of academic papers, online journals, and print journals. If submitting the manuscript to an online journal, the author guidelines indicate how the writer inserts figures and tables within the body of the paper.

Tables

Use **tables** to convey large amounts of information. Use the table tool for the word processor to create tables. Do not attempt to display data using the tab key. Oermann and Hays (2010, p. 280) suggest learning how to create tables and format them before embarking on writing, so that the process is not a distraction. They provide helpful comprehensive details for creating and formatting tables.

The trick to creating tables shown in the APA *Publication Manual* is using the tool for table border display. Display all borders when in the initial design process. Then, enter the data. When you are finished with the table, hide any borders to comply with APA style. The Borders tool is on the Home and Tables Formatting menus in Word. It is visible in the Tables Formatting menus for Writer and Docs.

Notice that the side borders of APA-formatted tables are invisible. To reiterate, first create the table showing all borders. Afterward, click on the borders that should not be visible and change the border properties to "No border." The process is simpler that it might first appear.

Repeating a Table Header Row. If a table spans across two pages, use the word processor menu to "repeat header rows." The first row of a table is the header row and includes column headings. When the **repeat header row** function displays, the header row will appear on the subsequent page(s). The Repeat Header Row tool is located in the Table Tools Layout menu. The Repeat Header Row feature is a default when you create a table using Writer. It is not yet available in Docs.

Embedding or Linking Table Data from Spreadsheets. When you create a report about data, the data may reside in a spreadsheet. You have a couple of options for displaying the data in the report. You could copy and paste (embed) the data from the spreadsheet into the word processing document or can use the linking feature. If you embed the data and the spreadsheet data changes, there is no associated change in the word processing document. However, when you use the **linking** feature, when the data in the spreadsheet changes, the change appears dynamically in the associated word processing document. Additional discussion on embedding and linking spreadsheet data is in Chapter 7.

Figures

Electronic documents continue to replace many of those in print. When designing electronic documents, you can use figures and media. The *APA Publication Manual* identifies five types of **figures**: graphs, charts, maps, drawings, and photographs (p. 151). APA defines graphs as displaying quantitative data for two variables using an x- and y-axes. A chart might be a flow chart or display of non-quantitative data. Maps show dimensional data. Drawings show information using pictures and photograph images captured using a camera.

To display an image in a regular document, use the Insert menu or drag and drop the image into place. When using more than one picture image, it is a good idea to control the display by first creating a table. Insert the image into a table cell and then hide the table borders when you are finished. If the word processing software does not have a menu item for inserting video, you can emulate the function by first inserting the image for the video and then inserting a hyperlink in the image to open the video source. Of course, the user would have to have an Internet connection to view the online video.

Conclusion

The conclusion provides a visual signal to the reader that the paper is ending. Summarize the information discussed throughout the paper in this last section. Restate important points of the paper in the conclusion.

References

References are the fourth section of an APA paper. References should follow the conclusion and, as noted earlier, be separated from the body of the paper using a page break. Like the rest of the document, references are double-spaced. APA style requires using hanging indent formatting for each reference. That means the first line of the reference is not indented but all of the subsequent lines are. Use the word processor paragraph formatting to automate hanging indent. Do not simulate the appearance using a tab key.

In Word, the Hanging Indent feature is available from the Paragraph Formatting window > Indent and Spacing > Indentation. Select "Hanging" from the Special drop-down menu.

There are many additional rules for formatting references, which is the reason it is so important to use the APA *Publication Manual*. Experienced authors rely upon using the APA *Publication Manual* and the *APA Style Guide to Electronic References*, sixth edition to verify correct formatting. If there is no access to the APA *Publication Manual*, consider using a reputable website such as the Purdue University Online Writing Lab (OWL) at https://owl.english.purdue.edu/owl/. Use the basic APA guidelines checklist in Table 5-2 to check your work.

APA Template

If you write a paper that uses APA sixth edition style, consider beginning with a predesigned template. A template is a preset guide for formatting a paper. To verify the APA template design, you should use the *APA Publication Manual* writing guidelines. Any well-designed template can save time, allowing you to concentrate on writing. For more information on APA templates and templates for word processors, go to http://thepoint. lww.com/sewell5e.

TABLE 5-2 Basic Checklist for an APA Paper	
Item	Check
Title page has appropriate page header.	
Abstract begins on separate page with a new header.	
Body of paper starts on a separate page.	
Spell and grammar checker used.	
Section paragraph headings formatted for the appropriate level.	
Reference citations formatted correctly and used appropriately.	
There is a summary/conclusion.	
References formatted using hanging paragraph and begin on a separate page.	

When editing each draft, you:
  Used grammar check.
  Used spell check.	

Read each paragraph to verify manuscript flow for the reader (checked transitions within and between paragraphs).	
Read aloud to check for meaning.	
Asked a secondary reader to review (if permitted by instructor).	
Spelled out the acronym the first time it was used, for example, electronic health record (EHR).	
Added and formatted tables and figures per author guidelines.	
Referred to every table and figure in the text.	
Numbered and titled all tables and figures.	

SPECIAL CONSIDERATIONS FOR SCHOLARLY PAPERS

You must recognize special considerations that differentiate academic papers from journal manuscripts.

Special Considerations for Academic Papers

Academic **scholarly writing** includes a variety of venues, for example, online discussion postings, master's theses, doctoral dissertations, and journal manuscripts. Criteria for preparation of academic paper depend upon the course or program.

If the paper were for a specific class, you should follow the instructor's instructions and grading rubric. If for a program, such as a master's or doctoral program, you follow the program guidelines for preparation. The paper preparation process may or may not allow for collaboration and peer review. It is important to use the instructor's guidelines.

Special Considerations for Journal Manuscripts

Perhaps you are to write a journal article as a simulation assignment for a class or the article as an expectation to disseminate information as a part of your research. In either case, begin with the end in mind. You need to select a topic pertinent for the reading audience of a journal. If you are learning how to write for publication in a peer-reviewed journal, there are learning resources that can assist with your success. Use faculty mentorship and master essential word processing skills to assure your success. The free quarterly newsletter, *Nurse Author & Editor*, has excellent articles about writing. It is an online at http://www.nurseauthoreditor.com/ and requires the user to create a log-in and password. The website includes resources, such as articles and downloadable booklets, with information for authors, editors, and reviewers.

The author(s) of a journal article should have expertise on the topic for the manuscript. Journal editors review the credentials of all authors when making the decision to have the manuscript peer reviewed (Berkey & Moore, 2012, p. 433). If there is more than one author, it is important to determine each author's responsibilities for writing. According to International Committee of Medical Journal Editors (ICMJE) (2013), all authors must meet all four of the following criteria (para 3):

- Make "substantial contributions" to the work in all aspects, such as the design, or obtainment and analysis of the information.
- Write and revise the work.
- Give final approval for publication.
- Agree to be responsible for the quality of the work.

Acknowledge the name(s) of contributors who mentored or assist with the preparation of the paper, such as proofreading. For example, if mentored by a faculty or committee, the author(s) should identify the faculty or committee name or committee member individual names (para 9).

When writing a journal manuscript, you should first identify the appropriate journal(s). Nursing journals all have a web presence. You can go to the journal homepage for the authors' guidelines. Since there are differences in journal author guidelines, write for the readers of the specific journal (Oermann & Hays, 2010; Webb, 2009).

Journal editors look for uniqueness in manuscripts. Editors want to avoid republishing either parts of or whole articles written by journal authors (American Psychological Association, 2011, p. 13). **Self-plagiarism** occurs when authors "present their own previously published work as new scholarship" (American Psychological Association, 2011, p. 16).

Tables in Journal Manuscripts

Print journal publishers use stringent requirements for typesetting the document. Usually, the journal author guidelines specify placing the tables at the end of the manuscript after the reference list. Use the table tool and the APA *Publication Manual* to format the table (see section on creating tables below). Note that the placement between paragraphs where you want the tables, boxes, or figures to display uses a callout. The callout displays the table number between the symbols < >, for example, <see Table 1>.

Figures in Journal Manuscripts

If you are using a figure previously published anywhere, such as a journal, textbook, or website, you must obtain the permission for use in your manuscript due to copyright law (American Psychological Association, 2011; Berkey & Moore, 2012; Oermann & Hays, 2010). If the figure was in a journal, you should contact the journal publisher, as opposed to the journal article author. When the publisher accepts a manuscript for publication, the associated images become the property of the publisher. The only exception for obtaining permission is if the image is from a government source, for example, the Centers for Disease Control and Prevention. In all cases, you must cite the source of the figure and include any necessary permission information. When using figures for a journal manuscript, use the author guidelines to guide you with the submission process. As with tables, use a callout such as <see Figure 1> to show where you want the figure displayed.

OTHER WORD PROCESSING TOOLS

Numerous word processing tools are available to assist the writer to create and edit documents.

Spelling and Grammar Check

Word, Writer, and Docs include **spelling check**. To avoid misspelled words, use the spell check tool. A squiggly red underline is a universal alert for a misspelled word. To make a spelling correction, right-click on word. Word, Writer, and Docs provide suggestions for correction or allow you to add the word to the dictionary. Spelling check find only misspelled words. It does not find words spelled correctly, but used incorrectly. An example is using the word *form* instead of *from* or *work* from *word*. Proofread the document to check for words used incorrectly.

Grammar check is a proofreading feature that alerts you of errors, such as subject/verb disagreement, run-on sentence, and split infinitives. A squiggly blue underline is the universal alert for grammatical errors. Word includes a grammar check, but you must activate the feature. Use the Options menu on computers with the Windows operating system (OS) or from the Tools menu on the Mac.

Grammar check is not a standard feature for Writer or Docs. However, when using Writer, you can download an extension for grammar check from *LanguageTool Style and Grammar Checker* at http://languagetool.org/. The LanguageTool is an open source proofreading software. The tool is not available for Docs, but you can copy and paste text into the LanguageTool website or download the software to your computer for use as a stand-alone app. There are several other free websites useful for checking grammar. To find them, do a web search using the terms "free proofreading software."

QSEN Scenario

You finished writing a paper about best practices for pressure ulcer prevention. How would you check for grammar and spelling errors with the word processor?

Page Ruler

Most word processors provide the ability to view a **page ruler**, which assists with formatting functions, such as modifying/setting tabs and creating a hanging indent used for the reference list. The ruler is available from the View menu in Word, Writer, and Docs.

Format Painter

Use the format painter option to modify text formatting. Format painter allows you to copy the text formatting from one place of the document to other places. Word and Writer display the format painter icon as a paintbrush. In Word, it is located on the Home menu in the clipboard section; in Writer and Docs, it is on the default menu. In Docs, the format painter icon looks like a paint rolling brush. To use the option, first, click anywhere on a text area with formatting you want to copy; second, click the paintbrush and then highlight the text you want to change. If you want to format text in more than one place in the document, double-click the format painter; when you are finished, tap the Esc key.

Automatic Bullets and Numbers

Word processors have features that allow you to outline something or generate a numbered or bulleted list. It is very useful when creating an outline for a paper or a multiple-choice test. Like most word processor features, you can select the feature before or after you enter the text.

If you enter the number 1, a period, and a space and then enter text, some word processors assume you are creating a numbered list and will enter a number 2, a period, and space when you tap the Enter key automatically. To stop the automation, click the numbering tool. Automatic numbering saves the effort of entering the numbers when you want to create a list. It is valuable when reordering items in the list because the numbers change automatically, so they remain in sequence. That is, if item 4 is moved to the line after item 1, the number 4 automatically becomes number 2, and the former number 2 becomes number 3, and so on.

To create a hierarchal multilevel list, change the format of the numbering feature. You can change the format to multilevel lists before or after you enter any numbers and text. The feature is on the Home ribbon in Word. It is available from the Format menu in Writer and More on the main menu in Docs.

Find and Replace

Find and Replace is a useful tool for editing documents. Find will locate every instance of a set of characters, which is usually a word or phrase. This feature is available in most application programs, including web browsers and e-mail packages. The Find and Replace feature can replace one set of characters with another. Suppose a user types the word "nurse" rather than "Registered Nurse." By accessing Find and Replace on the Home tab in Word (Edit menus in Writer and Docs), you can tell the word processor to find every instance of "nurse" and replace it with "Registered Nurse." The replacement can be automatic or the user can decide which occurrences to replace.

Table of Contents

Automatic generation of a table of contents is another powerful word processing feature in Word (not yet available for Writer or Docs). A **table of contents** includes the main headings used in the paper and the associated page numbers. Word processors use the paragraph headings to create the table of contents. The feature is available in all of the popular word processors. Some provide the ability to choose a template for the display. To use the feature, insert a blank page where you want to display the information and then select "table of contents" from the menu. You can update an automated table of contents to reflect corrections for paragraph heading and page numbers changes. Use the Help menu for additional assistance.

Footnotes and Endnotes

Footnotes and endnotes are different features, but you access and enter each one the same way.

Footnotes are notes located at the bottom of a page. **Endnotes** are notes displayed at the end of the document. Footnotes and endnotes convey additional information that might be a distraction in the table or paragraph, for example, an explanation.

Use the word processor footnote and endnotes tools to insert the placement of the number for the note in the text and automatically number the notes at the bottom of pages or end of the paper. When you remove or insert a footnote, the word processor renumbers the footnotes automatically, after the change. You can display footnotes and endnotes using Word (see Add Footnotes and Endnotes at http://office.microsoft.com/en-us/word-help/add-footnotes-and-endnotes-HA102809783.aspx) and Writer (see Using Footnotes and Endnotes at https://wiki.openoffice.org/wiki/Documentation/OOoAuthors_User_Manual/Writer_Guide/Using_footnotes_and_endnotes). Doc displays only footnotes from the Insert menu. Note: APA *Publication Manual* recognizes footnotes, but not endnotes.

Track Changes Tool

Use the review feature when collaborating with others to **track changes** and provide specific document feedback. When collaborating, it is helpful for the author to see proposed changes while maintaining the ability to see the original document. Track changes in Word uses electronic markups of suggested revisions for the document. Collaborative authors use track changes when editing a document together. If using Word, turn the feature on from the Review menu > Track Changes and select track changes from the drop-down menu. With Track Changes on, edited additions display using a different color. Edited word deletions are displayed using strikethrough lines.

The tracking and change choices provide a variety of functions. Show markup displays a listing of edits. Final displays the documents if the author accepts all of the suggested edits. Original displays the original file without the edits. The Changes menu allows the author to accept or reject changes.

Neither Writer nor Docs provides review tools as in Word. In Writer, if you and another person are working on a document, you must save the original and save changes with different file names. To compare the two documents, click Edit from the menu > Compare Document. Docs emulates track changes with shared editing and the ability to see history revisions (File > See Revision History).

Collaboration

Google Drive Docs and Microsoft OneDrive are examples of cloud computing resources that provide synchronous collaboration on word processing documents. Writers can collaborate in real time, even when working at a distance. Users can collaborate *asynchronously* using e-mail or a shared cloud computing workspace.

Mail Merge

Mail merge is a word processing feature that takes a set of data and places the different pieces into the desired place in a document, not just a letter. You can use mail merge for a variety of reasons. For example, you could use it to send print surveys to postal addresses as well as print labels. You could use it to send a website address of an electronic survey using e-mail addresses. You can also use it to send personalized letters to postal and e-mail addresses. It is indispensable tool for sending personalized mass e-mail, for example, invitations to a conference or a meeting.

To use names and merge data in a form document, the user first creates a set of data that includes fields, such as title, first name, middle name, last name, street address, city, zip code, and e-mail address. The data for the document can be a spreadsheet, a database table, or a word processing table.

After entering the data, you create the word processing document you plan to use for the mail merge. Word processing software includes a wizard to guide the user with the steps of the merge process. Mail merge is available for many popular word processing software, such as Word, Writer, and Docs. Use the word processing Help menu for additional information.

Language Translation

Given today's global culture, there are times you might need to translate text into a different language. Some word processors, such as Word, have a built-in translator feature. A variety of language translators are also available on the web, such as Google Translator and Bing Translator. The quality of computer translators varies, so use them carefully. When translating a document, such as manuscript you are preparing for publication into a different language, be sure to have a native speaker of the language to assist you.

Word processors make it possible to write characters in another language, such as an "e" or an "a" with an accent ("or," respectively) or adding an umlaut to a "u" (ü). You can change the keyboard language to write in languages that use special letter characters and diacritics. If you need to write in a language other than the default on your computer, use the Help feature.

LEARNING NEW WORD PROCESSING SKILLS

Continuous changes in technology challenge our ability to master word processing skills. Use the information in Box 5-1 to self-assess your skills

---

BOX 5-1 Word Processing Skills

Basic Word Processing Skills: Use Standard Features	Demonstrate basic word processing skills with one application.
Add basic text format—font size, color, and style.	Format lines, words, bullets, and line spacing.
Align text—center, left, right, and justify.	Identify spelling and grammatical errors.
Create a new document.	Insert clip art.
Create bookmarks.	Insert hyperlinks (URLs), e-mail addresses, and other places in the document.
Create headers and footers.	Insert page numbers.
Customize the menu.	

BOX 5-1 Word Processing Skills (*continued*)

Make changes—undo/redo.

Move and copy text—cut/paste, copy/paste, and drag/drop.

Name documents.

Obtain the word count information for a document.

Print documents—print preview and change printer settings.

Use Help menu.

Use search and replace.

Use tab key to indent.

Use the menu and quick access toolbar.

Use the ruler.

Intermediate Word Processing Skills: Modify Word Processing Features

Add readability statistics to the menu.

Autocorrect and styles

Change margins and bullets.

Change paragraph setting—hanging indent.

Collaborate with others using the Review tool in Word.

Collaborate with others using a cloud computing website (e.g., SkyDrive, Google Drive).

Create an index.

Create a paper.

Create a table.

Create a table of contents.

Create and format (styles, shadow effects, shape, and arrangement of) text.

Create citations, insert citations into a paper, and create an associated reference list with the citation and bibliographic manager.

Create new documents from a template.

Demonstrate word processing skills with two to four applications.

Design your own custom template.

Edit tab settings.

Format text with themes and styles.

Insert line breaks.

Make changes—adding, deleting, and moving text.

Modify and position graphics in a document.

Modify text alignment.

Modify text font style, color, size, and case.

Modify text using the format painter.

Modify the menus and toolbars.

Use APA citation style, abstract, and a reference page.

Use mail merge.

Use readability statistics to modify a document.

Use search and replace.

Use wizard—letter, envelopes, and labels.

Create a table auto-header.

Advanced Word Processing Skills: Create New Features and Teach Others

Create forms.

Create lists of figures, captions, table of contents, and index.

Create long documents—connecting several documents into one.

Create new functions with macros.

Create new style sets.

Create newspapers, brochures, and other print media using desktop publishing tools.

Create templates.

Create word files with embedded multimedia, such as PowerPoint, video, and sound.

Demonstrate word processing skills with three or more applications.

BOX 5-2   Word Processor Skill Development Learning Resources

Apache OpenOffice Tutorials: http://www.tutorialsforopenoffice.org/

Goodwill Community Foundation (GCF) LearnFree.org, Microsoft Word, and Google Docs: http://www.gcflearnfree.org/word

HP Learning Center: http://h10120.www1.hp.com/expertone/whats_learning_center.html

iWork Pages Tutorials: http://www.apple.com/findouthow/iwork/

Microsoft Training, Word: http://www.microsoft.com/learning/

Google Docs Tutorials: https://sites.google.com/site/gdocswebquest/

---

to identify new opportunities to gain new skills. There are three skill levels. Those with basic skills *use* word processing features. Intermediate-level users are competent *modifying* word processing features. Advanced-level users *create* new features and are able to teach others. It is difficult to apply information on using word processing software as a tool for effective communication without having the knowledge.

See Box 5-2 for examples of free learning resources to enhance word processing skills.

SUMMARY

Nurses use writing as an essential communication tool. Word processing software provides an assortment of features that facilitate writing requiring a stringent writing style, such as APA. This chapter provided examples of tools for writing scholarly documents using Word, Writer, and Docs word processing software.

Nursing education programs and some journals use APA style. When writing using APA style, you create defaults for the style initially. Afterward, you use the style to create section heading that guides the reader to understand the information.

Word processors have many features that not only make tasks easier but also make them economically feasible. Examples include using tables to organize data and mail merge for personalized print and electronic communication. Before beginning the writing process, you should practice technical skills that might distract from writing.

In order to gain competence learning new skills, you should use a word processing self-assessment checklist. With the rapid changes in software, mastering word processing competencies is a lifelong learning process.

APPLICATIONS AND COMPETENCIES

1. Self-assess your word processing skills using Box 5-1. After completing the skills inventory, identify at least two goals to improve your competencies. Discuss the results of the inventory and your skills development plan.

2. Reflect on scholarly papers you wrote for schoolwork. Discuss how manuscripts written for peer-reviewed nursing journals differ.

3. Compare commercial word processing software, such as Word, with a free software solution. Can you identify any similarities and differences? Summarize your finding with specific examples.

4. Format a sample paper using APA style that includes a title page, abstract, body of paper, and reference list. Include at least two paragraph headings, citations, and references.

5. Discuss the rationale for using paragraph headings.

6. Replicate the design of a table with APA style formatting. Explain the word processing tools used to format the table.

REFERENCES

American Psychological Association. (2011). *Publication manual of the American Psychological Association* (6th ed.). Washington, DC: Author.

American Psychological Association. (2012). *APA style guide to electronic references*. Washington, DC: Author.

Berkey, B., & Moore, S. (2012). Preparing research manuscripts for publication: A guide for authors. *Oncology Nursing Forum, 39*(5), 433-435. doi:10.1188/12.ONF.433-435.

International Committee of Medical Journal Editors (ICMJE). (2013). *ICMJE: Recommendations for the conduct, reporting, editing, and publication of scholarly work in medical journals.* Retrieved from http://www.icmje.org/

Norquist, R. (2014). *Paraphrase—Definition and examples of paraphrases.* Retrieved from http://grammar.about.com/od/pq/g/paraphterm.htm

Oermann, M. H., & Hays, J. C. (2010). *Writing for publication in nursing* (2nd ed.). New York, NY: Springer Pub. Co.

Stoddard, S. (2014). *Things people said.* Retrieved from http://rinkworks.com/said/yogiberra.shtml

The Biosemantics Group. (2007). *Jane: Journal/author name estimator.* Retrieved from http://biosemantics.org/jane/

Things people said: Yogi Berra. (2011, January 21). Retrieved from http://rinkworks.com/said/yogiberra.shtml

Webb, C. (2009). *Writing for publication.* Retrieved from http://www.nurseauthoreditor.com/WritingforPublication2009.pdf

CHAPTER 6

Authoring Scholarly Slide Presentations

OBJECTIVES

After studying this chapter, you will be able to:

1. Self-assess presentation competencies to identify opportunities to learn new ones.

2. Compare the differences between the lecture support model and lecture replacement model for slide designs.

3. Apply principles of best practice slide design for slideshows.

4. Discuss copyright licensing issues associated with using images with slide presentations.

5. Employ appropriate principles in creating handouts.

KEY TERMS

Background layer

Cognitive load theory

Content layer

Crop

Evidence-assertion order (assertion-evidence order)

Extraneous cognitive load

Germane cognitive load

Gradient background

Intrinsic cognitive load

Layout layer

Lecture replacement model

Lecture support model

Lessig style

Normal view

Outline view

Prezi

Progressive disclosure

Slide sorter

Slideshow view

Speaker notes

Storyboard

TED (Technology, Entertainment, Design) style

Theme

Visual literacy

You skipped today's lecture because you could get the slide presentation from the course website. Now, you are looking at these slides and wondering how the pieces of information fit together—should you memorize all the bullet points? How will you apply them? How can you make this information meaningful?

Many face this dilemma when reviewing class slides and handouts from online slideshow presentations. Most of us find ourselves frustrated in using information from slides only, or from handouts of slides only, even if we took notes along the sides of the slides. Slideshows may help us as presenters to outline our talk, but when slideshows stand alone, do they help those on the receiving end understand the information that we are trying to communicate?

Today, we use computer slideshows to supplement oral presentations or stand-alone slideshows with voice-over or notes. The key to developing useful slideshows is knowledge about how to create them so that they enhance the presenters' messages. Poorly designed slides are boring and distracting. Have you experienced slideshows that either detracted from or upstaged the speaker? The computer slideshow is the presenter's partner. It should enhance the communication of a message.

This chapter discusses the theoretical and pedagogical use of visuals in a presentation. It includes information on how to design slideshows to enhance learning. You will see the terms *presentation software* and *slideshow* as well as *slides* and *visuals* used interchangeably. Understanding the educational purposes for visuals is essential to the design of an effective presentation. The design of slides is dependent upon several factors including the type of presentation (lecture support or lecture replacement), audience, presentation style, and presentation setting. Slideshow design must also take into consideration the use of special effects as well as the necessity for designing handouts.

Reflect on past presentations that you thought were excellent. Compare the excellent presentations with ones that bored you. That information will assist you to self-assess your presentation skills. You should be able to identify opportunities to gain new skills. Box 6-1 identifies a listing of skills for basic, intermediate, and advanced users.

USING ELECTRONIC SLIDESHOWS IN NURSING

A slideshow, when effectively designed, conveys key points that the presenter wants to make to the audience. Did a PowerPoint slideshow design cause the explosion of the space shuttle Columbia on February 1, 2003? Evidence proves that it was a contributing factor (Kunz, 2012, March 21; Tufte, 2005). It seems that the National Aeronautics and Space Administration had become too reliant on using PowerPoint to present complex information instead of narrative technical reports. The nesting and subnesting of complex points caused those who had to make decisions about the safety of Columbia to misunderstand the true picture. One then must ask, "Could depending on PowerPoint slides to communicate information create a healthcare mistake?"

Principles for All Presentations

There are a few design principles for all presentations. For example, every presentation must have a purpose that is stated clearly, include slides with additional details to address the purpose, and end with a summary slide. To avoid plagiarism when using material from another source, include citations and references. If the topic is broad and complex, such as congestive heart failure or chronic renal failure, chunk the learning into smaller components, each with a separate slide presentation lasting 5 or 10 minutes. Chunking information prevents cognitive overload of the learner.

To assist the learner with applying new knowledge, consider interspersing short slide presentations with critical thinking practice questions that include correct answers and rationales. Slideshows using slide branching, or the ability to jump to a given slide using the number of the slide, can include multiple-choice questions that allow the audience to select answers and receive feedback from both incorrect and correct answers. A discussion about a choice of an incorrect answer can reveal misconceptions that the viewers are unaware that they have. The instructor might also use the questions to assist learners how to approach selecting the correct answer from response distractors.

The ability to interpret the meaning of visual images (Visual Literacy Standards Task Force, 2011) is an important skill for both the designer and audience. Before the advent of the printing press, ideas were conveyed by paintings and images. Today, however, we may not be as adept with visual skills as before printing became universal. Therefore, when planning a slideshow, you

BOX 6-1 Presentation Skills

Basic Presentation Skills
- Design a simple presentation.
- Apply a template to the background.
- Insert a new slide.
- Apply the use of different slide layouts.
- Use spell-check.
- Save a presentation.
- Add shapes to a slide.
- View a slideshow.
- Print a presentation.

Intermediate Presentation Skills
- Customize the presentation menu.
- Create handouts.
- Add clip art to slides.
- Add SmartArt to slides.
- Move and resize objects.
- Incorporate multimedia (audio, graphics, animation, and video) into slide design.
- Modify multimedia used for presentations, for example:
  - Compress photos (right-click) to reduce file size.
  - Edit photos/graphics for resolution, fit, and web use to use in a presentation.
- Demonstrate competency using two presentation software applications.

- Save a presentation in different file formats for use with other software applications.
- Share/collaborate with others on presentation design.
- Apply pedagogical principles to presentation design (purpose, visual clarity, consistency, readability).
- Print out a slide presentation handouts (more than one slide/page).

Advanced Presentation Skills
- Design on-screen navigation.
- Customize presentation toolbars.
- Embed/edit a spreadsheet.
- Create a macro.
- Add slide transitions.
- Add slide sections.
- Design slide animations.
- Demonstrate advance text and graphic editing techniques.
- Build custom slide masters.
- Build custom handout masters.
- Build custom notes masters.
- Create a presentation template.
- Publish and distribute presentations.
- Demonstrate competency using more than two presentation software applications.

need to consider how your audience will view a visual and think about what image it will convey to them. Besides slide design, there are principles to consider when planning a presentation. Two important factors are the visual literacy of the viewer and the cognitive load that the presentation places on the viewers.

Visual Literacy

Anytime you use visuals, you need to be aware of the **visual literacy** of the viewers. "Visual literacy is a set of abilities that enables an individual to effectively find, interpret, evaluate, use, and create images and visual media" (Association of Colleges and Research Libraries, 2011, para 2). Culture,

which also affects visual literacy, can pertain not just to what we usually think of in terms of culture such as nationality but also the background of the viewers. An image might convey information to one group of healthcare professionals although professionals of other disciplines might find it confusing.

Cognitive Load Theory

Sweller (1988) first described **cognitive load theory** in seminal work on learning. According to cognitive load theory, the brain has limited short-term memory and unlimited long-term memory. In simple terms, complex decision making adds to cognitive load. It is difficult for the brain to process reading words on a slide while listening to a presenter unless the two are congruent.

Van Merriënboer and Sweller (2010) identified three types of cognitive load: intrinsic, extraneous, and germane. **Intrinsic cognitive load** relates to the difficulty of problem solving or making sense of the learning material. **Extraneous cognitive load** relates to unnecessary information delivered in the design of instruction. **Germane cognitive load** relates to thought processes or schemas that organize categories of information for storage in long-term memory. Slide design should have minimal text and appropriate visual images and facilitate learners to process information (San Diego State University Department of Educational Technology, 2012).

> ## QSEN Scenario
> You are designing a slide presentation to use for an in-service on preventing blood-borne catheter infection using new protocols. What slide design features should you use?

Computer Slide Models

Today, computer slides are used to convey information in many settings. Two models of slide presentations exist—a lecture support and a lecture replacement. The **lecture support model**, or presentation supplement model, can guide audiences to follow the oral presentation, while the **lecture replacement model** requires text or narration to guide the audience viewer.

Lecture Support Model

When supplementing an oral presentation, the slides should help an audience keep track of ideas and illustrate points. The entire talk should not be on the slides. If using bullet points, use them to focus the listeners' attention. Set up the slide so that bullets display when they are discussed; otherwise, the viewer will read ahead and not hear you. (See the discussion of progressive disclosure later in this chapter, in the "Animation" subsection.)

Viewers, as well as presenters, need to realize that slides alone are only an outline of a talk.

Lecture Replacement Model

A slideshow used as a stand-alone source such as for an online course or "flipped classroom"

is designed differently. A flipped classroom is a teaching method in which the instructor provides learning content, such as a slideshow, as a homework assignment and then uses application activities in the classroom setting. A stand-alone slideshow, such as an interactive tutorial, can provide a self-learning function. Because the tutorial replaces a lecture, not only must the learning objectives be explicit to the viewer, but the information must also be far more detailed than when used to supplement a lecture. Designers of stand-alone presentations, such as for self-running kiosks, lecture supplementation, or tutorials, need to explain and elaborate on slide text and visuals using voice-over narration or adding the slides notes section to the presentation.

Presentation Styles

A traditional presentation style uses slides with the standard slide title and bullet design for other slides. However, new presentation styles and slide designs have emerged over the last decade. These slide designs use innovative technologies for creating visual images. They may take advantage of the ability to design and view slides online with mobile devices, such as tablets and smartphones. Examples of the newer design styles include TED (Technology, Entertainment, Design) style, assertion-evidence order, **PechaKucha**, Lessig style, and Prezi (Alley, 2013). The design of these presentations reduces the viewer's cognitive load.

TED Style

TED-style slide design uses commanding images with or without a few words to convey meaning (TED, 2013). Each slide conveys a message. The shortcoming of the TED-style design is the time that it takes to find or create appropriate high-impact images. An example of a before and after TED-style slide designs is online at http://www.slideshare.net/garr/sample-slides-by-garr-reynolds. TED-style guidelines are available online at http://www.ted.com/pages/tedx_presentation_design.

Evidence Assertion

Evidence-assertion order design replaces each slide title with a short sentence (Alley, 2013). A slide with visual evidence precedes a slide with the assertion or statement of meaning. The evidence might be a graph, image, or photograph. Evidence-assertion order is termed assertion-evidence order when the assertion slide appears before the evidence slide. Evidence-assertion order can convey complex information, such as engineering and medicine topics (Alley, 2013; Issa et al., 2011; O'Connor, 2010). A video about the assertion-evidence design is online at http://www.youtube.com/watch?v=xNW84FUe0ZA.

PechaKucha

Similar to TED-style and evidence-assertion order designs, PechaKucha slides are primarily images. A **PechaKucha** presentation does not use text. Instead, the viewer sees 20 image slides, each of which is visible for 20 seconds (PechaKucha, 2013). The slides appear automatically during the presentation, which is coordinated with the images. Research shows that learning retention from slides using the PechaKucha design is comparable to traditional PowerPoint slides (Alisa et al., 2013; Levin & Peterson, 2013). Examples of PechaKucha slide presentations are online at http://www.pechakucha.org/watch.

Lessig Style

The **Lessig style** is a fast-paced style used when the content is not detailed (Finkelstein, n.d.). The style name originated with Lawrence Lessig, a Stanford University law professor. As with other emerging presentation styles, the slides use text visuals of a few words or quotes to engage the viewers. The presenter spends only 15 seconds on each slide (ETHOS3, n.d.). An example of the Lessig style is online at http://randomfoo.net/oscon/2002/lessig/free.html.

Prezi

Prezi (http://prezi.com) is presentation software that uses zooming to navigate to images on a single canvas. The slide, referred to as a canvas, can include text, graphics, and hyperlinks. The free version of the software requires online design and viewing. Presentations created with the free version of Prezi are public by default. The free version also provides the user with online presentation file storage. Commercial versions of the software allow the user to remove the Prezi logo, share work privately with others, and use the software offline (Prezi, 2013).

There are pros and cons of Prezi presentations. Advantages include the fact that a free version is available and that the navigation, unlike most other slide presentations, is not linear. A possible disadvantage is that participants might complain of motion sickness when viewing poorly designed zooming features. To view an excellent example of a Prezi presentation, go to http://prezi.com/experts/presentationshow/.

Presentations with Embedded Polling

You can create a presentation with embedded questions using polling software. Questions serve to both engage the audience participants and provide feedback to the presenter. Embedded polling can be used for live or online presentations. Examples of free online polling software are:

- Micropoll http://www.micropoll.com/
- Polldaddy http://www.polldaddy.com/
- Poll Everywhere http://www.polleverywhere.com/

Live audience members can respond to polling software questions embedded into slide presentations using smartphones. Distance audience members can respond to questions embedded into online lectures. In both instances, the audience has the ability to see the results of the polling afterward. With this type of presentation, presenters do not have to tell the audience everything. Viewing collective responses as well as deducing or inducing answers can allow targeted coverage of only those topics that are confusing to the group, spur critical thinking, and result in greater retention of information. When polling is anonymous, participants can express honest beliefs and views different from others.

PRESENTATION SOFTWARE

Slideshow software is designed specifically for creating presentations. Slideshow software is often bundled with other office suite software. Like components of other office suite software discussed in this textbook, there are numerous types of slideshow software. Besides Prezi discussed above, examples include Microsoft PowerPoint, Apple iWork Keynote, Apache OpenOffice Impress, and Google Drive Presentation. PowerPoint and Keynote are full-featured commercial slideshow software. Apache OpenOffice is a free office suite for the desktop computer. Google Drive Presentation is a free cloud computing software solution.

Commercial presentation software packages include features that may not be available with free versions. Examples include the ability to narrate, galleries of graphic samples, and the ability to import and export presentations from other software programs. Additionally, they allow custom handouts and the inclusion of interactive help files that include videos and tutorials. If you do not have slideshow software on your computer, begin learning with free software, which will allow you to experiment with slideshow features and functions.

Compatibility of Software

Most slideshow software is compatible with other slideshow software. For example, you can import slides developed with PowerPoint into Keynote for the Mac and Google Drive Presentation. Although the slides import, the added special effects, like sound, transitions, and animations, may not import. The same drawback might occur when viewing the slides on a version of the slideshow software earlier than the one where you created the presentation.

PowerPoint files provide the option of saving the file as a PowerPoint Show (.pps or .ppsx), which can be viewed on any computer. The user does not need PowerPoint software to view a PowerPoint Show file. A .ppsx file will open in the presentation view rather than the normal view used to design the slides. In contrast, Keynote works only on Mac computers. There is no equivalent for PowerPoint Show; however, you can save Keynote files as PowerPoint files.

Collaborating on Slideshow Software Design

Some slideshow software supports real-time collaboration where two or more individuals can work on a slideshow at the same time. For example, PowerPoint users can save and share files for collaborative design using OneDrive. You can also share Google Drive Presentation files for collaborative work. Keynote files do not support real-time collaboration—only the ability to share with others as e-mail attachments.

BASICS OF SLIDE CREATION

Slideshow software is similar in all application programs that use a graphical user interface. The slideshow menu includes many of the same features as word processing menus, for example, font style and size options and ability to create tables and insert graphics and multimedia. The implementation of specific slideshow features varies by software type and version. All packages have more similarities than dissimilarities. They all have different views of the slides from the show view to handouts view. Additionally, they all operate with layers that are like pieces of transparent paper that are overlaid on each other, starting with the background layer, then the layout, and finally the content layer.

Views of the Slides

Slideshow software allows users to look at their slides in many ways. In PowerPoint, each of these views is accessed from icons on the lower right corner of the screen. In Apache Presentation, the views are available from tabs near the top of the left side of the screen.

The view that audiences see is the **slideshow view**, which is only for viewing, not editing. The **normal view** is the default creation mode. In normal view, the left-hand side of the screen has a column with thumbnail view of several slides. The right has a view of the slide under construction. Some presentation software provides an **outline view** and **speaker notes**. The normal, outline, and speaker notes views allow the user to enter and edit information. With PowerPoint, you can also create handouts that have both speaker notes and slides by converting the slides and notes to Word. In PowerPoint, select Save & Send from the file menu and then Create Handouts.

The **slide sorter view** shows many slides on one screen and is used for viewing and rearranging all the slides in the slideshow. This view is especially useful when copying slides from one presentation to another. To rearrange slides, use the click and drag feature. If slides are copied to another presentation, they take on the style of the new slideshow. Slides can be copied or deleted one by one or as a whole. To select more than one, after clicking on the first one, hold down the Control

(Ctrl)/Command key as you select the others. If the slides you wish to select are contiguous, select either the first or the last slide then hold down the Shift key as you select the other end of the group.

Layers

To provide consistency in the design, a slide is composed of three layers: background, layout, and content. Each is independent of the other, yet works together as a whole.

The Background Layer

The **background layer**, sometimes called the master layer, holds the design of the slides, or the theme. A **theme** is a predesigned combination of background colors, font style, size, and color.

The background layer is important because it keeps all the slides in the presentation consistent in looks. This layer has place keepers for the title and subtitle for the title page and for bullet points, graphics, and other items for subsequent slides. Because the place keepers are located in different places in different backgrounds, if you change the theme on the background layer after you have designed the slides, you need to check to be sure that all your slides are still intact.

A gallery of themes is included with most presentation software. Some of these include illustrations. Keep in mind that any graphics on your background layer will show on all slides, regardless of the layout selected. Although the graphic maybe interesting, it may interfere with your message, or even cause attention to be deflected from your message.

Designers can either modify or accept a selected theme. More background designs are often available on the website of the vendor of the slide program, or you can create your own. Keep in mind that just because a theme or background is available, it does not necessarily indicate the design is good or that it will add to your presentation.

When selecting a background for an oral presentation, it is helpful to know the kind of presentation room lighting. Borrowing from the days of 35-mm slides, when rooms were dark, many people still choose a dark background that is very appropriate with a dark room, but which allows content to get lost in a room that is lighted. Contrast is important, and having the background

match the lighting in the room is a good principle to follow. Design experts do not agree on the background color for presentations that are projected (Tufte, n.d.). However, consider using a light background for light rooms and dark background for dark rooms (Prost, n.d.).

To change the background for only one slide, right-click on a blank place in the slide and select "Format Background" from the menu. The Format Background menu provides the option of changing the background for all slides, too. Since consistency of colors and fonts is an essential component for good slide design, you should only change a slide background for an essential point of emphasis such as accommodating a graphic.

The Layout Layer

The **layout layer** builds on the background layer in the number and types of placeholders it has for different layouts. Opening up a document to create a new presentation will present you with a title page layout. The title slide layout has placeholders for a title and a subtitle. By default, the next slide layout will be bulleted text. Use bullet points only if they are an appropriate communication method for your message. Use the Tab key to create a lower level and the Shift+Tab to move back to a higher level just like you would do when using the outline feature of a word processor.

If you need a different layout, in PowerPoint, right-click anywhere outside of a placeholder and select Layout from the menu. In Apache OpenOffice Presentations, select the layout from the properties menu on the right side of the screen. Take the time to view all the various layouts available; bullet points may not be the most effective communication method. As you plan your presentation, avail yourself of some of the presentation styles that were discussed above. They may very well be a better choice to communicate your information. As you plan your presentation, think visually versus textually.

The Content Layer

Use the **content layer** to enter text or other objects, such as images, tables, and charts. Layout themes have boxes visible only in the normal view to guide the user in placing text. If the default font size or color employed by the master layer is not appropriate for an individual slide, you can use the text format menu to change these. Be careful not to introduce to many variations to one presentation. Also, be sure to use the spell-checker when finalizing the presentation!

CREATING THE PRESENTATION

When faced with creating a presentation, most designers want to start right away with creating slides. A little planning before the first slide is created will save much time and result in a more organized presentation. Once you have an outline or storyboard, you are ready to create professional slides using the features that slide presentation software makes available.

Storyboarding

The concept of **storyboarding** originated with film. However, it is valuable in any presentation that involves visuals. A storyboard is a plan for the visuals. It forces you to organize your thoughts and allows you to assemble your ideas into a coherent presentation. As with all projects, planning saves time! With presentation software, you can outline your thoughts using a title and text on a slide. After you complete the first draft, use the Slide Sorter view to look at the presentation as a whole. This will help you to see where a rearrangement of slides would be helpful and make it easy to rearrange the order by dragging the slides to a new position. When you think things are in the correct order, go back to each slide and develop it into a meaningful communication tool. Expect to switch between the Slide Sorter view and the Design view many times while working on the actual visuals!

Content

Unlike physical slides or overheads, presentation software makes the creation of visuals easier, giving designers numerous tools to create content such as text, images, charts, and tables.

Text

A facet of presentation software that is both an advantage and a disadvantage is the number of fonts available. Many of the fonts are unsuitable

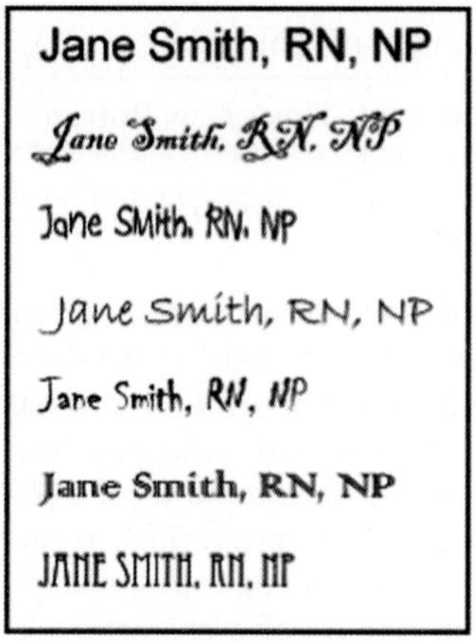

Which of the above fonts looks the most professional?

Figure 6-1. Different fonts elicit different emotional responses.

for text in a presentation slides. Even though one is always tempted to select a "jazzy" font in the hope that it will enliven a presentation, too often this choice creates readability problems. When selecting, remember that fonts can elicit an emotional response from the audience; thus, choose one that not only is visually appealing but also elicits the desired emotional response (Figure 6-1).

The background templates for presentation programs have preselected fonts that might be suitable for a presentation. You can change the font styles for an individual slide or for the entire presentation. However, changing a font after the completion of a presentation may disturb the layout on some slides because of the difference in size of the text in different fonts. For example, the font size of all the examples in Figure 6-1 is the same, yet you can see that the text is not all of the same size. The measurement unit for text size is points (Bear, 2014). There are about 72 font points in an inch. Point size, as you can see, is not always an accurate guide. Some fonts at 12 points, despite being one sixth of an inch in vertical height for capital letters (cap-height), are very difficult to read. The x-height, or the height of lowercase letters, causes the differences (Phinney, 2011). The stroke thickness, either horizontal or vertical, is also a factor. The smallest easily readable text size for computer slides is 24 points.

Sans-serif font: Arial	Generally easier to read online
Serif font: Times New Roman	Easier to read in a print format

Figure 6-2. Comparison of sans serif and serif fonts.

For projected visuals, use a sans serif (i.e., without serifs) font such as Arial or Helvetica (Figure 6-2). The fonts follow the basic rule in choosing a display font—that the letters appear crisp and clean. Some fonts (e.g., Garamond and Times Roman) have projections from the letter called serifs. These are fine strokes across the ends of the main strokes of a character. Serifs create softer edges to the characters, which add to readability on paper. However, serif fonts have a tendency to look fuzzy on projected slides.

You can add attributes to fonts just as you can in word processing. Bold text will emphasize a point as will italics. Italicizing, however, tends to make text more difficult to read; if it is used, give the audience more time to read the slide. Use this feature to your advantage when you want the audience to read more slowly. Avoid underlining text for emphasis; instead, use it to indicate hyperlinks. When using font effects, be consistent throughout the presentation, that is, always use the same attribute for the same type of information.

When placing text on visuals, include only the essential elements of a concept. You should state ideas as though they were headlines. Visual text serves as a focus to assist the audience in following the presentation. The information on a slide can also be helpful to the presenter as a guide to the oral presentation.

The audience should grasp the point of the visual text within the first 5 seconds after it appears. Some suggest that a presenter should be quiet for those 5 seconds to allow the audience to grasp the point. To avoid cognitive overload, limit the text on a slide. One way to determine whether you have too much information on the slide is to place the information on a 4 × 6 inches card and try to read it from a distance of about 5 to 6 feet. In oral and voice-over presentations, do not read the slide to the audience. Audience participants can read faster than a speaker can talk; therefore, they may become torn between reading ahead and listening. This practice can unwittingly encourage the speaker to pay more attention to the slides than to the audience and can lead the audience to ignore the speaker.

Images

Slideshow software provides ways to use images as part of a presentation. As you design your slides, think visually! Will a picture, graph, or table communicate your message better than words? Several sources of presentation quality images are available such as Clip Art in PowerPoint. There are also royalty-free photos and illustrations available on the Internet, or you can scan in an image, or create your own. Additionally, you can use the Internet to find images for noncommercial class presentations. Right-clicking on most images on the web will allow you to copy the image to the clipboard so you can place it in a presentation. Besides copy/paste, you can also use the Insert menu to add images to slides. Click and drag the image to move it to a location on the slide. When resizing an image, remember to click on the corner (not a side) to avoid stretching and skewing the image.

If you are using images, sound, or video for a presentation that you will give commercially, check the copyright permission and license terms of any objects that you use that you did not create yourself. Many types of clip art and other web images have copyright limitations. Before you purchase a package of clip art, read the fine print to be certain that the package is truly royalty free.

Drawing tools and image editing features assist in the slide design process. Slideshow software provides drawing tools that you can use to call out information in images or text or create illustrations. Also, you can **crop** images. Cropping allows the designer to move the sides of a picture inward to show only a smaller part of the image. The process does not delete any of an image, but it makes the covered part invisible. Because it does not change the size of the image or the file size, if you want to use only a small portion of an image, use a screen clip tool.

Occasionally, an image may not project well. To prevent this from marring a presentation, check the appearance of the slide in the Play or Show view before committing to using the visual in the presentation. Generally, if an image looks good in playback mode, it will project well. If possible, check how the image projects using the equipment that will be used to make the presentation.

Although using a scanned image, a clip art, or images from the Internet makes it possible to include very detailed pictures, there are several things that need to be considered. First, is the visual pertinent to your message or will it distract from your message? Second, is the image more complicated than needed to convey your meaning? For example, a presentation that includes an illustration of blood circulation through the heart could be confusing if were very detailed. Instead, using a schematic drawing that depicts only the four chambers and the veins and arteries leading into and out of the heart would make the information more understandable, allowing viewers to focus on the main points rather trying to separate them from the details. When adding images, remember that the point of visuals is to communicate a message to the audience. Use images only to enhance the presentation. While you may want a little variety to lighten a presentation, be careful. Be sure that an image used in this way is pertinent to the message, or you risk losing attention of the viewers.

Charts and Tables

A table or chart is often clearer in communicating meaning than text. You can import a graph or data directly from a spreadsheet as well as copy and paste it on slides. Be certain to use charts or tables to convey information accurately. (Chapter 7 includes information on the uses of the various types of charts.) When using a table, the slide limits the table size. If it is important to include a detailed chart or table in the presentation, include the information in a handout; do not include the information in a slide. Slides that are unreadable create viewer frustration.

Special Effects

Special effects such as color, sound, video, animations, and transitions can enhance slideshow presentations. However, use moderation when adding special effects to a presentation. You want the viewers to pay attention to your message, not the special effect. If you are giving a presentation that uses special effects, such as sound and video, test the presentation in the setting where viewers will see it.

Color

Although you can use color to draw attention to a feature, you should not use it as the only distinguishing characteristic. As with fonts, it is important to be consistent in using color. When viewers grasp the implications of a given color, the result is improved comprehension of the meaning of the visuals. Although the eye can perceive millions of colors, limit the number of screen colors from four to six.

Creators of slideshows also need to be aware that colors, like text fonts, have an emotional appeal (Um et al., 2012). Individuals can interpret red as exciting or as the color of passion, excitement, or aggression and green as calming or related to health or the environment. The meaning of colors varies with cultures. Purple may indicate spirituality and physical and mental healing in some cultures; in others, it may symbolize mourning or wealth (Kyrnin, 2010).

Select compatible color combinations that offer a strong contrast. Some color groupings, such as red on black, give a three-dimensional appearance that may make the red object appear closer than the black background. Additionally, objects sometimes appear larger in one color than in another. Reading accuracy is best when the colors used for background and text are on opposite sides of the color wheel. See http://www.colormatters.com/color-and-design/basic-color-theory for more information about combining colors. Keep this information in mind when selecting the theme for the background. Because different computers render color differently, check your color scheme on the presentation computer before the presentation, if possible.

Keep in mind that 8% of men and 0.5% of women have some kind of color perception problem or color blindness, usually a deficiency in discriminating red from green (Microsoft, 2015; Thomson, 2013). Individuals with color blindness see colors, but they see them differently from the rest of the population. Using sharp contrasts in colors assists these viewers in particular to read the text.

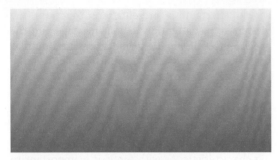

Figure 6-3. A gradient background.

Many slide backgrounds provided with presentation software use gradient backgrounds. Gradient backgrounds are gradually shaded from a lighter to a darker shade of the same color (Figure 6-3). When you use a **gradient background** on a slide, use a very sharply contrasting text color, and test the completed slide for readability.

Sound

You can insert sound into all commercial slideshow software and some free versions. Depending on the software, you may be able to insert audio from a file, Clip Art sounds, or record narration. Look for Insert > Audio in the slideshow menu. To record sound, you need a microphone and a sound card (available in all new computers). When recording narration, write out the information you want to record first. You can use a separate word processing document or the speaker notes section on the slide.

There are pros and cons for using the narration-recording feature built into slideshow software.

The pro is that recording narration is easy. However, there are several cons. The narration menu does not allow for audio editing. If you want to make changes, you must rerecord the narration. The second con is that presentation software, such as PowerPoint, may save recorded narration using an uncompressed file format. If you plan to save the file to a high-capacity flash drive or burn it to a CD, the file size may not be an issue. If you plan to use the file for podcasting and sharing with others on the Internet, the large file size is a major issue. Some slideshow software, such as PowerPoint 2013, allows you to optimize the file for media compatibility and to compress the media to decrease the file size.

You may want to consider prerecording narration and adding it to each slide. Some software applications allow you to use separate software to record the narration and to import the uncompressed or compressed file formats (Box 6-2). On a Windows PC, you can use the Sound Recorder that is included in the Accessories folder. Sound Recorder narration creates a Windows Media Audio (WMA) file, which is a compressed audio file. Sound Recorder saves only the WMA file format and does not include a sound editor. A second solution is to use Audacity (http://audacity.sourceforge.net/), a free cross-platform sound recorder and editor. Audacity provides a means to export audio files in numerous formats. If you want to save the file in the MP3 format, be sure to download the LAME MP3 encoder (http://lame.sourceforge.net/). If the purpose of the slideshow is to allow users to view and listen to the slideshow

---

BOX 6-2   Sound File Format Explanations

Uncompressed Formats
- WAV—used on Windows devices
- AIFF—used on Apple devices
- Au—designed by Sun Microsystems for use on LINUX systems

Compressed Formats
- MP3—used on Apple devices

- WMA (Windows media audio)—a designed for Windows Media Player
- Ogg (Vorbis off)—open source sound format similar to MP3

Others
- MIDI (Musical Instrument Digital Interface) for devices to play musical notes and rhythm

Source: Audio file formats explained in simple terms—http://www.makeuseof.com/tag/a-look-at-the-different-file-formats-available-part-1-audio/

on a portable media player, record the narration saved in a WMA or MP3 audio file format. Since slideshows with graphics and compressed audio can still be quite large, creating several small 3- to 10-minute slideshows rather than one that runs 15 to 30 minutes may be best for stand-alone purposes.

Video

Video clips are equally easy to insert. Many slide-show software allows you to insert digital video from a file or a website. You can use video from a camcorder, a webcam, most digital cameras, smartphones, and tablet devices. Some slideshow software includes a video editor. With Google Drive Presentation, you can select a video from YouTube.

When adding video to an oral presentation slideshow, as a rule of thumb, limit the video length to 45 to 60 seconds. Any length beyond that may distract the audience. As with sound, before using video in a presentation, check the presentation equipment. Make a copy of the presentation without video available in case the video portion of the presentation equipment fails on the day of the presentation.

Transitions

A **transition** is the way a slide makes an entrance. Presentation programs have a variety of transitions available. Some cause a slide to fade in, some cause the slide to appear first at the center and then expand, and others cause the slide to sweep across the screen. Transitions can be dramatic, enhance your message, or distract the audience. The best rule is to be consistent and use transitions sparingly. Avoid at all costs trying to dazzle the audience with multiple transitions.

Animation

The term **animation**, often referred to as Custom Animation, is available in some presentation software. Generally, animation takes the form of **progressive disclosure**, although some movement of objects is possible. Progressive disclosure is a technique in which items are revealed one at a time until all the items on a slide display. During your presentation, you can dim or convert bullets or images already discussed to a different color

while the current point takes center stage. You can make objects appear or disappear during a presentation using slide animation. Use of animation can reduce cognitive load for viewers. There are a variety of options available for progressive disclosure. Some of these options allow the item to slide in from any direction, bounce in, fade in, or even curve in. Like all special effects, use transitions judiciously and think hard about whether they are a distraction or a good addition.

You can also use animated GIFs (Graphics Interchange Formats—a type of image files from the web that show movement) with many presentation programs. If the animated GIF will be on the screen for a long time, it is a good idea to cover it up after a given time period—something you can set to happen automatically. Movement on a screen can become very distracting. When using animation, check the animation on the computer used for the presentation before the actual presentation. Unless you are using your own computer, it is best not plan a presentation around the movement in the image.

You can create a video simulation with slide-show software using a combination of motion path animation and stop motion. Stop motion is a technique where you simulate animation with progressive changes in the graphics on a group of slides (Stop Motion Works, 2008). Kuhlmann (2009) created a blog with the details about how to use this animation technique. The blog includes several narrated videos and graphics using the example of dissecting a frog using a scalpel and scissors. You might use this particular animation technique when creating tutorials on topics like starting an IV (intravenous) infusion or inserting a nasogastric tube.

Speaker Notes

As mentioned earlier, including speaker notes can help a speaker to remember information for a given slide. When the slideshow is projected, only the slide is visible to the audience. However, you can print speaker notes with the associated slides. Or you can use the speaker notes for recording narration or when rehearsing the presentation. If you use PowerPoint or Keynote software, you can view the slides with speaker notes on the presenter's computer while the audience sees only the slides from the overhead projector. The feature is available only on computers that support two monitors. Search the software help menu for additional information.

Creating a Show that Allows for Nonlinear Presentations

When giving a presentation, you should be somewhat flexible. Some audiences may ask questions; others will not. A presenter can also misjudge the time needed for the presentation. By using the computer for the presentation, you can manage the unexpected. With most presentation software, the presenter can prepare a hidden slide to show when an audience member asks a specific question or if time permits. Slideshow software also allows you to advance (or retreat) to a specific slide when the number of the slide is typed followed by the Enter key. To make it possible to use this feature, prepare a list of slide numbers and their corresponding titles so you will know what number to enter to show any slide.

THE PRESENTATION

Although creating good visuals is important, slides alone do not ensure a good presentation. To achieve that, you need to be sure that the visuals and the presentation reinforce one another. To reach that goal, it is necessary to plan the visuals and the presentation together. A good presentation provides the audience with an overview of what you will tell them, presents the information, and then provides a summary of the important points. Keep in mind that people will take away no more than five pieces of information from a presentation (Feierman, 2010). One suggestion for preparation is to write out your conclusion slide first, emphasizing your most important points, and build the presentation around that.

Handouts

As stated earlier, rarely is a printed copy of slides alone, even with space for the audience to take notes, a worthwhile reason to destroy trees. Preparing a word-processed document using your notes and inserting appropriate illustrations is a much better use of paper. You cannot reduce complex information to bullet points! To keep the audience's attention focused on your message rather than reading the handout, tell attendees at the beginning of the presentation that you will make a handout available after the presentation.

Professional conferences are transitioning from printed programs to online ones. For this reason, professional nursing conferences often require presenters to submit a copy of the slides or slide handouts before the conference. Sometimes, these are included in a printed program; other times they are placed online. Either format assists attendees to make selections of sessions to attend. They also minimize the need to take notes during the oral presentation.

Transferring to the Web

Although it is possible to transfer a computer slideshow designed for an oral presentation to the web as an html or a PDF file, it may not be a good idea. Remember that every medium is different. The difference between a live slide presentation and a stand-alone web presentation is huge. On the web, not only do the slides have to answer all questions, but they also need to be complete with all the information that readers need to have. Few slideshows meet this requirement. Bullet points do not! If you need to post the information to the web, think about how to best present it. You may need to add audio to the slides, or a narrative text with embedded illustration(s) for those who learn best by reading, or both. You may want to review the educational principles in Chapter 21 when considering posting something to the web.

The Oral Presentation

The moment has arrived; you have rehearsed the presentation until you know it cold. Despite this, hundreds of butterflies are tap dancing in your stomach, and you are wondering, "Will I remember what to say?" The title slide opens; you give the audience 5 seconds to read it—an eternity when you are the speaker (count to yourself from 1,001 to 1,005.). Then you read the title, and give the audience an icebreaker, maybe an anecdote about yourself. For example, you may share how you prepared for the talk, something light. Knowing that you want the audience to pay attention to the presentation, and not read ahead, you tell them that you will distribute handouts after the presentation. Your carefully designed handouts will provide the reader with information months or years after your presentation is complete. With the introduction out of the way, you open the next slide and start to communicate your message.

By the third or fourth slide, the butterflies are ending their dance, and the points on the slide remind you of the information you need to communicate. You make eye contact with various people in the audience, and the presentation is going smoothly—you are beginning to enjoy it. If someone asks a question that requires you to diverge from the planned presentation, and it is a point that you thought might come up, you switch to your nonlinear presentation. You can even take the time to jot down the present slide number to return to before you do this—audiences do not mind. If the question is something not planned for, but to which you need to respond, tap the letter "w" to make the screen white, or "b" to make it black, answer the question, tap Enter to bring back the screen, and go on with the presentation. Then, it is over! You made it—you are receiving thanks from the audience for sharing your knowledge. Enjoy! Keep in mind that it may take several presentations before you really feel comfortable with a presentation and that everyone has a first time presenting!

LEARNING NEW PRESENTATION SKILLS

Learning new presentation skills, like mastering new office software, is a lifelong journey. Software companies frequently release new versions. For example, Microsoft releases a new version of Microsoft Office every 3 years. Google and OpenOffice release updates presentation software, as they are available.

This chapter provided information common to presentation software. If you are a new user of presentation software and do not have it installed on your computer, consider using one of the free versions. If you have intermediate or advanced skills, work on gaining experience with more than one product platform and continue to mentor and share what you know with others.

There are free learning resources for using presentation software, including:

- Training Courses for PowerPoint 2013 (http://office.microsoft.com/en-us/powerpoint-help/training-courses-for-powerpoint-2013-HA104015465.aspx)
- Use Docs, Sheets, and Slides (https://support.google.com/drive/topic/2811739?hl=en&ref_topic=2799627)
- Mac Apps Support (http://www.apple.com/support/mac-apps/keynote/)
- Microsoft Office (http://www.gcflearnfree.org/office)

SUMMARY

The overuse of computer slides has led some to believe that we are dumbing down the message. Some believe that using bullet points forces presenters to "mutilate data beyond comprehension" (Thompson, 2003, December 14) and present disjointed information. Creating a good presentation means emphasizing the real message and using visuals to aid the message, not as a substitute for it. Well-thought-out visuals are important for all presentations, even small presentations given to a group of colleagues. As a nurse progresses up the career ladder, knowing how to give a presentation that conveys a solid message is an aid to advancement.

Presentation package software, including Apache OpenOffice Impress and Google Docs Presentations, have certain similarities. They facilitate the job of creating good visuals by providing a consistent background for the visual and tailored layouts. There are many options available, such as adding images or special effects such as sound, video clips, animation, and progressive disclosure. However, images and special effects must enhance the message. The same rule applies when selecting colors, fonts, backgrounds, and layouts. See Table 6-1 for a summary of the basic rules for creating and using visuals.

All presentations need planning and organizing. Handouts should reflect what the audience should take away from the presentation, not just the slides. Several issues are involved in creating a presentation: identifying key points, planning the visuals to be a partner, using good visual techniques, preparing a useful handout, and finally, rehearsing!

TABLE 6-1 **Basic Rules for Creating and Using Visuals**	
Text and Fonts	
Fonts	• Choose a sans serif font (e.g., Arial or Helvetica) for projected visuals. • Use no more than three font styles per presentation.
Font size	• Use font size ≥24 points.
Punctuation	• Be consistent. If using periods to end sentences or bullets, use them for all.
Colors	
Text and background	• Match slide lighting to presentation setting. Use light for light rooms and dark for dark rooms.
Font color	• Use strong contrast—opposite sides of color wheel.
For emphasis	• Match font color to reactions desired from the audience. Colors convey meaning (e.g., red is intense—use only for emphasis). • Avoid the use of red and green to assist viewers with color blindness.
Consistency	• Use same color for same meaning.
Number used	• Use no more than four to six colors per presentation.
Using Visuals	
Appropriateness	• Use images appropriately to enhance the learner's understanding of important information.
Presentation	• Use progressive disclosure for bullet points; for questions or information that does not pertain to the talk, blank out screen.
Audience reading	• Keep the narration focused on the slide in view. • If the audience needs to read an entire slide, give them time!
Screen manipulation	• To digress from the slides, tap the letter "w" to produce a white screen, or "b" for a black screen. • Hide mouse pointer: tap the A key (toggle) to turn mouse on/off. • Start presentation: tap the F5 key.

APPLICATIONS AND COMPETENCIES

1. Self-assess your presentation competencies using the information in Box 6-1. Identify your strengths. Also identify at least two areas where you can develop new competencies.

2. Compare the differences between lecture support and lecture replacement slide models. Identify best practice design techniques for each model.

3. Search the Internet for a slide presentation. Watch the presentation and analyze the slides for the following:

   a. Whether the text is readable.

      i. Background color shows text to best advantage.

      ii. Font used is easily readable.

   b. Whether the content is enhanced or lost with the slides.

   c. Whether the presenter uses the visuals as a partner.

      i. Slides do not upstage the presenter.

      ii. Slides do not present a message different from what is being said.

      iii. Slides make the presentation easy or difficult to follow.

      iv. Images add to the message.

   d. How you could use the slides as handouts that would aid your understanding a month from today.

   e. The type of presentation style.

4. Explore examples of at least two new presentation styles examined in this chapter. Analyze and summarize the differences. Which presentation style might you use and why?

5. Experiment with different backgrounds and decide why or why not they would be effective in a specific type of presentation such as a research report, a class project, or a welcome speech. If they are not appropriate, how could they be modified to be more useful for your purpose?

6. How could you use a cartoon in a visual? What are some of the things that you would have to consider if you choose to do so?

7. You need to teach a class about a physiological process. On the web, find some images to use in a noncommercial setting and insert them into a slide. Discuss the copyright licensing issues for the images (Search for "images of [the physiological process].")

8. Create a three- or four-slide presentation on a topic of your choice.

   a. Add a background.

   b. Create the slides using more than the title and bullet layouts.

   c. Use progressive disclosure (search for animation to learn how).

   d. Add an image.

   e. Add a video or sound.

   f. Use the principles of best practice design noted in Table 6-1.

   g. Create a handout that would be appropriate for an audience reference 6 months after the presentation.

9. Identify one or two new presentation skills that you would like to master. Create a four- to five-slide presentation that uses multimedia and employs the new skills. Create a handout for the presentation. What slideshow software did you use? Self-assess yourself and summarize what lessons you learned.

REFERENCES

Alisa, A. B., Catherine, G., & Julia, L. (2013). Comparing students' evaluations and recall for student Pecha Kucha and PowerPoint presentations. *Journal of Teaching and Learning with Technology, 1*(2), 26. Retrieved from http://jotlt.indiana.edu/article/view/3109/3051

Alley, M. (2013). *Rethinking presentation slides: The assertion-evidence structure*. Retrieved, from http://writing.engr.psu.edu/slides.html

Alley, M. (2013). *The craft of scientific presentations: Critical steps to succeed and critical errors to avoid* (2nd ed.) New York, NY: Springer.

Association of Colleges and Research Libraries. (2011). *ACRL visual literacy competency standards for higher education*. Retrieved from http://www.ala.org/acrl/standards/visualliteracy

Bear, J. H. (2014). *How many points in an inch?* Retrieved from http://desktoppub.about.com/od/faq/qt/pointsinaninch.htm

ETHOS3. (n.d.). *The Lessig method.* Retrieved from http://www.ethos3.com/design-tips/the-lessig-method

Feierman, A. (2010). *The art of communicating effectively: Tips from all aspects of pulling off the successful presentation!* Retrieved from http://www.presentation-pointers.com/showarticle/articleid/64/

Finkelstein, E. (n.d.). *Presentation styles—What style should you use?* Retrieved from http://office.microsoft.com/en-us/powerpoint-help/presentation-styles-what-style-should-you-use-HA102294769.aspx

Issa, N., Schuller, M., Santacaterina, S., et al (2011). Applying multimedia design principles enhances learning in medical education. *Medical Education, 45*(8), 818–826. doi: 10.1111/j.1365-2923.2011.03988.x.

Kuhlmann, T. (2009, January 13). *Why dissecting an e-learning course will improve your skills.* Retrieved from http://www.articulate.com/rapid-elearning/why-dissecting-an-e-learning-course-will-improve-your-skills/

Kunz, B. (2012, March 21). *The PowerPoint slide that brought down the space shuttle.* Retrieved from https://plus.google.com/113349993076188494279/posts/LhjCFJovjwV

Kyrnin, J. (2010). *Visual color symbolism chart by culture.* Retrieved from http://webdesign.about.com/od/colorcharts/l/bl_colorculture.htm

Levin, M. A., & Peterson, L. T. (2013). Use of Pecha Kucha in marketing students' presentations. *Marketing Education Review, 23*(1), 59–64. doi: 10.2753/MER1052-8008230110.

Microsoft. (2015). Creating accessible PowerPoint presentations. Retrieved from https://support.office.com/en-nz/article/Creating-accessible-PowerPoint-presentations-6f7772b2-2f33-4bd2-8ca7-dae3b2b3ef25

O'Connor, S. L. (2010). Creating effective slides. *AMWA Journal: American Medical Writers Association Journal, 25*(2), 57–61. Retrieved from http://www.amwa.org/journal

PechaKucha. (2013). *Frequently asked questions.* Retrieved from http://www.pechakucha.org/faq

Phinney, T. (2011, March 18). *Point size and em square: Not what people think.* Retrieved from http://www.thomasphinney.com/2011/03/point-size/

Prezi. (2013). *Choose your Prezi licenses.* Retrieved from http://prezi.com/pricing/

Prost, J. (n.d.). *8 mistakes made when presenting with PowerPoint and how to correct them.* Retrieved from http://www.frippandassociates.com/artprost2_faa.html

San Diego State University Department of Educational Technology. (2012). *Pecha Kucha and Lessig-style presentations.* Retrieved from http://edweb.sdsu.edu/courses/edtec470/fall12/resources/pechakucha.htm

Stop Motion Works. (2008). *Frequently asked questions.* Retrieved from http://www.stopmotionworks.com/faq.htm

Sweller, J. (1988). Cognitive load during problem solving: Effects on learning. *Cognitive Science, 12,* 257–285. Retrieved from http://onlinelibrary.wiley.com/doi/10.1207/s15516709cog1202_4/pdf

TED. (2013). *Great presentation design.* Retrieved from http://www.ted.com/pages/tedx_presentation_design

Thompson, C. (2003, December). *2003: The 3rd annual year in ideas; PowerPoint makes you dumb.* Retrieved from http://www.nytimes.com/2003/12/14/magazine/2003-the-3rd-annual-year-in-ideas-powerpoint-makes-you-dumb.html

Thomson, D. (2013). Eyesight and vision in the workplace. *Occupational Health, 65*(4), 27–30. Retrieved from http://www.personneltoday.com/occupational-health/

Tufte, E. (2005, September 6). *PowerPoint does rocket science: Assessing the quality and credibility of technical reports.* Retrieved from http://www.edwardtufte.com/bboard/q-and-a-fetch-msg?msg_id=0001yB&topic_

Tufte, E. (n.d.). *Recommended background for projected presentations.* Retrieved from http://www.edwardtufte.com/bboard/q-and-a-fetch-msg?msg_id=000082

Um, E. R., Plass, J. L., Hayward, E. O., et al (2012). Emotional design in multimedia learning. *Journal of Educational Psychology, 104*(2), 485–498. doi: 10.1037/a0026609.

Van Merriënboer, J. J., & Sweller, J. (2010). Cognitive load theory in health professional education: Design principles and strategies. *Medical Education, 44*(1), 85–93. doi: 10.1111/j.1365-2923.2009.03498.x.

Visual Literacy Standards Task Force. (2011). *ACRL visual literacy competency standards for higher education.* Retrieved from http://www.ala.org/acrl/standards/visualliteracy

CHAPTER 7

Mastering Spreadsheet Software to Assess Quality Outcomes Using Numbers

OBJECTIVES

After studying this chapter, you will be able to:

1. Identify differences between spreadsheet and word processing tables.
2. Use computer conventions to create mathematical formulas to analyze data.
3. Develop basic competencies to use spreadsheets to calculate numbers.
4. Discuss methods to eliminate errors in spreadsheets.
5. Design an appropriate chart to communicate a specific point.

KEY TERMS

Active cell	Chart	Pie chart
Area chart	Column	Spreadsheet
Bar chart	Combo box	Stacked chart
Cell	External reference	Workbook
Cell address	Freeze	Worksheet
Cell range	Line chart	

Numbers are often part of the information nurses need to manage. Computers, together with specialized software, provide freedom from the drudgery of manual calculations and make managing numerical information much easier. The first **spreadsheet** program, developed in 1979, greatly accelerated the acceptance of computers in the business world (Mattessich, n.d.). What is most remarkable about the first spreadsheet is that the design is so functional that it has not changed much over the years. Instead, there are many additional features, such as **charts** and components, which make it easier to enter formulas. The program design is intuitive and has remarkable similarities in spreadsheet vendor products.

Spreadsheets are not the only type of application program that simplifies managing numerical data. Other programs that assist in the management of numbers include financial management programs, tax preparation programs, and statistical software. Financial management software allows us to balance checkbooks and manage a personal budget, including help with categorizing items to facilitate tax preparation. Tax preparation software uses data from a financial manager or spreadsheet to create and print tax returns. Statistical software has preset statistical functions to analyze data. While there are a variety of number-crunching software packages available, this chapter focuses specifically on spreadsheet features useful for assessing quality outcomes in nursing. Examples of tutorials for learning new spreadsheet competences are included at the end of the chapter.

USES OF SPREADSHEETS IN NURSING

Spreadsheet skills are invaluable to all nurses. Because spreadsheet applications have many similarities with word processing and calculators, with a little practice, the use is almost intuitive. You can use spreadsheets to capture postal and email mailing addresses for use with the mail merge function in word processing. In clinical care, you can use spreadsheets to monitor and analyze quality outcomes. Examples include adverse drug events (ADEs), sepsis, stroke, ventilator-acquired pneumonia (VAP), and bloodstream infection (BSI). You can also use spreadsheets for administrative functions such as staff scheduling, time and attendance records, calculating nursing hours per patient day (NHPPD) for staffing decisions, budget analysis, and Failure Mode Event Analysis (FMEA). In the education setting, you can use spreadsheets to rank candidates for nursing program admission decisions, test item analysis, calculate course grades, calculate grade point averages (GPAs), and prepare research data for statistical analysis.

Every student and practicing nurse should demonstrate basic spreadsheet competencies (Box 7-1). Nursing educators, managers, and administrators should demonstrate intermediate or advanced spreadsheet competencies. Informatics nurse specialists should demonstrate advanced spreadsheet competencies because they develop new nursing applications and teach others.

As with any skill, learning the correct method is essential to maximize productivity and success. It is always easier to learn to do something correct than to unlearn and relearn. It is important to understand how to best display data for crunching, how to use the built-in powerful calculating functions, and how to display analyzed data with reports and charts. You can download a self-assessment skills list and samples of spreadsheets with features used in this chapter from the textbook website at thePoint (thepoint.lww.com/).

BOX 7-1 Essential Spreadsheet Competencies for Nurses

- Apply conditional formatting.
- Copy data to other cells.
- Create formulas using words.
- Create charts (graphs) from data.
- Create pivot tables.
- Insert date/time.
- Design a spreadsheet for efficient use.
- Use financial functions.
- Format cell data using font styles, font sizes, and color.
- Format cells using backgrounds and borders.
- Insert graphics.
- Manage text.
- Merge cells.
- Protect a workbook using a password.
- Resize a cell.
- Sort data.
- Use statistical functions.
- Use templates.
- Use wizards to guide you through complex calculation operations.

Nursing has lessons to learn from the business community. When searching the Web on the topic of spreadsheets, results include articles that associate spreadsheets with "heaven" or "hell," which should alert us that while spreadsheets offer benefits, they might be associated with risks. The European Spreadsheet Risks Interest Group maintains a website with spreadsheet "horror stories" that include a bad spreadsheet link causing a $6 million dollar error to the use of a wrong spreadsheet that omitted taxable property worth $1.6 billion (European Spreadsheet Risks Interest Group, 2013). Panko (2008) in seminal research on spreadsheet errors reported that 20% to 40% of all financial spreadsheets have errors. While it might be human to error, nursing needs to understand the nature of the errors and utilize solutions to mitigate them.

There are three types of quantitative errors in spreadsheets, which occur when data in a cell or formulas are incorrect: typing, logic, and omission errors (Panko, 2008). A typing error is a data entry error or a formula that addresses an incorrect cell. A logic error is a bug in the program, such as a cell formula, that causes it to work incorrectly.

An omission error occurs when essential data are missing.

TIPS FOR BETTER SPREADSHEETS

There is no doubt that spreadsheets have value in nursing practice, administration, and education settings. We need to leverage what we know from business and apply the knowledge in nursing by developing and using spreadsheets correctly. Follow the tips given in Box 7-2. Take advantage of the built-in calculating capabilities of spreadsheet software, and avoid using a spreadsheet like a word processing document with a table.

As when working with other computer applications, it is important that you first identify the problem you want to solve. Designing a spreadsheet that effectively communicates does not happen by adopting a casual approach. You should carefully design and organize spreadsheets so that they are useful.

When first using spreadsheet software, it is often most efficient to first draft out the design with a pencil and piece of paper. The paper and

---

BOX 7-2 Rules for Creating and Using Spreadsheets

1. Begin the spreadsheet development process with a clear purpose and carefully thought out design.

2. Use data validation tools with input and error messages for cells that might have repeating data.

3. Use conditional formatting tools to create assist users to interpret data.

4. Use charts to assist users to interpret aggregate data.

5. Treat the spreadsheet development as you would treat a major written paper, with footnotes and a bibliography (Ansari & Block, 2008).

6. Use formulas rather than entering precalculated numbers into cells to avoid data entry errors.

7. Check, recheck, and validate each formula and formula output.

8. If you reuse a formula, copy and paste the validated formula and then recheck the results.

9. Write out and analyze complex formulas prior to entering them into cells.

10. Use cell protection to prevent users from inadvertently changing a formula or data.

11. If the spreadsheet is "mission critical," meaning it affects the financial or patient outcome bottom line, there should be explicit guidelines, rules, and testing policies for developers.

12. Be a smart consumer of spreadsheet information. Scrutinize the quality of the spreadsheet data; do not assume that it is correct.

pencil design assists the user to identify parts of the spreadsheet. Use the computer to calculate values from cell data. If you need to sort the data needed for analysis, make sure you enter only one value into each cell. For example, if you need to sort by last name, create separate headers for the first name and the last name. Increase the row height rather than leaving blank rows between data. This tip is particularly important when formulas are with a range of cells.

It is best to use a separate **worksheet** for each table in a **workbook**. If you design a worksheet to include more than one table, make sure that an inserted new row or column does not change or corrupt other parts of the spreadsheet data. Name each spreadsheet to identify the purpose or topic.

While designing a complex spreadsheet or workbook, include a table of contents with hyperlinks to the appropriate sections. Include explanations of any logic or assumptions on the first worksheet. Provide clear labels and instructions that all users will be able to understand. Other users rarely have the same viewpoint as the creator. When using a complex formula, especially one that references the results of other formulas, carefully test the formula with simple numbers. This is particularly important if you will use the spreadsheet with different values.

SPREADSHEETS

A spreadsheet is an electronic version of a table consisting of a grid of rectangles (cells) arranged in columns and rows. You can uniquely format each cell to display numbers, text data, and formulas. Spreadsheet software is similar to word processing tables, but the design of spreadsheets is to crunch numbers and analyze data. Competency in the effective use of spreadsheets is an invaluable skill for nurses and other healthcare providers when assessing quality outcomes. Anytime you need to crunch and analyze numbers, the electronic spreadsheet is the software of choice.

Spreadsheet software, like word processing, is commonly bundled with other office software. Commercial examples include Microsoft Office Excel and Apple iWork Numbers. Numerous free versions are also available such as Apache

OpenOffice Calc and Google Drive Spreadsheets. What is the difference? The integrated office products work together seamlessly with software bundles. Commercial spreadsheet software includes features that may not be available in free versions. Examples include samples of images, print formatting with custom headers and footers, formula wizards, dragging a cell data to copy data to other cells, and tools to expedite creating a series of numbers or words, such as the months of a year or a series of quarters of a year.

If you do not have spreadsheet software on your computer, begin learning with a free version to visualize the features and functions. This chapter has examples from Microsoft Excel 2013 because Excel is the most popular spreadsheet software. However, it includes information on iWork Numbers, Apache OpenOffice Calc, and Google Drive Spreadsheet. Most spreadsheet software is available for Windows and Mac computers, tablets, and smartphones. An exception is iWork Numbers, which is only available for Apple devices.

The Spreadsheet Window

The spreadsheet window is similar in all application programs associated with a graphical user interface (GUI), which uses windows, icons, menus, and a mouse. At first glance, the main difference between a spreadsheet and a word processor seems to be that the document screen in a spreadsheet is only a table. Many of the features used in word processing are the same, such as file and edit. Some important differences, however, are, for instance, formula and chart functions built into the menu options. By default, each spreadsheet file is actually a workbook containing one or more spreadsheets. The tabs at the bottom of each spreadsheet allow the user to provide meaningful names and differentiate between multiple spreadsheets in a workbook.

Spreadsheet Basics

The vocabulary of spreadsheets is simple. A **cell** refers to the rectangles in the table. A row is a horizontal group of cells, and a **column** is a vertical group of cells. The **cell address** is the name given to a cell. It uses the letter of the column and the row where it is located (similar to a street map).

The **active cell**, analogous to the insertion point in other programs, is the location where you enter data. Besides being visible in the table by bold lines, the formula bar, which is located above the letters for columns, mirrors the contents of the active cell. A **cell range** is a group of contiguous cells, for example, B11:D13. To express the range of A2–B3 (Figure 7-1), type A2:B3. The formatting may depend on the spreadsheet application publisher. Users can name ranges of cells and use this name in commands instead of the cell location to create formulas.

Worksheet and workbook are terms that might be confusing initially. The terms worksheet and spreadsheet mean the same. A worksheet refers to one spreadsheet, whereas a workbook consists of one or more worksheets. Workbooks allow the user to have many worksheets open at the same time. Click on the tab name at the bottom of the worksheet to identify it. You can change the order of the sheets, add, or delete sheets from a workbook.

The number of columns and rows allowed in a worksheet varies according to the spreadsheet software publisher and version. For example, the size of a Microsoft 2013 Excel worksheet can be 16,384 columns by 1,048,576 rows (Microsoft, 2014a). In contrast, Apache OpenOffice 3.x Calc allows for 1,024 columns by 65,536 rows with a maximum of 67,108,864 cells per sheet (Apache OpenOffice Wiki, 2008, November 26) and iWork Numbers allows for 255 columns and 65,000 rows (Apple, 2012, August 17). Google Drive Spreadsheets will allow for 256 columns or 400,000 cells with a maximum file size of 20 MB (megabytes) (Google, 2013).

Design the size of a spreadsheet for optimum use. When working on a project, keep the spreadsheet size as small as possible. A worksheet with data in 256 columns may be more manageable if it is broken down into several worksheets. The content of a spreadsheet can include pictures (graphics) and charts. You can create charts (graphs) from data for analysis purposes. You have heard that a "picture is worth a thousand words"; charts can paint an impressive picture to assist in the analysis of complex data.

You can save spreadsheets as template files for reuse. A template provides a pattern of content for software applications. Spreadsheet software

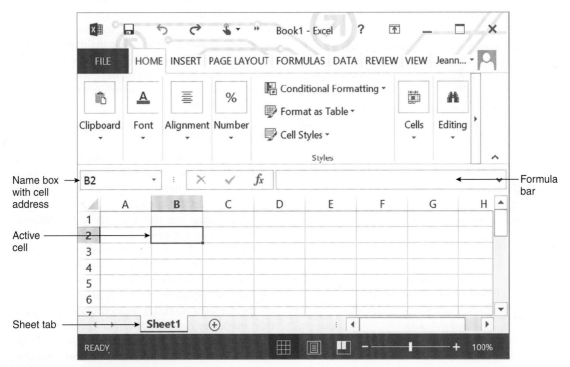

Figure 7-1. Spreadsheet basics.

	A	B	C	D	E
1	Employee #	Hourly Salary	% Raise	Salary Increase	New Salary
2	4567	20	0.03	=B2*C2	=D2+B2
3	7865	22.3	0.03	=B3*C3	=D3+B3
4	9876	21.5	0.03	=B4*C4	=D4+B4
5					

Figure 7-2. Relative formula.

often includes predesigned templates, either with the program or as a download from the associated website. For more information on the use of spreadsheet templates, check the software Help menu.

Spreadsheet Power

The real power of a spreadsheet is from the ability to organize and edit data and from its ability to recalculate when a number in a referenced cell is changed. A referenced cell refers to a formula. For example, in Figure 7-2, the cell E2 contains a formula. It references the cells D2 and B2. Any changes made to the contents of either of these cells will cause the number in cell E2 to change. Notice that the formula is visible in the formula bar.

Formulas

A spreadsheet formula is a mathematical equation that provides instructions to the computer for processing the data. Formulas can be either relative or absolute. When you copy a relative formula to another cell or range of cells, it adjusts to the move by changing the referenced cells (Figure 7-3). An

Values View

	A	B	C	D	E	F
1	Employee #	Hourly Salary	Salary Increase	New Salary		% Raise
2	4567	$20.00	$0.60	$20.60		3%
3	7865	$22.30	$0.67	$22.97		
4	9876	$21.50	$0.65	$22.15		
5						
6						

Formulas View
(Press Ctrl + ` [grave accent])

	A	B	C	D	E	F
1	Employee #	Hourly Salary	Salary Increase	New Salary		% Raise
2	4567	20	=B2*F2	=C2+B2		0.03
3	7865	22.3	=B3*F2	=C3+B3		
4	9876	21.5	=B4*F2	=C4+B4		
5						

Figure 7-3. Absolute formula.

absolute formula uses the dollar sign ($) to signify that it will retain the specific column and/or row cell when moved. For example, in Figure 7-3, $F references column F, $2 references row 2, and F2 references the specific cell address F2.

The equals (=) sign indicates a formula in a cell. Errors can creep into a spreadsheet when entering formulas into cells. Use the point and click method for entering cell addresses to prevent cell address entry errors. After entering the symbol to indicate formula entry, put the mouse pointer on the first cell addressed by the formula and then click with the left mouse button. The cell address will appear in the formula. Enter the necessary mathematical symbol, then point and click the next cell needed. When the formula is complete, tap the enter key. The formulas viewed in Figures 7-2 and 7-3 demonstrate the symbols used to enter the formulas.

An expression refers to the algebraic formula that contains symbols and characters to complete the formula operation. Functions refer to common predesigned formulas used in spreadsheet applications. Both commercial and free spreadsheet software include functions to expedite the accuracy of the formula entry. Arguments are the specific values required by the formula. In computer terms, argument means the data that the user furnishes to calculate the formula value. To view or hide the formula view in the spreadsheet, tap the Ctrl + grave accent mark key (`), which is usually located above the tab key.

Creating Formulas

The principles and symbols of formula calculation are identical in all spreadsheet software. The characters used to communicate that the computer performs a specific calculation, such as multiplying or dividing, are not necessarily the same as used on paper. An asterisk (*) is used to denote multiplication. If you use the familiar x, the computer is unable to distinguish the character "x" from a multiplication symbol. A computer formula for the multiplication of 5 times 50 is 5*50.

The forward slash (/) located under the question mark key denotes division. To use the computer to divide 10 by 5, the formula is 10/5. The results of division are not always a whole number (integer). Excel formats numbers as "general" in decimal format by default. To format a number as an integer (whole number), format the number with zero decimal places. The integer is a rounded number, whereas a decimal provides accuracy to the specified decimal point.

The caret (^) symbol located over the number 6 on the keyboard represents an exponent (raises a number to another power). Calculation of body mass index (BMI) is an example of an exponent used in nursing. The formula for BMI, when using pounds and inches, is to divide the weight in pounds by height in inches squared and multiplied by a conversion factor of 703 (Centers for Disease Control and Prevention, 2011, September 13). For instance, if a person weighed 150 pounds and was 65 inches tall, the formula = ((150/65^2)*703) would result in a BMI of 24.96. As seen in the formula for calculating a BMI, use parentheses to identify and nest calculations. As in all mathematical formulas, the number of leading parentheses must balance the number of trailing ones.

Order of Mathematical Operations

In performing arithmetical computations, computers follow the order of operations for mathematics. Three factors determine the order to perform mathematical procedures:

- The kind of computation required
- Nesting or the placement of an expression within parentheses
- Left-to-right placement of the expressions in the command

The computer performs operations using algebraic protocols in the following order:

- Anything in parentheses first
- Exponentiation next
- Multiplication and division in left-to-right manner
- Addition and subtraction last

All application packages that allow calculations, including spreadsheets, statistical packages, and databases, use the rules. When using the acronym (or mnemonic) given in Table 7-1, remember that when two mathematical operations are equal, such as multiplication and division, the calculations are completed from left to right. There are a number of excellent review sites about the order of mathematical operations. An example is the About.com: Mathematics website at http://math.about.com/library/weekly/aa040502a.htm (Russell, 2013).

Formatting Cells

Spreadsheet software provides a number of ways to format cells. Contents in a spreadsheet cell are of two different types: numbers and text. Depending on what they reference, you can format numbers in different ways. You can also format each cell in a spreadsheet uniquely. The cell default format is the type of data entered.

Format the font or content alignment of a particular cell using Excel or Calc by right-clicking on any cell to view the options (use Format menu in Google Drive Spreadsheet). To format a group of cells, row, or column, highlight the section using the mouse and right-click to use the Format menu. You can use the same technique to merge two or more cells and to change the color or the border of a cell or range of cells.

Spreadsheet software allows for the following formatting: rounded or decimal, financial, scientific (exponents), currency, percent, date, and time. To format a cell data type, right-click on the cell. Excel includes custom formatting for zip codes, telephone numbers, and social security numbers.

A rule of thumb is to use a "number" for anything used in a calculation, for example, added, subtracted, multiplied, or divided. Therefore,

TABLE 7-1	Acronym to Remember the Order in Which Computers Perform Calculations					
Please	Excuse	My		Dear	Aunt	Sally
		Equal (Left to Right)			Equal (Left to Right)	
Parentheses	Exponentiation	Multiplication		Division	Addition	Subtraction

format numbers used for medical record numbers (MRNs), admission numbers, zip codes, social security numbers, and telephone numbers as text.

Since you can use date and time for calculation, format them as numbers. In fact, if you enter a date such as "4/3" (with no parentheses) into a cell, the spreadsheet will automatically display the data as a date defaulting to the current year. To enter a time, enter it using a colon, for example, 4:00 AM or 14:00. If you want to change the way that the date or time is displayed, right-click on the cell(s).

Spreadsheet software will also allow you to enter a date and time into a single cell. These data and time features are very useful in nursing, when calculating a time difference for an event that begins one day and ends the next, for example, the visit time of a patient admitted to the emergency department (ED) on 1/2/2012 at 10:00 PM and discharged at 1:25 AM the next day. When you enter a formula calculating the difference into a cell, the calculation will appear as a number. In the example of ED's length of stay (LOS), the calculation is 0.14236111111. To get the decimal number to display as a time difference, format the cell as short time, meaning only hours and minutes. The reformatted cell will display 3:25.

Conditional formatting is a powerful spreadsheet feature. Conditional formatting allows for a simple, quick analysis of data. For example, if you had a spreadsheet to monitor grades in a program of study, you could use a conditional format to highlight a font or background of a cell for a grade of "D" or "C" in a course. The conditional formatting feature is not case sensitive, meaning that the software will recognize both a "d" and "D" when entered. You can use conditional formatting for numbers and text. Figure 7-4 is an example of the conditional formatting display. You can access the conditional formatting feature from the Home menu in Excel and from the Format menus in Google Drive and OpenOffice Calc.

Text to Columns

Consider this scenario. You created a spreadsheet with the names and addresses for all of the employees on your nursing unit before reading the section "Tips for Better Spreadsheets" in this chapter. The problem is that you included the first name and the last name in a single cell. You are unable to sort

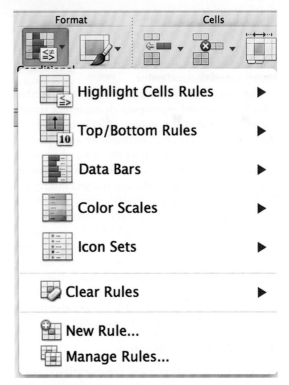

Figure 7-4. Conditional formatting.

the names by last name because you entered the first name before the last name. Is there a solution? Yes, you can use the text to columns feature to separate the names. Simply insert a blank column next to the column that you want to change. If the name includes a middle name of initial, insert two blank columns. In the Excel and Calc menus, select Data > Text to Columns, and follow the wizard to make the changes (possible but not easily done in Google Drive Spreadsheet). The text to columns feature is extremely useful for analyzing data queried and extracted from a hospital information system. Data imported from other information systems may have complex data in column row cells, which need to be in separate row cells for analysis or an import into database software.

Freezing Rows and Columns

When there are more rows or columns in a spreadsheet you can view on a computer screen, it is difficult to know what information is represented. Spreadsheets provide a way to **freeze** either the rows or columns or both. The term "freeze" means that you can keep one part of the spreadsheet visible while scrolling to another area on the spreadsheet. The freezing rows and columns feature is important for accurate data entry when the data refer to a heading in a column or row. To learn how to accomplish this task, use the spreadsheet Help menu. The name of the feature varies slightly according to the publisher but usually refers to "freezing" rows, windows, or panes.

Using Automatic Data Entry

Sometimes, spreadsheet design requires sequential data such as numbering 1 to 10, days of the week, months of the year, or quarters in the year. Excel includes a feature that allows the user to make a few entries and then have the computer complete the series. The feature works with a series of skipped numbers such as 2, 4, and 6. The term for this feature varies according to the spreadsheet software publisher, but usually refers to "fill."

Data Validation

Spreadsheet software includes features to validate data type. Data validation can be as simple as defining a rule for the spreadsheet software to verify that the text entered is the required number, text, or date. You can enter instructions and error messages to guide the user and ensure correct data entry.

Spreadsheet software allows you to create a list to validate data that will appear from a drop-down menu (**combo box**). For example, you can limit data entry for a column heading of gender to two choices, male and female. A quick and easy way to select data using a combo box in Excel 2013 is to right-click on the data field and select "*Pick from Drop-Down List.*" You will find the data validation feature in the spreadsheet data menu.

As you learn new spreadsheet features, you may find that you designed spreadsheets that include repeating data, such as unit names, or state abbreviations but with no data validation. The lack of data validation results in omission of some data when you attempt to sort it. Examples of data with the same meaning but entered differently include *NY, N.Y.,* and *New York.* If you were sorting the data for a column state named New York, you may

overlook the entries with the abbreviations for New York. You can use the Remove Duplicates feature in Excel to create a unique list. Highlight the column with the repeating values and copy that data to another place on the spreadsheet or a new worksheet. With the data still highlighted, select Remove Duplicates from the Data menu. A listing of unique values will appear. Go back to the data validation menu and point to the location of the unique values to use for a validation list. If you are using spreadsheet software without the Remove Duplicates feature, you will have to use the Search and Replace function to make the corrections.

Forms

Some spreadsheet software provides features such as forms to view and enter data. Database features in spreadsheet software may not as robust as a true database, but they are functional for many simple operations. The forms view is not a default menu in some spreadsheet software, such as Excel. However, you can customize the menu to add the feature. Use the Microsoft tutorial at http://support.microsoft.com/kb/291073 for specific directions (Microsoft, 2014b).

The form feature in Google Drive is very different from other spreadsheet software. The Google Drive Spreadsheet form uses data entered in a Google Drive Form to create a spreadsheet. To create the form, click on forms in the Google Drive menu. A wizard guides you to create form questions and answers. Answers can be text, multiple choice, paragraph, list, check boxes, grid, or scale. You can email or share the finalized form. You can use the Google Drive Form for an online quiz or survey. Data entered into the form display as aggregate data on a spreadsheet.

Formatting a Spreadsheet for Use in a Database

You can import spreadsheet, or any range of cells, to most database software for more extensive data manipulation. You can import or export any data structured in a listing format, whether a spreadsheet, a table in a word processor, a statistical package, or database from program to program. A listing format contains only column headings and the associated data.

Linking Cells and Worksheets from Other Sources

There are times when you want to reference (link) to a cell or a cell range in a spreadsheet located in another workbook. Use of an **external reference** to the workbook is prone to less error than trying to check the other sheet, copy the value(s), and enter it into a formula. Values changed in a linked cell change the referenced cell in another workbook. You can link entire spreadsheet tables in Microsoft Word for Windows; however, the feature is not available in Microsoft Office for the Mac, Google Drive, or OpenOffice.

This feature is easy to use and is a very powerful tool to ensure data consistency using Microsoft Word and Excel for computers with the Windows operating system. A quick way to use the linking feature is to highlight and copy the table data in Excel, navigate to the place in the Word document where you want to display the data, then right-click and select one of the two options for linking (icon with a link). One of the link icons maintains the spreadsheet source formatting and the other uses the destination formatting style. When you change values in the linked Excel document, the change displays dynamically in Word. Use the spreadsheet Help menu for more information on this feature.

Data Protection and Security

In healthcare, we often use spreadsheets to provide data protection and/or security. Data protection refers to locking cells to prevent the user from changing the cell value. This feature is very helpful to prevent accidental changes to cell text, numbers, or formulas. Security means that the user has to provide a password(s) to view and/or to edit the spreadsheet. Do not use free online spreadsheets such as Google Drive Spreadsheet to store confidential data since the spreadsheets are stored online in a public domain. Use spreadsheets to enter confidential data only if there is a way to provide security. Only password-protected or password-encrypted spreadsheets should be stored on public domains such as the shared healthcare agency or educational agency–shared server. Check with your Health Insurance Portability and Accountability Act (HIPAA) security official if you have any questions about the security of your file(s).

CHARTS

A chart (graph), terminology used in spreadsheet software, is a graphical presentation of a set of numbers. Charts provide a means to interpret the relationships of quantitative and categorical data in a table (Few, 2007). Use charts to communicate meaning visually that is difficult to understand from a raw set of numbers. Research shows the viewer's expertise and understanding of the purposes of the different chart formats affect the ability to interpret charts (Ancker et al., 2006). Avoid designing charts with distracting designs, fonts, and lines.

It is easy to create charts using a spreadsheet software. A computer can create any type of chart, whether or not it communicates anything meaningful. Using charts appropriately involves knowing the message you need to communicate and selecting the type of chart that best accomplishes the goal accurately and efficiently (Few, 2004a, September 4). Although other software packages facilitate the creation of charts, spreadsheets have the most powerful chart creation tools. Perhaps the biggest plus for creating charts in a spreadsheet is that if the numbers in the cells used to create the chart change, the chart automatically reflects the change.

Chart Basics

To construct a meaningful chart, it is necessary to understand the chart basics vocabulary. Table 7-2 includes chart terminology and the meaning. It is important to use the types of charts appropriately. The chart should assist the viewer to understand data, but not ever distort the meaning of data.

Types of Charts

Spreadsheets take the drudgery out of creating charts. There are options for creating many different types of charts, including making them three dimensional, changing the orientation for the horizontal (x) axis to that of a vertical (y) axis

TABLE 7-2 Chart Basics

Term	Meaning
x-axis	The horizontal axis (line) of a bar, line, or scatter graph, generally represents time values, categories, or division
y-axis	The vertical axis (line) of a bar, line, or scatter graph, most often used to represent amounts
Data	Numbers without meaning; those that are unprocessed
Data series or set	A set of numbers represented in the chart, usually on *y*-axis, or a group of items represented on *x*-axis
Axis title	The title for the information displayed on an axis
Chart title	A description of the graph used to title the chart
Legend	The visual representation of each item in the data series. Maybe a color, shape, or both
Data point	The plot point of a number. It is the intersection of its value on the *x*- and *y*-axes.
Data labels	Labels that show the actual value of specific data or the data points
Two-dimensional chart	A chart that represents data on the *x*- and *y*-axes
Three-dimensional chart	A chart that adds a third axis, referred to as the *z*-axis. Can be very misleading, use only when there is need to communicate an added dimension.

position, and combinations of all these factors. Each of these features can emphasize objects in the chart that may misconstrue the true meaning of the base numbers. Compare the two- and three-dimensional charts in Figure 7-5. Which figure most accurately depicts the data? You can use most of the variations in all charts. When using variations, be certain that they reflect the point you want to communicate. As a user of charts, be aware that these distortions exist. Although spreadsheet software provides many different chart types including pie, column, bar, line, combination, stock, surface, doughnut, bubble, surface, radar, and sparklines, this section will focus on the four main types of charts: pie chart, column chart, bar chart, line chart, and sparklines.

Pie Charts

Use **pie charts**, classified as **area charts**, to communicate the proportion of various items in relation to the whole. They are "part-to-whole" charts designed to show percentages, not amounts. A pie chart uses only one data series. You can also use a pie chart to show a proportional relationship between a slice and a whole. To communicate percentages clearly, use seven or less sectors (Microsoft, 2014c). Color and shading of the pie sectors should emphasize the chart message.

	January	February	March
# Falls	10	8	7
# Falls in Compliance	7	7	7

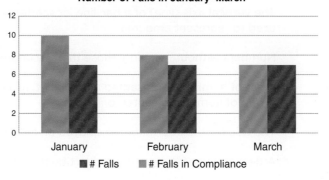

2-Dimensional Chart
Number of Falls in January–March

■ # Falls   ■ # Falls in Compliance

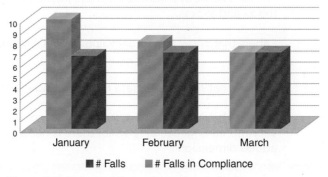

3-Dimensional Chart
Number of Falls in January–March

■ # Falls   ■ # Falls in Compliance

Figure 7-5. Two- and three-dimensional charts.

Figure 7-6 illustrates different types of pie charts. All of the pie charts represent the same data, for example, percentage of patient falls by shift. Notice how the exploded view chart looks larger than the three-dimensional and simple pie views. The explosion view can distort the viewer's perception of the data. Without the percent values, it is difficult to determine which slice is largest in both the exploded wedge and the three-dimensional pie. Few (2007), a well-known expert on information design, advises us to refrain from using pie charts, because our visual perception does not allow us to easily perceive the quantitative differences in the slices of the pie. However, some experts disagree with Few's view about the use of pie charts (Clark,

2007, January 14; Gabrielle, 2013, March 18). If you believe that a pie chart does best depict your data, be sure to limit the number of slices and include percentages as labels.

Column and Bar Charts
Use **column charts** to depict to show comparisons when using rows and columns to organize table data (Microsoft, 2014c). Place values on the vertical y-axis to depict changes in amounts. Use the horizontal x-axis to depict categories. If the category is time, such as quarters, place the earliest time on the left and time elapses to the right. To prevent a distortion of value, it is best if the longitudinal y-axis starts with a zero. If the y-axis

Shift	# Falls
Day	12
Night	30

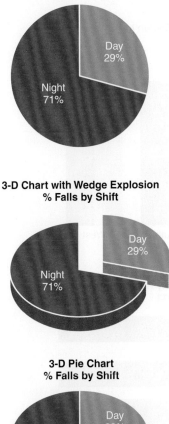

Simple Pie Chart
% Falls by Shift

3-D Chart with Wedge Explosion
% Falls by Shift

3-D Pie Chart
% Falls by Shift

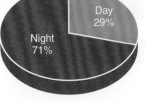

Figure 7-6. Pie charts.

does not start with a zero, include an explanation in the chart.

Bar charts are generally associated with comparisons of amounts. You can display data in a bar chart either vertically or horizontally. A clustered bar chart provides a visual comparison of amounts for a given time period, such as a month or quarter. Figure 7-7 depicts several types of bar charts that compare the percentage of all smokers, using

2-year intervals between 1997 and 2008. The simple bar chart compares smoking habit changes for all smokers. The clustered bar chart compares the percentage of smokers, aged 18 and older by income. It is clear that while the percentage of smokers decreased over the 12-year period, the percentages of persons in the poor and near-poor income continue to be higher than nonpoor.

The classification of a stacked bar chart, like the pie chart, is a part-to-whole chart. Percentage is usually the unit of measurement. In a **stacked chart**, each data set uses as its baseline the previous data set. For a 100% stacked chart, each data set is a percentage of the whole. You can use stacked bar charts to compare differences in groups of clustered data. However, a stacked chart is more difficult to understand than a simple bar chart or clustered bar chart.

When displaying column and bar charts in color, use bright and darker colors to emphasize key data. When possible, avoid the use of Fill patterns, as they can distract from the data. If all of the bars are bright and/or dark, the message will be confusing (Few, 2004b).

Line Charts

There are two types of **line charts**, one that communicates changes in elapsed time period data and one that shows data trends. Place the category data on the horizontal axis and the data values on the vertical axis. When communicating changes in data over time, use lines to connect individual data points. Figure 7-8 shows a line chart comparison of same smoking data used for the bar charts. When comparing more than one data set, consider using line colors or point markers to show differences in the data.

A chart with a trendline can be used for two-dimensional line or unstacked bar or column charts. A trendline can be straight or curved. For example, a straight trendline shows a linear regression whereas a curved might show a bell curve. The default trendline in Excel is linear regression. To learn more about trendlines in Excel, tap the F1 key for Help and type "trendline."

Sparklines

Sparklines are "simple, word-sized" graphics first described by Tufte (2013), a renowned American statistician and professor. Sparklines are a new chart feature introduced with Excel 2010. It is available as a free add-in for earlier versions of

	2010	2011
Northwest	17.4%	17.3%
Midwest	21.8%	21.8%
South	21.0%	20.7%
West	15.9%	15.0%

Year	Percent
2010	19.3%
2011	19%

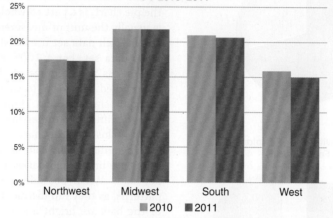

Bar Chart
Comparison of Smokers by Region in US
FY 2010–2011

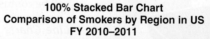

100% Stacked Bar Chart
Comparison of Smokers by Region in US
FY 2010–2011

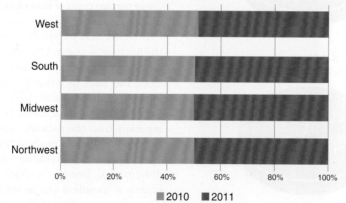

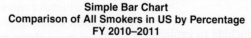

Simple Bar Chart
Comparison of All Smokers in US by Percentage
FY 2010–2011

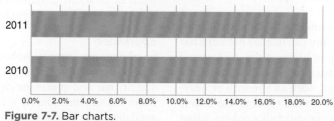

Figure 7-7. Bar charts.

	Males	Females
1970	26.40%	21.60%
1980	27.50%	24.10%
1990	24.20%	21.60%
2000	24.60%	21.90%
2009	24.60%	21.00%

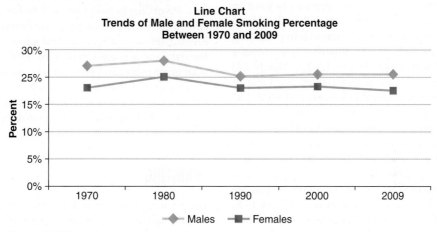

Figure 7-8. Line charts.

Excel from http://sparklines-excel.blogspot.com/. Sparklines show comparisons of data from individual data criteria in a single cell. Figure 7-9 is an example of sparkline depicting glucose value variances for a hypothetical patient on an insulin drip. In other words, you could view data trends using a single spreadsheet cell. You can use sparklines with data in the electronic medical record (EMR) to display variances visually in laboratory or vital signs. Like other standard chart features, you can add markers to depict specific periods.

the chart tool and select the types of chart that will best represent those data. Excel provides chart suggestions and a preview of how the chart will look before making the final selection. If you do not like the chart, delete it and begin again. Both commercial and free spreadsheet software provide a way to create and edit the chart title and legends. Spreadsheet software includes the ability to modify fonts and colors used in the chart. Once you have clicked on the icon to indicate that you have finished, the chart appears on the spreadsheet. You can always resize, move, or edit a completed chart. To edit the chart, right-click the object you want to change to obtain a drop-down menu of choices.

QSEN Scenario

You are designing a spreadsheet with a chart for the ICU nurses to show progress on preventing ventilator-acquired pneumonia over the last 12 months. What type(s) of chart should you use? Why?

Creating the Chart

Computer application programs allow the creation of many types of charts. The first task in creating any chart is to select the cells that represent the data. After selecting the appropriate cells, click on

Time	Glucose Value	
1/5/2016 13:45	98	
1/6/2016 13:00	128	
1/7/2016 13:45	151	
1/8/2016 14:00	132	
1/9/2016 13:45	126	
1/10/2016 13:30	100	

Figure 7-9. Sparkline example.

Dashboards

Dashboards provide a snapshot of trends from multiple data resources. A dashboard is simply a worksheet with multiple charts depicting the data located in a table. Both Excel and Google Drive Spreadsheet provide a way to display dashboards. A dashboard, similar to the control panel instruments used to drive a car, allows the user to visualize data from multiple sources to guide decision-making. Creating an executive-looking dashboard may require advanced Excel skills. Moore (2013, March 14) designed an easy-to-read tutorial on the topic at http://sites.psu.edu/nikkemoore/2013/03/14/creating-an-interactive-excel-dashboard/.

You can create a dashboard using Google Drive Spreadsheet from the chart menu. Unlike Excel, Google Drive Spreadsheet allows you to create a "gauge" using spreadsheet data. The gauge has a default range of 0 to 100. If, for example, you are monitoring compliance of a process or procedure to achieve 100%, consider using a gauge chart. The chart type reflects data similar to that of a car speedometer.

Pivot Tables and Pivot Charts

The term pivot tables is a good description of the function. Use a pivot table to change the data to view data in an aggregated format. It is an interactive view of aggregate data that allows the user to analyze the numerical data in different views. It is especially useful to analyze very large data sets. For example, you could analyze numbers of infections by nursing unit, and then drill down to infection types.

Data for pivot tables must be in the list formatting, which means that the data are organized using only column headings, which is not the standard way to display data in Excel. To create a Pivot Chart in Excel 2013, choose Pivot Chart from the Insert menu (Recommended PivotTables). If you are using another spreadsheet software, use the Help menu for instructions. You may find the tutorial designed by French (2012, June 1) at http://spreadsheets.about.com/b/2012/06/01/excel-2007-pivot-table-tutorial-2.htm helpful to learn this powerful data analysis tool.

Excel 2010 introduced two new pivot table features, Slicer and PowerPivot. Slicer is an enhanced pivot table filter. PowerPivot is a free add-in that you can download to use with Excel. It allows for integration of data from multiple sources and improved manipulation of very large data sets. To learn more about Excel features, including PowerPivot and Slicer, go to http://www.dummies.com/how-to/computers-software/ms-office/Excel/Excel-2013/Pivot-Tables.html.

PivotCharts are charts generated from data sets. PivotCharts look identical to bar charts discussed earlier in this chapter. The difference is that PivotCharts are interactive and allow you to filter the data and analyze differences. To develop skills with pivot tables and pivot charts, consider downloading one of the many data sets available from the Health Resources and Services Administration (HRSA) at http://www.hrsa.gov/data-statistics/report-downloads/index.html.

PRINTING

The printing function in Excel provides a number of alternatives. In Excel, if the printout is in multiple pages and there are columns and row headers, set up the pages to print both on every page using Page Layout > Print Titles (Format > Print Ranges in Calc). You can create page headers and footers from the Page Setup menu. Use print preview to set up and view the printout, especially if you are printing a large data set. Excel, OpenOffice Calc, and Google Drive Spreadsheet allow you to print out a single spreadsheet or the entire workbook.

The Google Drive Spreadsheet print function is slightly different. You can print Google Drive Spreadsheets only to PDF or HTML file formats. To learn more about the print function in Google Drive, use the Help menu.

LEARNING NEW SPREADSHEET SKILLS

Like other office software, learning new spreadsheet skills is a lifelong journey. Although there are few changes in the basic functionality of spreadsheet software, emerging vendors and new versions of software provide novel features for data manipulation, analysis, and display. Features in Microsoft Excel, OpenOffice Calc, and Google Drive Sheet are useful for nurses assessing quality outcomes.

BOX 7-3   Spreadsheet Skills

Basic Spreadsheet Skills
- Design a simple table.
- Name a worksheet tab.
- Apply a template.
- Insert a new worksheet.
- Create a simple formula (add, subtract, multiply, divide).
- Use basic functions (SUM, AVG, MIN, MAX, COUNT).
- Resize columns and rows to display data.
- Sort cell data.
- Use search and replace.
- Freeze rows and columns.
- Use automatic data entry.
- Use spell-check.
- Use a chart.
- Save a workbook.
- Print a worksheet.

Intermediate Spreadsheet Skills
- Customize the spreadsheet menu.
- Design spreadsheets using data validation features.
- Customize spreadsheets using conditional formatting features.
- Use simple data analysis tools.
- Create/modify a chart.

- Import/export data in text format.
- Link spreadsheet data from other sources.
- Apply principles of effective spreadsheet design.
- Create complex formulas.
- Create/modify a pivot table.
- Create a form.
- Create a report.
- Link and embed tables into word processing documents.
- Use data protection.
- Password protect a workbook.
- Demonstrate competency using two spreadsheet applications.
- Share/collaborate with others on a spreadsheet design.

Advanced Spreadsheet Skills
- Create formulas that use logical and statistical operations.
- Use advanced data analysis tools.
- Create a dashboard.
- Create a new template.
- Create macros.
- Create new functions using Visual Basic expressions.
- Demonstrate competency using more than two spreadsheet applications.

Spreadsheet skills range from beginner to advanced (Box 7-3). If you are a novice, begin working with a single solution software. Both OpenOffice Calc and Google Drive Sheet are free and serve as excellent tools for users who do not have Microsoft Excel. If you have intermediate or expert skills, learn to use spreadsheets from more than one vendor and mentor and share what you know with others. Capitalize on the advantage of using formulas for crunching data.

There are many resources to use when developing new competencies. The purpose of this chapter was to provide an overview of spreadsheet features useful in the nursing setting. There are free online tutorials, many of which include videos available. Some examples are as follows:

- Microsoft Training (http://office.microsoft.com/en-us/training/)
- Google Drive Support (https://support.google.com/drive/topic/2811739?hl=en&ref_topic=2799627)
- Goodwill Community Foundation International LearnFree.org (http://www.gcflearnfree.org/office)

■ HP Learning Center (http://h10120.www1.hp.com/expertone/whats_learning_center.html)

If you have Microsoft Excel 2013 and a Microsoft log-in and password, you can download an app for the Excel menu with video tutorials. To learn more, go to http://office.microsoft.com/en-us/templates/excel-video-tutorials-app-TC104116147.aspx. After you finish downloading the tutorial, it will appear in the Insert menu > Apps for Office > Excel Video Tutorials.

SUMMARY

Spreadsheet programs have taken much of the drudgery out of calculations. Spreadsheets deserve a place on every nurse's desktop. In order to make a difference in improving care quality outcomes, nurses should all demonstrate essential spreadsheet competencies (see Box 7-1). Spreadsheets have much in common with other office application programs including word processing, presentation software, and database software. The basic structure in a spreadsheet is a table, with a column of numbers on the left side and a row of letters at the top. The letters and numbers provide a way for each cell to have a corresponding name. The principles and symbols for formula calculation are the same as all other computer programs.

Although spreadsheet software can make managing numbers easier, poorly designed spreadsheets create a great amount of misinformation. Users should use spreadsheets to perform calculations from data. Scrutinize formulas for accuracy to avoid misinterpretation of data. As with all computer use, nurses should use common sense when interpreting computer numerical and chart outputs; this includes understanding the assumptions that various models use. Given thoughtful use, spreadsheet software that calculates numbers can assist all healthcare professionals in managing information. Data protection and security features are especially important in healthcare. Users should be knowledgeable about how to protect cell data and formulas from inadvertent changes. Users should also know how to password protect confidential spreadsheet information.

Spreadsheet competencies and skills are valuable assets for all nurses.

APPLICATIONS AND COMPETENCIES

1. Identify at least three differences between a word processor table and a spreadsheet.

2. Use spreadsheet software to calculate a baby's gestational age at the time of the mother's prenatal visit. Copy the column headers and dates below into cells A1:B5. Type the formula in C2 and then copy the formula to cells C3:C5.

	A	B	C
1	Prenatal Checkup Date	Baby's Due Date	Baby's Gestational Age (Weeks)
2	1/1/2015	9/1/2015	=((B2–A2)/7)
3	9/2/2015	2/20/2016	
4	4/1/2014	9/1/2014	
5	1/20/2016	2/20/2016	

3. Calculate the BMI using the data in the table below. Copy the column headers and data below into cells A1:B4. Type the formula in C2 and then copy the formula to cells C3:C4. Format the BMI to one decimal point.

	A	B	C
1	Weight (pounds)	Height (inches)	BMI
2	110	67	=((A2/B2^2)*703)
3	150	60	
4	200	70	

4. Calculate the ages of patients on admission to your nursing unit. Copy the data from the table below onto a spreadsheet. Format the cells C2:C4 as YY. Type the formula in C2 and then copy the formula to cells C3:C4. Type the formula noted in cell C5 to determine the average age of the patients.

	A	B	C
1	Admission Date	Birth Date	Age (Years)
2	9/16/2014	11/10/1985	=(A2–B2)/365
3	4/5/2015	11/17/1971	
4	4/27/2016	4/27/1950	
5			= AVERAGE (C2:C4)

5. You recently implemented a new intervention to prevent patient falls. Copy the data noted below on a spreadsheet. Use the Fill feature to create columns with the months of the year. Design a chart to show the changes in the number of falls. Use the Help feature when necessary.

	January	February	Mar	April	May	June
Number of Falls	25	31	35	10	12	30

6. You want to show the percentage of all visits to your ED during each shift. For the month of May, you had 600 visits on the day shift, 1,000 visits on the evening shift, and 400 visits on the night shift. Design a chart depicting the data.

7. You want to show the changes in the number of pounds gained each month of pregnancy from month 3 to month 5. You have the average number of pounds gained in each month (2 pounds in month 3, 5 pounds in month 5) for 300 pregnant women. Design a chart to show the changes over time.

8. Reflect on information from this chapter, the literature, and your experiences using spreadsheet software. Discuss how errors might be mitigated using spreadsheet software.

REFERENCES

Ancker, J. S., Senathirajah, Y., Kukafka, R., et al. (2006). Design features of graphs in health risk communication: A systematic review. *Journal of the American Medical Informatics Association, 13*(6), 608–618. doi: 10.1197/jamia.M2115.

Ansari, S., & Block, R. (2008, May 14). Spreadsheet *"worst practices."* Retrieved from http://ww2.cfo.com/technology/2008/05/spreadsheet-worst-practices/

Apache OpenOffice Wiki. (2008, November 26). *What's the maximum number of rows and cells for a spreadsheet file?* Retrieved from https://wiki.openoffice.org/wiki/Documentation/FAQ/Calc/Miscellaneous/What%27s_the_maximum_number_of_rows_and_cells_for_a_spreadsheet_file%3F

Apple. (2012, August 17). *HT3779 file too large.* Retrieved from https://discussions.apple.com/message/19305170#19305170

Centers for Disease Control and Prevention. (2011, September 13). *About BMI for adults.* Retrieved from http://www.cdc.gov/healthyweight/assessing/bmi/adult_bmi/index.html

Clark, J. (2007, January 14). *In defense of pie charts.* Retrieved from http://www.neoformix.com/2007/InDefenseOfPieCharts.html

European Spreadsheet Risks Interest Group. (2013). *EuSpRIG original horror stories.* Retrieved from http://www.eusprig.org/horror-stories.htm

Few, S. (2004a). Common mistakes in data presentation. *Perceptual Edge.* Retrieved from http://www.perceptualedge.com/articles/ie/data_presentation.pdf

Few, S. (2004b). Elegance through simplicity. *Intelligent Enterprise, 7*(15), 35. Retrieved from http://www.informationweek.com/software/information-management/elegance-through-simplicity/d/d-id/1027686?

Few, S. (2007). *Save the pies for dessert.* Retrieved from http://www.perceptualedge.com/articles/08-21-07.pdf

French, T. (2012, June 1). *Excel pivot table tutorial.* Retrieved from http://spreadsheets.about.com/b/2012/06/01/excel-2007-pivot-table-tutorial-2.htm

Gabrielle, B. (2013). *Why Tufte is flat-out wrong about pie charts.* Retrieved from http://speakingppt.com/2013/03/18/why-tufte-is-flat-out-wrong-about-pie-charts/

Google. (2013). *Google drive spreadsheet, sheets, and slides size limits.* Retrieved from https://support.google.com/drive/answer/37603

Mattessich, R. (n.d.). *Spreadsheet: Its first computerization (1961–1964).* Retrieved from http://www.j-walk.com/ss/history/spreadsh.htm

Microsoft. (2014a). *Excel specifications and limits.* Retrieved from http://office.microsoft.com/en-us/excel-help/excel-specifications-and-limits-HA103980614.aspx

Microsoft. (2014b). *How to use the forms control on a workbook in Excel.* Retrieved from http://support.microsoft.com/kb/291073

Microsoft. (2014c). *Available chart types.* Retrieved from http://office.microsoft.com/en-us/excel-help/available-chart-types-HA102809710.aspx

Moore, N. (2013, March 14). *Creating an interactive Excel dashboard.* Retrieved from http://sites.psu.edu/nikkemoore/2013/03/14/creating-an-interactive-excel-dashboard/

Panko, R. (2008, May). *What we know about spreadsheet errors.* Retrieved from http://panko.shidler.hawaii.edu/SSR/Mypapers/whatknow.htm

Russell, D. (2013). *Order of operations.* Retrieved from http://math.about.com/library/weekly/aa040502a.htm

Tufte, E. (2013, November). *Sparkline theory and practice.* Retrieved from http://www.edwardtufte.com/bboard/q-and-a-fetch-msg?msg_id=0001OR&topic_id=1

CHAPTER 8

Databases: Creating Information From Data

OBJECTIVES

After studying this chapter, you will be able to:

1. Explain the role of databases for improving patient care outcomes.
2. Describe the process for creating a simple database to assess patient care outcomes.
3. Differentiate methods of viewing data in a database.
4. Use Boolean tools to search a database.
5. Describe methods of discovering knowledge in both relational and large databases.

KEY TERMS

Atomic level

Attribute

Boolean logic

Data

Database

Database Management System (DBMS)

Database model

Data mining

Data warehouse

Entity

Field

Flat database

Foreign key

Form

Hierarchical database

Lookup table

Network model

Normalization

One-to-many relationship

Parameter query

Parent–child relationship

Primary key

Query

Record

Relational database

Report

Scope creep

Structured Query Language (SQL)

Table

D oes hospitalization of patients whose diabetes is newly diagnosed prevent future hospitalizations for diabetic complications? Do certain approaches to pain management shorten hospital stays? Is the incidence of preventable illnesses lower in children whose mothers received postpartum visits from a nurse? The literature can provide some answers to these questions, but true evidence-based practice requires clinical **data**. The clinical data that could be used in conjunction with the literature to answer these questions are recorded, but are very infrequently used to answer these questions.

This chapter provides a brief overview of **database** concepts and the associated terminology. It includes types of software available for the personal computer that you can use to create a database. The chapter also covers concepts common to all databases including web-based databases and those used in education and healthcare settings, including the electronic medical record. Although someone taking a course on database design might need an in-depth book on that topic, a novice should be able to create a simple database by applying the concepts found in this chapter. Nurses can use knowledge of database concepts to direct others with design expertise to create or modify a complex database, such as a clinical information system. The Access database used as an example in this chapter is available at http://thepoint.lww.com/sewell5e.

USES OF DATABASES IN NURSING

As nurses, we want to improve patient care outcomes. In the past, we used our experience and experts to help us. The world in which we live, learn, and work is increasingly using digital databases to search, retrieve, organize, and analyze information. Nurses use a variety of digital databases to access data for nursing education and practice. Examples of databases we commonly use include Web search engines, library databases (as discussed in Chapter 10), the electronic patient record, as well as an assortment of others in the education and healthcare settings.

The electronic patient record allows us to use patient documentation data. Although a paper medical record provides a wonderful individualized record for one patient, the lack of data structure makes it difficult to retrieve the data. Therefore, comparisons with similar patients are difficult. As a result, we are not aware of the richness that lies embedded in patient care data.

The electronic patient record, however, changes this equation. With electronic records, we can retrieve data that will provide answers to the questions at the beginning of this chapter and many others. When we gain an understanding of how a database works and how to manipulate data, we have a way to explore patient care outcomes. This chapter provides a beginning view of the principles behind storing, retrieving, and manipulating data that could be used to create knowledge from data in an electronic record. Experimenting with and expanding on these ideas in a real database will further your ability to employ evidence-based care.

In nursing education, students often use databases to track their clinical requirements, such as immunizations or cardiopulmonary resuscitation certifications. Nursing students may also use databases to create e-portfolios with examples of learning and/or technical competencies. Databases may be used to schedule clinical lab experiences.

In the healthcare setting, nurse educators may use databases to track licensure and clinical competencies. They may also be used for scheduling nursing unit staffing. In nursing administration, databases may be used to track patient adverse events, such as falls, Code Blue events, and pressure ulcers. In risk management, databases are used to track incident reports for medication errors and other risk incidents.

Data access is included as an essential competency for all beginning nurses in the American Nurses Association Nursing Informatics: Scope and Standards of Practice (American Nurses Association, 2015). Entry level staff nurses should be able to use database software proficiently. Skills for use of information management tools for monitoring care processes are identified as essential by the QSEN Institute (2014) for prelicensure nurses. However, once a nurse has some proficiency with practice, there may be opportunities to assist in the design of databases for clinical practice settings. Certainly, master's- and doctoral-prepared nurses should have essential competencies in data management (American Association of Colleges of Nursing, 2006, 2008, 2011; QSEN Institute, 2014). In all cases that require the use of databases, it is very important for nurses to understand how the databases work.

ANATOMY OF DATABASES

Let's review the overall anatomy of a database. A database is a collection of related objects: tables, forms, queries, and reports. Queries, forms, and reports are abstractions of data from tables. This makes it possible to use a piece of data many times, even though it has only been entered once. This concept also underlies healthcare information systems, although their data storage is more complex.

Tables

Tables contain all of the data. Each table contains records located in rows with unique data. Table data serve as a foundation for the database. Each table in a database has a particular relationship to another table in that database. The table has field names (column names) for the records. Each field name has attributes that instruct the database about the type of datum. For example, a field attribute may be a date, time, currency, number, or text. Database software uses strict rules to manipulate the data correctly. Because a form is based upon a table or query, the tables must be designed first and include at least some sample data.

Queries

A **query** is used to ask questions of one or more related tables or other queries. The output of a query looks identical to a table, but it provides a custom view of the data. Queries are one of the characteristics that make databases powerful. The ability to create information from the data in a database is limited only by the ingenuity of the query creator. Because querying is such a powerful and important tool in all electronic databases, not just relational ones, we will look at searching, which is a type of querying.

With the progression from paper to electronic library catalogs as well as Web search tools, most of us have had experience with some type of database searching. You have probably searched the Web for something or needed references on a specific subject and used an electronic bibliographic catalog to find them. When you entered keywords for a search, you created a query, or a set of conditions that the located records should meet. When you clicked the Search button, the search tool looked for references that met the criteria you stated in the query.

Boolean Logic Querying

When searching in any database, you use **Boolean logic**, which is named after the 19th-century mathematician George Boole (School of Mathematics and Statistics, 2004). It is a form of algebra in which matches are either true or false. That is, the data in the field either match or not. There are three concepts that make up Boolean logic: "AND," "OR," and "NOT." "AND" searches require that all specified terms be returned. If you specify both database AND healthcare (Fig. 8-1), you are using the Boolean "AND" to narrow the search. If you use the Boolean "OR," all records with both terms, but also those in which only one term appears, will be returned. If you want to exclude a return, such as veterinary from healthcare, use the Boolean "NOT."

Record Requirements

There are record requirements for database searches. The data should be organized by categories, which is a structured format. The field names of a table identify the structure format. A field name may be a date indicating that all records for that field name should display a date. If you have filled out a form online that asks for demographic data, you may have noticed that each piece of data you enter is stored in a field with the associated label. Another record requirement is that there must be a field for the data. For example, if you are searching for a birth date, there has to be an associated field for birth date in the database. Finally, the database terminology must be standardized for successful searches. For example, if you are searching for a patient who is taking aspirin and the data are entered as "aspirin," your search will be unsuccessful if you enter the search term "ASA."

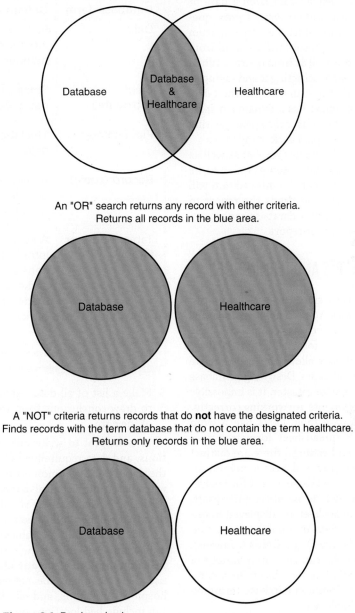

An "AND" search returns only records in which **both** criteria are met.
Returns only records in the blue area.

Database

Database
&
Healthcare

Healthcare

An "OR" search returns any record with either criteria.
Returns all records in the blue area.

Database

Healthcare

A "NOT" criteria returns records that do **not** have the designated criteria.
Finds records with the term database that do not contain the term healthcare.
Returns only records in the blue area.

Database

Healthcare

Figure 8-1. Boolean logic.

Forms

Forms are used to add, edit, and view data from a table or query. Although stored in a table, data entry is not confined to the table view. You can enter data from a form view that shows all the fields related to that record for which data must be entered, regardless of the base table in which the data are stored. Forms are not only useful for data entry, but you can use them to view or print data.

Reports

A **report** is used to display data from a data or query. A database can contain many forms, queries, and reports, all of which are derived from table data. Reports can present information from more than one table as well as from queries. When you run a report after constructing it and saving it, it displays all data that are currently in the table. In other words, the report has a dynamic display of the most recent data. Thus, time spent creating a well-designed report is paid back many times.

Reports may include charts (graphs) as well as permit calculations on data. Reports should be designed in such a way that the information will be easy for the person who needs the report to understand. The design of a database report can replicate the look of a paper report.

DATABASE CONCEPTS AND TERMINOLOGY

You should master basic spreadsheet skills prior to working with databases. You can apply many of the spreadsheet functions, such as formula construction, sorting, and data formatting, to database design. Database software allows the user to relate data located in different tables. Designing a database without data is a recipe for disaster. It is impossible to see that the components are working correctly.

Although a database table looks like a word processing table or spreadsheet formatted as a list with only column headings, there are distinct differences. Whereas a spreadsheet is helpful for crunching numbers, a database is best for analyzing data that may include numbers (Microsoft, 2014). Data in a spreadsheet are displayed in different cells, whereas data in a database are connected with **records** (rows) and **fields** (columns). Spreadsheet workbooks can contain a variety of unrelated worksheets, but the objects in a database are all related. Common database terminology is displayed in Table 8-1.

There are three important steps in the database design process:

1. Identify the purpose of the database. Consider what data will be included as well as data that will be excluded.
2. Identify the questions or queries that aggregated data can answer.

TABLE 8-1   **Database Phenomena**

Database Term	Definition
Data	Facts without meaning, for example the number 37
Field (**attribute**)	Smallest structure in a database
Field name	The label applied to a field
Record (tuple)	All the information about a single "member" of a table
Table (**entity** or file)	A collection of related information. A table consists of records, and each record is made up of a number of fields

Note: Words in parentheses are the names that database professionals use for these items.

3. Make a list of all data requirements necessary to draw conclusions from the questions asked of the data.

It is helpful to write out the purpose, questions, and data requirements before constructing the database. A common error that novices make when designing a clinical database is to replicate a paper form. The database should contain only the data that will be aggregated for analysis.

The relationship of tables in a database is important. You will see the terms "**one-to-many relationship**" and "**parent-child relationship**" used. For example, one patient can have many hospital admissions, and one hospital admission can include bed locations on many nursing units. Each record (row) of the data table uses a unique key to identify the location. Each table is identified with a primary key. The **primary key** is represented in the related table as a **foreign key** to link related tables. There is a foreign key in the "many" or "child" table relating the data with the "one" or "parent" table.

Use of consistent terminology (naming conventions) is required for efficient database design. This applies to column headings and names of tables, forms, queries, and reports. Consistent terminology also applies to primary and foreign keys. For example, the medical record number (MRN) is the primary key of a patient table and is represented as the foreign key in the admission table. If the term MRN is used for the patient table's primary key, MRN, not MR#, should be used for the foreign key in the admission table.

Databases use normalization rules to organize, aggregate, and display data (Chapple, 2014). Each table represents a category of data, and each field should be unique to the database. For example, the patient's name is located in the patient table but in no other table. The primary and foreign keys allow the name to be associated with the data in related tables.

Learning the correct database design method is essential to maximize productivity and success. It is important to understand how to best design the database for efficient analysis, how to use the built-in powerful query functions, and how to display analyzed data with reports and charts.

DATABASE MODELS

The term "**database model**" refers to the way data is organized. Several models exist: flat, hierarchical, network, relational, and object oriented. Each has advantages and disadvantages. The choice for which model to use is the tasks that the database must perform. Today, most business and personal computer databases use the relational database model.

Flat Database

A **flat database** has all of the data located in one table. A spreadsheet worksheet is the simplest flat database model. The address book in a word processor is another example of a flat database. Flat databases are very simple to construct and use, but they have limitations when it comes to tracking items that belong in a record when there are more than one of the same item. For example, if you wanted to track the infections that occurred in a unit using a flat database, you would need to enter two records

for each patient who had more than one pathogen causing the infection. This duplicates data and wastes memory but, more importantly, creates errors in data manipulation when the person doing data input does not enter identical information for the same field in the new record. Another limitation is that flat databases provide only one view of the data, even if there are multiple users.

A Microsoft Excel table is an example of a flat database. Excel allows for the use of a few sophisticated database concepts. For example, if the data are organized as records for each row with associated column heading labeled with field names, you can instruct Excel to format the data as a database from the Home menu. Excel tables formatted as a database give you the ability to sort and filter with each column heading. You can also provide data integrity using standardized terminology for data entry from the Data > Data Validation menu.

Hierarchical Database

The **hierarchical database** was an early database model. This type of database (Fig. 8-2) is a database with tables that are organized in the shape of an inverted tree, like an organizational chart. In this organizational plan, often called a tree structure, records are linked to a base, or root, but through successive layers. In Figure 8-2, the Record Number table is the root table. The Demographics table would be a child of the root, as would the length of stay (LOS) table. Nursing Diagnosis and Surgery would be the children of the parent LOS table and the grandchild of the Record Number. Each child in a hierarchical database can have only one parent, whereas a parent may have none, one, or many children. The difficulty with the hierarchical structure is that it is hard to link data from one branch of the tree with another (e.g., Nursing Diagnosis with Demographics). Because of its structure, this model is complex and inflexible (Oppel, 2009).

Network Model

The **network model** is similar to the hierarchical model, but the trees can share branches. If Figure 8-2 was a network database, you would see a line indicating a relationship between Demographics and all the tables at lower levels. Because of the data structure, the network model is complex and inflexible (Oppel, 2009).

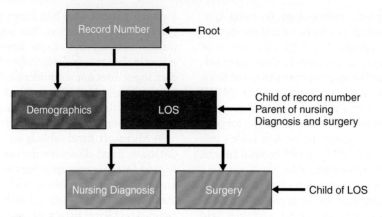

Figure 8-2. Hierarchical database model.

Relational Database Model

A **relational database** is more flexible than the hierarchical and network models. In a relational database model, there can be two or more tables that are connected by identical information in fields in each table that are called key fields. This allows the data in a record from one table to be matched to any piece or pieces of data in records in another table. The related key field in the related table is the foreign key. The relationship of tables is displayed in Figure 8-3. The 1111 MRN from the tblPatient table, which is the master table, is matched to the 1111 MRN in the tblUTI table, likewise is true for MRN 1122.

In Figure 8-3, the MRN is the primary key for tblPatient. MRN is the foreign key for tblUTI. The primary key for tblUTI is CaseID. The CaseID in tblUtI will automatically populate with a unique number each time a record is added. Fields that populate themselves do not need to be visible in a form view of a record. However, including one

in the table design for child tables is an excellent idea because it preserves the ability to develop the database. Databases have a habit of "**scope creep**." That is, when those who want information see what they can learn from the data, they ask for more information. A good database designer will anticipate this reaction and provide for expansion in the original design (Table 8-2).

The table shown in Figure 8-4 is an example of a query that matched the Patient table (tblPatient) and the UTI table (tblUTI)tblA from the UTI database using the key fields. This query created a flat table from the two tables to answer the question: What patients had antibiotics, a Foley catheter, and/or UTI on admission and what was the admission and discharge date?

You can use queries as a basis for a report with the relational model. Like reports, queries always produce their information based on the current data in the tables, not the data that were there when they were created. For queries for which you

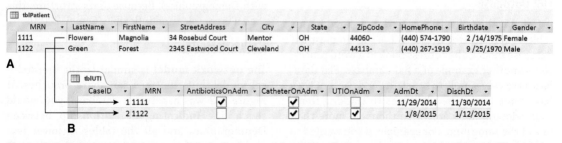

Figure 8-3. Relational database model. **A:** Demographics table. **B:** Drug reactions table. (Used with permission from Microsoft.)

TABLE 8-2   Relational Database Terms

Term	Definition
View	A look at the data; these vary according to the requirements of the user. Tables, forms, queries, and reports are all different views of data.
Database Management System (DBMS)	A software application that provides tools for creating a database, entering data, retrieving, manipulating, and reporting information contained within the data.
Form	A view of data that often shows only fields from one record. Very useful for data entry. Can be printed
Query	Search function for a relational database.
Parameter query	A query that when run asks the user to specify data for a given field so that only records that match that "parameter" are returned.
Report	Often used for printing information from data in a table(s) or query, it provides data organized to fulfill user need.
Primary key	The key field in the master (parent) table
Foreign key	A field that contains data identical to that in the master table, but is in the detail (child) table.
Validation table (**lookup table**)	A table that provides a list of allowable entries for a field that is linked to that field. The data in the drop-down boxes in the Google Advanced Search are an example.

will want information at routine intervals, such as monthly, have a query answer a question using specific criteria in a given field. For example, let's say you wanted to answer the following question: What were the medical diagnoses for a specified nursing diagnosis in January 2015? To find out, design a query to ask the user to specify criteria for a field, such as the month and year for the date field. Queries that require the user to enter a constraint to define data output are called **parameter queries**. For example, to print out monthly reports, create a parameter query that asks for the dates to include. In this way, we can use the same report every month, but instead of showing all the data in the table, it will show only the information for the identified time period entered when the report is run.

When designing a database, each field must contain atomic level data. **Atomic level** data are data that cannot be reduced. First name is at the atomic level, as is the systolic blood pressure. When the systolic and diastolic are in one

qryPatient Query								
MRN	LastName	FirstName	AntibioticsOnAdm	CatheterOnAdm	UTIOnAdm	AdmDt	DischDt	
1111	Flowers	Magnolia	✔	✔		11/29/2014	11/30/2014	
1122	Green	Forest		✔	✔	1/8/2015	1/12/2015	

Figure 8-4. Query from two tables (tblPatient and tblUtI). (Used with permission from Microsoft.)

field, the data are not at the atomic level, nor is a combination of the first and last name in one field at the atomic level. This is one aspect of a guide to database design that is called **normalization**. The complete process involves what are termed "five forms," each one building on the one below it. At the level of our UTI database, we need to be concerned only with the following:

1. Each value in a table is to be represented once and only once. With the exception of the key fields, a piece of data should never be repeated in another table.
2. All data should be at the atomic level.
3. Each record (row) in a table having a field should have unique data in the form of a key field—that is, it is not repeated in that table in that field.

Anytime it is possible for data that belong in a field to have more than one entry for a field, you should create a lookup table or lookup list (discussed later in this chapter). Given the fact that many people have more than one phone number—cell, home, and business—designers of databases that contain demographic data need to create a special table for phone numbers with fields designating the type of phone and the number. Anticipating when creating special tables is required is often a difficult task and requires the people who input the data to be those who actually enter, use, or, ideally, both enter and use the data.

To summarize, the relational database model consists of two or more tables that are related through primary and foreign key fields. When the datum in a key field of a record in one table matches the datum in a key field in another table, the data in the records are related—that is, able to be looked at as if they are one record. It is this principle that makes it possible to use one piece of data in many different ways. A rule of database design is that users are never required to enter the same piece of data more than once. One entry of the data has many uses!

Object-Oriented Model

The true object-oriented model combines database functions with object programming languages, making a more powerful tool (Barry, 2014). Because it provides better management

of complex data relationships, it is more suited to applications such as hospital patient record systems, which have complex relationships between data. To create such a database requires knowledge of programming languages and is not suited to the application software in an office suite. Data from this type of database, however, can be exported and used in a relational database from the professional version of office suites to analyze data.

DATABASE SOFTWARE SOLUTIONS

There are two main categories of database software: enterprise and personal computer. Enterprise database software is used to deploy databases across an organization. Examples of enterprise software include Oracle and Microsoft SQL Server. Examples of personal computer database software include Microsoft Access, FileMaker Pro, Apache OpenOffice Base, and Zoho Creator. The design principles for enterprise and desktop database software are similar. This chapter focuses on use of Microsoft Access.

If you don't have database software on your computer, begin learning with a free version, such as Apache OpenOffice Base, to visualize the features and functions. You can use Base to open Access database files. Base allows you to create tables, queries, forms, and reports.

CREATING A SIMPLE DATABASE

Databases are tools that assist nurses and other healthcare personnel in uncovering knowledge in data from an information system or in managing information. For the purpose of the example in this section, we will work together to create and use a database to accomplish these aims. When you start Microsoft Access, you have a choice of creating a blank database or using a template. When you select a blank database, you are prompted to give it a name and choose where it will be filed. The default is to open Table1 in a datasheet view, which looks identical to a spreadsheet grid, but without the row numbers or column letters. As noted earlier, each row is called a record. All data entered into a row should relate to that specific

explanations for the field names and to customize the way data should be entered.

The very first step in creating a database is to identify the question that the data need to answer so that you can draw conclusions. In our example, the nurse manager wants to answer the following questions each month: How many patients arrive with a UTI, and how many develop one after they arrive? After the question or questions have been decided, you can identify the data needed to answer them. After conferring with the nurse manager, you develop a purpose for the database and identify what is needed to provide the answers to the questions. The result of the efforts can be seen in Box 8-1.

The first step is to create two tables—one table for the patient data and the second table for the admission with UTI data. When you create a table, use the design view of which is seen in Figure 8-5A. Notice that in this view, there is a name for each field, designated its type, and provided a description of the data that this field will contain. The data entry view is seen in Figure 8-5B. Note that each table name is preceded by the suffix "tbl." It is a good practice in a database to precede each object with a prefix designating its type. After completing the design of the table, to test the assumptions of the data needed, enter some data into the table itself.

record. It is best to switch from the datasheet view to design view when creating a new table. Use the Access menu and click the View icon to toggle between the design view and the datasheet view. The design view allows you the ability to provide

tblPatient

Field Name	Data Type	Description (Optional)
MRN	Short Text	Primary key for relating tables
LastName	Short Text	Patient's last name
FirstName	Short Text	Patient's first name
StreetAddress	Short Text	Street address
City	Short Text	City
State	Short Text	State
ZipCode	Short Text	Zip code for the address
HomePhoneNumber	Short Text	Home phone number
Birthdate	Date/Time	Birthdate
Gender	Short Text	Gender

A

tblPatient

MRN	LastName	FirstName	StreetAddress	City	State	ZipCode	HomePhone	Birthdate	Gender
⊞ 1111	Flowers	Magnolia	34 Rosebud Court	Mentor	OH	44060-	(440) 574-1790	2 /14/1975	Female
⊞ 1122	Green	Forest	2345 Eastwood Court	Cleveland	OH	44113-	(440) 267-1919	9 /25/1970	Male
⊞ 1212	Day	Summer	4562 Maple Street	Aurora	OH	44204-	(442) 987-1234	5 /11/1999	Female
⊞ 1234	Shore	Sea	3491 Beach Drive	Mentor	OH	44060-	(440) 574-1111	11/21/1990	Female
⊞ 1331	Coyote	Will	12 South Woods Street	Medina	OH	44256-	(443) 654-2222	10/30/1989	Male
⊞ 1357	Farmer	Jersey	45678 Barn Street	Avon Lake	OH	44012-	(444) 777-0000	9 /25/1969	Male

B

Figure 8-5. Master Patient (tblPatient) table in (**A**) design view and (**B**) data entry view. (Used with permission from Microsoft.)

The patient table (tblPatient) will have the following fields and field attributes or data type. The field attributes are displayed with parentheses.

- MRN (short text—primary key)
- LastName (short text)
- FirstName (short text)
- StreetAddress (short text)
- City (short text)
- State (short text)
- ZipCode (short text)
- HomePhoneNumber (short text)
- Birthdate (date/time)
- Gender (lookup wizard—type in the values > Female; Male; Unknown [Limit to list])
- Race (lookup wizard—type in the values > American Indian or Alaska native; Asian; Black or African American; Other Race; White [Limit to list])

To facilitate data entry and prevent entry errors, create a **lookup list** using the **Lookup Wizard** (Data Type > Lookup Wizard > [I will type in the value that I want]) that has these entries and relate this table to that field in the design view. When this is done, a data enterer selects from a drop-down menu list instead of typing in an entry. Whenever possible, the designer should create a list of possible data entries using a lookup list. An alternative for typing in values is to create a lookup table. You would create the relationship between the table with the lookup value and the lookup table using the Data Type Lookup Wizard. This makes it easier for the data enterer and ensures that correct, identical data will be entered in the field.

The UTI (tblUTI) table will have the following fields:

- CaseID (autonumber—primary key)
- MRN (short text)
- AdmittedFrom (short text)
- AntibioticsOnAdm (yes/no)
- CatheterOnAdmission (yes/no)
- UTIOnAdm (yes/no)
- AdmDt (date/time)
- DischDt (date/time)

In Access, the design view of the tables has a column labeled "Data Type." Notice that the information in this column is not the same for all fields. The data type tells the database how to process or

handle the data in that field and limits the type of data that the field will accept. The data type in the table, tblUTI, is AutoNumber, where the computer generates a number for each new record that is automatically entered into the table each time a new record is created. Letting the computer number the records saves the data enterer from the trouble of entering the data for a key field as well as preventing any duplication of key field data. The AutoNumber field should be a primary key field, a unique field for which there will never be an identical entry in that field (column) in that table. Naming fields using brief text words with no spaces is an example of a naming convention. You certainly want your database to be people friendly, so use Field Properties > General tab > Caption to write out the meaning for each field name. The caption will be displayed in the datasheet view and for all forms and reports. Also, write a short description for each field. Notice that the text field type in the primary key field for tblPatient matches the text field type for tblUTI. Fields that are related must be of the same type, and a numeric field that contains only long integers matches the AutoNumber type of field.

A text field can contain any type of data, but is limited to 255 characters, including spaces. If a field will contain more than 255 characters, use a long text (memo field). Date/Time fields allow "date calculations." In this database, the Date fields will allow us to calculate the LOS when the time and the date are entered in this field. The "Yes/No" field type is a logical field—that is, only yes or no can be entered.

If you added a third table that is related to tblUTI, since the primary key for tblUTI is an autonumber, the key would be displayed as a foreign key with a numeric field type in the related table. Numeric fields serve other purposes too. Because a database can do "date arithmetic," you decide to have a field for the date admitted and the date discharged and let the computer calculate the LOS. To calculate the LOS, you would add a new column to the tblUTI with a field name of LOS with a calculation field type. Once you select calculation, an expression window opens, which allows you to enter the calculation for LOS (Fig. 8-6). You simply click the names of the fields and mathematical symbols to write the formula for the expression.

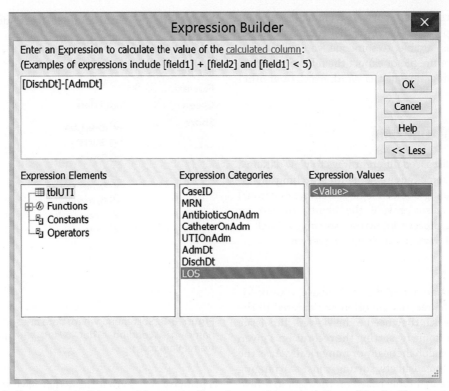

Figure 8-6. Expression builder used to create formulas used in calculations. (Used with permission from Microsoft.)

Unlike Excel, you do not precede the formula with an equals sign.

The type of relationship shown in Figure 8-7 is a one-to-many relationship. In other words, a record in the main, or Master Infections, table, may have anywhere from none to an infinite number of matching records in the antibiotics table. This type of relationship is symbolized in the relationship window by the infinity symbol (∞) next to the Antibiotics, or subordinate, table.

SAVING DATA IN A DATABASE

Unlike other office application programs, Access saves a data entry as soon as the insertion point is moved from the record in which the data were entered. This has several implications. Once you make a change to a record and leave it, consider the change permanent. It is possible to undo only the last change made. Deleting a record, however, is permanent; there is no undo. When using a database, the only things that you need to save are objects such as a table, query, or form after you create them. The only time you need to save is after you create an object or after you make a change to the object in the design mode. When you close this object, you will be prompted to save. Some databases, including Access, save all the objects such as

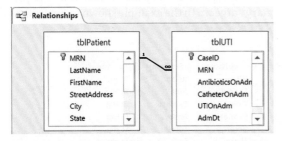

Figure 8-7. Relationship between two tables (tblPatient and tblUTI). (Used with permission from Microsoft.)

tables, forms, and reports as one file. If you want to send a piece of a database that you have created, such as just a table, to someone, you will need to send the entire file or export the table or query to another program, such as Word, Excel, or another database.

MANIPULATING DATA

We have discussed different ways to view data in a table and some requirements for searching a database including Boolean logic searching. Relational databases also provide the ability to reorder records, a process known as sorting, as well as additional ways of searching, or querying.

Sorting

When data are entered in a database, a record is created. The records are often not entered in the order in which they need to be viewed. This issue can be overcome by sorting the records on a given field, either alphabetically or numerically. As is the case with spreadsheets, sorting is just rearranging the records in a table based on the data in a field or fields in a table. The simplest **sort** is a primary sort; that is, the records are resorted based on one field. An example would be reordering records in a database based on last name to produce a table similar to the records shown in Figure 8-8. You have probably used the sort feature if you made a purchase online. For example, if you purchased slacks, you may have searched first by price and then by color.

Databases are not limited to sorting on just one field. One can have primary, secondary, tertiary, and even further levels of sorts, each built on the groupings provided by the sort one level above it. In a tertiary sort, the records will first be sorted in

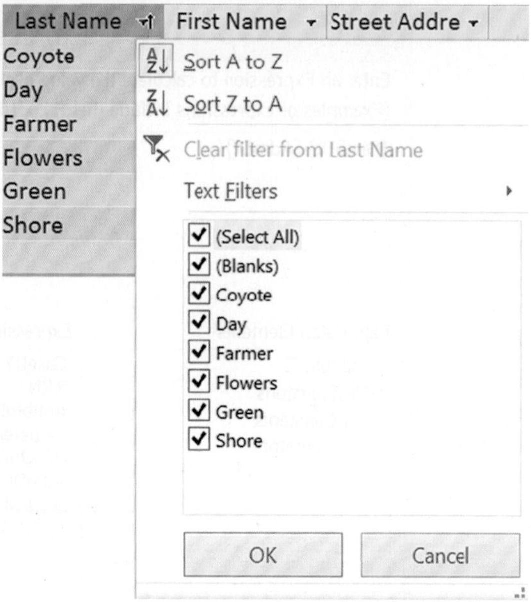

Figure 8-8. Sort menu where data are sorted on last name in ascending order. (Used with permission from Microsoft.)

a primary sort so that those that have similarities in the sort field are listed together. Then, another sorting is done on another field on records in each group created from the primary sort (the secondary sort); finally, a tertiary sort can be performed on another field of each group from the secondary sort. For example, a primary sort is performed on all patients in a hospital by the type of surgery; then, the records are reordered within each type of surgery in a secondary sort so that those from the same unit within each type of surgery are together. For a tertiary sort, the records are further reordered so that the records on a given unit for each type of surgery are reordered by the primary surgeon. In the example shown in Figure 8-9,

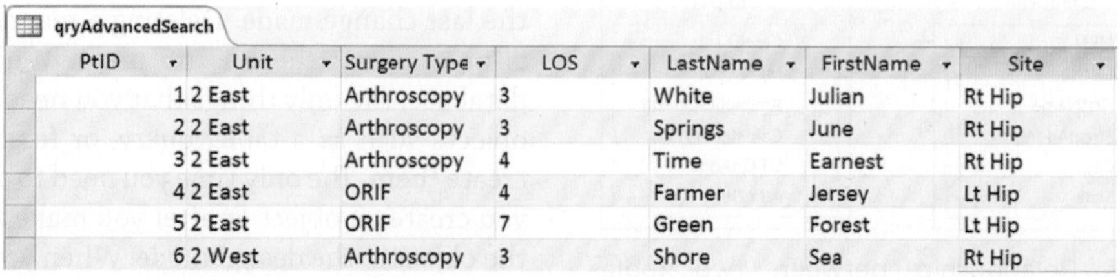

Figure 8-9. Primary, secondary, and tertiary sort for unit, surgery type, and length of stay (LOS). (Used with permission from Microsoft.)

Surgery Type by Unit

Unit	Surgery Type	LOS	LastName	FirstName	Site
2 East					
	ORIF	7	Green	Forest	Lt Hip
	ORIF	4	Farmer	Jersey	Lt Hip
	Arthroscopy	4	Time	Earnest	Rt Hip
	Arthroscopy	3	Springs	June	Rt Hip
	Arthroscopy	3	White	Julian	Rt Hip
2 West					
	Arthroscopy	3	Light	Tiffany	Lt Hip
	Arthroscopy	3	Shore	Sea	Rt Hip

Figure 8-10. Report view of surgery type by unit. (Used with permission from Microsoft.)

the primary sort is the patient unit, the secondary sort is the type of surgery, and the tertiary sort is the LOS. This type of grouping is most useful in producing reports that need to look at a given characteristic within various groups. The report shown in Figure 8-10 was produced by a primary sort of the records into the type of facility from which the patient was admitted.

TABLE 8-3 Mathematical Operators for Querying

Operator	Query Criteria in Age Field	Returns from a Table with Data in the Age Field
> (greater than)	>50	Records in which the entry in the age field is greater than 50
< (less than)	<50	Records in which the entry in the age field is less than 50
<> (not equal to)	<>50	Records in which the entry in the age field is any number but 50
≥ (greater than or equal to)	≥50	Records in which the entry in the age field is greater than or equal to 50
≤ (less than or equal to)	≤50	Records in which the entry in the age field is less than or equal to 50
Between	Between 30 and 40	Records in which the entry in the age field is between 30 and 40 (inclusive)
Null, or blank (field is empty)	Null (or blank)	Records in which the entry in the age field is empty
Count, sum, average, standard deviation, minimum, maximum, and others	Make a selection from a drop-down list	Does a calculation based on the term selected. For text fields, only the count function, which counts the number of times a given term appears, is available. Numeric fields are open to all types of calculations.

Querying

A query is the most powerful tool in a database. You have seen the results of a Boolean query in databases. There are many other ways that queries can be used to manipulate data. Queries can produce a subset of records based on fields that meet given criteria, or they can report on the entire database. Additionally, queries can be performed on the results of another query. The only limiting factors are the data available, the user's imagination, and the ability to use the criteria selectors of Boolean algebra and the symbols referred to as mathematical operators. (This is not as complicated as it sounds, keep reading! ☺.)

The mathematical operators in Table 8-3 may be used in combination with each other or with Boolean logic. A query of the surgery type table that contains the surgery types by nursing unit allows the nurses to see the number of surgery types by nursing unit. To accomplish this, you use the "count" function and create the query shown in Figure 8-11. You also want to see the average LOS and standard deviation for each of these patients. Using those functions on the LOS field, you create the query shown in Figure 8-12.

It is possible to use and manipulate data downloaded from a large information system to answer questions such as those above. Although some of the examples used in this chapter included identifying information about fictitious patients to help clarify the examples, data downloaded from a healthcare agency database should not contain any data that would allow individual patients to be identified.

Effective querying involves not necessarily the technical skill to construct a query, but instead the cognitive component that allows us to see the possibilities. When we can communicate exactly what information we want from data, a technical person can construct the query. One way to incorporate this cognitive component is to create and use small databases. Using data that you have entered, or a database that you have designed, creates a situation in which you can see more of the possibilities for getting answers.

qryCount

Surgery Type	CountOfSurgery Type
Arthroscopy	5
ORIF	2

Figure 8-11. Query that uses the count function. (Used with permission from Microsoft.)

qryAvg_StdDev

Unit	AvgOfLOS	StDevOfLOS
2 East	4.2	1.6431676725155
2 West	3	0

Figure 8-12. Query that displays average length of stay (LOS) and standard deviation for two nursing units. (Used with permission from Microsoft.)

One caveat: When you design a query, always test it with a subset of data for which you know the answers to test if it actually works as desired. Include in this subset outliers that might or might not conform to your query. The best way to learn how to query is to play with the data by querying. You may have to try several times to get the desired answer. This is not unusual, as the author has seen database professionals work hard to enter just the right criteria to produce the answers they needed. Because ultimately the database designer is responsible for answers that are produced, testing a query with a small subset of data is especially important when someone else who is unfamiliar with the data will be constructing the query.

QSEN Scenario

You are using a database with patient data with the MRN, age, fall date, and unit name. You want to analyze data for all patients older than 65 years. What database function(s) will you use?

SECONDARY DATA USE

In this chapter, we looked at the use of health information for purposes beyond direct patient care, a process known as **secondary data use**. This usage permits the analysis of all aspects of care for which data are available. Secondary use of healthcare data can greatly improve healthcare by increasing our knowledge of diseases and treatments. It can improve nursing care by enabling us to access empirical evidence to support our practice. The use of secondary health data, however, has ethical implications. It is critical to verify that safeguards are in place to be sure that the data is fully deidentified—that is, all identifiers such as the name of the patient, record number, or social security number are removed.

Ideally, a statistician will determine that there is only a very small chance that secondary data can be combined with public sources of information to identify an individual. For clinicians to learn answers to clinical care questions, it is necessary for agencies to create policies that safeguard patients' rights while also providing for the secondary use of data. Before this happens, clinicians must communicate the importance that secondary data can have in improving patient care. A first step toward this goal is to become knowledgeable about the questions that can be answered using secondary data.

DISCOVERING KNOWLEDGE IN LARGE DATABASES

The methods described in this chapter are very useful for gaining answers from a relational database. Relational databases, however, are limited to a relatively small set of data when compared with a hospital information system. In the relational database example, we had limited fields (which could be thought of as variables), and we knew what type of questions we wanted answered. To answer these types of questions, we can engage in ad hoc querying, or querying in a situation in which we know enough about the data to know what questions to ask. Electronic healthcare records contain a huge number of records and variables. Although we can ask for a subset of these data to analyze with a relational database, to pinpoint more information requires more powerful tools such as **data mining**, online analytical processing (OLAP), and structured query language (SQL).

Data Mining

Large clinical databases possess an inordinate amount of information that is not amenable to this type of relatively simple querying. To uncover this knowledge requires what is called "knowledge discovery in databases" (KDD). Using a process known as data mining, it is possible to extract from data potentially useful information that was previously unknown. Like ad hoc querying, data mining can find relationships only between the data to which it has access (Vararuk et al., 2008).

Originally developed to process corporate sales and production data, data mining is very relevant to healthcare. It has been successfully used to uncover fraud in many areas, including healthcare, and is useful in uncovering hidden relationships in patient care. There are three types of data mining applications: classification, regression, and clustering (StatSoft Inc., 2014a). Data mining is a form of research, but research in a retrospective manner using existing data to see what, if any, relationships are present. It uses complex statistical techniques to uncover hidden relationships that are predictive of some outcome.

Data mining can be used to predict diseases, understand the relationships of symptoms, and identify where to target treatment (Jaret, 2013, January 14). For example, Massachusetts Institute of Technology (MIT) has a research partnership with a hospital to predict patients who are likely to crash in order to allow early intervention and thwart the bad outcome (Health Data Management, 2010, May 1). Data analysis is done with data from the critical care monitoring system and the electronic medical record. This is a strong incentive for nurses to use standardized terminology to ensure that not only medical information but also independent nursing actions and outcomes are included in data that will be analyzed.

Data mining requires the use of specialized software. Two data mining software packages that you may be familiar with are SAS Business Analytics and IBM SPSS. Both are statistical software packages commonly used in statistics and nursing research courses.

Although it is possible to do data mining against a regular large electronic database, it is more effective when done on a "**data warehouse**." A data warehouse is a comprehensive collection of clinical and demographic data on large populations (Lyman et al., 2008). Developing a data warehouse involves processes that extract the data, then clean and date it. It is not a process that is done in a vacuum. It is imperative that this be done with someone who is familiar with the data. Barriers that impede the large-scale use of data mining in healthcare are the lack of integrated medical data repositories, such as those that can be made possible by regional health information organizations (RHIO), guidelines for the secondary use of medical data (Lyman et al., 2008), and differing work processes among healthcare facilities that make it difficult to maintain clean and useful data.

Online Analytical Processing

OLAP, or fast analysis of shared multidimensional (FASM) information, performs real-time analysis of data stored in databases. Despite the name, one does not have to be online to use it. Not nearly as powerful as data mining, it is a faster way of analyzing information. OLAP provides a multidimensional analysis of various types of data as well as the ability to do comparative or descriptive summaries of data (StatSoft Inc., 2014b). For example, OLAP can be used with patient records to discover the degree of disease within sets of patient groups (Ordonez & Chen, 2009). When combined with geographical information system (GIS), OLAP can analyze climate changes and the effects on the health of the associated population (Bernier et al., 2009). The final result can be as simple as frequency tables, cross tabulations, or descriptive statistics, or more complex such as the removal of outliers, or other forms of data cleansing (StatSoft Inc., 2014b).

Structured Query Language

Structured Query Language (SQL) is the name of the coding that is used for querying in many databases. It is an ANSI (American National Standards Institute) standard computer language for retrieving and updating data in a database. It is used by Microsoft Access as well as with the more powerful Oracle relational DBMS. Many different versions of SQL are available, but to comply with the ANSI standard, they must support such major query keywords as Select, Update, Delete, Insert, Where, and others (w3schools.com, 2014). In Microsoft Access, if you click View when Queries are the active object, one of your choices is SQL View. Clicking that will show you the code that is executed when you run that query.

SUMMARY

Databases underpin all healthcare information systems. Data at the atomic level are the basis for the tables that are the structure on which a database is built. The different database models are hierarchical, network, object oriented, flat, and relational. The databases that come in the professional version of office software suites are a hybrid combination of the object-oriented and relational models, but they primarily use the relational model. In a relational database, the records in tables are related by a key field that is present in both tables. Getting data into a database, including a healthcare information system, is one of the most difficult tasks involved with databases. This is why a database designer should try to make it as simple as possible with forms and entry selections.

Information is produced from a database by querying. Boolean and mathematical operators can be used with criteria either singly or in combination. Before trusting query outcomes, results should always be tested with a subset of data for which the answers can be visually determined. When conclusions are drawn from the data, it is advisable to consider whether all the data needed for that conclusion are present in the database.

Effective databases are planned on paper before being created on the computer. The first step is to identify what outcomes the database should provide. By using that information, the data necessary to meet these needs are determined, along with the methods for manipulating and reporting those data. These steps are iterative; it is often necessary to make corrections or additions to a prior step as planning progresses.

A well-designed database, whether a small one such as the UTI example or a large electronic patient record system, can perform many tasks. As electronic patient records become more prevalent, we will move beyond just using patient care data in a primary way (i.e., only for the care of one patient) to secondary data use (i.e., for purposes other than the primary one for which it was collected). For example, the Health Information Technology for Economic and Clinical Health (HITECH) Act (discussed in detail in Chapter 17) requires eligible healthcare providers to use certified electronic health records (EHRs) that allow for secondary data use (Hogin & Daniel, 2011, May 18; HealthIT.gov, 2014, February 24). To use EHRs and secondary data, nurses need the skills for effective querying.

One difficulty with today's electronic patient records is the lack of nursing data that is identifiable and retrievable in an aggregated form and in which we can link problems, interventions, and outcomes. This puts nursing at a disadvantage because it can stall improvements in our practice as well as prevent nursing data from being considered in planning healthcare. As was pointed out in this chapter, if data are not in the database, the database cannot be used to answer questions. Missing data lead to erroneous conclusions.

APPLICATIONS AND COMPETENCIES

1. How can nurses use databases to improve patient care outcomes? Search the Internet and online library, or draw from clinical practice experience. Provide specific examples and cite your sources.

2. Create a simple database with two related tables. Explain the process.

3. What are the different methods for viewing data in a database? Use examples you found when reading the chapter.

4. Search the Internet or online library for a resource that expands your understanding of Boolean logic. Summarize your findings and provide an example for each of the Boolean terms.

5. Describe the methods for discovering knowledge in both relational and large clinical databases.

6. Discuss the limitations of a database.

7. Evaluate the data that are collected by an information system for identifiable nursing-sensitive data.

8. What questions could you ask of a database with the following data? Which of the Boolean or mathematical operators would you use for the query?

First Name	Last Name	Primary Diagnosis	Medical Diagnosis	Nursing Diagnosis

REFERENCES

American Association of Colleges of Nursing. (2008). *The essentials of baccalaureate education for professional nursing practice*. Retrieved from http://www.aacn.nche.edu/education-resources/essential-series

American Association of Colleges of Nursing. (2011). *The essentials of master's education in nursing*. Retrieved from http://www.aacn.nche.edu/education-resources/essential-series

American Association of Colleges of Nursing. (2006). *The essentials of doctoral education for advanced nursing practice*. Retrieved from http://www.aacn.nche.edu/education-resources/essential-series

American Nurses Association. (2015). *Nursing informatics: Scope & standards for practice* (2nd ed.). Silver Spring, MD: Author.

Barry, D. (2014). *Object-oriented database management system (OODBMS) definition*. Retrieved from http://www.service-architecture.com/object-oriented-databases/articles/object-oriented_database_oodbms_definition.html

Bernier, E., Gosselin, P., Badard, T., et al. (2009). Easier surveillance of climate-related health vulnerabilities through a Web-based spatial OLAP application. *International Journal of Health Geographics*, 8, 18.

Chapple, M. (2014). *Database normalization basics: Normalizing your database*. Retrieved from http://databases.about.com/od/specificproducts/a/normalization.htm

Health Data Management. (2010, May 1). *Mining ICU data for early-warning signs*. Retrieved from http://www.healthdatamanagement.com/issues/18_5/mining-icu-data-for-early-warning-signs-40168-1.html#Login

HealthIT.gov. (2014, February 24). *HITECH programs for Health IT adoption*. Retrieved from http://www.healthit.gov/policy-researchers-implementers/health-it-adoption-programs

Hogin, E., & Daniel, J. G. (2011, May 18). *The many uses of health information technology*. Retrieved from http://www.healthit.gov/buzz-blog/meaningful-use/meaningful-health-information-technology/

Jaret, P. (2013, January 14). Mining electronic records for revealing health data. *Health data management*. Retrieved from http://www.nytimes.com/2013/01/15/health/mining-electronic-records-for-revealing-health-data.html?_r=0

Lyman, J. A., Scully, K., & Harrison, J. H., Jr. (2008). The development of health care data warehouses to support data mining. *Clinics in Laboratory Medicine*, 28(1), 55–71, vi. doi: 10.1016/j.cll.2007.10.003

Microsoft. (2014). *Top 10 reasons to use Access with Excel*. Retrieved from http://office.microsoft.com/en-us/excel-help/top-10-reasons-to-use-access-with-excel-HA010264081.aspx

Oppel, A. (2009). *Databases: A beginner's guide*. New York, NY: McGraw Hill.

Ordonez, C., & Chen, Z. (2009). Evaluating statistical tests on OLAP cubes to compare degree of disease. *IEEE Transactions on Information Technology in Biomedicine*, 13(5), 756–765.

QSEN Institute. (2014). Quality and safety education for nursing. Retrieved from http://qsen.org/

School of Mathematics and Statistics. (2004). George Boole. Retrieved from http://www-history.mcs.st-andrews.ac.uk/Biographies/Boole.html

StatSoft Inc. (2014a). *Data mining techniques—OLAP. Electronic statistics textbook*. Tulsa, OK. Retrieved from https://www.statsoft.com/Textbook/Data-Mining-Techniques/button/1

StatSoft Inc. (2014b). *Statistics glossary: On-line analytic processing (OLAP) (or Fast Analysis of Shared Multidimensional Information—FASMI)*. Retrieved from https://www.statsoft.com/Textbook/Statistics-Glossary/O/button/0#Olap

Technology Informatics Guiding Education Reform (TIGER). (2007, February 26). *The TIGER initiative: Evidence and informatics transforming nursing: 3-Year action steps toward a 10-year vision*. Retrieved from http://www.himss.org/ResourceLibrary/ResourceDetail.aspx?ItemNumber=8772

Vararuk, A., Petrounias, I., & Kodogiannis, V. (2007). Data mining techniques for HIV/AIDS data management in Thailand. *Journal of Enterprise Information Management, 21*(1), 52–70.

w3schools.com. (2014). *Introduction to SQL*. Retrieved from http://www.w3schools.com/SQL/sql_intro.asp

Information Competency

John Paul Getty once said, "In time of rapid change, experience could be our worst enemy" (GoodQuotes.com, 2010). Healthcare continues to stay in the midst of rapid change. As a result, nurses have an obligation to use information and health literacy skills, as well as computer technology skills, proficiently. These skills are a part of the nurse's personal and professional growth. Nurses in clinical practice must maintain current knowledge. Nurses must have information literacy skills to guide patients and families in accessing quality healthcare information from Internet sites. Information literacy is a lifelong journey that requires repeated practice to obtain proficiency. Skills required for information literacy include critical thinking and the ability to find new, valid, reliable information pertinent to clinical practice, as well as computer skills.

Chapter 9 opens this unit with an exploration of evidence-based practice (EBP) using the millions of resources found on the Internet. It focuses on the essential skills for discovering valid and reliable health information in the literature and on the Internet. Information in Chapter 10 guides the user to develop the essential information search competencies necessary to discover knowledge embedded in online library resources and digital databases. Chapter 11 focuses on the use of mobile devices, such as tablets and smart phones, in educational and healthcare settings.

CHAPTER 9

Information Literacy: A Road to Evidence-Based Practice

OBJECTIVES

After studying this chapter, you will be able to:

1. Identify three obstacles that interfere with the adoption of evidence-based resources in nursing practice.

2. Interpret the relationships between information literacy, clinical reasoning, and information technology skills.

3. Discuss use of the PICO framework when investigating evidence-based practice information needs.

4. Discuss how to use information literacy skills to find and evaluate healthcare information on the Internet.

5. Differentiate scholarly nursing articles, from those in magazines, newspapers, newsletters, and websites.

KEY TERMS

Best research evidence	Information literacy	Peer-reviewed article
Clinical expertise	Information technology skills	PICO (PICOT, PICOTT)
Clinical reasoning	Nursing knowledge	Scholarly nursing journal
Evidence-based nursing	Open access journals	
Evidence-based practice (EBP)	Patient values	

There was a time when you found scholarly health information only in printed journals, textbooks, and brick and mortar libraries. The brick and mortar libraries, still essential resources for healthcare knowledge and EBP, now include access to the electronic resources, such as library catalogs, journals, magazines, newspapers, e-Books, as well as other Internet websites. Sackett, Haynes, & Rosenberg (2000) defined **evidence-based practice (EBP)** as "the integration of best research evidence with clinical expertise and patient values" (p. 1). **Best research evidence** is clinically relevant research. It includes outcomes and effectiveness of patient care (Sackett, 1997). **Clinical expertise** means the ability to use clinical skills and past experience to rapidly identify each patient's unique health state and diagnosis, individual risks and benefits of potential interventions, and personal values and expectations (Institute of Medicine, 2001, p. 47, para 2). **Patient values** "refers to the unique preferences, concerns, and expectations that each patient brings to a clinical encounter" (p. 147, para 4) that are used when making clinical decisions.

The IOM EBP definition expounds upon the original definition of evidence-based medicine by Sackett et al (1996). Sackett (1997) initially defined evidence-based medicine as "the conscientious, explicit, and judicious use of current best evidence in making decisions about the care of individual patients" (p. 71, para 2). The updated IOM definition includes the concepts of safety and patient values. Since the definition applies to a multitude of healthcare disciplines, we use the terminology, evidence-based practice (EBP).

There was a significant increase in awareness about patient care outcomes and the associated factors beginning in the 1990s for medicine and nursing. Richardson et al. (1995) introduced the **PICO** process for asking a research question, without using the PICO acronym. The PICO process is a standard used today to investigate evidence-based care in medicine and nursing (Boudin et al., 2010; Caldwell, Bennett, & Mellis, 2012; Yensen, 2013).

- P—patient, problem, or population (e.g., age, ethnicity, or gender, type of clinical problem)
- I—intervention (the types of clinical intervention)
- C—comparison (a comparison of interventions)
- O—outcome (the type of patient care outcome)

Over the years, others modified the acronym to be PICOT, where the T meant time. The time variable is not required, though.

In this day of digital information, we are data resource rich and information poor due to the volume and ever-expanding growth of resources. Technologies are constantly changing. As a result, the development of information skills is a life-long learning process. The focus of this chapter is using information literacy skills and use of the PICO process to discover valid and reliable health information for **evidence-based nursing** practice.

INFORMATION LITERACY COMPETENCIES FOR NURSES

In 2007 Pew report, not yet updated, of the 85 million Americans who searched for health information, only 15% stated that they always check for the source and date of the information (Fox, 2007). In essence, the public is turning to the Internet for health information but most need assistance to evaluate and effectively use the information. If the public is learning to be information literate, it behooves those of us in the healthcare profession to stay one-step ahead. We must be able to guide healthcare consumers to make decisions about the care that they receive. Healthcare providers must develop information literacy and information technology skills to identify valid and reliable health information on the Internet and interpret the findings to improve patient care outcomes.

Information literacy refers to the awareness that there is "a need to know" information, the ability to find it, analyze it for validity and relevance, and interpret it for use. Information literacy is a learned competency that requires repeated practice over time to develop expertise. Another definition is "…knowing when and why you need the information, where to find it, and how to evaluate, use and communicate it in an ethical manner" (CILIP, 2013). **Information technology skills** refers to the ability to use computers, computer software, and peripherals to access electronic information efficiently.

The Association of College and Research Libraries (2013) approved the Information Literacy Competency Standards for Nursing. The document consists of five major standards, indicators, and outcomes. It serves as a framework for undergraduate and graduate nursing education. An overview of the standards is noted below.

- Standard 1: Identifying the PICO, the types, formats, location, scope of information resources, and the cost–benefit for information retrieval. For example, "what question do I need to ask to assess a practice issue and where are the information resources?"
- Standard 2: Retrieving the information using PICO search strategies, as well as using and managing the appropriate resources. For example,

"what is the problem I am trying to solve and what are the appropriate resources to use?"

- Standard 3: Synthesizing, summarizing, and evaluating the information retrieved to assure where or not information needs are met. For example, "how good is the information I found? Do I need to search for more?"
- Standard 4: Using the information to address the clinical practice problem and sharing the findings with others.
- Standard 5: Demonstrating awareness of the socioeconomic, ethical and legal issues for access and use of the information.

Impact of the Healthcare Professional's Information Literacy

Health literacy is a requisite for using and generating nursing research. Nursing research is the scientific foundation for practice used to promote health, prevent diseases, manage illness symptoms, as well as assist with care for persons receiving palliative care and at the end of life. Nursing research addresses individuals, as well as populations (American Association of Colleges of Nursing (AACN), (2016, March 13); National Institute of Nursing Research (NINR), 2014). According to AACN, students in baccalaureate nursing programs learn the research process and can interpret and use research findings in their clinical practice. Students in Master's nursing programs can evaluate research findings and use the research to develop EBP guidelines. Students in doctor of nursing practice programs conduct nursing research and work with others in the research process.

Besides the AACN and the NINR, a number of other nursing organizations emphasize the importance of information and technology skills. A position paper, *Preparing the next generation of nurses to practice in a technology-rich environment: An informatics agenda,* by the National League for Nurses (NLN) (2008) supports the use of information and healthcare technologies. The Technology Informatics Guiding Education Reform (2007) (TIGER) report as well as the Quality and Safety Education for Nurses (QSEN) (2010) address the importance of information literacy skills. Because of these recommendations, nursing programs are teaching information literacy skills and accessing evidence-based nursing resources. Information literacy is essential for evidence-based nursing practice.

Synthesizing the results of a literature search is an important tool for improving the quality of patient care as well as the first step in any research study. Research shows that using information provided by literature searches changes clinical decisions. Literature findings provide information to justify, question, and improve patient care. Synthesis of literature leads to new knowledge, design of solutions, implementation, and evaluation methods. Knowledge from literature findings allows the nurses to empower the healthcare consumers to become partners in their own care. The positive patient care outcomes from nursing and medical research support.

Unfortunately, there is a translation of research into practice gap. The gap is evident with the example of using PICO to define a research question. Richardson recommended using PICO is 1995; however, wide use of the process in nursing is relatively recent. A limited number of nursing journal articles identify using PICO. It takes about 17 years for translation of research into practice (Morris et al., 2011; Westfall et al., 2007).

Teaching Information Literacy Skills

There is a longstanding need to improve the health literacy skills with nursing students and practicing professionals. With lack of knowledge about specialized library databases with nursing literature citations, how to search the databases, and how to appreciate and understand research articles, students and practicing nurses prefer to consult with colleagues and/or search the Internet using a search engine, such as Google (Beke-Harrigan, Hess, & Weinland, 2008; Ross, 2010; Pravidoff, Tanner, & Pierce, 2005). To address the need, faculty members are teaching information literacy skills in a variety of ways.

For example, Flood, Gasiewicz, and Delpier (2010) integrated information literacy across the five-semester curriculum of a baccalaureate nursing program with a systematic approach. They used the TIGER report and QSEN knowledge, skills, and attitude competencies as resources for teaching information literacy. The design of the assignments was for novice, intermediate, and advanced users.

During the first semester, students worked with a university librarian to find and evaluate physical and digital library resources. Afterward, the student worked in pairs using preset criteria to analyze a scholarly article related to care of the patient with diabetes. The students submitted a written report of the findings for grading. At the intermediate phase, student learned to use literature to implement an intervention. In the first phase, groups of students researched and designed a teaching brochure for a patient with a new diagnosis of diabetes. The group project was a graded assignment. In the second intermediate user phase, the students compared literature review findings with an organizational policy or procedure related to diabetes. The written comparison was a graded assignment. At the advanced phase, students learned about role development. In the first phase, students worked in teams to research a specific health problem for patients with acute care complex health problems. The focus of the research was acute care and home health providers. Students presented their research findings during a team conference and submitted a reflective paper for a grade. In the second part of the advanced user phase, students completing an externship explore and identify examples for using informatics and healthcare information in the clinical setting. The students submitted a written reflection of their findings for a grade. The novice to advanced user approach is one that other nursing programs might consider adopting into their exiting curriculum.

Jeffrey and colleagues (2011) identified low self-confidence or anxiety as a barrier for the development of information literacy skills. To address the barrier, they designed 10 two-hour workshops with four higher education institutions. Students were encouraged to collaborate and share while learning using a trial and error approach. The students used self-directed learning and personal goals to achieve the workshop outcomes. Faculty assessed learning from the students' reflective journaling. Student met the learning outcomes for the workshops while demonstrating improved confidence, motivation, and excitement in the learning process.

Brettle and Raynor (2013) compared student information literacy learning outcomes for students enrolled in an online tutorial with one provided in a 1-hour face-to-face session. Learning activities included search techniques using keywords, Boolean operators, truncation, and synonyms. The results of the study demonstrated improved knowledge acquisition in both settings and no difference in the learning outcomes. The sample size was small (77 students), but the results are not surprising.

The results of the different studies indicate that we cannot develop information and health literacy skills by reading a book or listening to a lecture. Active learning must take place. Nurses must have domain knowledge, clinical experience, functional understanding of search skills, and be able to analyze, integrate, and apply knowledge to practice. We learn information literacy skills best with repeated practice, using a variety of search settings over time.

Critical Thinking and Clinical Reasoning

Information literacy is an integral component for critical thinking. Critical thinking is a difficult concept to define. It is a little like good nursing care, we know it when we see it, but defining it in objective terms is complex. Consequently, the definition is the result of several different perspectives. Some say it is thinking about thinking. Others believe critical thinking is purposeful, goal directed, and that it requires the use of cognitive strategies to increase the probability of a desired outcome.

Breivik (1991) is responsible for seminal research on information literacy. She saw information literacy as a foundation for using critical thinking skills. Breivik stated, "In this information age, it does not matter how well people can analyze or synthesize; if they do not start with an adequate, accurate, and up-to-date body of information, they will not come up with a good answer" (1991, p. 226).

Critical thinking has two components: skill sets to process and generate information and the intellectual commitment to use those skills to guide behavior. Critical thinkers approach a problem logically from multiple angles. A vital part of critical thinking includes asking questions, knowing when one needs more information, developing and applying a plan for acquiring this information, and using the plan to generate knowledge. The plan can encompass searching for information in established databases, creating a database for information and knowledge, or both. The result improves outcomes based on information and knowledge. **Clinical reasoning** uses critical thinking skills. Clinical reasoning considers all factors influencing patient preferences by nurse care provider (Benner, Hughes, & Sutphen, 2008). The nurse uses clinical reasoning to determine pertinent factors to assist the patient to maintain or attain health.

Knowledge Generation

Integrating evidence-based literature with clinical information results in new **nursing knowledge**. Knowledge generation has two parts. In terms of clinical informatics, it refers to the knowledge that is developed from converting nursing data into information and reinterpreting it. The design of clinical information systems includes decision support systems that automate knowledge generation from clinical data. From the research perspective, knowledge generation starts with the application of the steps of information literacy—identifying, retrieving, appraising, and synthesizing nursing literature to solve nursing problems in new and better ways. Recognition of the nurse's role as a knowledge worker evolves from understanding both parts and their relationships to nursing practice. Information literacy and informatics are keys to knowledge work and generation.

Knowledge Dissemination Activities

The process of changing data from information into knowledge results in value across practice settings when knowledge is shared with others in the profession. Knowledge sharing allows nurses to influence nursing, drive health policy, and guide interdisciplinary health practices. The computer is a tool that facilitates knowledge dissemination in multiple ways. In a broad sense, raw data transferred between settings facilitate use of data with different nurse groups in a variety of ways.

After interpreting knowledge from data information, the findings are ready for publication and dissemination across the profession. Using the following types of software facilitates the process:

- Word processing to create a manuscript.
- Presentation and graphics programs to develop drawings or create a presentation or poster presentation.
- Spreadsheets to aggregate data and create charts.
- Databases to query, aggregate data, and create reports.
- Web development software to create web documents.
- Statistical software to analyze quantitative data.
- E-mail to collaborate and share nursing knowledge.
- Wikis and blogs to interact using web-based professional collaboration on nursing knowledge.

The maturation of professional nursing practice is dependent on the development and dissemination of nursing knowledge. Whether sharing information between two nurses or across the entire profession, use of information technology speeds the dissemination process.

INFORMATION TECHNOLOGY SKILLS

Information technology skills are necessary to support the application of information literacy. Information literacy is concerned with information seeking, access, content, communication, analysis, and evaluation, while information technology is concerned with an understanding of the technology and skills necessary for using it productively. Information technology skills require three kinds of knowledge: current skills, foundational concepts, and intellectual abilities (Association of Colleges and Research Libraries, 2000).

Current skills imply the ability to use up-to-date computer applications such as desktop applications and search tools. Foundational skills refer to understanding the underlying principles of computers, networks, and information. Current and foundational skills provide insight into the abilities as well as limitations of this technology in information management. The skills also provide the raw material for adapting to new information technology. The ability to apply information technology for problem solving requires intellectual capabilities that encompass abstract thinking about information and how data manipulation produces new understandings. Information technology skills combined with information literacy enable individuals to cope with unintended and unexpected problems when they occur.

DISCOVERING AND EVALUATING HEALTH INFORMATION ON THE INTERNET

Health information on the Internet is growing in abundance. Unfortunately, many of the websites have misleading and incorrect information. All Internet users must approach searching for health information through a systematic analytical review process. The evaluation process for a health information website should use the same basic principles for evaluating general websites, but health information websites require a higher standard of review, since health information can involve life and death issues. The National Library of Medicine has a variety of resources including links to tutorials and journal articles to assist evaluating health information at http://www.nlm.nih.gov/medlineplus/evaluatinghealthinformation.html.

Table 9-1 shows essential information that you should validate when using a website for health information. You should approach health information on the Internet with a certain amount of skepticism. If the information sounds too good to be true, it is probably not true.

> ## QSEN Scenario
> You are using an Internet search engine to find EBP information on genomics. What criteria will you use to evaluate the online resources?

Website Source

When reviewing a website with health information, the first criteria to investigate is the website source or sponsor. You can usually locate this information at the bottom of the homepage window or in a link for "About" or "Contact us." Look for sponsors without strong political or social bias. Health information sponsored by nonprofit organizations are often good resources.

Website Authority

The credibility of the website author is the second criteria to investigate when assessing sources of health information. Is the website author a recognized health information resource? Examples include the American Heart Association, The American Cancer Society, The American Diabetes Association, the Centers for Disease Prevention and Control (CDC), and the National Library of Medicine. Some healthcare provider practices sponsor websites with health information. If so, look for the names and credentials of the healthcare providers and the physical location of the office practices.

Many nursing organizations host websites with health information. Examples include the Oncology Nurses Society (ONS), The American Nurses Association (ANA), and the Emergency Nurses Association. In all cases, including websites sponsored by organizations and individuals, there should be a way to contact the author and make corrections or comments.

Website Funding

Funding is the third criteria to consider. Is the website sponsor a nonprofit or for-profit organization? Generally, websites with nonprofit support have less bias. The American Heart Association is an example of a nonprofit organization. The web address is http://www.heart.org. The ".org" usually refers to nonprofit status. You can also investigate the tax deductibility code. The tax code designation for nonprofit organizations is 501(c).

If the sponsor of the website is a commercial organization, consider the following questions. Do the advertisements have labels? Do the advertisements interfere with viewing the site? Do the advertisements represent any conflict of interest? An example of conflict of interest is if the website sponsor serves to gain a profit from advertisements. For the most part, it presents the reviewer's judgment call.

Website Validity and Quality

The fourth criterion to consider is the website validity and quality. Health information often changes, so look for a last update date. If you do not see the last update date specified, look at the copyright date. Abandoned websites usually have copyright years that are not current.

Look to see that a qualified editor reviewed the health information. For example, if you look at any

TABLE 9-1	Health Information Website Checklist	
Piece of Information	**Questions to Ask**	**Check**
1. Source	• Who is the website sponsor? Who is the website owner?	
2. Authority	• Who is the author? Are the author's credentials noted? Is the author an expert in the subject area? Is the author qualified to write the information? • What is the author's affiliation? • Is there a link that will allow the user to contact the author?	
3. Funding	• Is the site a not-for-profit site? • Is there any commercial funding? • Are there any potential conflicts of interest? • Are there any advertisements on the site, if so, are they clearly labeled?	
4. Validity and quality	• Is the site last update date specified? • Is there a clear statement of the website purpose? • Is the information accurate and referenced to current scholarly nursing and medical resources? • Is the information current? • Is the information peer reviewed or verified by a qualified editor? • Is the site free from content and typing errors? • Is the information free from bias and opinion? • Are all the links to quality reputable resources?	
5. Privacy and disclosure	• Does the site include an easy to understand privacy statement or nondisclosure agreement? • Does the site meet a recognized privacy standard, such as "Health on the Net" (http://www.hon.ch/)?	

website topic at MedlinePlus (http://www.nlm.nih.gov/medlineplus/), you will see a last update date posted at the bottom of the window. If you click on a specific subtopic for a condition, you can see the name of the content reviewer posted at the bottom of the website window.

Also, assess the ability to navigate the website easily. When clicking on a link that opens a different website, does a new window open? Is the menu the same for each page of the website?

Finally, look for confusing writing, spelling errors, and broken links. Editors review high-quality websites. The website should be error free.

Website Privacy and Disclosure

Finally, consider the website privacy. Is there a privacy statement that most visitors will understand? Look for a "Privacy" link at the bottom or top of the webpage. Read the privacy information. A credible website should state that the site does not collect any personally identifiable information. You can anticipate that websites will collect anonymous analytical data that assist the website sponsors to make improvements to the website. See the MedlinePlus privacy statement at http://www.nlm.nih.gov/medlineplus/privacy.html as an example.

The Health on the Net Foundation (http://www.hon.ch/) is a recognized privacy standard for websites with health information. The HONcode icon certifies website health information quality. The types of codes/icons vary by user status, patients or individuals, medical professionals, and website publishers. The HONsearch feature allows you to search for reliable and trustworthy websites with health information. The HONcode toolbar allows you to download a toolbar to add to the Internet Explorer and Firefox web browsers. After installing the toolbar, the HONcode toolbar icon is gray for noncertified HONcode website. It turns changes to blue, red, and white colors for HONcode-certified sites. Many excellent health information websites do not have the HONcode certification; however, the code assists users because it signals verification of quality.

NURSING INFORMATION ON THE INTERNET

Nursing information on the Internet is a subset of health information. Nursing information addresses resources that enhance professional nursing expertise. Examples include websites with clinical practice information, print and online scholarly journal resources. Other online resources cover laws, rules, and regulations related to nursing practice. You can also find information about nursing education programs; government sponsored and not-for-profit health and disease specialty organizations; nursing professional organizations and continuing education resources; and evidence-based nursing resources. This list serves to provide the wide scope of resources designed to enhance nursing practice.

Clinical Practice and Informatics

Information literacy, knowledge generation, and knowledge dissemination activities are integral parts of all nursing roles. Few nurses will become informatics nurse specialists, but all nurses need an awareness and general understanding of the potential of the various applications. The nurse as a knowledge worker should embrace role-appropriate activities and processes.

Evidence-Based Practice for Nursing

STTI defines **evidence-based nursing** as "an integration of the best evidence available, nursing expertise, and the values and preferences of the individuals, families, and communities who are served" (Sigma Theta Tau International, 2005, para 5). The Institute of Medicine identifies use of EBP as a core competency for healthcare professionals (Greiner & Knebel, 2003). The Internet includes many resources that explain evidence-based nursing as well as evidence-based care guidelines. The Internet, however, is not a primary source for evidence-based nursing research. Although there are several excellent evidence-based nursing websites, STTI is striving to become a global leading source of information on evidence-based nursing. The "Resources" section of the STTI website http://www.nursinglibrary.org/vhl/pages/resources.html is an excellent place to begin searching the Internet for evidence-based guidelines and other evidence-based nursing resources.

PICO: Defining the Clinical Question

Use the PICO process to answer clinical questions with no definitive answers. Use the process to explore knowledge gaps in care practices and serves as a foundation for many translational research studies. For example, what is the best way to treat otitis media in children under the age of 5? How do symptoms of angina compare between women and men after the age of 65. Write out the PICO question.

Map the terms used in the PICO question with terms used in the library database. Ask a librarian for assistance as needed, because there are differences in search terminology for individual databases. Avoid using medical abbreviations and acronyms, such as PICC line or PEG, to avoid limiting searches. Computer databases are not able to make interpretations about the meaning of abbreviation, so always write out the meaning.

MEDLINE/PubMed, sponsored by the National Library of Medicine, is available at no charge from any computer with an Internet connection. You can search MEDLINE/PubMed using the PICO tool at http://pubmedhh.nlm.nih.gov/nlmd/pico/piconew.php (Figure 9-1). Yensen (2013) described using the MEDLINE/PubMed PICO search engine in an article for the Online Journal

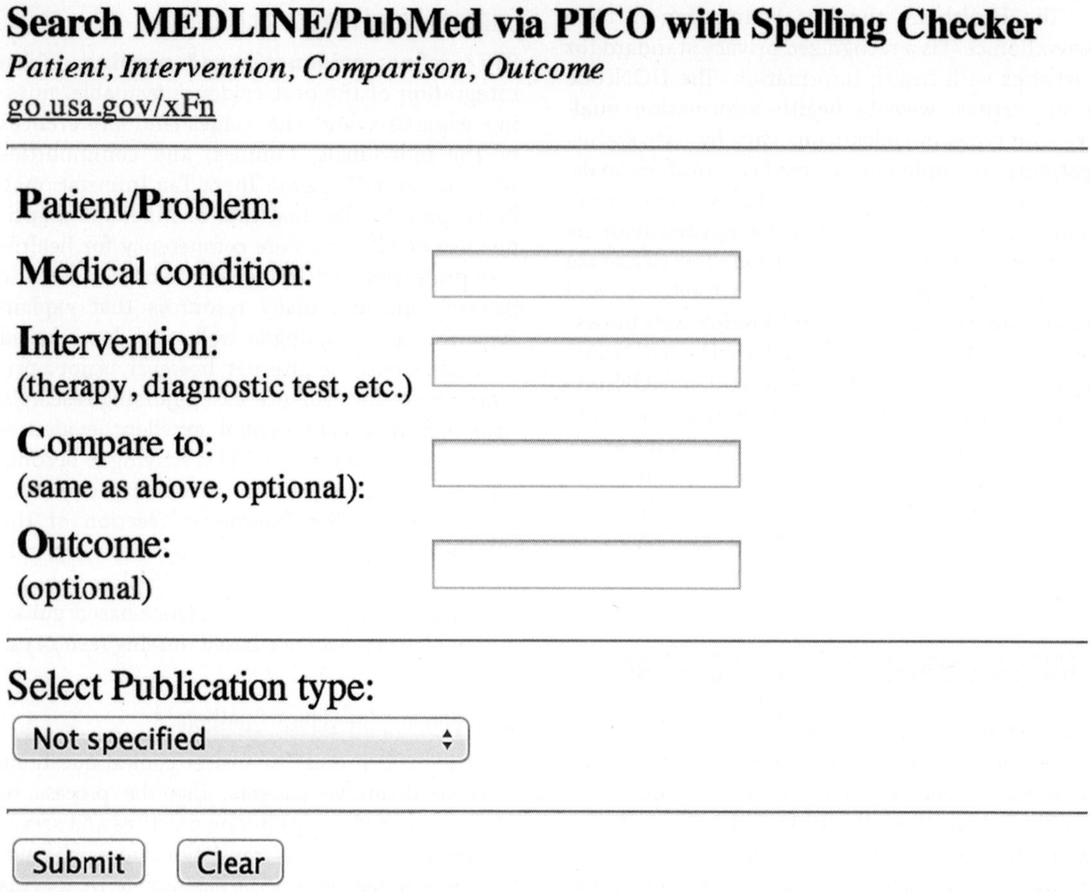

Search MEDLINE/PubMed via PICO with Spelling Checker

Patient, Intervention, Comparison, Outcome

go.usa.gov/xFn

Patient/Problem:

Medical condition:

Intervention:
(therapy, diagnostic test, etc.)

Compare to:
(same as above, optional):

Outcome:
(optional)

Select Publication type:

Not specified ▲▼

Submit   Clear

Figure 9-1. MEDLINE/PubMed PICO search tool. (Reprinted from National Library of Medicine.)

of Nursing Informatics (OJNI) at http://ojni.org/issues/?p=2860. The article includes screen shots and visuals on how to use the PICO search tool. The PICO search engine allows you to select a research study type, which are levels of evidence. There are seven levels of research evidence (Melnyk & Fineout-Overholt, 2011). Figure 9-2 collapses the seven levels into five, where expert opinion is the lowest level, and systematic reviews (and meta-analyses) are the highest level of research evidence. Systematic reviews involve a critical analysis of a grouping of research studies addressing a specific research question to inform healthcare decision making (Green et al., 2011). The systematic methods used minimize bias of the reviews. The Cochrane Library (http://www.thecochranelibrary.com), discussed in Chapter 10, is the gold standard when searching for systematic reviews that support EBP.

Notice that the levels of evidence in the MEDLINE/PubMed PICO search tool are not in order according to levels of evidence. For more information on research studies and levels of research evidence, go to http://nnlm.gov/training/evidencebased/PICO/PICOunderstandingresearchstudies.pdf

The National Library of Medicine has several tutorials on using PICO to define clinical questions and EBP. Since updates for the resources are ongoing, go to http://www.nlm.nih.gov/ and enter the search term "PICO" into the search window to find the most current instructional information.

Innovations to Support Translational Research

In nursing education, the PhD (doctorate of philosophy) students conduct new investigative research

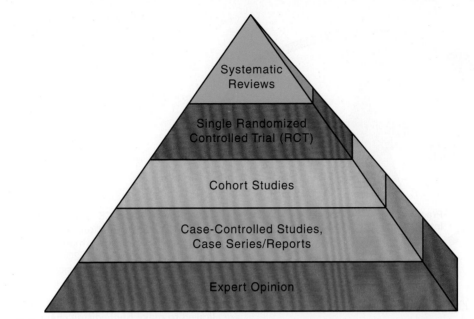

Figure 9-2. Levels of research evidence. (Reprinted from Nield-Gehrig, J. S., & Willmann, D. E. (2012). *Foundations of periodontics for the dental hygienist* (3rd ed.). Baltimore, MD: Lippincott Williams & Wilkins, with permission.)

studies that serve as a foundation for translational studies. The doctor of nursing practice (DNP) students apply the investigative research findings in the clinical practice settings. The outcome for translational research is to translate or facilitate implementing research finding into the practice setting.

As noted earlier, it takes almost a couple of decades for the translation of research findings into practice. The purpose for the creation of NCATS (National Center of Advancing Translational Sciences) in December 2011 was to speed the process implementing research findings into practice. NCATS has teams of investigative scientists. It provides grants to support innovation.

Mulnard's translational research is an example of nursing research supported by NCATS. Mulnard (2011) wanted to know whether estrogen replacement therapy might benefit women with mild-to-moderate Alzheimer disease. At the time of the study, some providers were prescribing estrogen use as a preventative measure. The outcome of the study was that there was no benefit from estrogen replacement therapy. After

publication of the negative results, support for use the estrogen replacement therapy declined.

Nursing Evidence-Based Practice and the ACE Star Model of Knowledge Transformation

The ACE Star Model of Knowledge Transformation seen in Figure 9-3 (Stevens, 2012) depicts EBP as a cyclical process of moving knowledge from original research into patient care. (ACE is short for the Academic Center for Evidence-Based Practice at the University of Texas Health Science Center San Antonio.) To begin this process, the discovery step involves a synthesis of original research studies, which produces an evidence summary. The goal of an evidence summary is to provide the best evidence of effectiveness by summarizing an entire body of studies. The process involves identifying pertinent research evidence through a critical appraisal of original studies using defined questions. Best practice guidelines use translation of evidence clinical settings. After integration of the guidelines, they can be evaluated in terms of patient outcomes, health status, efficiency, satisfaction, and economic factors. Conclusions from the evaluation stage may lead to more research.

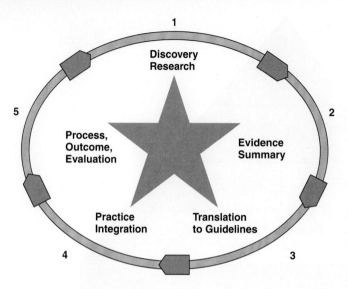

Figure 9-3. ACE Star Model of knowledge transformation. ACE Star Model of Knowledge Transformation. (Copyrighted material [Stevens, 2012]. Reproduced with expressed permission.)

Scholarly Journal Articles

Although academic libraries provide the most comprehensive nursing and medical knowledge, many nursing and medical journals and full-text scholarly journal articles are also available on the Internet. Most print journals have an online presence. Online journals with no print version also exist.

It is important to differentiate a scholarly article from news or magazines. Scholarly articles usually have an abstract and include references. The name and credentials of the author(s) are listed in the article. When using a library database, you can limit your search options to include resources that are peer reviewed. The search findings will indicate that the article was peer reviewed. The Sojourner Truth Library of the State University of New York New Paltz provides an excellent resource to assist users to identify scholarly articles at http://library.newpaltz.edu/assistance/scholar.html.

Only qualified nurses with expertise in the subject area write scholarly journal articles for publication in **scholarly nursing journals**. The peer review process for scholarly journals is rigorous. Once received by the editorial office, the journal's editor screens each article. If the editor considers the subject matter appropriate for the journal readers, the editor sends a copy with the author(s) name(s) removed (sometimes called a blind review) to two or more nurse experts for review to assure the validity, quality, and reliability of information. If the article receives approval for publication, the author(s) is/are allowed to make final editing changes based on the comments of the reviewers and editors.

Online Journals

True online journals publish all of their articles online with no print version. They feature **peer-reviewed articles** and maintain an archive of the articles. Bibliographic databases, such as Cumulative Index to Nursing and Allied Health Literature (CINAHL) and Medline, index some online journals. Most online journals feature articles in HTML format or portable document format (PDF), which requires Adobe Acrobat Reader to view. The number of free online nursing journals continues with a slow growth.

In June 1996, Kent State University College of Nursing Faculty in conjunction with the American Nurses Association (ANA) first published the *Online Journal for Issues in Nursing* (OJIN) (http://nursingworld.org/OJIN/). ANA now sponsors OJIN. The focus of OJIN is to provide different views on current topics relating to nursing practice, research, and education. OJIN is peer reviewed and indexed in both CINAHL and Medline. The *Online Journal of Nursing Informatics* (OJNI) at http://www.ojni.org/current.html focuses on topics relating to nursing informatics. OJNI is peer reviewed and indexed in CINAHL. Healthcare Information and Management Systems Society (HIMSS) now sponsors OJNI.

Several factors affect online journals. One difficulty with online journals is the perception that the quality of their content is lower than that of print journals. A few bibliographic indexes still categorically refuse to index such journals. Part of this perception may result from the great variability in online journals; part is a belief among some academics that only print journals have peer-reviewed articles. This perception is changing as the realization that online journals can be, and often are, peer-reviewed permeates the understanding of faculty.

Writing for publication in an online journal can present a dilemma, given that most writers are members of academic faculties who need publication in recognized journals to gain promotion and tenure. The number of articles published and the reputation of the publishing journal are important considerations for many promotion guidelines. This makes publishing in an online journal risky for faculty who are seeking tenure. These perceptions can affect the quality of writers who write articles in online journals and therefore the quality of the articles these writers produce.

Another difficulty with online journals that are not indexed by a service such as EBSCO or Embase is nurses' lack of awareness that the journals exist. Although nurses in all specialties need to be information literate, many are not. A person who has not learned how to use the web is limited to print journals. In addition, search engine results do not necessarily make a distinction between a scholarly print journal with a web presence and a true online journal, magazine, or newspaper. The user might simply conclude that no online journals exist because the results of an Internet search are overwhelming and lead to many false links.

Unlike print journals, which are the product of a publishing company, most online journals started with little financial or organizational support. As a result, the lifecycle of some online journals is short. Although it may seem easy to run an online journal, a large amount of work is involved in producing one of high quality. The journal staff must find writers, reviewers, and persons to coordinate the progress of articles; someone to convert the articles to an online format; and staff to market the journal. The journal overhead includes staff salaries and office expenses. All these tasks and responsibilities take time and money. Without a strong financial backing, sustaining publication of the journal can become insurmountable.

Open Access Journals

Open access journals publish peer-reviewed articles with no user fees. Many open access journals have limited copyright/licensing restrictions and allow anyone with an Internet connection to download, copy, and distribute the articles. BMC Nursing, at http://www.biomedcentral.com/bmcnurs/ is a peer-reviewed online open access journal that publishes research on topics relating to nursing research, training, practice, and education. Access to full text articles from other medical journals is available from Free Medical Journals at http://freemedicaljournals.com/, BioMed Central at http://www.biomedcentral.com/browse/journals/, and the Directory of Open Access Journals (DOAJ) at http://doaj.org/. The MERLOT Journal of Online Learning and Teaching (JOLT) at http://jolt.merlot.org/ is a peer-reviewed journal, with articles about the scholarly use of multimedia resources in education.

Some open access journals charge processing fees to author(s) to cover publishing costs. In fact, some high-quality journals may charge several thousand dollars to publish an article. As a result, the publication setting shifts from high-priced journal subscriptions/copies of journal articles to one where there is high-priced publication costs for the author(s). The pay to publish issue is currently under ethical debate. Those that support open access publication state that people have the right to have access to current research, thus facilitating scientific progress (Parker, 2013; Willinsky & Alperin, 2011). Research is available to low-income areas in the world. It is unethical to limit access to high-quality research due to the cost of publisher fees required to read the articles.

Those who are against open access journals suggest that the high costs for publication for the author create an economic divide where authors who cannot afford the costs of publication lose out against others who can (Parker, 2013; Willinsky & Alperin, 2011). There is no proof that access to current research on open access journals fosters further high-quality research more quickly. Another ethical issue is that open access publishing has spurred the growth of numerous questionable open access journals. Beall maintains a listing of questionable open access journals and the criteria that determines which journals are included in that list at http://scholarlyoa.com/individual-journals/.

Open Access Journal Articles Resulting from Grant Funding

Beginning in 2005, several research funding organizations began to mandate unrestricted open access to publications resulting from grant funding (MIT Libraries, 2014). As a result, many high-quality research articles published in peer-reviewed print and open access journals are available. The trend for mandating open access to publications from grant funding continues to grow in the United States (US), Canada, United Kingdom, and Europe. For example, in 2007, President Bush signed a bill requiring that NIH (National Institutes of Health) mandate open access to publications resulting from NIH funding. As of 2013, U.S. federal agencies granting more than $100 million had to mandate publications resulting from research funding open access and available within 1 year. As a result of the mandates, much high-quality peer-reviewed research is available from the U.S. National Library of Medicine PubMed website at http://www.ncbi.nlm.nih.gov/pubmed/.

Print Journals with a Web Presence

Full-text digital versions of print journal articles are often available online as a personal subscription benefit of the printed journal or a small fee for nonsubscribers. For more information on how to download full-text articles, go to the print journal website. The journal website includes instructions with how users with a personal subscription can activate their online subscription accounts. The online presence of print journals also allow nonsubscribers who want to purchase and download articles, how to set up an account where they can purchase the journal articles.

Articles from Internet Search Engine Results

Internet search engines such as Google (http://google.com) or Google Scholar (http://scholar.google.com/) may reveal many journal articles. When searching for journal article resources using the Internet consider using Google Scholar. On the Google Scholar homepage, you can select the met-

rics icons and Health and Medical Sciences from the opening window to view the journals that the search engine uses. If you select the preferences icon on the Google Scholar homepage, you can set preferences for the search engine to search up to five other library links (Open World Cat is the default library). In addition, if you use a reference manager, Google Scholar allows you configure the search engine to show links so that you can directly import the citations into your reference manager.

The search engines can find free full-text journal articles from websites such as Medscape (http://www.medscape.com/) and FindArticles (http://findarticles.com/). Medscape, sponsored by WebMD, is free but requires a login and password. The FindArticles website includes a few nursing journal articles and some from magazines and newsletters. When researching for scholarly papers, consider using a search engine, such as Google Scholar, in addition to academic library searches, but never in place of academic searches.

Scholarly Article Versus Magazine, Newsletter, Newspaper, or Website

Most online magazines and newsletters are available without charge because of advertising support. Generally, they address current topics such as career information, jobs, and news items of interest to their audience. Only a few magazines maintain archives. Magazine information on sites with no archives has a very short life. Users must be extremely cautious when using a search engine because many of the results link to magazines and other websites that are not scholarly resources. It is critically important for nurses to be able to differentiate a scholarly nursing article from an article in a magazine, a newspaper, or a website.

In contrast to the peer review process of scholarly articles, reporters write magazine, newsletters, and newspaper articles. Nurses or reporters may write magazine articles. Reporters are not required to be nurses or to have any expertise in nursing practice. Editors review and approve content to publication. Magazines and other news media may not cite specific references. Examples of magazines include ADVANCE for Nurses (http://nursing.advanceweb.com/), ADVANCE for Nurse Practitioners (http://nurse-practitioners-and-physician-assistants.advanceweb.com/), and

ALLnurses (http://allnurses.com). The information in online magazines and newsletters varies in quality, which is why nurses should carefully scrutinize websites using a checklist such as the Health Information Checklist (see Table 9-1).

Government and Not-for-Profit Health and Disease Specialty Organizations

Government-sponsored and not-for-profit health and disease specialty organizations include quality information that enhances nursing knowledge. Information for a few popular sites follows. The National Institutes of Health (NIH) (http://www.nih.gov/) has links to the associated 28 specialty institutes and centers providing information to the latest research, clinical trials, and grants to promote health. The Centers for Disease Control and Prevention (CDC) (http://www.cdc.gov/) provides statistical data, information about diseases and disease control, and online disease control and prevention journals. CDC Wonder (http://wonder.cdc.gov/) provides searchable online databases with public health data, morbidity tables, and Healthy People 2020. The Agency for Healthcare Research and Quality (http://www.ahrq.gov/) provides information on EBP, grants, research, and quality and patient safety issues. Finally, the Centers for Medicare and Medicaid Services (CMS) (http://www.cms.gov) provides access to manuals, Medicare coverage database, CMS forms, communication of policy changes, and Medicare Learning network resources.

Professional Nursing Organizations

Each professional nursing organization has a website with general information for the public and password-protected information for its members. For example, the ANA website, http://nursingworld.org/, includes membership information and links to purchase the nursing code of ethics and the scope and standards of practice for nursing specialties. The ANA also includes links to information on continuing education modules, individual and Magnet certification; ANA-sponsored nursing journals and books; healthcare policy and much more.

Sigma Theta Tau International (STTI) honor society for nursing (http://www.nursingsociety.org/) has membership information, links to STTI-sponsored journals and books, and continuing education modules. One distinctive factor for the STTI website is the link to the Virginia Henderson Global Nursing eRepository (http://www.nursinglibrary.org/vhl/). The eRepository includes an online comprehensive nursing resources. Examples of resources include grants, research, full text journal article and data sets, doctor of nursing practice final projects, theses, and learning objects created by faculty.

Laws, Rules, and Regulations

Several sites relate to laws, rules, and regulations. The National Council of State Boards of Nursing (NCSBN) (https://www.ncsbn.org/index.htm) includes links to all U.S. state boards of nursing and includes information about the National Council Licensure Examination (NCLEX). Each state board of nursing site includes clearly stated laws, policies, and rules and regulations. The state boards of nursing websites also provide services for license verification and license renewal online. Other regulatory websites include The Joint Commission (http://www.jointcommission.org/), the Centers for Medicare and Medicaid (CMS) (http://www.cms.hhs.gov/), and individual state departments of health and human services.

Online Evidence-Based Resources

The Internet has an abundance of information about evidence-based care resources. As with other healthcare information found on the Internet, the variation in quality is tremendous. The first step toward approaching a search for evidence-based care is to determine what you want to learn. You can find some of the most comprehensive websites in libraries and educational EBP centers. Clinical practice guidelines are available from government and educational websites in the United States, Canada, England, and Australia. Table 9-2 provides a starting point for nurses and healthcare professionals beginning to learn about EBP.

SUMMARY

Nurses and healthcare providers have an obligation to become proficient in the use of information and health literacy skills as well as information

TABLE 9-2 Evidence-Based Practice Information on the Internet	
Evidence-Based Practice Topic	**Websites and URLs**
Definition and history	• *Crossing the quality chasm: A new health system for the 21st century* (2001), Chapter 6: http://www.nap.edu/openbook.php?isbn=0309072808
Core competencies	• *Health professions education: A bridge to quality* (2003), Chapter 3: http://www.nap.edu/catalog.php?record_id=10681
Education resources	• EBP (Interactive Tutorial): http://www.biomed.lib.umn.edu/learn/ebp/ • Center for Evidence-Based Medicine: http://ktclearinghouse.ca/cebm/
Evidence-based nursing	• Sigma Theta Tau International: http://www.nursing-society.org/
Clinical practice guidelines	• AHRQ Clinical Practice Guidelines Online: http://www.ahrq.gov/professionals/clinicians-providers/guidelines-recommendations/index.html • The Community Guide: http://www.thecommunityguide.org/ • Nursing Best Practice Guidelines (Registered Nurses of Ontario): http://rnao.ca/bpg • Joanna Briggs Institute: Best Practice Information Sheets: http://wacebnm.curtin.edu.au/information/
Types of research (how to read, evaluate, and use)	• What is critical appraisal?: http://www.medicine.ox.ac.uk/bandolier/painres/download/whatis/What_is_critical_appraisal.pdf • Nursing research: Show me the evidence (The St. Joseph Hospital blog): http://evidencebasednursing.blogspot.com/

technology skills for several reasons. Nurses should be able to guide the patients and their families to obtain health information using the Internet. The standards for health information on the Internet must meet a much higher standard than any other types of information because inaccuracies have the potential to impact patient injury, illness, and death.

Undergraduate nursing programs must introduce information literacy skills. As with all skills, nurses must practice it in a variety of settings over time. Expertise in health literacy depends on the development of nursing domain knowledge, experience, information technology skills, critical thinking, and knowledge dissemination skills. Information literacy is an integral component of evidence-based nursing practice.

The Institute of Medicine and professional nursing organizations recommend using EBP to improve patient care outcomes. In theory, EBP is widely accepted, but practice of EBP is not universal in all education and clinical practice settings. Knowledge deficits about how to access, search, and synthesize literature findings has slowed implementation. Moreover, nurses in some clinical settings prefer to consult colleagues seen as having clinical expertise rather than analyze clinical and literature findings.

The good news is that abundant health information and EBP resources are available on the Internet. The Internet opens endless learning opportunities to nursing and healthcare providers who use analytical skills to scrutinize online resources for value.

APPLICATIONS AND COMPETENCIES

1. Identify any obstacles that interfere with the adoption of evidence-based resources in nursing practice in your clinical or healthcare agency work setting. Discuss how nurses can successfully address those obstacles.

2. Discuss the differences between the relationships between information literacy, health literacy, and information technology skills. Give examples of each and describe the significance to nursing.

3. Identify a resource(s) for writing a clinical research question using PICO. Write the question using the components of PICO. Use the MEDLINE/PubMed PICO search tool. Summarize the PICO process and research finding results.

4. Identify a website with nursing knowledge and identify the essential elements for validating the knowledge.

5. Find healthcare examples for each of the following and discuss the differences:

   a. online scholarly nursing article

   b. article in a nursing magazine

   c. newspaper

   d. newsletter

   e. Website

6. Identify one EBP nursing resource you found by searching the Internet. Discuss how you used information literacy skills to find and evaluate healthcare information you found.

REFERENCES

American Association of Colleges of Nursing. (2006, March 13). *Position paper: Nursing research*. Retrieved from http://www.aacn.nche.edu/publications/position/nursing-research

Association of College and Research Libraries. (2013, October). *Information literacy competency standards for nursing*. Retrieved from http://www.ala.org/acrl/standards/nursing

Association of Colleges and Research Libraries. (2000). *Information literacy competency standards for higher education*. Retrieved from http://www.ala.org/ala/mgrps/divs/acrl/standards/standards.pdf

Beke-Harrigan, H., Hess, R., & Weinland, J. A. (2008). A survey of registered nurses' readiness for evidence-based practice: A multidisciplinary project. *Journal of Hospital Librarianship, 8*(4), 440–448. doi: 10.1080/15323260802382794.

Benner, P., Hughes, R. G., & Sutphen, M. (2008). Clinical reasoning, decisionmaking, and action: Thinking critically and clinically. In R. G. Hughes (Ed.), *Patient safety and quality: An evidence-based handbook: AHRQ Publication No. 08–0043*. Retrieved from http://www.ncbi.nlm.nih.gov/books/NBK2643/

Boudin, F., Nie, J. Y., Bartlett, J. C., et al. (2010). Combining classifiers for robust PICO element detection. *BMC Medical Informatics and Decision Making, 10*, 29. doi: 10.1186/1472-6947-10-29.

Breivik, P. S. (1991). Information literacy. *Bulletin of the Medical Library Association, 79*(2), 226–229. Retrieved from http://www.pubmedcentral.nih.gov/picrender.fcgi?artid=225527&blobtype=pdf

Brettle, A., & Raynor, M. (2013). Developing information literacy skills in pre-registration nurses: An experimental study of teaching methods. *Nurse Education Today, 33*(2), 103–109. doi: 10.1016/j.nedt.2011.12.003.

Caldwell, P. H., Bennett, T., & Mellis, C. (2012). Easy guide to searching for evidence for the busy clinician. *Journal of Paediatrics and Child Health, 48*(12), 1095–1100. doi: 10.1111/j.1440-1754.2012.02503.x

Chartered Institute of Library and Information Professionals (CILIP). (2013, July 15). Information literacy - definition. Retrieved from http://www.cilip.org.uk/sites/default/files/documents/Information%20literacy%20skills.pdf

Flood, L. S., Gasiewicz, N., & Delpier, T. (2010). Integrating information literacy across a BSN curriculum. *Journal of Nursing Education, 49*(2), 101–104. doi: 10.3928/01484834-20091023-01

Fox, S. (2007, October 8). *E-patients with a disability or chronic disease*. Retrieved July 30, 2011 from, http://www.pewinternet.org/Reports/2007/Epatients-With-a-Disability-or-Chronic-Disease.aspx

GoodQuotes.com. (2010). *In times of rapid change e ... by J. Paul Getty*. Retrieved from http://www.goodquotes.com/quote/j-paul-getty/in-times-of-rapid-change-experience-co

Green, S., Higgins, J. P. T., Alderson, P., et al. (2011). Cochrane handbook for systematic reviews of interventions. In J. P. T. Higgins & S. Green (Eds.), *Chapter 1: Introduction: The Cochrane collaboration*. Retrieved from http://handbook.cochrane.org/

Greiner, A. C., & Knebel, E. (Eds.). (2003). *Health professions education: A bridge to quality*. Washington, DC: National Academy Press.

Institute of Medicine (U.S.). Committee on Quality of Health Care in America. (2001). *Crossing the quality chasm: A new health system for the 21st century*. Washington, DC: National Academy Press. Retrieved from http://www.nap.edu/openbook.php?isbn=0309072808

Jeffrey, L., Hegarty, B., Kelly, O. et al. (2011). Developing digital information literacy in higher education: Obstacles and supports. *Journal of Information Technology Education, 10*, 383–413. http://www.jite.org/documents/Vol10/JITEv10p383-413Jeffrey1019.pdf

Ku, Y., Sheu, S., & Kuo, S. (2007). Efficacy of integrating information literacy education into a women's health course on information literacy for RN-BSN students. *Journal of Nursing Research, 15*(1), 67–77.

Melnyk, B. M., & Fineout-Overholt, E. (2011). *Evidence-based practice in nursing & healthcare: A guide to best practice* (2nd ed.). Philadelphia, PA: Wolters Kluwer Health// Lippincott Williams & Wilkins.

Melnyk, B. M., Fineout-Overholt, E., Stillwell, S. B., et al (2010). Evidence-based practice: Step by step: The seven steps of evidence-based practice. *American Journal of Nursing, 110* (1), 51–53. doi: 10.1097/01.NAJ.0000366056.06605.d2.

MIT Libraries. (2014). *Research funder policies and related legislation*. Retrieved from http://libraries.mit.edu/scholarly/publishing/research-funders/#OAUK

Morris, Z. S., Wooding, S., & Grant, J. (2011). The answer is 17 years, what is the question: Understanding time lags in translational research. *Journal of the Royal Society of Medicine (JRSM), 104*(12), 510–520. doi: 10.1258/jrsm.2011.110180.

Mulnard, R. A. (2011). Translational research: Connecting evidence to clinical practice. *Japan Journal of Nursing Science, 8*(1), 1–6. doi: 10.1111/j.1742-7924.2011.00184.x.

National Institute of Nursing Research (NINR). (2014). *What is nursing research?*. Retrieved from http://www.ninr.nih.gov/

National League for Nursing. (2008). *Position statement: Preparing the next generation of nurses to practice in a technology-rich environment: An informatics agenda*. Retrieved from http://www.nln.org/aboutnln/PositionStatements/informatics_052808.pdf

Parker, M. (2013). The ethics of open access publishing. *BMC Medical Ethics, 14*, 16. doi: 10.1186/1472-6939-14-16. Retrieved from http://www.biomedcentral.com/1472-6939/14/16

Pravikoff, D. S., Tanner, A. B., & Pierce, S. T. (2005). Readiness of U.S. nurses for evidence-based practice. *American Journal of Nursing, 105*(9), 40–51. Retrieved from http://journals.lww.com/AJNOnline/pages/default.aspx

Quality and Safety Education for Nurses. (2010). *Project overview/QSEN—Quality & safety education for nurses*. Retrieved from http://www.qsen.org/overview.php

Richardson, W. S., Wilson, M. C., Nishikawa, J., et al. (1995). The well-built clinical question: A key to evidence-based decisions. *ACP Journal Club, 123*(3), A12–A13. Retrieved from http://acpjc.acponline.org/

Ross, J. (2010). Information literacy for evidence-based practice in perianesthesia nurses: Readiness for evidence-based practice. *Journal of Perianesthesia Nursing, 25*(2), 64–70. doi: 10.1016/j.jopan.2010.01.007.

Sackett, D. L. (1997). Evidence-based medicine. *Seminars in Perinatology, 21*(1), 3–5.

Sackett, D. L., Haynes, B., Rosenberg, W., et al. (2000). *Evidence-based medicine: How to practice and teach EBM* (2nd ed.). Edinburgh, SA: Churchill Livingstone.

Sackett, D. L., Rosenberg, W. M. C., Gray, J. A. M., et al. (1996). Evidence based medicine: What it is and what it isn't. *British Medical Journal, 312*, 71. http://www.ncbi.nlm.nih.gov/pmc/articles/PMC2349778/

Sigma Theta Tau International. (2005, July 6). *Evidence-based nursing position statement*. Retrieved from http://www.nursingsociety.org/aboutus/PositionPapers/Pages/EBN_positionpaper.aspx

Stevens, K. R. (2012). *ACE Star Model of EBP: Knowledge transformation*. San Antonio, TX. Academic Center for Evidence-Based Practice. The University of Texas Health Science Center San Antonio.

Technology Informatics Guiding Education Reform. (2007). *TIGER phase II—collaborative report*. Retrieved from http://www.tigersummit.com/uploads/TIGER_Collaborative_Exec_Summary_040509.pdf

Westfall, J. M., Mold, J., & Fagnan, L. (2007). Practice-based research—"blue highways" on the NIH roadmap. *Journal of the American Medical Association (JAMA), 297*(4), 403–406. http://dx.doi.org/10.1001/jama.297.4.403 doi: 10.1001/jama.297.4.403.

Willinsky, J., & Alperin, J. P. (2011). The academic ethics of open access to research and scholarship. *Ethics and education, 6*(3). Retrieved from http://www.tandfonline.com/doi/abs/10.1080/17449642.2011.632716

Yensen, J. (2013). *Online Journal of Nuring Informatics (OJIN). 17*(3), 1, Retrieved from http://ojni.org/issues/?p=2860

CHAPTER 10

Finding Knowledge in the Digital Library Haystack

OBJECTIVES

After studying this chapter, you will be able to:

1. Compare nursing knowledge found in online library databases with that found using the Internet.
2. Discuss library bibliographic databases useful to nurses.
3. Demonstrate effective literature search strategies to support evidence-based practice.
4. Describe the use of personal reference management software.

KEY TERMS

Advanced search

Evidence-based care

Factual database

Federated search

Index

Keywords

Knowledge-based database

Medical subject headings (MeSH)

Meta-analysis

Personal reference manager

Randomized controlled trials

Research Information Systems (RIS)

Research practice gap

Seminal work

Stop words

Subject heading

Systematic review

Given the vast amount of published information, it is impossible to know everything applicable to nursing practice. Library online resources provide a pivotal gateway to knowledge discovery. To improve patient care and promote the scholarship of nursing, all nurses and healthcare providers must proactively develop and practice information search competencies. Without these, knowledge remains embedded in the digital haystack.

To assist with information searches, library vendors (indexing services) provide digital **indexes** of the literature. The literature indexes produce bibliographic databases, which you can search electronically. Bibliographic databases are replacements for the legacy print card catalogs and annual print indexes of the periodical literature. Electronic databases, not limited by paper, are generally more flexible and provide more information than print indexes. A user can retrieve information from electronic databases in the form of citations, abstracts and, in some cases, even full-text journal articles or full-text books. Online databases include many types of information and media resources.

DIGITAL LIBRARY BASICS

There are two types of digital databases: knowledge based and factual. **Knowledge-based databases** index published literature. **Factual databases** replace reference books with searchable and updatable online information—for example— drug and laboratory manuals. Knowledge-based databases focus on areas such as health sciences, business, history, government, law, and ethics. Furthermore, each database is specialized by the number and type of resources (e.g., journal or book names) indexed, the span of years indexed, and the words that the database uses to describe the resources for searching purposes.

Libraries purchase electronic databases from library vendors. Library vendors market and package their databases into bundles containing two or more separate databases. Libraries, therefore, may offer different electronic resources depending on the vendor and the database bundle that the library purchased. Each bundle of databases comes with a search interface window that identifies the vendor name. A few examples of library venders that package health science databases are EBSCO, Ovid, and ProQuest. Access to databases is essential for clinical nurses, nursing students, and faculty to stay current in the profession and to provide **evidence-based care**. Nurses should discuss their needs with their librarian to ensure access to the specific health science databases that allow them to improve clinical practice.

All healthcare professionals must be able to search online bibliographic databases. An index system used to file or catalog references provides the mechanism for library searches. You can search electronic databases using many different attributes such as title, author name, and year. There are many other ways to search an online bibliographic database. You can search for **keywords** found in a title, abstract, the text, or all of these. You can limit searches to finding sources by language, by age of subjects of a research article, by type of article, and by years of publication and in some databases to finding only those sources that provide full text. There may be times when it is helpful to conduct a **federated search**, which is a type of search that allows you to search several databases simultaneously. As an example, if you use EBSCOhost, look for a link, *Choose Databases by Subject*, located just above the Find field on the basic search screen.

Most search windows allow you to select a citation format and to save the search results. If there is an option for saving with a specific citation format, there will be a drop-down menu with the common formats such as the American Psychological Association (APA), the Modern Languages Association (MLA), and the American Medical Association (AMA). You can save search findings using print, e-mail, export to a **personal reference manager**, and/or save as a file onto the personal computer.

REFERENCE MANAGEMENT SOFTWARE

You can often export search findings into personal reference manager. A personal reference manager refers to database software that allows the user to create a personal collection of citations. Most digital library database interfaces include an export feature that allows the user to download citation information into reference management software. Other common reference manager features include the ability to store digital copies of full-text articles and the ability to cite sources and automatically generate a formatted reference list while writing with word processing software.

There are a number of commercial reference management products available—for example, Citavi (https://www.citavi.com/), EndNote (http://endnote.com/), Reference Manager (http://www.refman.com/), and RefWorks (http://www.refworks.com/). The citation information in reference managers can include hyperlinks to the associated resources on the computer, such as digital versions of articles, websites, or graphics.

There are several free reference managers comparable to commercial products. Zotero (2013) (http://www.zotero.org) is an open-source reference manager (see Chapter 2 for more on open source). Many free reference managers provide free cloud storage (see Chapter 4 for more on cloud computing) and the ability to share and collaborate with others. Mendeley (http://www.mendeley.com/) and CiteULike (http://www.CiteULike.org/) are two other popular free reference managers. Both are online personal cloud storage solutions for reference managers that allow users to store, organize, and share citation information (CiteUlike, 2014; Mendeley, 2014). Users must register for an account with a log-in and password. You can also import and export references from Mendeley and CiteULike to other personal reference management software. Wikipedia (2014) provides a comprehensive comparison of reference managers at http://en.wikipedia.org/wiki/Comparison_of_reference_management_software.

Personal reference managers that include the import/export feature provide an efficient means of managing citation information. However, reference managers integrated into word processing software may not be capable of importing citations from a digital library database. For example, Microsoft Word 2013, 365, and Apache OpenOffice Writer both include personal reference manager features; however, you must key in each citation separately.

LIBRARY GUIDES AND TUTORIALS

Even the most experienced library patrons can benefit from library guides and tutorials because the technology development for library resources continues to change rapidly. Lifelong learning for professional nursing must begin with demonstrated competencies in the use of digital library searches to discover new nursing knowledge. Nurses must integrate nursing knowledge, including evidence-based practice (EBP) findings, into clinical practice quickly to improve patient outcomes. Fortunately, there are numerous library guides and tutorials available on the Internet. The most efficient way to develop/improve library competencies is with the assistance of a librarian. Qualified librarians have a master's or doctoral degree with a specialization in an area of library science. The focus of their expertise and continuing education is to assist users in accessing and utilizing library resources.

To learn how to use a library facility, use the Internet to find the library's homepage. Information on a library web page generally includes the hours of operation, links to services and departments, information on how to find books and journals, and links to help resources such as guides and tutorials. Just-in-time learning using online library guides and tutorials is also an efficient way to develop/improve library information competencies. The guides and tutorials address how to use the specific library facility, how to search using subject headings including medical subject headings (MeSH) terms, how to use a vendor search interface, and how to use a specific database.

Subject Headings

Subject headings refer to standardized terms used to index or catalog reference materials. Each library chooses a standard subject authority or thesaurus for all of its cataloging. Libraries using the National Library of Medicine (NLM) classification use the "medical subject headings" or MeSH (http://www.nlm.nih.gov/mesh/).

Searching Using MeSH Terms

Each library database also uses a "controlled vocabulary" of terms (subject headings) to index the materials for database searches. **Medical subject headings (Mesh)** refers to the controlled vocabulary of terms used to index materials in PubMed and MEDLINE databases. Cumulative Index to Nursing and Allied Health Literature (CINAHL) subject headings follow the MeSH structure (CINAHL, 2014). Since CINAHL and MEDLINE are two primary databases with nursing literature, it is important to understand the search term structure. MeSH differs from many other subject-heading lists because the basis is a hierarchal structure, as shown in Box 10-1. Because of this structure, you can search on a broad subject that includes the narrower subjects in the MeSH tree structure. This search method as "explodes" the broader term to include all of the terms in the hierarchy.

Take a few minutes to understand how to use subject headings and MeSH terms before using a

Neoplasms
Neoplasms by site [C04.588]
   Abdominal neoplasms [C04.588.033] +
   Anal gland neoplasms [C04.588.083]
   Bone neoplasms [C04.588.149] +
   Breast neoplasms [C04.588.180]
     Breast neoplasms, male
   [C04.588.180.260]
     Carcinoma, ductal, breast
   [C04.588.180.390]

Reprinted from http://www.nlm.nih.gov/mesh/mbinfo.
html

search interface. The National Library of Medicine (NLM) provides a helpful online tutorial on using MeSH terms: http://www.nlm.nih.gov/bsd/disted/meshtutorial/introduction/.

Using a Search Interface

Taking time to review a search interface guide and tutorials before embarking on a literature search may prevent hours of frustration and disappointing results. To use a vendor search interface, use the Help menu. You will often find embedded tutorials and guides for its use. It is very important to understand that the search features for each library vendor differ. For example, the EBSCOhost includes a link to Help in the main menu at the top of the search window. The Help website has a very comprehensive listing of Help files that range from general information on database searching to online Flash videos and PowerPoint tutorials. The Ovid search window help provides training specifically for Ovid users, using interactive 1-hour web-based workshops on numerous topics. Ovid also provides an online self-paced tutorial. Table 10-1 provides the web pages for the tutorials for some of these bibliographic search tools.

When searching for nursing knowledge, be familiar with the way the vendor search engine handles Boolean terminology (AND, OR, and NOT). (See Chapter 8 for more information on Boolean searching.) Truncation and wildcards with the asterisk (*) and question mark (?) can be used with some search engines. Use truncation for searching spelling variations. For example, a search for nur* would result in citations with the words nurse and nursing. Use the question mark with a wildcard to replace a single unknown character or letter anywhere in the word. For example, a search for hea? results in citations with the words heat and head. Search engines generally do not search for **stop words**, such as articles and prepositions, unless they are a part of a phrase enclosed with quotes. Users should be aware of stop words ignored by the search engine (e.g., Box 10-2). For more information about stop words, go to http://nlp.stanford.edu/IR-book/html/htmledition/dropping-common-terms-stop-words-1.html.

Some vendor search engines, such as EBSCOhost, Ovid, or ProQuest, allow the user to

TABLE 10-1	Online Search Help Resources
Interface Help	**URL**
EBSCOhost	EBSCOhost research databases—http://support.ebsco.com/help/ Tutorials—http://support.epnet.com/training/tutorials.php
Ovid	OvidSP training—http://www.ovid.com/webapp/wcs/servlet/content_service_Training_13051_-1_13151
ProQuest	ProQuest Quick Start Reference Overview—http://www.proquest.com/assets/downloads/products/qsg_np.pdf
	ProQuest User Guide—http://www.proquest.com/assets/downloads/products/userguide_np.pdf

BOX 10-2	Examples of Stop Words			
After	Be	Like	Said	Through
Also	Do	Make	Should	To
An	Each	Many	So	Use
And	For	More	Some	Was

restrict online searches to peer-reviewed articles in scholarly journals, articles with references, articles with abstracts, research articles, or full-text articles. Peer-reviewed articles are excellent resources to support nursing knowledge. A journal is a scholarly publication that provides peer-reviewed articles. (See Chapter 9 for more information on the peer review process.) In contrast, articles in magazines, newsletters, and newspapers serve as points of information and entertainment, but you should never use them to support nursing knowledge.

BIBLIOGRAPHIC DATABASES PERTINENT TO NURSING

There are numerous databases with information pertinent to nursing. Essential ones with a focus on nursing and health-related topics are CINAHL, MEDLINE/PubMed, Cochrane Library, and PsycINFO/PsycARTICLES. Although there may be some overlap in the journals and resources these databases index, there are important differences that may affect the search outcome. Furthermore, there are variations for each of the databases for each library system: Some include only citations and abstracts and others contain varying numbers of full-text documents. Unless you are an experienced researcher, consult with a reference librarian to assist with refining your search question and selecting the best databases to search. See Table 10-2 for a list of databases according to nursing topic. The databases discussed in this table are commonly available through most medical and academic libraries.

Most vendor search interfaces and online libraries provide links to guides and tutorials for specific databases within the collection. Unfortunately, currently, there is no universal standard for indexing

health science search terms; each library database is unique. Unless you have expertise in using a particular library database, it is critical that you review a guide and tutorials first. The nuances in the search terminology and methods can be very tricky, especially for novice student nurses who are in the process of learning terminology. Table 10-3 provides the location of the tutorials for many of the bibliographic indexes that nurses need.

CINAHL

When researching a nursing topic, the CINAHL database is an excellent place to start. The CINAHL Complete database includes information for more than 50 nursing specialties and searchable cited references for more than 1,460 journals (CINAHL, 2014). CINAHL Plus with Full-Text database includes full-text articles in addition to citations and abstracts. The subject headings use the NLM MeSH structure. To identify search terms, click CINAHL Headings in the Menu bar and enter the word or phrase you are searching to get a list of the associated subject headings. CINAHL may also include selected full-text documents such as nursing journal articles, evidence-based care sheets, book chapters, newsletters, standards of practice, and nurse practice acts.

MEDLINE/PubMed

When researching a biomedical research topic that crosses healthcare disciplines, use MEDLINE in addition to CINAHL. MEDLINE, a service made available through the NLM, is unique from proprietary library databases because it is also a free service that is accessible on the Internet through PubMed. The NLM is the largest medical library in the world. MEDLINE provides access to over 5,600 journals worldwide and includes a comprehensive collection of citations from biomedical articles dating back to 1946 (National Library of Medicine, 2013, February 20). You can access MEDLINE through PubMed on the Internet at http://www.ncbi.nlm.nih.gov/PubMed/. PubMed includes citations to literature not yet included in MEDLINE in addition to other services. PubMed Central allows access to free full-text articles (PubMed Central, 2014).

PubMed provides a variety of free services. NLM Mobile at http://www.nlm.nih.gov/mobile/ provides software mobile apps. PubMed for

TABLE 10-2 Discovering Nursing Knowledge in Library Databases

Topic of Search Question	Examples of Databases to Search	Topic of Search Question	Examples of Databases to Search

Nursing	CINAHL
	Cochrane Library
	
	ProQuest Nursing and
	    Allied Health Source
	MEDLINE/PubMed
		Patient teaching	MedlinePlus
			HealthSource:
			    Consumer Edition
			Consumer Health
			    Complete
			Micromedex CareNotes

Biomedical research	MEDLINE/PubMed EMBASE CINAHL	Psychosocial	CINAHL PsycINFO PsycARTICLES
Education	ERIC CINAHL		Sociological Abstracts Sociological Collection
Legal/ethical	LexisNexis Academic CINAHL MEDLINE/PubMed	CINAHL	Cambridge Scientific Abstracts

Management
Oncology
	ABI/INFORM
	MEDLINE/PubMed
	National Cancer
	    Institute and
	    Physician Data
	    Query (PDQ)
	CINAHL
			CINAHL

TABLE 10-3 Online Help for Specific Library Databases

Online Help for Specific Library Databases	URL
CINAHL	http://support.ebsco.com/training/tutorials.php
Cochrane Library	http://www.thecochranelibrary.com/view/0/index.html
PsycINFO	http://scientific.thomson.com/tutorials/psycinfo2/
MEDLINE/PubMed	http://www.nlm.nih.gov/bsd/disted/pubmedtutorial/
	http://www.nlm.nih.gov/bsd/viewlet/search/subject/subject.html
	(MeSH) http://www.ncbi.nlm.nih.gov/sites/entrez?db=mesh

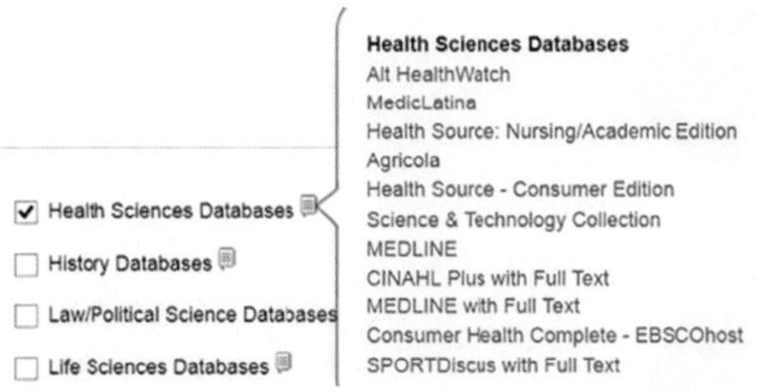

Health Sciences Databases
Alt HealthWatch
MedicLatina
Health Source: Nursing/Academic Edition
Agricola
Health Source - Consumer Edition
Science & Technology Collection
MEDLINE
CINAHL Plus with Full Text
MEDLINE with Full Text
Consumer Health Complete - EBSCOhost
SPORTDiscus with Full Text

☑ Health Sciences Databases
☐ History Databases
☐ Law/Political Science Databases
☐ Life Sciences Databases

Figure 10-1. PubMed4Hh app for handhelds. (Courtesy of the National Library of Medicine.)

Handhelds (PubMed4Hh) at http://pubmedhh. nlm.nih.gov/nlm/ is a website designed specifically for use with handheld computers. PubMed4Hh is also a free app for iOS and Android mobile devices (Figure 10-1). My National Center for Biotechnology Information (NCBI) at http://www. ncbi.nlm.nih.gov/entrez/cubby.fcgi? provides the ability to save users' information and preferences, search and store searches, as well as set email alerts of updates to saved searches (National Center for Biotechnology Information, 2014). My NCBI is free but requires new users to register and create a log-in and password.

> ## QSEN Scenario
>
> You are working on a nursing research paper on nanotechnology using the PubMed database. What search techniques should you use to find peer-reviewed literature on the topic?

Cochrane Library

When researching for a **systematic review** about a research question, use the Cochrane Library. Cochrane reports are useful to nursing students, practicing nurses, and nurse researchers. Nursing students and practicing nurses may not have the confidence and experience to analyze research without assistance of faculty or nurse researchers. The Cochrane Library, available through Wiley InterScience, is a gold standard for synthesis of medical research (Sackett et al., 1996).

In 2001, the Institute of Medicine (IOM) (Institute of Medicine & National Academy of Sciences, 2001) challenged healthcare providers to implement "systematic approaches to analyzing and synthesizing medical evidence for both clinicians and patients." The IOM recognized the Cochrane Collaboration, founded in 1993 by Dr. Archie Cochrane, as a model for synthesizing evidence to inform healthcare decision making.

Access to the library may be through the library digital database listing or by using a log-in and password provided by your local library. The Cochrane Library is online at http://www. thecochranelibrary.com. The Cochrane Library is available free in certain locations. For example, it is available free in many "low- and middle-income countries" (The Cochrane Library, 2013).

The design of a systematic review reduces three types of bias inherent in individual research studies: selection, indexing, and publication (South African Medical Research Council, 2013). The basis of selection bias is the person's point of view or knowledge. The cause of indexing bias is searches that use limited databases or search terms. Publishing bias results when searches are limited to certain publications or languages.

There are several types of literature reviews. Examples include meta-analysis, clinical inquiry, and integrative reviews. **Meta-analysis** is the process of systematic reviews. Researchers use systematic reviews to carefully review and analyze the results of multiple, similar research studies. Researchers conduct clinical inquiries when questioning and evaluating practice (American Association of Critical Care Nurses, 2014). The results may provide a basis for changes in practice. Integrative literature reviews address research questions using diverse research procedures and methods for retrieving, analyzing, and synthesizing literature (Im & Chang, 2012; Whittemore & Knafl, 2005). All types of reviews contribute to evidence-based nursing knowledge.

PsycINFO and PsycARTICLES

When researching a research question relating to psychology, behavior, and/or mental health, consider searching psychosocial databases, such as PsycINFO and PsycARTICLES, which are services of the American Psychological Association (APA). Both databases provide the most complete pertinent resources for knowledge discovery. PsycINFO provides citations and abstracts for psychology and psychosocial aspects of other disciplines (American Psychological Association, 2014a). PsycARTICLES provides access to full-text articles (American Psychological Association, 2014b).

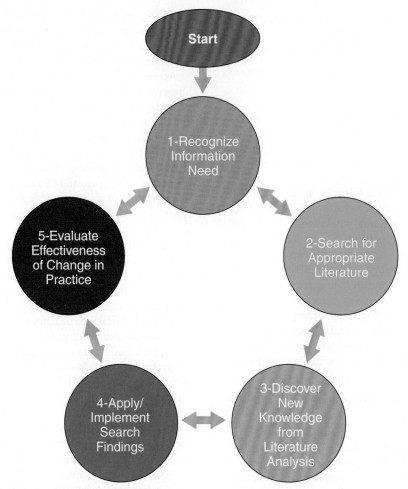

Figure 10-2. Knowledge quest.

EMBARKING ON THE QUEST FOR KNOWLEDGE

The quest for knowledge is a five-step process (Figure 10-2). The process is cyclical and iterative rather than linear. In other words, the researcher may go back and forth through the steps. Because the generation of new knowledge is continual, the quest process never stops.

Step 1: Questioning Practice: Recognizing an Information Need

The first step in the quest for knowledge is recognizing an information need. Questioning practice may be difficult, but we must find new means

for providing cost-effective care. A case in point is Medicare nonpayment for higher costs of care resulting from preventable hospital-acquired injuries such as patient falls and infections from medical errors (Centers for Medicare & Medicaid Services, 2013). Healthcare practices must change to make patients safe, and nurses must be involved in searches for solutions to improve care practices.

As an example of a quest for knowledge, consider conducting a literature search for information on prevention of patient falls. The search question is "How can patient falls be prevented in nursing?" Notice that the broad topic, patient falls, is narrowed using the terms prevention and nursing. A common search mistake is searching a very broad topic. Take a few moments to write out the search question to focus on the topic.

Although it is best to carefully define the information need before beginning the search, it is possible to allow the search engine to assist by allowing you to choose terms from a list of search terms.

Step 2: Searching for Appropriate Evidence

The literature search process is an essential skill that nursing professionals must learn and practice. It is vital to discovering nursing knowledge and developing EBP. The quest for new nursing knowledge involves discovering, understanding, analyzing, and applying findings from literature. The process for conducting a literature search must be systematic and comprehensive. To develop search strategies that lead you to the most useful information on your search question, use subject headings. Although ideas for changes in clinical practice may come from regular reading of the literature, it is supported by other articles and warrants a change in clinical practices (Price, 2009).

While searching, first determine the library databases that are most appropriate for the evidence for which you are searching and then identify the search terms that match that database. Selecting the most appropriate database(s) is just as important as the search strategy. If you are looking for peer-reviewed scholarly literature, use the online databases for libraries serving populations engaged in healthcare and education, and search databases and indexes such as CINAHL, MEDLINE, Cochrane Library, and Education Resources Information Center (ERIC). If you

are looking for patient teaching resources, use the online library databases and the Internet. Consider using MedlinePlus (http://www.nlm.nih.gov/medlineplus/), which is an NLM resource designed for healthcare consumers.

It is important to remember that a comprehensive search must never be limited to the Internet or online library full-text resources. Although you can find a wide range of information resources online, libraries, librarians, and bookstores are vital to help borrow or purchase the knowledge-based resources needed for nursing education and practice. If you cannot locate the resource in your library, you might be able to locate it using interlibrary loan.

The patient fall example uses the PubMed Advanced Search Builder window (http://www.ncbi.nlm.nih.gov/pubmed/advanced). After opening the PubMed database, select the **Advanced Search** option (Figure 10-3). (See your librarian if you need help gaining access to the database.) The advanced search option allows users to enter multiple search terms as well as define fields to narrow the search further. You can use the *Show index list* link for assistance with search terms. In this example, we used patient falls with double quotes to find only "patient falls" along with 'prevention' and 'nursing' (see Figure 10-3). A goal for an effective search is a return of 50 or less results.

The initial search on preventing patient falls for nursing, run in 2014, resulted in 144 citations; the most recent publication date was 2014. When the search was limited to academic journals, clinical

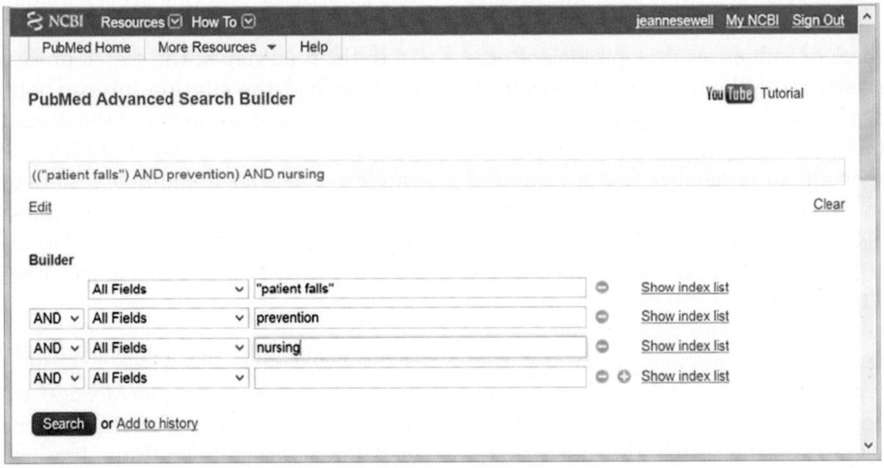

Figure 10-3. PubMed Advanced Search Builder—selecting search terms. (Courtesy of the National Library of Medicine.)

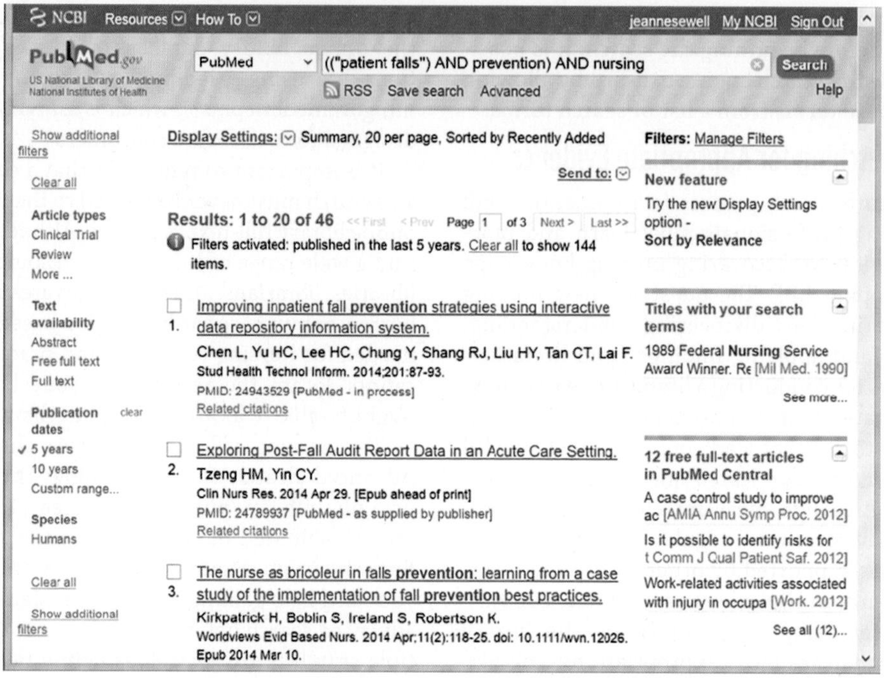

Figure 10-4. PubMed filter narrowing the search to publication dates within the last 5 years. (Courtesy of the National Library of Medicine.)

trials, or reviews from 2010 to 2014 (Figure 10-4), the result was 46 citations. The publication dates for the first four citations were in 2014. A rule of thumb is to use the most current citations for sources published within the past 3 to 5 years. A search for a classic journal article, for example, one that documents **seminal work** on a particular topic, may require searching into much older resources. Seminal work refers to work frequently cited by others or influences the opinions of others. The Sackett article about evidence-based medicine, cited in the section on the Cochrane Library in this chapter, is an example of seminal work.

It is important to remember that a computer determined the results of the search based on search terms. Although critical thinking is required for each step in the search process, it is especially important to analyze the information from the search results to make sure that it provides the appropriate evidence to answer the information need. Is the purpose of the search to advance nursing knowledge, advance EBP, or both? In order to set further limits on the search, the journal category was limited to nursing journals (Figure 10-5).

The search result was 26 citations and 8 were published between 2013 and 2014.

In the fall prevention example, the initial search used keywords. If the initial search is too narrow, you can expand it by modifying the filters. When narrowing the search once again by searching only the past 3 years of literature, the result was 21 articles. Filtering provides a quick method to limit and assist with analysis of the findings.

In the final step of the search process, you save or download the citation information for use in the analysis and summary of the literature search. By clicking *Send to* in the PubMed search return window, you can add multiple results to a file, collection, order, citation manager, clipboard, e-mail, or My Bibliography (Fig. 10-6). You can send the search to *My Bibliography* if you have an NCBI account.

Export to Reference Management Software

You can use *Send to Citation Manager* to export the search findings into any personal reference manager (e.g., Citavi, EasyBib, EndNote, ProCite, Reference Manager, or Zotero). The **Research Information**

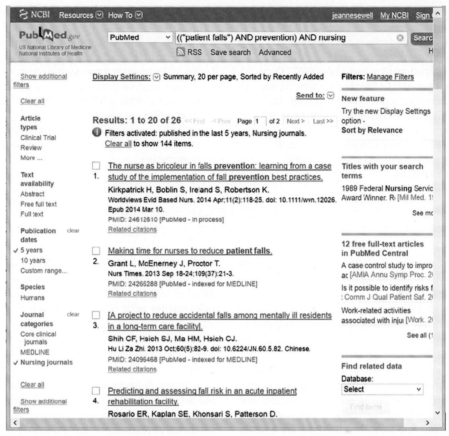

Figure 10-5. PubMed filter narrowing the search to nursing journals. (Courtesy of the National Library of Medicine.)

Systems (RIS) format is a standardized tag used by citation programs for data exchange (Reference Manager, 2011). When you click on the *Create File* button, a new window should open. Use the default program or choose another more appropriate application. The default export settings may vary by other library databases. Click the *OK* button to automati-cally export the citation metadata from PubMed into your citation manager. Metadata refers to all of the descriptors used to organize data for citations. For example, for a journal article, it includes the author(s), article title, journal name, volume, and issue number, year of publication, DOI (digital object identifier), and abstract.

Step 3: Critically Analyzing the Literature Findings

Critical analysis of the literature findings is the point in the process where you discover new knowledge. The first step is to select citations for articles that are possibly relevant to the information need and then obtain a full-text version of the articles. Review of the article abstract, reference list, and journal name are helpful to determine

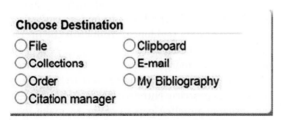

Figure 10-6. PubMed Save to destination choices. (Courtesy of the National Library of Medicine.)

> **BOX 10-3** Rating System for the Hierarchy of Evidence
>
> Level I: Evidence from a systematic review or meta-analysis of all relevant randomized controlled trials (RCTs) or evidence-based clinical practice guideline based on systematic review of RCTs.
>
> Level II: Evidence obtained from at least one well-designed RCT.
>
> Level III: Evidence obtained from well-designed controlled trials without randomization.
>
> Level IV: Evidence from well-designed case–control and cohort studies.
>
> Level V: Evidence from systematic reviews of descriptive and qualitative studies.
>
> Level VI: Evidence from single descriptive or qualitative study.
>
> Level VII: Evidence from the opinion of authorities and/or reports of expert committees.
>
> Reprinted from Melnyk, B. M., & Fineout-Overholt, E. (2015). *Evidence-based practice in nursing & healthcare: A guide to best practice* (3rd ed). Philadelphia, PA: Wolters Kluwer Health/Lippincott Williams & Wilkins, with permission.

which articles to read. Consult a librarian if you need assistance in finding full-text printable versions of the articles.

The next step is to read each article to analyze the findings critically. Highlight key points pertinent to the search question. Identify any gaps in knowledge. For example, were any age groups of patients omitted? Was there an omission of any practice settings? Look for agreements and differences in research findings using the literature review, discussion, and conclusion sections of the research articles. Assess whether or not the literature findings are current and relevant to answer your search topic question.

Finally, assess the quality of the evidence. Analyze the literature using the seven-level rating system for hierarchy of research evidence (Melnyk & Fineout-Overholt, 2015) (Box 10-3). The highest priority or evidence is derived from meta-analysis of **randomized controlled trials** (RCTs) and evidence-based clinical guidelines based on systematic reviews of RCTs. When searching and reviewing the literature, look for the search terms systematic review and meta-analysis. (See Chapter 23 for more detailed information on research.) Be aware that the lowest forms of evidence are from the opinion of authorities and/or reports from expert committees.

Step 4: Applying/Implementing the Search Findings

EBP is about using rather than doing research. It is an outcome-focused tool for clinical decision to improve healthcare delivery. Its purpose is to bridge the gap between research and clinical practice. In EBP, the nurse systematically records clinical observations without bias and synthesizes the information with original research that has been subject to a systematic review. The healthcare team with a patient-centered focus should practice EBP collaboratively.

The IOM recommends application of EBP to healthcare delivery to reduce the time between the scientific discovery of effective forms of treatment and their implementation (Institute of Medicine & National Academy of Sciences, 2001). Sackett et al. (1996, p. 71), credited for one of the earliest definitions of EBP, said, "Evidence-based medicine is the conscientious, explicit, and judicious use of current best evidence in making decisions about the care of individual patients." Current definitions of EBP recognize the importance of clinical expertise to assess, diagnose, and plan care. They also emphasize the importance of patient-centered care that encompasses the patient's values, beliefs, concerns, and expectations.

The emphasis on outcomes and efficiency in the healthcare changes the focus from data gathering to the use of data (evidence) from both the literature and the clinical documentation. A **research practice gap** emerges when there are differences between clinical practice and the research on effective clinical practice. Nurses must expedite closing the research practice gap in order to make dramatic, needed improvements to our healthcare delivery system.

Step 5: Evaluating the Result and Effectiveness of Practice Changes

Although expedient implementation of quality search findings is vital, it is not the final step in the quest for improved care based on knowledge and research evidence. We must evaluate the result and effectiveness of practice changes. The process of evidence-based care is cyclical and iterative. Once we implement changes, we must be cognizant of the need for additional information. Related and new questions will emerge from the practice change. We must explore the new questions.

CHALLENGES TO THE ADOPTION OF EVIDENCE-BASED NURSING

Although EBP is widely accepted today, originally, there was initial criticism of the concept. Those critical believed that it was impractical to implement and served to only reduce costs and limit clinical freedom (Sackett et al., 1996). Critics believed that EBP was a cookbook approach to medicine that eliminated their clinical decision-making skills. Findings from nursing research suggest that challenges to wide adoption of EBP in nursing persist. The problem is complex, ranging from access to knowledge resources, attitudes toward research, and information literacy knowledge and skills (Pravikoff et al., 2005). Other barriers to evidence-based nursing include lack of time, lack of sufficient staff, and difficulties in interpreting statistics and research writings (Gerrish & Cooke, 2013; Hannes et al., 2007; Yip Wai et al., 2013; Thompson et al., 2005).

Access to resources is a challenge. The Joint Commission requires facilities to have knowledge resources available in the healthcare facility; however, access to digital libraries resources is not universally available 24 hours a day, 7 days a week. Recommendations from the IOM and professional nursing organizations agree upon the definition of EBP as being the best evidence currently available, yet there is no universal recommendation about what constitutes resources (e.g., library databases) of best practice. As a result, the available library resources for nursing programs and healthcare providers vary. While there is continued improvement for access of information and knowledge resources, there are no universal requirements for all nursing programs and clinical settings. The Cochrane Library is the gold standard for systematic reviews and meta-analysis research findings, but access to all of the Cochrane Library resources is not free for most libraries or users.

The culture of clinical practice settings may not support or value information-seeking practices and current research. Culture of clinical practice refers to situations where management, physicians, and other nurses do not value or support information seeking and research. Another challenge to the adoption of EBP is that nurses prefer to obtain their information from another colleague, especially if they see that person as a nursing expert. Often in the fast pace of providing healthcare, nurses prefer to ask another nurse whose opinion they value rather than search for answers themselves.

A classic study by Pravikoff et al. (2005) revealed 10 personal barriers to the adoption of EBP; the most significant was the lack of value in clinical settings for research. The other nine barriers are related to access of research resources, lack of research skills, lack of information literacy skills, and lack of information technology competencies. The study revealed six different institutional barriers; the primary one was the presence of goals with a higher priority. Other organizational barriers are related to staffing issues, budget, organizational perceptions about nurses' preparation for EBP, and organizational perceptions about the unrealistic use of research.

SUMMARY

The two types of library databases—knowledge based and factual—provide an essential gateway to knowledge discovery. Information search competencies and the use of a personal bibliographic reference manager are essential skills for all nurses who use online library databases to extract nursing knowledge. Effective use of online library databases provides unlimited opportunities to discover knowledge that will improve patient care.

The CINAHL, MEDLINE/PubMed, Cochrane Library, and PsycINFO/PsycARTICLES databases are just a few knowledge-based databases vital to nursing knowledge discovery. The process of searching for knowledge is a skill that requires repeated practice. The process is cyclical and iterative but not linear. There are five steps in this process: (1) defining a search topic based on an information need, (2) searching for evidence embedded in the literature, (3) critically analyzing and summarizing the literature, (4) implementing the findings into practice, and (5) evaluating the results of implementation by asking additional questions or discovering new questions.

Improving patient care and reducing health-care errors require that nursing and hospital administrators, clinicians, educators, and nursing students adopt a culture of care that uses evidence-informed nursing practice. To this end, nurses must be proactive in breaking down the challenges and barriers to adopting EBP. It also requires that nurses self-assess their knowledge needs in locating and evaluating research and identify strategies for gaining the skills needed for competency in this area. Additionally, administrators must see that clinicians have the necessary time, training, support, and access to knowledge resources needed for EBP.

APPLICATIONS AND COMPETENCIES

1. Search the Internet and an online library database, such as CINAHL, for nursing knowledge about a topic of your choice. Compare the quality and quantity of the results. What search engine did you use? What library database did you use? Summarize the findings of the lessons you learned.

2. Explore and compare two databases pertinent to nursing discussed in this chapter using a nursing topic. Identify any strengths and weaknesses for the databases you noted your search. Discuss and summarize the findings.

3. Conduct a literature search for evidence-based practice on a topic of your choice. Identify citation examples for relevant translational literature, evidence summaries, and original research. What nursing outcomes does the evidence-based practice information in the literature address? Discuss how the cited publications might help you prepare a clinical guideline to facilitate needed changes in practice.

4. Search for personal reference management software. Summarize your findings using information from the criteria noted below.

   a. Read recent articles and reviews discussing personal reference management software, both online and journal articles that you retrieved with the search.

   b. Identify pertinent online tutorials and support for users of the personal reference management software.

   c. Based on your research, identify a personal reference management software that best meets your needs.

REFERENCES

American Association of Critical Care Nurses. (2014). *The AACN synergy model for patient care.* Retrieved from http://www.aacn.org/wd/certifications/content/synmodel.pcms?menu=certification

American Psychological Association. (2014a). *PsycINFO.* Retrieved from http://www.apa.org/pubs/databases/psycinfo/index.aspx

American Psychological Association. (2014b). *PsycARTICLES.* Retrieved from http://www.apa.org/pubs/databases/psycarticles/index.aspx

Centers for Medicare & Medicaid Services. (2013, May 1). *Evidence-based guidelines for selected and previously considered hospital-acquired conditions.* Retrieved from https://www.cms.gov/Medicare/Medicare-Fee-for-Service-Payment/HospitalAcqCond/Downloads/Evidence-Based-Guidelines.pdf

CINAHL. (2014). *CINAHL Complete.* Retrieved from http://www.ebscohost.com/academic/cinahl-complete

CiteUlike. (2014). *CiteULike frequently asked questions.* Retrieved from http://www.citeulike.org/faq/faq.adp

Gerrish, K., & Cooke, J. (2013). Factors influencing evidence-based practice among community nurses. *Journal of Community Nursing, 27*(4), 98–101. Retrieved from http://www.jcn.co.uk/

Hannes, K., Vandersmissen, J., De Blaeser, L., et al. (2007). Barriers to evidence-based nursing: A focus group study. *Journal of Advanced Nursing, 60*(2), 162–171. doi: 10.1111/j.1365-2648.2007.04389.x

Im, E-O, & Chang, S. J. (2012). A systematic integrated literature review of systematic integrated literature reviews in nursing. *Journal of Nursing Education, 51*(11), 632–640.

Institute of Medicine & National Academy of Sciences. (2001). *Crossing the quality chasm: A new health system for the 21st century*. Washington, DC: National Academies Press. Retrieved from http://www.nap.edu/openbook. php?isbn=0309072808

Yip Wai, K., Mordiffi, S. Z., Liang, S., et al. (2013). Nurse's perception towards evidence-based practice: A descriptive study. *Singapore Nursing Journal, 40*(1), 34–41. Retrieved from http://www.sna.org.sg/site/singapore-nursing-journal/index.php

Melnyk, B. M., & Fineout-Overholt, E. (2015). *Evidence-based practice in nursing & healthcare: A guide to best practice* (3rd ed). Philadelphia, PA: Wolters Kluwer Health/Lippincott Williams & Wilkins.

Mendeley. (2014). *Mendeley portal*. Retrieved from http://support.mendeley.com/

National Center for Biotechnology Information. (2014). *Welcome to NCBI*. Retrieved from http://www.ncbi.nlm.nih.gov/

National Library of Medicine. (2013, February 20). *MEDLINE fact sheet*. Retrieved from http://www.nlm.nih.gov/pubs/factsheets/medline.html

Pravikoff, D. S., Tanner, A. B., & Pierce, S. T. (2005). Readiness of U.S. nurses for evidence-based practice. *American Journal of Nursing, 105*(9), 40–51. Retrieved from http://journals.lww.com/AJNOnline/pages/default.aspx

Price, B. (2009). Guidance on conducting a literature search and reviewing mixed literature. *Nursing Standard, 23*(24), 43–50. Retrieved from http://rcnpublishing.com/doi/abs/10.7748/ns2009.02.23.24.43.c6829

PubMed Central. (2014). *Pubmed Central homepage*. Retrieved from http://www.ncbi.nlm.nih.gov/pmc/

Reference Manager. (2011, October 6). *RIS format specifications*. Retrieved from http://www.refman.com/support/risformat_intro.asp

Sackett, D. L., Rosenberg, W. M., Gray, J. A., et al. (1996). Evidence based medicine: What it is and what it isn't. *British Medical Journal, 312*(7023), 71–72. doi:10.1136/bmj.312.7023.71

The Cochrane Library. (2013). *Free online access*. Retrieved from http://www.thecochranelibrary.com/view/0/FreeAccess.html

Thompson, C., McCaughan, D., Cullum, N., et al. (2005). Barriers to evidence-based practice in primary care nursing—Viewing decision-making as context is helpful. *Journal of Advanced Nursing, 52*(4), 432–444. Retrieved from http://onlinelibrary.wiley.com/journal/10.1111/%28ISSN%291365-2648

Whittemore, R., & Knafl, K. (2005). The integrative review: Updated methodology. *Journal of Advanced Nursing, 52*(5), 546–553. doi: 10.1111/j.1365-2648.2005.03621.x

Wikipedia Contributors. (2014, July 27). *Comparison of reference management software*. Retrieved from http://en.wikipedia.org/wiki/Comparison_of_reference_management_software

Zotero. (2013, May 17). *Quick start guide [Zotero Documentation]*. Retrieved from http://www.zotero.org/support/quick_start_guide

CHAPTER 11

Mobile Computing

OBJECTIVES

After studying this chapter, you will be able to:

1. Discuss the uses of mobile computers in healthcare.
2. Describe the strengths and weaknesses of smartphones and tablets.
3. Discuss data security issues associated with the use of mobile computers.
4. Identify mobile software appropriate for nurses to use in the clinical setting.
5. Identify mobile software appropriate for nurses to use in the learning setting.

KEY TERMS

Beaming

Bluetooth

Cell phone

eBook

Flash memory

Handheld computer

Hot spot

Personal information management

Piconet

QWERTY keyboard

Random-access memory (RAM)

Read-only memory (ROM)

Smartphone

Synchronization

Wi-Fi

The development of wireless technology has radically changed the way we do business worldwide. With continued growth of mobile technology communications, Wi-Fi and cellular services are replacing phone communication that used wired telephone outlets. Batteries supplement electricity requirements. As a result, nurses and other healthcare providers can use mobile devices such as smartphones and tablet computers at the point of need.

Most mobile devices come with an assortment of **personal information management** software, such as contact information, a calendar, and a clock. The large storage capacities of mobile devices allow for storage of a variety of software applications (apps), electronic books (**eBooks**), reference material, graphics, videos, and other data files. Connectivity using **synchronization** (sync) software, **beaming**, **Bluetooth**, **Wi-Fi** (wireless fidelity), and cellular services allows for transfer of information from mobile devices to personal computers (PCs) or health information clinical systems. The possibilities for effective use of handheld mobile computing in nursing education and healthcare are endless. Emerging disruptive innovations in mobile technology challenge us to stay current. This chapter covers the basics of mobile computing and its use in nursing.

MOBILE-COMPUTING BASICS

Mobile computers, such as smartphones and tablets, are all small computers. All mobile devices use an operating system (OS), and most allow the use of third-party software applications. The **cell phone** is a shortwave wireless communication device that has a connection to a transmitter. The word "cell" refers to the area of transmission. Cell phones, like landline phones, require a paid subscription to the transmission service provider. **Smartphones** are cell phones with Internet connectivity. The common term "**handheld computer**" used in this chapter refers to all handheld mobile devices. The information presented for each device includes differences in features as well as examples of the uses of these devices in educational and healthcare settings.

HISTORY OF MOBILE COMPUTING

The Psion Organiser was the first personal digital assistant (PDA) concept and developed in the early 1980s (Medindia, 2014). The first PDA design was primarily as personal information managers (PIMs) that included electronic telephone books and appointment calendars. The Newton MessagePad, developed by Apple in 1983, was the first popular PDA that featured a touch screen and handwriting capabilities (Bort, 2013). However, the PalmPilot, introduced by U.S. Robotics in 1996, was lightweight, fit in the palm of the user's hand, and featured Graffiti handwriting recognition software. It also had much better handwriting recognition than the Newton. As a result, it quickly dominated the market by 1999. Apple discontinued production of the Newton in 1998.

The Rocket eBook was one of the first eBook readers (electronic readers for books) and released in 1998 (Pence, 2012; Rothman, 2009). However, the market was not prepared for a replacement for the print book. The cost of the eBook reader was $250, and it could hold up to 10 books.

IBM introduced the first smartphone, known as "Simon," in 1993. The smartphone combined features of the cellular telephone and personal information management software. It cost $900 and weighed 1 kg (2.2 pounds) (PC World Staff, 2013). In 1999, Qualcomm released the pdQ, which featured a cell phone and the Palm organizer (Qualcomm, 1999, September 22).

The smartphone had not yet captured the attention of the market when Microsoft introduced the Pocket PC PDA in 2000. The Pocket PC offered a compact version of the Windows OS (Tilley, 2014). It gave users the privilege of having more than one application open at the same time. They could also view or edit Microsoft Office documents. The Pocket PC grew in popularity with users, capturing the market with 54.2% of the OS shipments in the second quarter of 2006 (Gartner, 2006). PDAs began to lose popularity beginning in 2007 with the introduction of the Amazon Kindle eBook reader, Apple iPhone and, later, the Google Android smartphone.

The iPod, a music player introduced by Apple in 2001, dominated the music player market with more than 100 million devices sold in less than 6 years (Apple, 2007). The iPod used Apple iTunes software to transfer music, video, or other applications from a PC quickly to the device. In 2007, Apple released the iPod Touch, an updated version of the iPod, and the iPhone. The iPod Touch provided a screen size close to the width and length of the device including touch screen icons and Wi-Fi access to the Internet. In 2008, T-Mobile released the first Android phone (German, 2011, August 2). As of December 2013, there is a significant waning of the popularity for the iPod (Gedeon, 2014) because today's smartphones also serve as music players.

Amazon released the first Kindle eBook reader in 2007 at the cost of $399 US (Patel, 2007). In 2009, Amazon released the Kindle 2 eBook reader. The same year, Barnes & Noble released their eBook reader, the Nook. eBook readers were no longer a novelty. December 2013 was the first time in history when eBooks outsold print books (Kozlowski, 2013). Apple released the iPad tablet computer and iBookstore in 2010. Apple sold two million iPads in less than 60 days after they were released (Apple, 2010). The first iPad tablet triggered innovations of an array of tablets by a variety of manufacturers. Microsoft joined the tablet market with the release of Microsoft Surface in 2012. As of 2014, manufacturers are releasing a variety of clones of the Microsoft Surface tablet; some have the Windows OS and others have the Android OS or a combination of the two.

UNDERSTANDING MOBILE COMPUTER CONCEPTS

There are similarities and differences between personal computers and mobile computers. Mobile computers do not necessarily have the same OSs as PCs do. Although the OSs differ, the design of mobile-computing software is for interoperability (the devices work together). There are hardware differences between mobile computers and PCs, and it is important to understand them. Hardware variations include display, battery, memory, synchronization and connectivity, and data entry devices. Synchronization and connectivity using beaming, Bluetooth, Wi-Fi, and cellular services are data transfer functions common to mobile computers.

Smartphones and Tablet Devices Defined

The modern smartphone is a miniature computer that includes multiple software programs (apps), documents, music, video, Internet access capability, a forward- and rear-facing camera, and a telephone. Smartphones provide Internet access using cellular services, or Wi-Fi, or both. All smartphones require a subscription to a cellular service provider. Smartphones are popular with users who do not want to carry a computer and cell phone as separate devices. Smartphone features are very similar. Many smartphones, such as the iPhone (Figure 11-1), allow

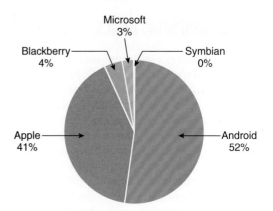

Figure 11-2. Smartphone market share (Data from Protalinski, 2014).

for navigation using a touch screen, an on-screen keyboard, video, flash for the camera, and editing tools for photographs and video (Erdley & Hansen, 2012). Others include a keyboard either below the viewing screen or as a slide- or flip-out. In 2013, Android smartphones had the majority of the smartphone market share (Protalinski, 2014) (Figure 11-2).

Tablet devices are also miniature computers with most of the capabilities of smartphones with the exception of the traditional telephone service, although there are apps that emulate telephone communication, such as Skype, FaceTime (iOS7+), and FaceTime Audio (iOS7+). All tablet devices have Wi-Fi for Internet access. Some also provide access to cellular services with a monthly subscription fee. Tablet devices are more popular for reading eBooks. Tablets come in a variety of screen sizes, ranging from 5+ to 11+ inches. For detailed information, go to *Tablet PC Dimension and Case Sizes* at http://en.wikipedia.org/wiki/Tablet_PC_dimensions_and_cases_sizes. Because tablets are lightweight and easily portable, many nurses use tablets instead of laptops or desktop computers.

Wi-Fi Mobile Computer Operating Systems

For smartphones and other mobile devices, OSs determine the functions and software capabilities. Examples of these OSs include Apple iOS, BlackBerry Research in Motion (RIM), Google Android, Linux, Symbian, and Windows. The Google Android OS, released in 2008, is a modified version of Linux kernel—an open software platform designed to rival the Apple iPhone.

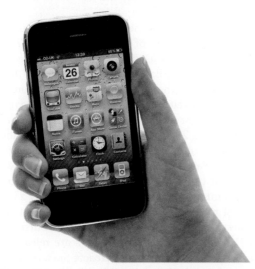

Figure 11-1. iPhone (http://www.shutterstock.com/sgm).

The Android is the OS used by numerous mobile device manufacturers. Unlike the Apple iOS, the Android OS and Windows OS support the use of Adobe Flash for streaming audio and video. In 2014, smartphones and tablets using the Android OS (Lunden, 2013) were outselling those with the Apple iOS. Mobile devices with the Windows OS and BlackBerry RIM OS had less than 5% of the market share. To provide a perspective about market shifts, in 2010, the BlackBerry RIM had the largest market share, followed by the iPhone and Windows smartphones. Tablets as we know them today did not gain popularity until after 2010.

There are thousands of nursing and medical apps for the popular mobile-computing OSs. Many of the apps are free or have a nominal fee for purchase. For example, apps for mobile devices using the Android OS are available from the Google Play store and the Amazon Appstore. The Apple App Store has apps for mobile devices using the Apple iOS. BlackBerry apps are available from the BlackBerry World store.

Display

Mobile computers have a liquid crystal display (LCD) like laptop PCs. Many mobile computers also provide a touch screen for data input. The screen display size and resolution differ from PCs. The diagonal screen display size on mobile computers ranges from 3.5 to 11+ inches. Resolution is an important consideration—the higher the number, the sharper is the image. A sharp screen image is a factor to consider if the user needs to view video of, for example, physical assessment or nursing procedures.

The display for mobile devices designed primarily as eBook readers differs from the LCD display. eBook readers use E Ink, which replicates the look of the printed paper. The MIT Media Lab developed E Ink (Hidalgo, 2014). E Ink is proprietary now and owned by Prime View International, a Taiwanese firm. There are advantages and disadvantages for use of E Ink. The advantages include reduced eye strain when reading, lower power consumption requirements, and the resemblance to reading text on printed paper. The disadvantages of the initial E Ink include the lack of support for color and video and the lack of backlighting, which makes it difficult to read

eBooks using E Ink in dim settings. Research is underway to address E Ink limitations.

Battery

All mobile computers operate using battery power. (See Appendix A for more information about batteries.) Most mobile devices use rechargeable batteries. Innovations in mobile technology continue to improve battery life. Factors that shorten battery life are multitasking features, increased memory, audio, screen brightness, push and fetch email features, location services, and Bluetooth/Wi-Fi/cellular service connections. Always use the latest software updates, as they may include ways for improved battery life performance.

Memory

Mobile devices use three types of built-in memory—**read-only memory (ROM), random-access memory (RAM)**, and built-in **flash memory**. Flash memory is also available as expansion cards, as shown in Figure 11-3. The ROM stores the OSs and standard applications such as contacts, calendar, and notes. The RAM stores all of the add-on applications and data files and requires a small amount of continuous battery power. RAM memory is volatile; hence, all of the data stored in RAM are lost with the depletion of the battery life. Most mobile devices use flash memory instead of RAM because flash memory is nonvolatile, meaning that the applications and data will not disappear after the loss of battery power. (See Appendix A for more information about flash memory.)

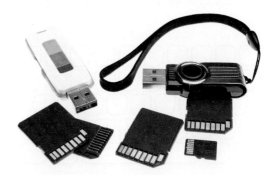

Figure 11-3. Flash memory (http://www.shutterstock.com/Sergio Stakhnyk).

Many mobile digital devices have expansion slots for removable flash memory cards for software and data storage. Removable memory, commonly used by mobile devices, includes Secure Digital (SD) cards, Compact Flash cards, and Memory Sticks. A few mobile devices also accept a universal serial bus (USB) flash drive. Flash memory cards are useful for storing eBooks, photographs, video, and music. The price of flash memory has plummeted. Today, you can purchase an 8-gigabyte (GB) SD card for less than $10.

Data Entry

Most tablets and smartphones have a touch screen for data entry. Some devices allow the use of a stylus. **QWERTY keyboard** data entry is available in all smartphones and tablets (Figure 11-4). QWERTY refers to a keyboard layout common to the PC and typewriter that comprises the first six letters on the top row of letters. Most tablets and smartphones include a microphone, audio recorder, and forward- and rear-facing cameras with a zoom lens for capturing pictures and video clips.

Unless there is a separate keyboard especially designed for the mobile device, it is easier to enter large amounts of data using a PC, rather than the mobile device, and then synchronize the file with the mobile device. It is simple, however, to enter data such as a new appointment or contact on a mobile device. Office software such as Documents to Go or Office Mobile (for Windows phones and iPhone/Android phones with eligible subscription for Office 365 subscriptions) allows users to create or edit Microsoft Word, Excel, and PowerPoint files on the mobile device. Google Drive app allows for word processing, spreadsheet, and presentation

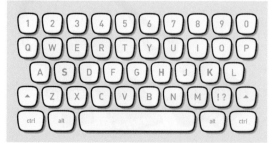

Figure 11-4. QWERTY keyboard (http://www.shutterstock.com/Alhovik).

solutions (http://docs.google.com/m) on mobile devices. Apple iWork Pages, Numbers, and Keynote are apps for the iPhone and iPad. Microsoft OneDrive and OneNote work on Apple and Android mobile devices. Evernote (https://evernote.com/) is a cloud computing note taking app that works on all smartphone and tablet devices.

Synchronization (Sync)

Most smartphones and tablets do not require syncing with a PC because of the ability to update apps automatically when there is an Internet connection and the ability to backup data to online cloud storage (see Chapter 2 for more on cloud computing), such as OneDrive (Microsoft), G Cloud (Android), or iCloud (Apple devices). However, mobile devices can sync with PCs using proprietary software so that all of the files on the two computers coincide. Windows Mobile devices use Windows Mobile for data transfer between the mobile device and the PC. The Apple devices use iTunes, a free download for Macs and Windows PCs, to transfer data. There are syncing apps for the Android devices, too. An example is SideSync.

Connectivity

Depending on the mobile device, these devices can connect in several ways with other devices or the Internet. Connectivity features include beaming, Bluetooth, Wi-Fi, and cellular services. Bluetooth and Wi-Fi expansion cards are available for those devices that have an expansion card slot but do not have this built-in feature of connectivity.

Beaming

Beaming allows for wireless, very short-ranged (4 inches to 3 feet), transmission of information to other beam-enabled devices with the same OS using infrared (IR), Bluetooth, or near field communication (NFC) on Android devices (Figure 11-5). AirDrop provides beaming sharing features for the Mac, iPad, and iPhone with iOS7+ (Nations, 2015). The type of file you share depends on the mobile device, the sharing feature, or beaming app(s) that the mobile device is capable of using. (See Appendix A for more information about IR ports.) Check an Internet source for the exact procedure to use with your device.

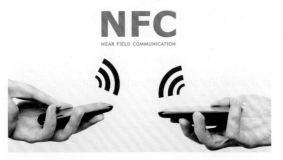

Figure 11-5. Smartphone using NFC communication (http://www.shutterstock.com/Piotr Adamowicz).

Bluetooth

Bluetooth allows for a wireless, short-ranged (32 feet), low-powered radio frequency connection to other Bluetooth-enabled devices (Franklin & Layton, 2014). When you have Bluetooth enabled on the mobile device and paired with another Bluetooth device, it creates a personal area connection or a **piconet** (Webopedia, 2014). There are several uses of Bluetooth. You can use Bluetooth to use an external keyboard, share files, synchronize a mobile device with a PC, or print to a Bluetooth-enabled printer. Bluetooth headphones allow the user to listen to music, podcasts, and other audio media. Bluetooth headsets provide hands-free use of smartphones for phone calls. Security is always a potential issue for wireless use, and so, it is a good idea to turn Bluetooth off when it is not used.

Wi-Fi

Wi-Fi networking is another means of mobile device connectivity. Wi-Fi is an industry standard (Brain et al., 2014; Mitchell, 2014). It uses a router that supports Wi-Fi standard 802.11 a, b, g, n, or ac to form a local area network. The 802.11 n standard is very common and inexpensive. The newer 802.11 ac is the most recent standard that improves the speed of the wireless connection and reduces interference (Brain et al., 2014). Wi-Fi networking is popular with family homes because it allows multiple users to access wireless printers and the Internet. Wi-Fi networks are simple to set up using a software wizard that comes with the purchase of a wireless router.

Hot spot is a term used to identify a Wi-Fi–enabled area so that you can use your Wi-Fi–enabled mobile device to connect to the Internet. You can find Hotspots at public libraries, most colleges and universities, coffee shops, airport terminals, and hotels. Not all Hotspots are public; many hot spots use encryption for security reasons and require the user to enter an access code or pay a fee for use. Wi-Fi security, like Bluetooth, is an important issue. For example, hospitals that use Wi-Fi have very secure encrypted systems. Setup information for routers used in home wireless networks includes methods to address security issues.

Smartphones and tablets with cellular capability can connect to the Internet using regular cellular services. Cellular service users should be aware of their "connection package" agreement to avoid paying high fees for large data downloads. Users who need to access the Internet using the cellular service, as opposed to Wi-Fi, should have unlimited minutes as part of their cellular service agreement.

ADVANTAGES AND DISADVANTAGES OF USING MOBILE DEVICES IN NURSING AND NURSING EDUCATION

There are benefits and shortcomings of the use of handheld computers in nursing, although many argue that the advantages far outweigh the disadvantages. Time-saving and time management are often mentioned in the literature as positive outcomes after infusing handheld computers in nursing education and clinical settings (Temple University, 2011; Wyatt & Krauskopf, 2012). Instead of looking up information in several printed textbooks, nurses and nursing students can query the handheld mobile device, which can hold numerous textbooks. Patient safety and error reduction are also benefits. The ease of looking up reference information (Table 11-1) improves confidence and decreases errors in the clinical setting. Unlike the printed counterpart, you can update reference eBooks and renew subscriptions. Finally, the handheld computers are

TABLE 11-1   Library Websites Designed for Handheld Computers

Library Sites Designed for Mobile Computers	Website Address
American University Library	http://www.library.american.edu/mobile/
Ball State University Libraries	http://www.bsu.edu/libraries/mobile/
New York Public Library	http://m.nypl.org/
Boston University Medical Center Mobile Library	http://medlib.bu.edu/mobile/
Harvard College Library	http://hcl.harvard.edu/mobile/
National Library of Medicine	http://pubmedhh.nlm.nih.gov/nlm/
Fondren Library, Rice University	http://m.library.rice.edu/

easy for nursing students and other healthcare professionals to use when answering patient questions at the point of care.

Concerns about patients having a negative perception of nurses' use of handheld computers are not validated by research (Lee, 2007). There have been no recent studies on patients' perception of handheld use, perhaps because the use of computers by care providers, patients, and their families is so pervasive today. Patients see nurses using a computer and bar code medication administration as standard practice. They also see physicians and nurse practitioners explain radiology and laboratory findings with hand-held computers. As patients become more aware about the benefits of accessing online and eBook resources with handheld devices, they may have an expectation that we use mobile devices at the point of care.

Imagine a scenario in which a nursing student, with an instructor, is preparing to administer a combination of regular and NPH insulin. The student removes a small mobile device from a uniform pocket and taps the screen several times to pull up insulin on the drug eBook. The student verifies the procedure for mixing the two types of insulin before proceeding to prepare the injection. This type of use of mobile devices in education

is a growing trend. Some of the issues that have prevented widespread adoption of mobile devices include faculty and nursing students' attitudes toward technology, costs, and rapid change of technology.

Although mobile computers offer benefits, there are also shortcomings. The rapid change in technology could be a problem, because there is no guarantee that the manufacturer of a given mobile device will continue to manufacture and offer support. The expense of the mobile device is a common concern (Doyle et al., 2014; Phillippi & Wyatt, 2011). Some nursing programs require the students to purchase the device, whereas others use grant money or incorporate the cost as a laboratory fee. The time involved with the selection and preparation of the devices for use is another worry. There is a potential for misuse of mobile devices using the camera, scanner apps, and social media (see Chapter 4 for more information on mobile devices and social media). Students and practicing nurses must never take unauthorized photos or make copies of any patient information with mobile devices. Doing so breaches patient privacy and confidentiality. Finally, there are occasional issues with faulty devices and short battery life. Despite the shortcomings, advances in technology are easing the adoption of mobile devices for students in nursing education and for students, registered nurses (RNs), and advanced practice RNs in clinical practice settings.

Use in Nursing Education

Swan et al. (2013) reported the findings about using tablets in a small qualitative study of one focus group with eight faculty members and three focus groups with fourteen students. The study participants received tablets (iPad2) 4 weeks prior to the beginning of classes. Both faculty and students agree that they needed additional time to master the technology before using in a classroom setting. Some faculty believed that they received insufficient training prior to preparation of learning activities. Students identified additional challenges, for example:

- The ability to multitask (email and Facebook) was distracting.
- The iPads did not support their learning styles.
- The iPad did not fit into lab coat pockets, but there was no place to store them safely in the hospital setting.
- Internet connectivity was lost when taking online exams.
- The design of some eBooks was not optimal use on tablet computers.
  - Inability to bookmark.
  - eBook page numbers did not correspond to the print book page numbers that were in the instructors' assignments.

The Swan study revealed positive findings, too. Students indicated that they enjoyed the ability to take and review class notes, to watch videos, and to have multiple books on one device. They saw the potential for tablet use in the nursing education setting. As a result of the study, faculty recognized that the benefits outweighed the negatives. Faculty made decisions to select eBooks optimized for use on the iPad. They also worked to improve technical and instructional design support for students and faculty.

The use of mobile devices as a tool continues to grow in nursing curricula. Proficiency with technology skills for the delivery of nursing care is an expectation of nursing students. For example, nursing students learn how to set up intravenous administration pumps, administer medications using bar code patient identification, and record patient care using the electronic health record (EHR). Nursing students must have proficient technology skills to use computers to write care plans using a word processor, draw concept maps with concept map software, use online learning management systems to submit assignments, take quizzes, and participate in online discussion forums.

Use of Mobile Devices in Clinical Practice
General Nursing Clinical Practice Use

When nurses discover better ways to deliver patient care, they quickly adopt the new ways. The nursing literature has an abundance of information on how to purchase and use handheld computers. Nurses find handheld computers affordable and indispensable in various nursing practice clinical settings including the medical–surgical nursing unit, the operating room, and the emergency department. A growing number of clinical information systems incorporate the use of handheld computers for point-of-need documentation. Wireless synchronization allows for real-time documentation in the electronic medical record (EMR).

Personal Handheld Computers for Clinical Use

Many nurses in clinical practice purchase their own handheld computers to use electronic references to provide point-of-need information for decision making in practice. References commonly used by a clinical nurse include a nursing drug book, a medical dictionary, a nursing procedure's manual, a handbook of diagnostics tests, and a health assessment handbook (Table 11-2). Two popular tools used in nursing are drug references and medical calculators (Wyatt & Krauskopf, 2012). The cost of the electronic references is comparable to the print version. The advantage of the electronic format is that when updates are available, they can be downloaded and saved to the mobile device so that the information is available at the point of care.

The best way to find apps and eBooks for clinical use is to search for them using the mobile app store or bookstore for the device. Some print nursing handbooks include app store information, so if you have a copy of the print book, you are able to download updates from an online store with resources for mobile devices. Some books for

TABLE 11-2 Examples of Mobile Computer Reference Resources	
Examples of Handheld Reference Resources	**Website Address**
Skyscape Drug books, medical dictionaries, laboratory and diagnostic test books, NCLEX (National Council Licensure Examination for Registered Nurses) review manuals, and nursing procedure manuals	http://www.skyscape.com
Handango Many healthcare and office applications	http://www.handango.com/
Centers for Disease Control and Prevention Podcasts and sexually transmitted disease (STD) treatment guidelines	http://www2a.cdc.gov/podcasts/
Epocrates Rx Drug database (free)	http://www.epocrates.com/
Lexicomp Clinical reference resources for nurses and advanced practice nurses	http://www.lexi.com/
Pepid Reference resources for clinical nursing, oncology, and critical care	http://www.pepid.com/
Shots by STFM (free) Immunization schedules for children and adults	http://www.immunizationed.org/ http://www.immunizationed.org/
Statcoder An assortment of clinical apps (free)	http://www.statcoder.com
Unbound Medicine Clinical references resources for nurses and nursing schools	http://www.unboundmedicine.com/

mobile devices provide a preview. Potential buyers can also review user comments and ratings for the resources prior to making a purchase.

Handheld Computers for Clinical Information Systems

The use of handheld computers for bar code administration of medications is prevalent. Visualize a scenario. The nurses arrive for report from the 7 AM to 7 PM shift on the cardiac nursing unit. After the walking rounds report, each nurse picks up a wireless handheld computer, logs into the device, and uses a stylus to select assigned patients from the list of patients on the nursing unit. While planning medication administration for the shift, the nurse uses the real-time electronic medication administration record (MAR) to review the scheduled medications for each patient in preparation for organizing care. When administering the medication, the nurses follow the six rights of medication administration (right drug, right patient, right dose, right time, right route, and right documentation) using bar coding technology by first scanning the bar code on the drug. In addition to asking the patients their names, the nurse also scans the identification band to verify that the correct patient is administered the medication. Afterward, the nurse charts the drug administration by clicking a checkbox on the handheld computer MAR.

Handheld computers with a secure wireless connection to the clinical information system are used in many healthcare facilities for medication administration. Because the device is wireless, the patient data are always up to date. As soon as a patient is admitted to a room, the patient's name shows up on the list of patients for that unit. When a medication is ordered and verified by the pharmacy, it shows up on the list of scheduled medications for administration. The medication name and information disappear when discontinued. The handheld computer eliminates the need to push heavy drug carts with attached computers or other computers on wheels. If the physician or advanced practice nurse checks the electronic chart on a remote computer, they can view the medication charted seconds ago.

Advanced Practice: Nurse Practitioner Use

Nurse practitioners have quickly adopted the use of handheld computers into their practices. In addition to references used by the clinical nurse, nurse practitioners can monitor and evaluate patient progress. Patient Tracker is a program used by physicians and nurse practitioners for patient care management. The free version allows user to enter up to ten patients. For additional fees, users can access a pain assessment, blood sugar assessment, and an unlimited number of patients. Some of EMR/EHR office systems, for example, eClinicalWorks, OneTouch EMR, and drchrono EHR, have associated handheld mobile-computing solutions for practitioners.

The practice setting for nurse practitioners can be extremely busy. Prescription writing and coding for reimbursement of care can be automated with handheld software. Prescription writing software such as Allscripts ePrescribe is available for handheld computers in addition to patient care management software. Although the mobile app is free, the user must have a paid subscription account for the software. There are also numerous software packages to identify ICD-9 and ICD-10 (International Classification of Diseases) and CPT (common procedural terminology) codes for billing of care. Search the mobile app stores using the terms "ICD" and "CPT."

> ### QSEN Scenario
>
> **You work as a nurse at a rehabilitation center that specializes in the care of geriatric patients. You want to have mobile resources to use with a smartphone. What kind of resources might you use from the American Geriatrics Society?**

Use of Mobile Devices in Nursing Research

Handheld computers are useful for the research process. Users can take web-based research surveys with a handheld computer. The data from the surveys are stored on the researcher's web server for aggregation and analysis. Researchers can use the audio recorder on the handheld computer to record focus group interviews and then later download the recordings for data analysis. The camera on the handheld computer could be used to take pictures to document changes that occurred as a result of a research treatment.

The mobility of a handheld computer makes it an excellent tool for accessing and collecting research data. Many online evidence-based resources are designed specifically for handheld computers. (See Chapters 9 and 23 for more information.) The Agency for Healthcare Research and Quality includes the National Guideline Clearinghouse (http://www.guideline.gov/resources/pda.aspx), which has links to evidence-based clinical practice guidelines specifically designed for handheld devices. The website also has a comprehensive listing of links to pocket guidelines from multiple medical societies, such as the American

College of Cardiology, the National Institutes of Health, and the Centers for Disease Control and Prevention (CDC).

Use of Mobile Devices to Read eBooks

As noted earlier, the popularity of eBooks continues to grow. Users access eBooks with eBook readers or they can download and read eBooks on any mobile device with eBook reader apps. There are many eBook reader apps. They vary by the file types and kinds (for purchase or free) of the books.

Online bookstores that sell eBooks also sell eBook readers specific for the eBook file types in their stores. For example, Barnes & Noble sells the Nook and Amazon sells the Kindle. Both eBook readers use Wi-Fi to allow their users to purchase, download, and read eBooks sold in their stores. The recent Kindle has a color touch screen, has Internet access, and allows users to read books, listen to music, and watch video (Amazon, 2014). The recent Nook has color touch screen and allows for storage of more than 15,000 eBooks, as well as MP3 music files (Carnoy, 2014, January 14).

If you want to read an eBook on a smartphone or tablet, you may choose to have several eBook reader apps so that you can access eBooks from different stores, libraries, and websites that provide access. Search the app store for your mobile device to download the eBook reader apps. Examples of eBook reader apps for smartphones and tablets are:

- Bluefire Reader—to read books downloaded using Adobe Digital Editions from a library
- iBooks—to read books purchased from the Apple iBookstore on Apple smartphones and iPads. Also used to store and read PDF files
- Kindle—to read eBooks purchased from the Amazon bookstore
- Kobo—to read eBooks purchased from the Indigo books and Music and the Borders bookstore
- Nook—to read eBooks purchased from the Barnes & Noble bookstore
- Play Books—to read eBooks purchased from the Google Play store
- Stanza—to read any electronic content including eBooks, newspapers, and Web content on Mac devices

Most eBooks that you purchase or borrow from a library are protected by Digital Rights Management (DRM). DRM provides copyright protection for eBooks, as well as commercial movies and music. DRM prevents the ability for users to make copies of eBooks. DRM is the reason you can read borrowed eBooks from the library only with Adobe Digital Editions and that the eBook disappears from the app at the end of the expiration date. The Digital Millennium Copyright Act of 1998 made disabling DRM illegal in the United States.

However, not all eBooks are protected by copyright; some are free. Project Gutenberg (http://gutenberg.org) provides access to over 44,000 free eBooks without copyright protection. Examples of books for nursing include those written by Florence Nightingale's *Notes on Nursing*, Clara Barton's *The Red Cross in Peace and War*, and Louisa May Alcott's *Hospital Sketches*.

Many publishers now offer nursing textbooks in eBook format as an alternative to print textbooks. The advantages of textbooks in eBooks format include the ability to search, bookmark, and highlight content. Current technology provides opportunities for greater development and adoption of eBooks for nursing education. For example, eBooks can support embedded media, such as videos, embedded quizzes, and gaming.

Use of Mobile Devices for Library Searches

Your smartphone rings; when you glance at the screen, you note that you have received a text message—from the virtual librarian answering your question about when the library closes. Yes, libraries have changed from bricks and mortar to include websites, digital catalogs of books and journal citations, eBooks, e-mail notification, blogs, "really simple syndication" (RSS) feeds, chat, and text messaging. Libraries lend more than books; they also lend music CDs, movies on DVDs, and computer equipment, such as laptops and iPods. Many college and health science libraries have extensive handheld mobile resources designed to assist healthcare students and professionals.

You can use mobile computers to assist in finding and storing literature citations used for library searches. For example, users can access their personal reference managers on tablet devices using apps such as EndNote or PaperShip for Mendeley & Zotero. The portability of the references saves time when visiting the library to search for journal articles and books or storing the call numbers for the book locations in the library.

Most libraries have websites on the Internet, but only a few of those websites are tablet and smartphone friendly (see Table 11-1). The design of mobile-computing websites allows the content to fit the screen size without requiring horizontal scrolling. Additionally, the URL should be as short as possible to facilitate input, and the content should address what the mobile user needs.

The number of resources for mobile devices is growing exponentially every day. To discover new resources, search the Internet using the terms "mobile learning resources." Many universities value mobile learning. For example, the Tennessee Board of Regents, a system responsible for 45 institutions, hosts an innovative website designed to assist users with mobile devices at http://www.tbrelearning.org/.

DATA SECURITY ISSUES

Data security is a minimal issue if the mobile device is used only for reference resources. However, data security is always an issue with small wireless devices, and it can and must be addressed by the user. Because handheld computers are small, it is inevitable that they fall out of pockets, be misplaced, or stolen. All handheld computers with any type of clinical data must be secure or encrypted using a password or biometrics, such as fingerprint recognition. If passwords are used, they must be one that cannot be easily hacked (Microsoft, 2014). Other password considerations are as follows:

- Prefer longer passwords (7 to 10 characters).
- Use words or characters easily remembered, but that are not personally identifiable.
- The misspelled name of a fruit or flower, rather than the name of a family member or pet.
- The first letter of each word in a phrase.

- Replace letters of the word with number or other keyboard characters. For example, the letter A might be replaced with the @ sign and the letter O with the number 0. Also include other keyboard symbols.
- Be familiar with password strategies to avoid at http://www.microsoft.com/protect/fraud/passwords/create.aspx.
- Check the strength of the password using an online tool such as https://www.microsoft.com/protect/fraud/passwords/checker.aspx?WT.mc_id=Site_Link.

Most important of all, if there is a need to store patient data, users must follow the policies and procedures outlined by their healthcare agency. Check with the agency's Health Insurance Portability and Accountability Act (HIPAA) officer for questions.

FUTURE TRENDS

We would need to have a crystal ball to predict the future of handheld mobile devices in education and clinical settings; however, history has already set trends that we can expect to continue. We can expect mobile devices to be easier to use. The software will be more intuitive. Voice commands currently available to operate handheld computers can be expected to improve and become a primary method of data input. Mobile broadband, for high-speed transfer of data, will be an accessible and affordable feature for smartphones.

Medical devices are available and under development for integration with smartphones (TEDMED, 2009). The medical devices can be used by both care providers and patients for monitoring and diagnostic purposes. Patients will be able to share medical information from the devices with their care providers electronically. Topol, a cardiologist and geneticist, describes his vision of the future of medicine using technology in his book *The Creative Destruction of Medicine: How the Digital Revolution Will Create Better Health Care* (Topol, 2012).

We can expect smartphones and tablets to be the norm. Smartphones and tablets will continue to be appropriate for use in education, classroom, simulation clinical labs, and the clinical settings. As the popularity of mobile devices increases, the pricing will continue to drop.

As the future unfolds, healthcare will harness the use of technology to improve patient care and save lives. All healthcare agencies will ask the providers to log into their human resources information systems to input a cell phone contact number. In the event of a disaster, team notification will be done primarily using text messaging to smartphones. Clinical information systems will "push" text messaging alerts to healthcare providers, advising them to log in to the system to retrieve reports of critical values.

SUMMARY

Once technically savvy students and nurses learn how to use a handheld computer, the small mobile device becomes an essential clinical tool just as valuable as their stethoscope and patient care devices. Handheld computers allow nurses to discover essential knowledge in the palms of their hands. Synchronization software makes it very easy to update the handheld computer from the PC with calendar appointments, contact name, e-mail, phone numbers, and addresses. Users can store digital eBook nursing references to use in the classroom and clinical practice. Handheld computers with access to the Internet provide real-time access to e-mail, news, and other essential information resources.

Handheld computers provide added value to nurses in all settings. Nursing students should be expected to use handheld computers in the classroom and the clinical setting. Development of proficient technical skills improves time management and work efficiency. Knowledge gained from up-to-date information improves decision making and patient care outcomes and prevents unnecessary errors. The handheld computer, designed to integrate with clinical information systems, has the potential to improve accuracy of documentation and shorten the time between the delivery of care and documentation in the electronic medical record. Future uses of handheld computers in the nursing are limited only by our imaginations.

APPLICATIONS AND COMPETENCIES

1. Use a search engine, such as Google, to search for health science library PDA websites.

2. Check with your local library to see if they lend mobile-computing devices such as PDAs, iPads, and/or iPods.

3. If you have access to a PDA or a smartphone, discuss the connection resources. Does the device have Bluetooth, beaming, or Internet capabilities? Explain the advantages and disadvantages of each type of connection.

4. Set up a Skype account. Use the app to contact a friend or your instructor. Discuss the outcome. Identify the potential benefits for use of Skype in the nursing education setting.

5. Download a trial version of nursing reference software from the Internet. Use a search engine, such as Google, and enter the search terms: "nursing mobile software trial downloads."

6. Use the Internet to preview software that you might use on a mobile device. Discuss the similarities and differences between the printed book view and the electronic view.

REFERENCES

Amazon. (2014). *Kindle Fire HDX tablet*. Retrieved from http://www.amazon.com/gp/product/B00BWYQ9YE/ref=r_kdia_h_i_gl#tech

Apple. (2007, April 9). *100 million sold*. Retrieved from http://www.apple.com/pr/library/2007/04/09ipod.html

Apple. (2010, May 31). *Apple sells two million iPads in less than 60 days*. Retrieved from http://www.apple.com/pr/library/2010/05/31ipad.html

Bort, J. (2013, June 2). *The history of the tablet, an idea Steve Jobs stole and turned into a game-changer*. Retrieved from

Brain, M., Wilson, T. V., & Johnson, B. (2014). *How Wi-Fi works*. Retrieved from http://computer.howstuffworks.com/wireless-network1.htm

Carnoy, D. (2014, January 14). Barnes & Noble Nook. *CNET Reviews*. Retrieved June 6, 2010, from http://reviews.cnet.com/eBook-readers/barnes-noble-nook/4505-3508_7-33786175.html?tag=rnav

Doyle, G. J., Garrett, B., & Currie, L. M. (2014). Integrating mobile devices into nursing curricula: Opportunities for implementation using Rogers' Diffusion of Innovation model. *Nurse Education Today, 34*(5), 775–782. doi: 10.1016/j.nedt.2013.10.021.

Erdley, W. S., & Hansen, M. (2012). Overview of smart phone video essentials. *Computers, informatics, nursing: CIN, 30*(3), 119–122. doi: 10.1097/NXN.0b013e31824ef20b.

Franklin, C., & Layton, J. (2014). *How Bluetooth works.* Retrieved from http://electronics.howstuffworks.com/bluetooth1.htm

Gartner. (2006, August 7). *Gartner says PDA shipments reached record high in second quarter of 2006.* Retrieved from http://www.gartner.com/newsroom/id/495172

Gedeon, K. (2014, January 30). *The death of the iPod? Apple faces huge sales drop for popular music device.* Retrieved from http://madamenoire.com/345317/death-ipod-apple-faces-huge-sales-drop-popular-music-device/

German, K. (2011, August 2). *A brief history of Android phones.* Retrieved from http://reviews.cnet.com/8301-19736_7-20016542-251/a-brief-history-of-android-phones/

Hidalgo, J. (2014). *What is E Ink?* Retrieved from http://portables.about.com/od/newsandviews/f/E-Ink-FAQ.htm

Lunden, I. (2013, November 26). *Canalys: Half of all PCs shipped in 2014 will be tablets; Android 65%, Apple 30%.* Retrieved from http://techcrunch.com/2013/11/26/half-of-all-pcs-shipped-in-2014-will-be-tablets-cost-friendly-androids-65-of-them-apple-30-and-most-profitable/

Kozlowski, M. (2013, May 17). *A brief history of eBooks.* Retrieved from http://goodereader.com/blog/electronic-readers/a-brief-history-of-ebooks

Lee, T-T. (2007). Patients' perceptions of nurses' bedside use of PDAs. *Computers, Informatics, Nursing: CIN, 25*(2), 106–111. doi: 10.1097/01.NCN.0000263980.31178.bd.

Medindia. (2014). *History of PDA.* Retrieved from http://www.medindia.net/pda/pda_history.htm

Microsoft. (2014). *Tips for creating a strong password.* Retrieved from http://windows.microsoft.com/en-us/windows-vista/tips-for-creating-a-strong-password

Mitchell, B. (2014). *Wi-Fi—wireless fidelity.* Retrieved from http://compnetworking.about.com/cs/wireless80211/g/bldef_Wi-Fi.htm

Nations, D. (2015). What is AirDrop? How does it work? Retrieved from http://ipad.about.com/od/iPad_Guide/ss/What-Is-Airdrop-How-Does-It-Work.htm

Patel, N. (2007, November 21). *Kindle sells out in 5.5 hours.* Retrieved from http://www.engadget.com/2007/11/21/kindle-sells-out-in-two-days/

PC World Staff. (2013). *In pictures: A history of cell phones.* Retrieved from http://www.pcworld.idg.com.au/slideshow/194761/pictures_history_cell_phones/

Pence, J. H. (2012, July 13). *A brief history of e-publishing, pt. 2: The rise and fall of the Rocket Ebook.* Retrieved from http://wordservewatercooler.com/2012/07/13/a-brief-history-of-e-publishing-the-rise-and-fall-of-the-rocket-ebook/

Phillippi, J. C., & Wyatt, T. H. (2011). Smartphone in nursing education. *Computers, Informatics, Nursing: CIN, 29*(8), 449–454.

Protalinski, E. (2014, January 29). *Strategy analytics: Android smartphone shipments up to 78.9 (in 2013, iOS down to 15.5%, Windows phone at 3.6%).* Retrieved from http://thenextweb.com/mobile/2014/01/29/strategy-analytics-android-smartphone-shipments-78-9-2013-ios-15-5-windows-phone-3-6/#!tY0Th

Qualcomm. (1999, September 22). *Qualcomm announces the shipment of the pdQ smartphone to Israel.* Retrieved from http://www.qualcomm.com/media/releases/1999/09/22/qualcomm-announces-shipment-pdq-smartphone-israel

Rothman, D. (2009, February 13). *Rocket eBook, SoftBook and Gemstar machines revisited: A few lessons from history.* Retrieved from http://www.teleread.com/drm/rocket-ebook-softbook-and-gemstar-machines-revisited-a-few-lessons-from-history/

Swan, B. A., Smith, K. A., Frisby, A., et al. (2013). Evaluating tablet technology in an undergraduate nursing program. *Nursing Education Perspectives, 34*(3), 192–193. Retrieved from http://www.nln.org/nlnjournal/

Temple University. (2011, February 1). *Future nurses learn to provide better care using smart phones.* Retrieved from http://news.temple.edu/news/future-nurses-learn-provide-better-care-using-smart-phones

Tilley, C. (2014, April 26). *The history of Microsoft Windows CE—Index and humble beginnings.* Retrieved from http://www.hpcfactor.com/support/windowsce/

TEDMED. (2009, October). *Eric Topol: The wireless future of medicine.* Retrieved from http://www.ted.com/talks/eric_topol_the_wireless_future_of_medicine/

Topol, E. (2012). *The creative destruction of medicine: How the digital revolution will create better health care.* New York: Basic Books.

Webopedia. (2014). *Piconet.* Retrieved from http://www.webopedia.com/TERM/P/piconet.html

Wyatt, T. H., & Krauskopf, P. B. (2012, June). Using smartphones to enhance nursing practice. *Online Journal of Issues in Nursing, 16*(2). Retrieved from http://ojni.org/issues/?p=1706

UNIT IV

The Evolving Healthcare Paradigm

An electronic health record for every American by 2014 was a goal set by President George W. Bush in 2004—a wonderful goal, but one that is complicated. The steps involve both healthcare professionals and consumers. The change is part of a new paradigm in healthcare. Consumers are changing from patients to clients who make treatment decisions with healthcare professionals. The challenge for healthcare consumers is to take an active responsibility for their care. As this paradigm makes its perspective felt, professionals are finding that clients want reasons for treatments and that they will search the web for information to either support or refute the information that we give them. Clients also expect designated parts of their healthcare history to be available to all their healthcare providers. This requires decisions about who should have access to what information, what terms to use for this information, and the protocols needed to electronically exchange it.

This unit begins with Chapter 12, informatics benefits for the healthcare consumer. The chapter includes a discussion of benefits, current availability, and barriers to personal health records, along with the use of electronic communication. Chapter 13 looks at all aspects of the empowered consumer, the good, the not so good, and healthcare professionals' parts in assisting healthcare consumers. Chapter 14 explores interoperability, an elusive characteristic as it applies at the international and national levels. The last chapter in this unit, Chapter 15, looks at nursing's efforts to make nursing information interoperable through standardizing our data.

CHAPTER 12

Informatics Benefits for the Consumer

OBJECTIVES

After studying this chapter, you will be able to:

1. Differentiate between an electronic patient record, an electronic health record, and a personal health record.

2. Describe the various forms of a personal health record.

3. Discuss barriers to the establishment of personal health records.

4. Describe healthcare smart cards.

5. Construct a plan for electronic communication with healthcare consumers.

KEY TERMS

Confidentiality

Consumer informatics

De-identified data

Electronic health record

Electronic medical record

Flash drive

Health Insurance Portability
and Accountability Act
(HIPAA)

Interoperable

Nationwide Health Information
Network (NwHIN)

Patient portals

Personal health record (PHR)

Personal identification
number (PIN)

Privacy

Protocol

Security

Smart card

Unique patient identifier

USB port

As you help the paramedics wheel the unconscious patient into the emergency room, you notice something around his neck. Upon closer inspection, you see that it is an identification device with a universal serial bus (USB) connection. Quickly you remove the device and plug it into the **USB port** of a nearby computer. Immediately information appears on the screen that tells you his name and other identifying information including that he is on Coumadin and that he has congestive heart failure. You print this information and communicate it to the rest of the team. Does this scenario sound far-fetched? It is not. **Flash drives** designed to hold health information for use in emergencies exist today. **Smart cards**, discussed later in this chapter, are an example of another device designed to store health information.

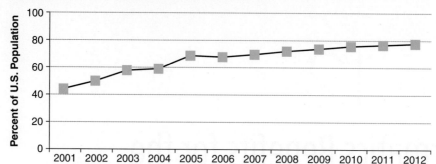

Figure 12-1. Growth of U.S. population online. (Data from *Internet World Usage and Population Statistics*. (2014). Retrieved from http://www.internetworldstats.com/am/us.htm and U.S. Census Bureau. (2014, January 31). *Computers and Internet Use*. Retrieved from http://www.census.gov/hhes/computer/publications.)

Information technology (IT) continues to change the face of healthcare. Between a public demanding more participation in their healthcare, providers looking for ways to improve the quality of healthcare, and communication technology that can access and transmit health information, we are seeing a transformation of healthcare. The Internet is at the heart of this revolution. In a little more than a decade, the percentage of the United States (U.S.) population who are online has increased to almost 80% (Figure 12-1). Worldwide usage has also increased, with 27.5% of Asians and 63.2% of Europeans online in 2012 (Miniwatts Marketing Group, 2014). With this trend, the pressure is on healthcare providers to use the Internet responsibly for their healthcare, as the patient in the above scenario did when he purchased, entered data into, and wore the identification device. Further, as more and more "health care consumers" use the Internet to learn about their conditions, you will see the relationship between the consumers and healthcare providers change. Healthcare providers become more of an advisor while patients become clients or consumers. The term "patient" used in this chapter indicates the person who is receiving healthcare. The terms "client" and "consumer" refer to the person who seeks and purchases the healthcare services. This chapter focuses on the informatics benefits for consumers.

IMPLEMENTING THE PROMISE OF THE INTERNET IN HEALTHCARE

There must be integration of all healthcare records before the full promise of the Internet in healthcare becomes a reality. Many other countries are ahead

of the United States in this endeavor, particularly those with a nationalized health service; however, none has yet reached the full potential. All countries have common **privacy** and **security** concerns for sharing health information. Privacy refers to the right of patients to control what happens to their personal health information (HRSA, n.d.). Security refers to the measures implemented to prevent unauthorized users access to the personal health information of patients. **Confidentiality** refers to authorized care providers maintaining all personal health information as secret, except to other care providers who need access to that information and to others that the patient has consented to allow access. Confidentiality is an important measure to maintain privacy and security of personal health information.

In the United States, the **Nationwide Health Information Network** (NwHIN; discussed further in Chapter 13) serves as a foundation for secure information exchange over the Internet using a "a set of standards, services, and policies" (HealthIT.gov, 2014a, para. 1). The effectiveness of the secure information exchange is dependent on each healthcare provider using electronic patient care records, these records being accessible by those designated by the patient anywhere in the United States, and patients having access to their healthcare records. There is a gradual build of components for the information, with full interconnectedness being the last step.

The Office of the National Coordinator (ONC) for Health IT, established in 2004, coordinates programs established by the Health Information Technology for Economic and Clinical Health Act (HITECH Act) (HealthIT.gov, 2014b). The ONC also facilitates the adoption of health IT programs in the United States. As of 2008 in the United States, the ONC agreed upon the terms used to identify the three parts of the patient's record: **electronic medical record** (EMR), **electronic health record** (EHR), and the **personal health record** (PHR). The ONC for Health IT continues to use the terminology (HealthIT.gov, 2014c). Figure 12-2 is a diagram depicting the integration of health information records.

■ The EMR is a digital healthcare record created by healthcare providers or agencies, such as a hospital. EMRs that meet national standards for interoperability will be able to share health information with the EHR.

■ The EHR is an **interoperable** electronic healthcare record that can contain data from the EMRs of all healthcare providers, including care facilities, clinicians, laboratories, and pharmacies involved with the patient's care. The EHR provides real-time information and includes evidence-based decision support tools. Interoperable means that the data can be shared electronically.

■ The PHR allows users to maintain/manage their own health information and communicate the information with authorized providers. If the PHR conforms to interoperability standards, it can contain data from the EHR, but still controlled by the individual. PHRs tethered (can communicate) with EHRs are private, secure, confidential, and protected by the **Health Insurance Portability and Accountability Act (HIPAA).** Stand-alone PHRs are not HIPAA protected.

Electronic Medical Record

EMRs are the focus of most healthcare agencies today. The institution or provider that creates EMRs owns and manages them. As healthcare agencies merge and form large corporations, those with the required authorization often combine these EMRs so that information from all member agencies and providers is accessible. Many agencies refer to their EMR as EHR, but an electronic record that cannot interface with outside

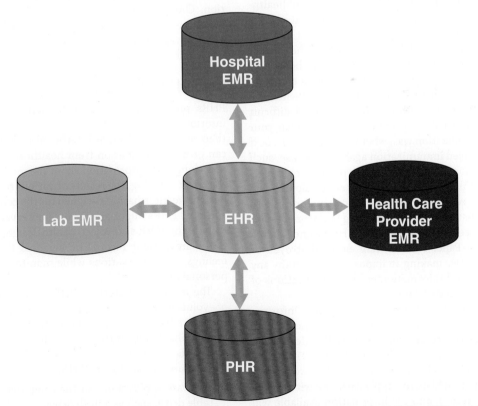

Figure 12-2. Integration of a patient's health information with different providers' EMRs, EHR, and PHR.

agencies is not a true EHR. (Chapter 16 includes additional information about EMRs.)

Consumers have access to their own health information in EMRs. For many years, a person's healthcare record, whether in a hospital or clinic, was the property of the agency providing the care. Patients had no permission to see their records. In fact, it was improper to share health information such as a temperature or blood pressure with a patient. HIPAA, passed in 1996, changed this by giving patients the right to see their own healthcare records (U.S. Department of Health and Human Services, 2014a, 2014b). Difficulties arise however, because in many cases, pieces of a patient's medical history are scattered in many different locales.

Electronic Health Record

When babies born in the United States are 2 months old, they might have healthcare records in at least two places: the hospital where they were born and in the pediatrician's office. As the babies grow, the number and location of their healthcare records also grow. The current record system, whether paper or electronic, makes it difficult for individuals to have access to their healthcare records. Additionally, it handicaps healthcare providers by preventing them from having complete information about a person. Individuals who have not kept their own health records find it difficult to remember details. Try to remember what your last immunization was, where you received it, or if you received immunization against a disease, such as tetanus. Remembering all one's surgeries is more difficult, as one grows older, let alone being able to remember one's medical history. These problems can be life threatening in an emergency, as was seen in the aftermath of Hurricane Katrina in 2005. Paper records were either destroyed or inaccessible, making it impossible to obtain any past medical information or list of medications of people in need of care.

Under the EHR model, one's health information is available from any location where there is Internet access and a health information exchange (HIE) exists (HealthIT.gov, 2014d). The accessibility makes it easier for patients who visit multiple providers to supply each one with an up-to-date record, and the information available will usually be more than what a referring provider sends. It also provides safer care in the advent of an emergency when regular records may not be available. A record of all the consumer prescriptions can minimize adverse drug effects. Additionally, data from HIEs can assist in identifying those who abuse prescription drugs using multiple pharmacies so that the users can obtain assistance. Having healthcare data in an electronic format allows use of **de-identified data** in an aggregated form to assess patterns of disease, quickly identify potentially dangerous side effects of medications, and detect disease outbreaks. De-identified data contain no personal identifiers, such as name, birth date, and zip code.

Although change is evolving, the results of a 2010 Harris Interactive poll revealed that less than 10% of Americans used electronic health information or email communication with their providers (Harris Interactive, 2010). The percentage is increasing; however, there is no update of the study, available. Many Americans still do not understand the rationale for use of electronic health information. Only 78% thought their physicians should have access to the electronic information. Twenty-eight percent thought that their physicians used an electronic record (Figure 12-3).

Personal Health Record

PHRs provide clients access to their healthcare information and may allow clients to enter data into their records. A PHR that is tethered with the EHR can provide information from healthcare encounters along with information about the medications the client is taking, the results of various tests, and healthcare information designed for the consumer. Tethered PHRs might also include observations of daily living (ODLs) (Project HealthDesign, 2012). ODLs are patient records of personal thoughts, feelings, and observations while monitoring their personal health.

The initial computerized PHRs were in a state of evolution, with no one agreeing on exactly what they were (Halamka et al., 2008). Today, ONC certified PHRs that meet the national interoperability standards can share data with the EHR. There are three main formats for the PHR:

■ Software applications for the computer or portable drive, such as a flash drive.

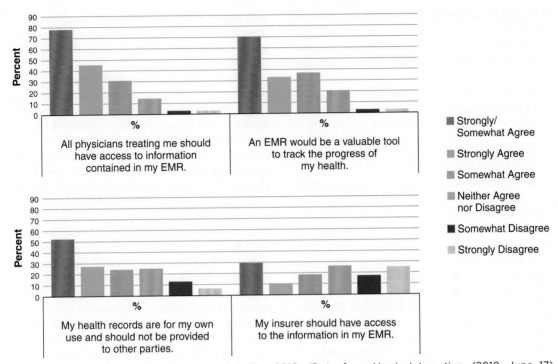

Figure 12-3. Americans' attitudes toward EMRs—2010. (Data from Harris Interactive. (2010, June 17). *Few Americans using 'e' medical records.* Retrieved from http://www.harrisinteractive.com/NewsRoom/ HarrisPolls/tabid/447/mid/1508/articleId/414/ctl/ReadCustom%20Default/Default.aspx.)

- Web portals that store the information on another computer remotely.
- Hybrid PHRs that allow for remote storage of the health information, as well as the ability to store the information on a personal computer or portable drive.

In 2004, Dr. David Brailer, as ONC national coordinator, outlined the strategic framework for the ONC (HITECHAnswers, 2014). The report advocated for consumer empowerment, personalized care, and the consumers' ability to select healthcare based on their values and information. Consumer empowerment has the ability to affect the rising rate of health plan costs by incorporating economic consequences for low-quality care. It can also improve healthcare by providing consumers with data such as the cost and quality of healthcare services along with information for self-diagnosis and referral to appropriate providers. At the same time, it can preserve the best elements of our present system of clinical support for those who suffer from acute illnesses, injuries, or chronic conditions.

Historical Perspectives of Consumer Empowerment

The term "consumer empowerment" means that patients have enough health information to make informed decisions. In other words, they can become consumers or clients, not patients. Consumer empowerment initiative started in the legal system in the early 1900s.

The initial legal case was a 1905 Illinois Court of Appeals decision that established that patients have the right to know in advance what surgery is going to be performed (Pratt v. Davis, 1905). The case resulted from a physician who performed a hysterectomy on an epileptic patient without her consent. According to the case, the physician obtained consent from the husband, instead of the wife, stating that the patient could not consent because of her mental condition, although the physician never established her incompetency.

Schloendorff v. Society of the New York Hospital (1914) is the seminal case that supported informed consent and patient empowerment. A woman consented to surgery to diagnose a thyroid tumor as benign or malignant, but she did not give consent to remove the tumor. After determining that the tumor was malignant, the surgeon removed it against the patient's wishes. Justice Benjamin Cardoza noted:

> Every human of adult years and sound mind has a right to determine what shall be done with his own body; and a surgeon who performs an operation without his patient's consent commits an assault for which he is liable in damages. (Schloendorff v. Society of the New York Hospital, 1914).

Although the courts supported patient rights to consent for treatment, medicine remained largely a paternalistic practice for many decades. Informed consent did not include the right to understand the personal medical condition, treatment options, risks associated with the options, or prognosis. The Patient's Bill of Rights approved in 1973 by the American Hospital Association stimulated a culture change in healthcare (Paasche-Orlow et al., 2009).

Further court cases in the 1970s affirmed the rights for patients to receive this information in plain English. Despite the slow beginning, today many consumers expect to receive understandable information about their health conditions and be full partners in their healthcare, not passive recipients. Consumers want to make intelligent decisions about healthcare based on cost and quality.

Patient Portals

Patient portals provide patients access to their EHR data. Common portal communication functions include the ability to make routine appointments, renew prescriptions, or receive alerts. Examples of alerts include sending notifications for appointments, flu shots, or immunizations. Some portals allow patients to upload blood glucose results and then provide feedback on glucose control. Assisting diabetic patients to manage their chronic condition has the potential of saving healthcare dollars (Paylor, 2010) and improving their quality of life.

This type of personalization of information is successful, especially in the care of patients with chronic diseases such as diabetes and heart disease. Most patient portals contain some type of decision support using computerized prompts. Some provide secure email messaging features. Using patient portals is one way to meet the needs of consumers who expect personal attention. Consumers desire the same services that the financial industry provides, namely, personalized information individually targeted for them.

Although the number and types of patient portals are growing, the usage as of 2010 was less than 10% (Harris Interactive, 2010). The percentage for use of patient portals is greater if the consumer has a health insurance plan that provides a patient portal. For example, 50% of patients who had Kaiser and 30% of patients who had United Healthcare reported that they had a PHR. What is interesting is that the 2010 Harris Interactive poll indicated that only 30% of the population believed that insurance companies should have access to their health information, although most believed that an electronic record would be valuable to track their health progress (see Figure 12-3).

Currently, many nongovernmental groups sponsor PHRs; some are commercial, and some are nonprofit. Examples of free resources include Microsoft HealthVault (http://www.healthvault.com/), MyPHR by AHIMA (http://www.myphr.com/), WebMD Personal Health Record (http://www.webmd.com/phr), and MyMediConnnect Personal Health Records (https://www.mymediconnect.net/phr.php). Microsoft HealthVault allows users to store and share emergency information. Users can also give permission to healthcare services and providers, such as pharmacies, hospitals, labs, and clinics, to send information to the users' HealthVault records. Users with devices, such as blood glucose, blood pressure, or heart rate monitors, can import the data into their HealthVault accounts. In addition, users can track and share fitness goal achievements.

The MyPHR website is not a PHR, rather, it provides information about PHRs, as well as providing links to PHR resources, based upon the user's needs. WebMD Personal Health Record allows users to collect, store, and manage personal and health history information, as well as share it with authorized others. My MediConnect Personal Health Record is similar to HealthVault and WebMD, allowing users to collect, store, and manage health information from authorized providers and services.

Before recommending a PHR resource, the healthcare provider must thoroughly evaluate it. If the PHR resource depends on advertisements for support, the information and links provided must be bias free and complete. Users should always read the privacy statement.

The U.S. government provides several free resources for PHRs. Examples are My Family Health Portrait sponsored by the U.S. Surgeon (https://familyhistory.hhs.gov/), My HealtheVet sponsored by the Veteran's Association (https://www.myhealth.va.gov/index.html), MyMedicare.gov (https://mymedicare.gov/) sponsored by Medicare.gov (2014), and Blue Button Connector (HealthIT.gov, 2014e) sponsored by HealthIT.gov (http://www.healthit.gov/bluebutton). The U.S. government PHRs all allow users to collect, store, and manage personal and family history, medications, provider information, and more. Healthcare providers, when authorized by the PHR owner, can access the personal health information, too.

Similar efforts to provide personal health information are underway in other countries. Australia launched the Personally Controlled Electronic Health Record (PCEHR) in 2012 (http://www.ehealth.gov.au/internet/ehealth/publishing.nsf/content/home). England provides a Summary Care Record with information about medications, allergies, and adverse reactions (http://www.nhscarerecords.nhs.uk). The Summary Care Record is used when patients are seen after hours in places other than their primary care provider, such as the emergency department, urgent care, or hospital admission. Scotland uses an approach similar to England, with the Scottish Emergency Care Summary (http://www.nisg.scot.nhs.uk/currently-supporting/emergency-care-summary).

Benefits of PHRs

PHRs will further collaborative care—that is, care in which there is a partnership between the patient and their healthcare providers. When the healthcare provider and a consumer view an individual's PHR together, instead of the healthcare provider giving orders, which the patient may or may not understand or accept, the healthcare provider can help the patient to understand his or her condition and work together with this individual to achieve an agreed-upon goal. Consumers can also collaborate in the creation and maintenance of the healthcare record.

Another benefit of PHRs is the ability to manage one's disease treatment more effectively. For example, those with a chronic disease, such as diabetes or hypertension, can track their disease together with their healthcare provider, which can lower the communication barrier between consumer and provider and empower the consumer (HealthIT.gov, 2014f). A PHR tethered with the EHR permits the provider share individualized information with the client; thus, providing more personalized as well as higher-quality care. The improved communication that results will lead consumers to a better understanding of their healthcare responsibilities and disease management. A tethered PHR reduces administrative costs associated with electronic prescription refills and scheduling appointments.

> ### QSEN Scenario
> You are working with a small group of patients at a clinic that provides a web portal that allows patients to access health information, make appointments, and renew prescriptions. What resources might assist you to teach the patients about the benefits of a personal health record?

Barriers to Implementation of PHRs

Overcoming several barriers is necessary before the full PHR becomes a reality. The technology to create a full PHR is here, but the agreements, **protocols** (a system of rules for exchange of data by computers), and procedures are still evolving. Barriers include provider reluctance to use PHR data. There is no unique identifier to connect EHR and EMR data. Other issues include concerns about privacy and security, interoperability, data presentation, and costs.

Provider Reluctance and Responsibility
A PHR and an EHR can threaten the autonomy of some healthcare providers who still want to practice in the traditional model (Wynia et al., 2011). The reluctance is dissipating with the rollout of reimbursement incentives (and penalties) associated with the 2009 HITECH Act "meaningful use" plan (meaningful use is discussed in Chapter 17). Despite the fact that patients can now get copies of their healthcare records, traditional agencies and healthcare providers may still see themselves as owners of this information, instead of guardians.

Historically, healthcare practitioners have had concerns about providing client access to information not designed for lay interpretation or that may contain information inappropriate to divulge to patients, such as psychiatric problems or diseases. Providers are also concerned about the effects on the patient, on the provider–client relationship, and on healthcare itself. There have been questions about a client's interest in reading and contributing to a healthcare record. Other concerns are that the patient, for litigious reasons, may use access to healthcare records. In addition, there are concerns about problems with client understanding of information in the records.

To mitigate liability risks, providers must share expectations with clients who can access and send communications to the provider using electronic healthcare systems (McGraw et al., 2013). Examples of decisions are listed below.

- Decide the providers that receive the communication, how to share the communication, and what to do in a medical emergency.
- Decide which problems the patient shares.
- Decide when the care provider receives and reviews the information.
- Decide storage resource for the information (medical device or patient portal)
- Decide how to format the information and the mechanism for teaching patients expectations for their use of communication.

Unique Patient Identifier

Besides an EMR, in theory, a full PHR requires that each citizen have a **unique patient identifier** (UPI) for his or her healthcare information regardless of where it is stored. Today, individual providers have their own method of identifying EMRs despite the fact that the 1996 HIPAA required the UPI. An UPI is a single source that links each patient with his or her individual health record. The vision for the use of the PHI was to allow authorized persons to file and obtain the patients' health records with accuracy. However, because of concerns about privacy for sharing health information, it has not been adopted (Hillestad et al., 2012; Montgomery & Zhang, 2013).

The Rand Corporation, a nonprofit research group, published a report noting that use of the UPI would improve efficient use of the electronic record and reduce errors (Hillestad et al., 2012). The RAND report also indicated that the cost for a UPI would be as much as 11 billion dollars. Privacy groups immediately rejected the report (Lauer, 2008). Privacy groups have lobbied against the use of the UPI vociferously since HIPAA became law, citing privacy and security concerns. The National Alliance for Health Information Technology (NAHIT) was another very strong proponent of the UPI. However, once NAHIT disbanded in September 2009 (Monegain, 2009), there has been little further discussion.

Data Privacy and Security

For consumers to feel comfortable with exchanges of their healthcare information, there must be assurances about protection of their data from those without permission to access it. This requires individual healthcare providers and agencies have the state-of-the-art security but also that there are protocols that govern access to data. Every healthcare practice must conduct a security risk analysis. A good resource with common myths regarding risk analysis is online at http://www.healthit.gov/providers-professionals/top-10-myths-security-risk-analysis. HealthIT.gov provides a gaming approach to educate providers on the topic at http://www.healthit.gov/providers-professionals/privacy-security-training-games.

Data Standards

Another barrier to implementation of PHRs has been the lack of data standardization. (See Chapter 14 for more information on this topic.) All agencies involved in healthcare, including pharmacies, must agree to record a defined set of data in a defined manner, that is, decisions need to be made about what information to record and the protocols used for recording and transmission. Identification of this core set of data elements requires participation by representatives of all healthcare record users including consumers. This barrier is currently being resolved by using the ONC certification process.

Data Presentation

It is one thing to provide consumers with access to their healthcare data, and it is another to present this in a useful, understandable manner. For example, how should information be grouped? What should a certain screen present? This area is one of the primary focuses in the field of **consumer informatics**. Data presentation is a concern for healthcare providers and falls into the category of usability.

Consumers

Clients need to think of themselves as healthcare consumers with a responsibility to participate actively in their healthcare. A client raised in an era (such as before 1950), in which one was a passive patient may have developed security in placing responsibility for health with others. Consumers may need assistance to understand new roles and responsibilities.

Costs

Financing of EHRs and PHRs is another barrier to implementation. Although the U.S. government is offering financial incentives to adopt electronic records for healthcare providers, like so many informatics advances, the expectation is often that healthcare agencies and healthcare providers will pay for them. Yet, the majority of advantages accrue to payers and patients. It is easy to say that electronic records will save money; these savings, however, generally come from the pocket of the healthcare agencies and healthcare providers who will lose business as patients do not require as many office visits, laboratory tests, or hospitalizations. Incentives such as values-based purchasing approach to motivating healthcare providers to promote value and quality in return of the dollars spent.

Smart Cards

Some providers use smart cards for patient identification. A smart card looks like a plastic credit card and, like a credit card, has embedded information that a smart card reader can read. In a smart card, however, the embedded data are on a computer chip and a contact plate, which is usually gold (Smart Card Alliance, 2012). See Box 12-1 for the contents of a smart card. The chip, which requires

---

| **BOX 12-1** | Basic Contents of a Smart Card |

- A microcontroller for managing data
- A secure encrypted microchip to store data
- A contactless radiofrequency (RF) interface
- A contact interface (usually gold colored)

---

the appropriate computer system and access code to read and write, encrypts the data on the card. The first introduction of smart cards was 1992 in France to combat fraud in telecommunications and banking (Chase Paymentech, 2014). Since then, many industries including healthcare use them.

Smart cards identify patients when making contact with the healthcare system and transmit information that will assist treatment by healthcare providers. A healthcare smart card has four subsets of data: data necessary to operate the card including privacy protection, data unique to the consumer, administrative data such as insurance carrier, and clinical data. Access, however, is not automatic; users must provide a password, a **PIN** number (**personal identification number** used to gain computer access), or both, and possibly a biometric, such as a fingerprint or digitized iris. Use of biometrics in emergency care might be difficult or impossible if the patient is unconscious.

A concern for use with healthcare smart cards is security (Madden, 2012). However, smart cards that use embedded intelligence, as well as its processing capability and standards-based cryptography, ensure adherence to the privacy requirements of HIPAA. Additionally, the smart card has built-in tamper resistance and the ability to store large amounts of data. Healthcare smart cards also aid in the portability provision of HIPAA. This provision is concerned with the ability of healthcare data to be portable, that is, to be able to send and receive data electronically in an understandable format, while protecting the confidentiality of the data. The objective is to simplify the administration of healthcare data.

Honnegowda et al. (2013) suggest that an electronic smart card will be the next generation smart card. The electronic card is battery powered. A combination of the contact plat, magnetic stripe emulator, and RF interface provide international interface standards for interoperability. The cons of the next generation smart card related to the lifespan, since the electronic card is powered using an embedded battery.

There are many advantages to health smart cards (Box 12-2). One benefit is that they provide information management, which ensures that security practices are followed, simplifying hospital admissions, and providing emergency healthcare data (Smart Card Alliance, 2012). Having

---

BOX 12-2   Advantages of Healthcare Smart Cards

- Require user identification and authorization
- Require employee credentials for strong authentication for HIPAA compliance and network security
- Provide immediate access to lifesaving information
- Provide data portability
- Guard against healthcare fraud, abuse, and misuse
- Resolve language issues associated with health record information
- Reduce administrative costs
- Support the NwHIN standards

Source: Smart Card Alliance. (2009, February). *A healthcare CFO's guide to smart card technology and applications.* Retrieved from http://www.smartcardalliance.org/resources/lib/Healthcare_CFO_Guide_to_Smart_Cards_FINAL_012809.pdf

---

patient information, such as allergies, prescribed medications, and medical conditions such as diabetes or congestive heart failure, readily available in emergency rooms and ambulances can greatly facilitate care. Additionally, smart cards can provide patients with the knowledge in situations where their healthcare data are not readily available.

SUMMARY

The use of Internet and web features in healthcare is changing the relationship of the provider and the client. The client can access information previously held only by the practitioner increases. EMRs that provide healthcare records for only one provider will morph into EHRs that provide access to records from many different agencies from one access point. Subsequently, a PHR that permits and encourages client access to their healthcare information is emerging. Work continues to overcome barriers for universal access including gaining provider compliance, an UPI, and changing consumer behavior.

The exchange of information between a healthcare provider and a client will become an expected mode of communication; one particularly involving nurses in telephone consultations of private practice. This will not happen without overcoming provider reluctance and planning that includes decisions such as what information to provide to clients and when. Nevertheless, tethered PHRs are becoming a normal part of healthcare delivery.

APPLICATIONS AND COMPETENCIES

1. Differentiate between an EMR, an EHR, and a PHR, as described in this chapter.

2. Search HealthIT.gov or other pertinent website for information that extends your understanding about selecting a PHR for yourself or other healthcare consumers. Describe the various forms of PHRs. Discuss the barriers to the establishment of PHRs. Cite the sources you used.

3. Conduct a search using a digital library resources and the Internet to extend your knowledge about healthcare smart cards. Would you use a healthcare smart card? Why or why not? Summarize the results of the research and cite the resources used.

4. Write a proposal for instituting email communication with clients in a specific practice such as primary care, obstetrics, or cardiology. Cite the resources used for the proposal.

5. Examine the pros and cons of a unique patient identifier. Create a listing of talking points and cite the resources you used.

REFERENCES

Chase Paymentech. (2014). *FAQ: EMV chip card technology.* Retrieved from https://www.chasepaymentech.com/faq_emv_chip_card_technology.html

Halamka, J. D., Mandl, K. D., & Tang, P. C. (2008). Early experiences with personal health records. *Journal of the American Medical Informatics Association, 15*(1), 1–7.

Harris Interactive. (2010, June 17). *Few Americans using 'e' medical records.* Retrieved from http://www.harrisinteractive.com/NewsRoom/HarrisPolls/tabid/447/mid/1508/articleId/414/ctl/ReadCustom%20Default/Default.aspx

HealthIT.gov. (2014a, February 9). *Nationwide health information network (NwHIN).* Retrieved from http://www.healthit.gov/policy-researchers-implementers/nationwide-health-information-network-nwhin

HealthIT.gov. (2014b, February 15). *About ONC*. Retrieved from http://www.healthit.gov/newsroom/about-onc

HealthIT.gov. (2014c). *What are the differences between electronic medical records, electronic health records, and personal health records?* Retrieved from http://www.healthit.gov/providers-professionals/faqs/what-are-differences-between-electronic-medical-records-electronic

HealthIT.gov. (2014d, February 12). *Health information exchange (HIE)*. Retrieved from http://www.healthit.gov/HIE

HealthIT.gov. (2014e, February 9). *About Blue Button*. Retrieved from http://www.healthit.gov/patients-families/blue-button/about-blue-button

HealthIT.gov. (2014f, February 4). *What are the different types of PHR models that are available today?* Retrieved from http://www.hrsa.gov/healthit/toolbox/HealthITAdoption toolbox/PersonalHealthRecords/modelsavailable.html

Hillestad, R., Dreyer, P., Greenberg, M.D., et al. (2008). *Identify crisis: An examination of the costs and benefits of a unique patient identifier for the U.S. health care system*. Santa Monica, CA: RAND Corporation. Retrieved from http://www.rand.org/pubs/monographs/MG753

HITECHAnswers. (2014). *History of EHR adoption*. Retrieved from http://www.hitechanswers.net/ehr-adoption-2/history-of-ehr-adoption/

Honnegowda, L., Chan, S., & Lau, C. T. (2013). Embedded electronic smart card for financial and healthcare information transaction. *Journal of Advances in Computer Networks, 1*(1), 57–60. doi: 10.7763/JACN.2013.V1.12. Retrieved from http://www.jacn.net/show-7-20-1.html

HRSA. (n.d.). *How can I maintain patient privacy in a health information technology system?* Retrieved from http://www.hrsa.gov/healthit/toolbox/hivaidscaretoolbox/securityandprivacyissues/howcanimaintainpat.html

Lauer, G. (2008, October 30). *Privacy advocates reject unique patient identifier study*. Retrieved from http://www.ihealthbeat.org/features/2008/privacy-advocates-reject-unique-patient-identifier-study.aspx

Madden, R. A. (2012, February 13). *Smart cards for healthcare: Can you carry your health records in your wallet? Advance for NPs & PAs*. Retrieved from http://nurse-practitioners-and-physician-assistants.advanceweb.com/Features/Articles/Smart-Cards-for-Healthcare.aspx

McGraw, D., Belfort, R., Pfister, H., et al. (2013, December 18). Going digital with patients: Managing potential liability risks of patient-generated electronic health information. *Journal of Participatory Medicine, 5(5)*, e41. Retrieved from http://www.jopm.org/perspective/narratives/2013/12/18/going-digital-with-patients-managing-potential-liability-risks-of-patient-generated-electronic-health-information/

Medicare.gov. (2014). *Medicare's Blue Button*. Retrieved from http://www.medicare.gov/manage-your-health/blue-button/medicare-blue-button.html

Miniwatts Marketing Group. (2014, February 4). *World Internet stats: Usage and population statistics*. Retrieved from http://www.internetworldstats.com/stats.htm

Monegain, B. (2009, September 25). *NAHIT disbands after seven years of advocacy. Healthcare IT News*. Retrieved from http://www.healthcareitnews.com/news/nahit-disbands-after-seven-years-advocacy

Montgomery, D., & Zhang, C. (2013). *The unique patient identification (UPI) debate: Implementing a U.S. patient identification standard*. Paper presented at the Southern Association for Information Systems Conference. Savannah, Georgia. Retrieved from http://sais.aisnet.org/2013/MontgomeryZhang.pdf

Paasche-Orlow, M. K., Jacob, D. M., Hochhauser, M., et al. (2009). National survey of patients' bill of rights statutes. *Journal of General Internal Medicine, 24*(4), 489–494. Retrieved from http://link.springer.com/article/10.1007%2Fs11606-009-0914-z

Paylor, M. (2010). Patient portals and health records in diabetes care. *British Journal of Healthcare Management, 16*(3), 142–145.

Pratt v. Davis. (1905). *118 Ill. App 161*. Retrieved from http://digitalcommons.law.yale.edu/cgi/viewcontent.cgi?article=3909&context=fss_papers

Project HealthDesign. (2012). *Observations of daily living*. Retrieved from http://www.projecthealthdesign.org/resources/observations-of-daily-living

Schloendorff v. Society of the New York Hospital. (1914). *211 N.Y. 125, 105 N.E. 92*. Retrieved from http://digitalcommons.law.yale.edu/cgi/viewcontent.cgi?article=3909&context=fss_papers

Smart Card Alliance. (2012, September). *Smart card technology in U.S. healthcare: Frequently asked questions*. Retrieved from http://www.smartcardalliance.org/resources/pdf/Smart_Card_Technology_in_Healthcare_FAQ_FINAL_096012.pdf

U.S. Department of Health and Human Services. (2014a). *Your medical records*. Retrieved from http://www.hhs.gov/ocr/privacy/hipaa/understanding/consumers/medicalrecords.html

U.S. Department of Health and Human Services. (2014b, February 7. *Summary of the HIPAA privacy rule*. Retrieved from http://www.hhs.gov/ocr/privacy/hipaa/understanding/summary/index.html

Wynia, M. K., Torres, G. W., & Lemieux, J. (2011). Many physicians are willing to use patients' electronic personal health records, but doctors differ by location, gender, and practice. *Health Affairs, 30*(2), 266–273. Retrieved from http://content.healthaffairs.org/content/30/2/266.full.pdf

CHAPTER 13

The Empowered Consumer

OBJECTIVES

After studying this chapter, you will be able to:

1. Analyze the effect of consumer empowerment on healthcare.
2. Describe approaches to guiding healthcare consumers to high-quality web-based health information.
3. Analyze the effects of health literacy and health numeracy on patient care and teaching.
4. Demonstrate finding and evaluating a web-based support group for a client with a specific condition.
5. Explore the potential for web-based health education.

KEY TERMS

Accessibility	Health literacy	Patient portal
Alt tag	Health numeracy	Readability
Braille reader	HONcode	Screen reader
Consumer informatics	Image map	Support group
Flesch Reading Ease	invisible/deep Web	Usability
Flesch-Kincaid Grade Level	Navigation bars	visible/surface Web

An imagined dialogue with Socrates, in Chapter 12 of the book *Consumer-Driven Healthcare*, asks why consumers who can intelligently purchase financial products, cars, and computers cannot do the same with healthcare (Hyde, 2004). The answer was that we never allowed consumers to do so. In the past, consumers did not have the knowledge that healthcare providers did, which resulted in a culture of paternalism. Healthcare providers expected patients (consumers) to accept prescribed care disregarding cost and labeled patients "noncompliant" if they did not. Additionally, there was an underlying flawed assumption on the part of payers and consumers that all healthcare was equal; hence, there was no concern about quality or cost.

The nonprofessional healthcare consumers were dependent on healthcare providers for all their information needs. The advent of the Internet in the 1990s leveled the playing field so that the consumer had access to much of the same information as the healthcare professional. The caveat is that the Internet empowers consumers to take ownership of their health without the benefit of advanced education and training to interpret the meaning of most of the information.

The Internet and the World Wide Web (WWW) make healthcare consumer empowerment progress possible. Consumers today can learn about the quality of care provided by many hospitals and find information about diseases that previously was available only to healthcare professionals. This move to consumerism in healthcare is permanently changing the face of the healthcare industry. Healthcare providers are evolving from being care providers to health and wellness brokers, a role that fits naturally with nursing. This chapter focuses on factors affecting the empowerment of healthcare consumers. (Use of the terms *consumers, clients,* and *patients* is interchangeable in this chapter.)

CONSUMER INFORMATICS

The easy availability of information on the Internet, the push for more cost-effective healthcare, and the desire of many consumers to take more responsibility for their health has resulted in the development of **consumer informatics**, a subspecialty in healthcare informatics. The goal is to improve the consumer decision-making processes and healthcare outcomes with electronic information and communication (American Medical Informatics Association, 2014). This field is an applied science using concepts from communication, education, behavioral science, and social networking. The design of consumer informatics provides consumers healthcare information, allows consumers to make informed decisions, promotes healthy behaviors and information exchange, and provides social support. Practitioners analyze consumer needs and information use and develop ways to facilitate consumers in finding and using health information. They also evaluate the effectiveness of electronic health information and study how this affects public health and the consumer–healthcare provider relationship.

The focus of consumer informatics is consumers, rather than healthcare providers, as end users. The hope is that intelligent informatics applications result in healthcare information that reaches consumers, creating a healthy balance between self-reliance and professional help. Full realization of consumer informatics potential depends on the features and breadth of information systems. Consumer informatics applications may include interaction with healthcare providers; however, others applications may not. Examples include websites, information kiosks, blood pressure kiosks, mobile health applications, and personal health records.

HEALTH/NUMERACY LITERACY COMPETENCIES FOR CONSUMERS

Literacy is an antecedent to health literacy. In 1992, the U.S. Department of Education surveyed over 26,000 adults using the National Adult Literacy Survey (Kirsch et al., 1993; National Center for Education Statistics, n.d.a). It was the second survey used to assess literacy; the first survey was done in 1985. The survey results revealed that 40 to 44 million people have very low literacy skills. To address the literacy issue and improve patient outcomes, the report recommended patient education materials be written at *no higher than a fifth grade* reading level ("Communicating with patients who have limited literacy skills. Report of the National Work Group on Literacy and Health," 1998; Wilson, 2009).

In 2003, the National Center for Education Statistics (n.d.b) sponsored the National Adult Literacy Survey with 19,000 adults who were 16 years and older, representing those living in their homes and in some prisons from all of the United States, including Washington, D.C. It was a landmark survey because it was the first to include questions on health literacy. The 2003 survey results showed that adults who were 65 or older had lower average literacy skills than any of the other age groups; 29% had below basic skills and 30% had basic skills (Kutner et al., 2006).

The benefit that consumers gain from all the information available today depends not only on its quality and availability but also on the ability of the consumer to understand it, or health literacy. **Health literacy** is not simply the ability to read but "to obtain, process, and understand basic health information and services need to make appropriate decisions" (Agency for Healthcare Research and Quality, 2013a, para. 2). It includes the capacity to understand instructions on prescription drug bottles, appointment slips, medical education brochures, doctor's directions, consent forms, and the ability to negotiate complex healthcare systems (Berkman, et al. 2011) (Box 13-1). **Health numeracy** is the

BOX 13-1 Skills Needed for Health Literacy

Patients may face complex health information and treatment decisions. Some of the specific health literacy requirements may include the following:

- Evaluating information for credibility and quality
- Analyzing relative risks and benefits
- Calculating medication dosages [and dosing intervals]
- Interpreting test results
- Locating health information

To accomplish these tasks, individuals may need to be

- Visually literate (able to understand graphs or other visual information)
- Computer literate (able to operate a computer)

- Information literate (able to obtain and apply relevant information)
- Numerically or computationally literate (able to calculate or reason numerically)

Oral language skills are important as well. Patients need to

- Articulate their health concerns and describe their symptoms accurately
- Ask pertinent questions
- Understand spoken medical advice or treatment directions

In an age of shared responsibility between physician and patient for healthcare, patients need strong decision-making skills. With the development of the Internet as a source of health information, health literacy may also include the ability to search the Internet and evaluate websites.

Adapted from National Networks of Libraries of Medicine (NNLM) (2013, October 2, para. 5). *Health literacy*. Retrieved from http://nnlm.gov/outreach/consumer/hlthlit.html

ability of a consumer to interpret and act on all numerical information, such as graphical and probabilistic information needed to make effective health decisions (Rothman et al., 2008). There is an association between health literacy, health numeracy, and education; however, the number of years in school does not assure high health literacy (U.S. Department of Health and Human Services, 2008). Much of the numeracy information that we expect of clients is quantitative—for example—calculating medication schedules, interpreting laboratory values and food labels, and understanding charts (Stagliano & Wallace, 2013).

In the 2003 National Assessment of Adult Literacy sponsored by the National Center for Education Statistics, 44% of high school graduates and 12% of college graduates had basic or below basic health literacy (U.S. Department of Health and Human Services, 2008). Results of a 2007 Dutch survey conducted with 5,136 adults revealed low education is associated with low health literacy (van der Heide et al., 2013).

The first report of the correlation between health literacy and poor health was in 1999 in the *Journal of the American Medical Association* (Ad Hoc Committee on Health Literacy for the Council on Scientific Affairs & American Medical Association, 1999). Health literacy is a greater predictor of health than age, income, employment status, level of education, or race. Health literacy is not static; it varies with context and setting. Healthcare costs are four times higher for persons with lower health literacy skills (National Patient Safety Foundation, 2014). Low health literacy is associated with a 50% risk for hospitalization and a 50% risk for medication administration errors. It is necessary to assess health literacy when working with clients face to face or by phone, when using a computer, or when designing educational materials.

The current health literacy movement evolves from history, when President George H. Bush signed the National Literacy Act (1991), which addressed reading, writing, and arithmetic, the foundations of functional literacy. President Bush commissioned the U.S. Department of Education to conduct the National Health Literacy Survey in 1992 (U.S. Department of Education, & Office of Educational Research and Improvement, 2002).

The survey results demonstrated a significant health literacy issue, with almost one fifth of the respondents having very low health literacy skills. President Clinton issued two executive orders (E.O.) that addressed literacy. Executive Order No. 12,866, 2 (1993) stated regulations must be "simple and easy to understand." Executive Order 12,988, 4731 (1996) stated that regulations must use "clear language."

In 2004, the Institute of Medicine reported that almost half of all Americans had difficulty understanding health information, resulting in unnecessary spending of billions of dollars (Nielsen-Bohlman & Institute of Medicine (U.S.), Committee on Health Literacy, 2004). Six years later, President Obama signed the Plain Writing Act (2010), which prompted significant revision of written resources about health information from federal government agencies.

ASSESSING HEALTH/NUMERACY LITERACY

There are several tools available to assess health literacy. Examples include the Rapid Estimate of Adult Literacy of Medicine (REALM), the Test of Functional Literacy in Adults (TOFHLA), the Newest Vital Sign (NVS), and Single Item Literacy Screener (SILS) (Dickens & Piano, 2013; Kandula et al., 2011). There are abbreviated versions of REALM and TOFHLA (S-TOFHLA), too. Although all of the tools are valid and reliable, the problem is the time necessary to administer the tools, as well as potential embarrassment of the patient.

Stagliano and Wallace (2013) conducted a health literacy study with 241 patients in a primary care setting. The researchers used a combination of the following tools:

- NVS (Weiss et al., 2005), in which the client reads an ice cream label and answers six questions: this tool tests both health literacy and numeracy literacy.
- A three-question health literacy screening tool developed by Chew et al. (2004, 2008) includes questions about how frequently the consumer has trouble understanding written material, how frequent has someone help them with this, and how secure he or she feels in filling out medical forms.

A two-question numeracy literacy tool has been developed by Woloshin et al. (2005), which focuses on consumers' self-assessment of their ability to understand medical statistics and their reliance on such information to make healthcare decisions. Analysis of the data compared with the short-form SOFHLA (S-SOFHLA) and REALM indicated that the Chew et al. health literacy screening item that asked about confidence filling out medical forms was the best predictor of limited and limited/marginal health literacy. Analysis of the data compared with the NVS indicated that the two questions used with the Woloshin et al. tool were strong predictors of numeracy literacy. The results of the Stagliano and Wallace study indicated that a brief assessment using three questions (question on confidence filling out medical forms from the Chew et al. health literacy screen and the two questions assessing numeracy literacy from the Stagliano and Wallace study) was a reliable predictor of health and numeracy literacy.

ADDRESSING HEALTH LITERACY ISSUES

There are numerous resources available to assist healthcare providers in addressing health literacy issues. The US federal government has several excellent online resources. For example, the Health Literacy Precautions Toolkit is available from the Agency for Healthcare Research and Quality (2013b). The toolkit is a comprehensive file with an array of resources to assist healthcare providers' practices to assess and address the health literacy issue. Use of the term *precautions* is analogous to universal precautions used to combat the spread of infection, because low health literacy may not be easy to recognize. Box 13-2 has examples of other health literacy online resources.

Oral Communication

It is easy for clients to misunderstand medical jargon. To help with this and other oral communication issues, healthcare professionals can turn to many excellent resources. As an example, the video Health Literacy and Patient Safety, Help Patients Understand (http://www.youtube.com/watch?v=cGtTZ_vxjyA; also available at www.ama-assn.org) shows several consumers talking

BOX 13-2   Health Literacy Online Resources

- Centers for Disease Control and Prevention—Health Literacy, http://www.cdc.gov/healthliteracy/
- Healthy People 2020, http://healthy-people.gov/2020/topicsobjectives2020/overview.aspx?topicid=18
- National Network of Libraries of Medicine—Health Literacy, http://nnlm.gov/outreach/consumer/hlthlit.html
- National Patient Safety Foundation—Ask Me 3, http://www.npsf.org/for-healthcare-professionals/programs/ask-me-3
- National Institutes of Health—Plain Language, http://www.nih.gov/clearcommunication/plainlanguage/index.htm
- Plain Language, www.plainlanguage.gov
- Pfizer Clear Health Communication, http://www.pfizerhealthliteracy.com/

about points of confusion, including a client who misunderstood the term *hypertension*, believing that the physician thought he was "hyper" or overactive.

The general rules for effective oral communication are as follows:

- Use eye contact.
- Speak slowly and use plain language.
- Limit the communication to 3 to 5 things that are essential to know.
- Repeat important information.
- Encourage questions.
- Use pictures, models, or drawings.
- Use "teach-back" technique, where you ask the client to explain what you said in their own words.

Written Communication

The ability to read and understand is an important component of the health literacy problem. Nurses and other healthcare professionals may attempt patient care teaching using printed educational literature or websites that the patients and families cannot understand. The Centers for Medicare and Medicaid Services (2012) has a toolkit for creating written material online.

Fortunately, there are several methods to test written information for **readability** including Microsoft Word and websites.

You can use Microsoft Word to calculate readability statistics with the Flesch Reading Ease and the Flesch–Kincaid Grade Level tests. You must activate the feature from the File > Options > Proofing menu. Readability statistics display after checking spelling and grammar in a document (Review > Spelling & Grammar menu). The **Flesch Reading Ease** calculates a value from a formula using the average sentence length and the average number of syllables per word. The recommended score is between 60 and 70; higher scores correlate with easier readability (Microsoft, 2014). The **Flesch–Kincaid Grade Level** test uses the average sentence length and average number of syllables to calculate a US school grade level. When you write patient education resources, write at the Flesch–Kincaid Grade Level score of six. Use the Microsoft Word Help menu (http://office.microsoft.com/en-us/word-help/test-your-document-s-readability-HP010148506.aspx) for more information.

Several writing strategies improve readability of documents. Examples include the following:

- Limit the number of word syllables. As examples, use "doctor" instead of "physician" and "drugs" instead of "medications."
- If possible, use plain language instead of medical terminology and jargon.
- Use bullets to highlight critical points.
- Use graphics with captions to reinforce the meaning of words.
- If you use sentences, keep the length as short as possible.
- Balance words with white space.

The website, How to Write Easy-to-read Health Materials (http://www.nlm.nih.gov/medlineplus/etr.html), published by MedlinePlus, outlines a four-step process for writing health materials and includes links to additional readability resources. The Harvard School of Public Health website, Assessing and Developing Health Materials (http://www.hsph.harvard.edu/healthliteracy/practice/innovative-actions/), includes links to other readability assessment tools.

Readability-score.com (https://readability-score.com) is an online solution to test readability. You can copy and paste text into a window to obtain readability statistics. To visualize how readability statistics work, consider the problem of asthma. Asthma is a common health problem affecting millions of people in the world. Nurses frequently need to teach patients and their families about the condition starting with a definition of asthma. A comparison of the results of different readability tools was done using the definition of asthma from MedlinePlus website at http://www.nlm.nih.gov/medlineplus/asthma.html.

The results using Readability-score.com were:

Readability Formula—Score

- Flesch–Kincaid Reading Ease—68.3

Grade Levels
Readability Formula—Grade

- Flesch–Kincaid Grade Level—6.9
- Gunning–Fog Score—8.5
- Coleman–Liau Index—12.5
- SMOG Index—6.2
- Automated Readability Index—7.6

A comparison of the results from the two tools shows similarities and differences. The lowest reading level was the SMOG with a grade of 6.2 and the highest reading level was the Coleman–Liau Index with a grade of 12.5. The average reading level was 8.3. It is important to understand that the website software uses computer algorithms (rules) to analyze the readability. The nurse must further analyze the results and must review the material to determine whether the client can understand the reading material and whether it is appropriate for use. Because MedlinePlus is an authoritative resource, sponsored by the U.S. National Library of Medicine, most nursing professionals would agree on using its definition of asthma in a teaching plan. The results of the readability statistics serve to alert the nurse that further explanation of the definition may be necessary.

QSEN Scenario

You are designing a brochure on hand hygiene to distribute to patients in your clinic. You want to make sure that the brochure has a readability score at the 5th grade level. How can you use word processing software to check the reading grade level?

Empowering the Healthcare Consumer for Self-Management

The Pew Foundation studied 3,014 adults in the United States between August and September of 2012. According to a 2013 report, 89% of adults in the United States (US) have Internet access; however, only 72% of those with chronic illness have Internet access (Fox & Duggan, 2013a). While the percentage of adults with Internet access continued to increase over the last decade, the 10% gap between adults with chronic disease and those without Internet access remains.

With the transformation of the healthcare provider–client relationship from a paternalistic approach in which the healthcare providers have all the knowledge to a more participatory approach in which clients take responsibility for their own care, there is an increased need for individuals to have valid health-related information. Searching for health information online has never been easier with use of the Internet. A search for a condition, such as diabetes, using the Google search engine produces not only a list of sites but also allows the selection of sites specific to either professionals or consumers. Clients can narrow their searches by selecting from categories such as treatments, tests, or alternative medicine using the consumer sites.

There is always concern about the quality of information on the web. Currently, the trend is not to criticize online resources but to guide users to evaluate the quality of online information. Although there is certainly inaccurate information on the web, one can argue that the accuracy of the information is comparable to many traditional sources such as pamphlets, acquaintances, and popular press articles.

Searching World Wide Web Resources

As more and more information is online, the WWW provides users with an encyclopedia in their computer. Unlike an encyclopedia, however, the documents that provide the needed information are located all over the world and are not always easy to discover. Additionally, the WWW provides an outlet to anyone who wishes to share personal views. Thus, the use of the WWW puts a burden on the user to become adept, not only at finding sources but also at evaluating the sources. If we are going to help consumers to find and analyze web-based sources, it behooves us to develop some expertise first. Discovery of quality resources requires us to understand the different types of search engines, how to find information buried in the invisible web, and to understand the criteria for scrutinizing the quality of the resources.

Using Search Tools

There are many search tools available on the WWW. The search tools are automated or human driven. Search tools fall into three general categories: crawler or spider, human-powered directories, or a combination. The popularity of specific search engines tends to fluctuate. Crawler or spider search engines visit each website, "read" each web page and the associated links, and then index or catalog the information in preparation for a search (Google, 2014). An interactive visual guide on how search engines works is online at http://www.google.com/intl/en_us/insidesearch/howsearchworks/thestory/.

Currently, crawler or spider search engines, such as Google (http://www.google.com/), Yahoo! (http://www.yahoo.com/), and Bing (http://www.bing.com/), have widespread use. Ask Jeeves (http://www.ask.com/) specializes in answering questions by using natural language. There are fewer human-driven directories available than electronic crawlers. The Open Directory (http://www.dmoz.org) and Yahoo! Directory (http://dir.yahoo.com/) are examples.

Many search engines are specialized. Although there is a default search engine built into each web browser, you can change the search engine. To do so using the Chrome web browser, click on the Customize and Control Chrome icon (icon with three orange horizontal bars) and then click on Setting from the menu. Click on the drop-down menu for Search settings to change the search engine choice (Figure 13-1). The Firefox web browser allows you to search for additional search engines to add to the drop-down menu. For example, the eBay search engine will look for sale items on the eBay website, Flickr will search for photos, and Internet Movie Database will search for movies. Find Articles will search print publications, including magazines and selected scholarly journals. The Combined Health Information Database (CHID) will search for medical topics.

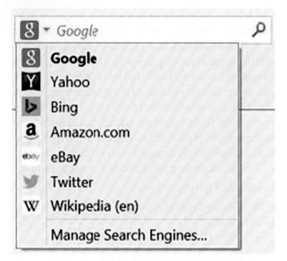

Figure 13-1. Change search engine in the Chrome web browser. (Google and the Google logo are registered trademarks of Google Inc., used with permission.)

Searching the Invisible Web

You can find only a small portion (about 0.3%) of websites on the **visible/surface web** using traditional search tools (Open Education Database, 2014). There are other websites available on the **invisible/deep web**. There are several reasons for documents to be invisible; one is that not all pages are static or permanent. Some websites are dynamic, that is, created on the fly in response to a question. An example is a schedule of flights required by a user or a list of resources in response to a question. Some sites require a password or login that keeps spiders, which cannot type, out.

Sometimes, the kind of web page prohibits discovery with a search tool. The programming of some search engines avoids any web page with a question mark in the web address. A question mark indicates that the web page is dynamic and runs a script. The rating of static web addresses by a search engine is higher than that of dynamic ones, so that the web addresses are higher up in the returns reported from the search (Webconfs.com, 2013).

Although thousands of online resources are invisible to standard searches, you can discover them with a little user ingenuity. Any of the specialized search engines noted above should identify invisible sites. Even if the search engine did

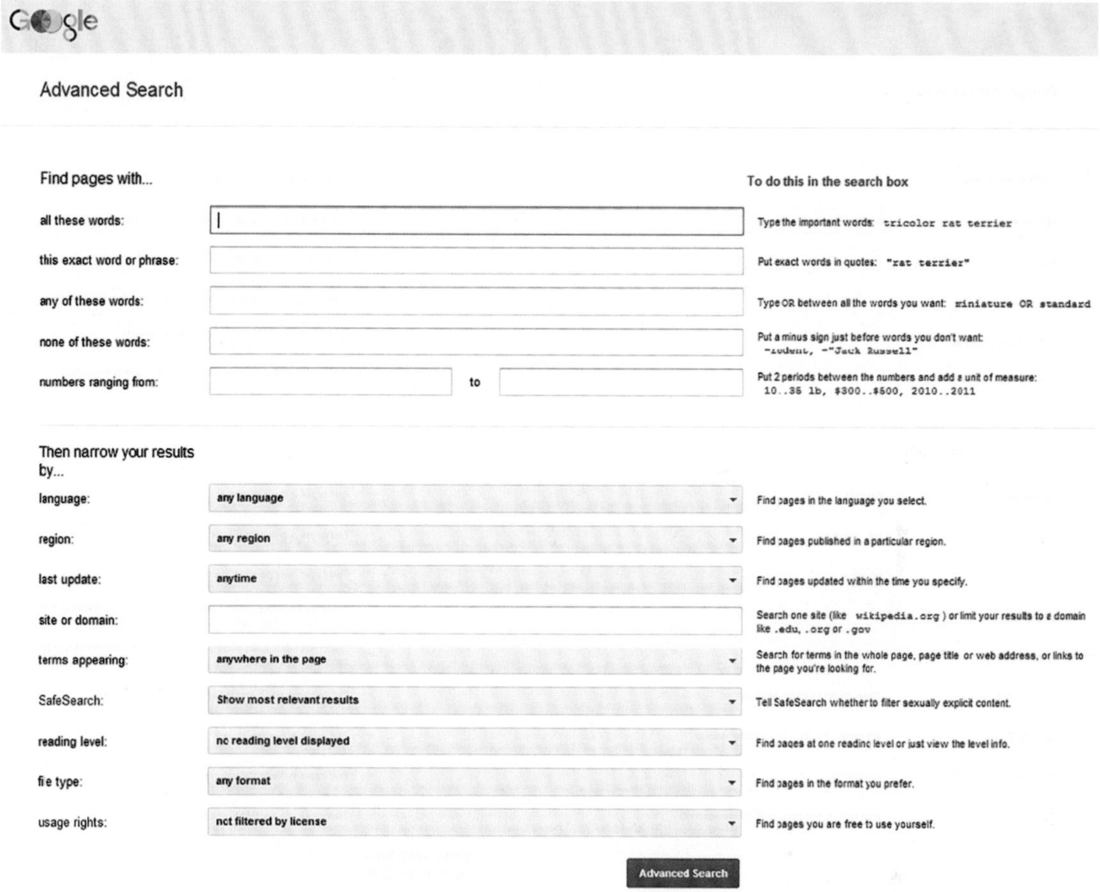

G●●gle

Advanced Search

Find pages with...		To do this in the search box
all these words:		Type the important words: `tricolor rat terrier`
this exact word or phrase:		Put exact words in quotes: `"rat terrier"`
any of these words:		Type OR between all the words you want: `miniature OR standard`
none of these words:		Put a minus sign just before words you don't want: `-rodent, -"Jack Russell"`
numbers ranging from:	to	Put 2 periods between the numbers and add a unit of measure: `10..35 lb, $300..$500, 2010..2011`

Then narrow your results by...

language:	any language	Find pages in the language you select.
region:	any region	Find pages published in a particular region.
last update:	anytime	Find pages updated within the time you specify.
site or domain:		Search one site (like `wikipedia.org`) or limit your results to a domain like `.edu, .org or .gov`
terms appearing:	anywhere in the page	Search for terms in the whole page, page title, or web address, or links to the page you're looking for.
SafeSearch:	Show most relevant results	Tell SafeSearch whether to filter sexually explicit content.
reading level:	no reading level displayed	Find pages at one reading level or just view the level info.
file type:	any format	Find pages in the format you prefer.
usage rights:	not filtered by license	Find pages you are free to use yourself.

Advanced Search

Figure 13-2. Advanced search feature in Google. (Google and the Google logo are registered trademarks of Google Inc., used with permission.)

make the discovery, you may not know it because of the thousands of returns. If you want a particular type of file format, click on Advanced Search from the Settings menu on the Google search page to use the advanced search features (Figure 13-2). As an example, advanced searches allow you to look for specific file types, reading level, and usage rights. Figure 13-3 shows an advanced search for health literacy resources with filters to annotate results with reading levels, in any file format, and usage rights that are free to use or share, even commercially.

There are specialized tools for searching the invisible web. Examples are Google Book Search (http://books.google.com/), ipl2 (http://www.ipl.org/), and Complete Planet (http://aip.completeplanet.com/).

To discover the latest information about revealing the invisible web, conduct your own search by using the search terms "invisible web search engines." Like any search of the literature, finding useful documents depends on the search strategy you use. For simple topics, using a one-word search may be helpful, but locating all of the pertinent information on many topics requires a good preplan, just like digital library searches.

Evaluating Web Resources
The freedom of publication on the Internet allows an airing of ideas, many of which are not in the mainstream. The authenticity that we count on in the print world with the reputations of various newspapers is not yet available on the WWW.

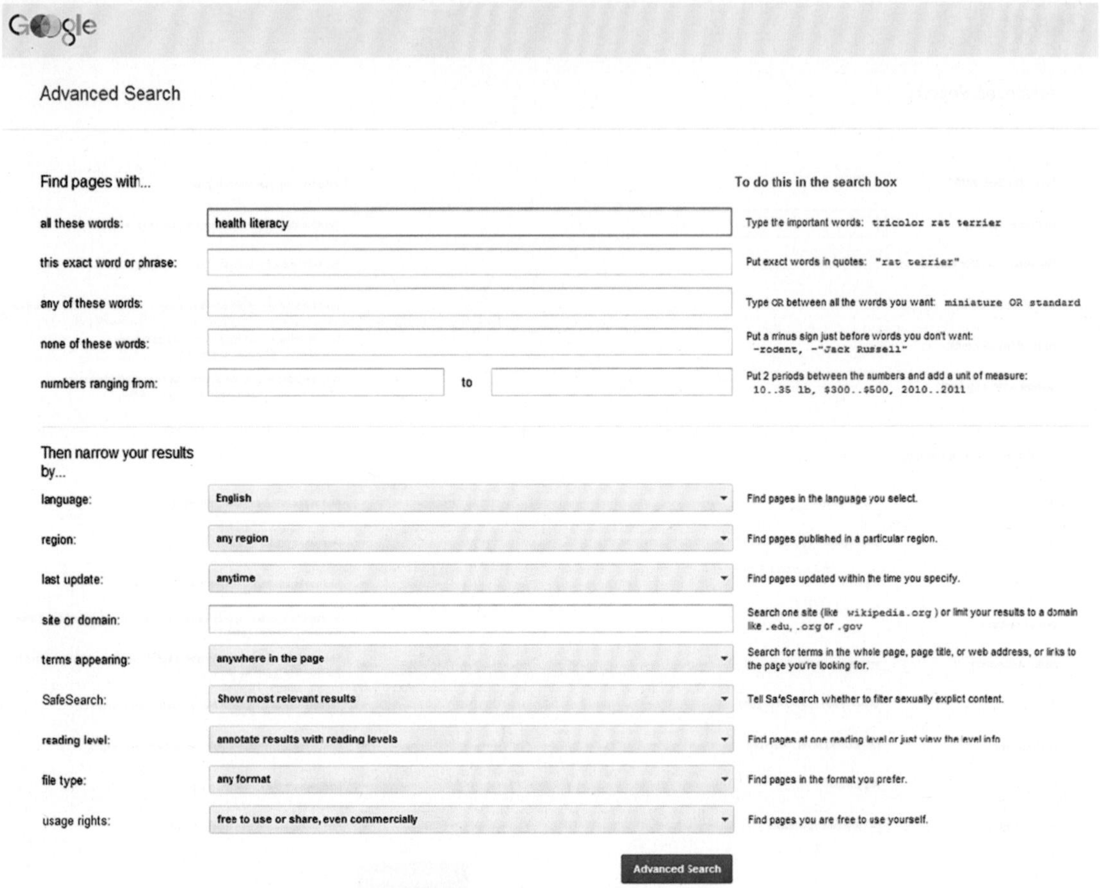

Figure 13-3. Example of using the Google advanced search feature. (Google and the Google logo are registered trademarks of Google Inc., used with permission.)

Although we may long for the security of a library in which all material is vetted to a degree, the fact that yesterday's "far out idea" may become today's newest knowledge makes it undesirable.

The variety of types of information on the web means that using only one set of yes/no criteria for web document evaluation is not valid. A rubric that allows rating the authority of the site, quality, currency, ease of use, privacy, and other resources provides a way to evaluate websites. The Medical Library Association has an online user's guide for finding and evaluating healthcare websites at http://www.mlanet.org/resources/userguide.html (Medical Library Association, 2014). The site includes a link designed specifically for healthcare consumers.

Certification from an authority, such as the Health on the Net Foundation, an international nonprofit organization, mitigates the need for personal evaluation of the site. The **HONcode** icon signifies certification of the website. Health on the Net Foundation provides a website online for professionals, patients, and individuals to use at https://www.hon.ch (Health on the Net Foundation, 2014). The Foundation also provides a downloadable search toolbar to assist users to find certified health information websites.

Teaching Clients How to Find and Evaluate Web-Based Information

You can guide clients to trusted websites for web-based health information. Government sites are trustworthy, as are many organizational sites. Be sure to emphasize the importance of looking closely at the last letters of the website address. For example, the site http://heart.com is a search engine for top shopping sites, and the site http://www.heart.org belongs to the American Heart Association. Chapter 9 contains detailed information about evaluating websites with health information.

Nurses should counsel clients to ask for assistance when searching the web for healthcare information. Advise clients to look at the following information to evaluate the quality of a health information website:

- Authority, qualifications, and credentials of the authors
- The About Us section of the site for:
  - Purpose of the site
  - A disclaimer that acknowledges that the website health information does not replace advice of the health professional
  - A privacy and confidentiality statement acknowledging that the website does not keep personal identifiable information for website users
  - A website contact email address
  - Funding resources information
- References for all medical information
- The last update date

MedlinePlus at http://www.nlm.nih.gov/medlineplus/ exemplifies the website evaluation criteria noted above. Although it is possible to find credible health information online, it is and always will be a "buyer beware" situation.

Assisting Clients With Health Information From the Web

It is impossible for healthcare providers to stay abreast of all recent developments. Additionally, most web-savvy clients will search the web for any information of their diagnoses or any condition they suspect they have. Unfortunately, only 57% of the people who find health information on the web discuss the information with their healthcare provider (Fox & Duggan, 2013, January 15). Clients may arrive for an office visit or hospitalization with information from online searches. The information might not be accurate or the healthcare provider might be unaware of it. Conflicts can arise when the client questions the provider and second-guesses treatment, resulting in a lack of trust in the provider.

When the client mentions suspect or new information, the healthcare provider has several options. Consider accessing the site web address noted by the client. Websites with personal accounts of a disease may have inaccurate information. Use the evaluation criteria stated above to assess the website. If no web address is available, attempt to duplicate the search with search information that the client used. Even if you are unsuccessful, you have demonstrated to the client that you respect the client and are interested in his or her well-being.

Always keep in mind if the information the client brings is new to you, or even refutes current practices or strongly held theories, it may be correct. For example, most hospitals and surgical centers still prescribe nothing by mouth after midnight before surgery, with no regard to the scheduled surgery time. A search of the web for preoperative fasting will reveal, however, that this is not necessarily the best practice (Crenshaw, 2011).

Whatever your decision about the information, you will need to discuss it further with the client. If the information is from a reliable source and contradicts what you "know," acknowledge it. You may discover that the client has unanswered questions, is frightened, needs more understanding of the underlying disease, or just needs more information. In many cases, especially if the information is suspect, working with the client might take a great deal of patience and tact, but it is vital in providing care. More troubling can be the clients who have accessed information about their condition and do not discuss it with their healthcare provider but use it in decisions regarding their treatment. Asking if a client has accessed information about his or her condition on the web may start a conversation that leads to better understanding on the part of you and the client.

Cyberchondria or Online Diagnosers?

Consumers searching for health information on the web has led to a new term: *cyberchondriac* (Cohen, 2007; Fergus, 2014; Starcevic & Berle, 2013). Cyberchondria is a term that describes people who become distressed and frightened after repeated and excessive web searches for health information (Starcevic & Berle, 2013). However, cyberchondria is an anxiety disorder and does not typify most consumer searches for health information.

A 2012 Pew Research survey reported that 74% of adults had searched online for health information and 60% had searched the previous month (Fox & Duggan, 2013a). The term *online diagnosers* was used for those who searched for online health information. The researchers also found that this information affected people's understanding of any health problems they had and improved their health management. The majority (90%) of the online diagnosers reported successful or somewhat successful searches. Most used search engines (69%) or medical websites (62%).

As a nurse, you can influence how patients are affected by any information they have found (from any source) by answering clients' questions about this information and clarifying any misunderstandings. In these discussions, always remember that a client may be accurate in self-diagnosis. More than one person has accurately diagnosed himself or herself from web information. In fact, the following online symptom checkers are from reputable sources:

- U.K. National Health Service Online Symptom Detector: http://www.nhs.uk/NHSDirect/Pages/Symptoms.aspx
- WebMD Symptom Detector: http://www.webmd.boots.com/symptoms/
- FamilyDoctor.org Symptom Detector: http://familydoctor.org/familydoctor/en/health-tools/search-by-symptom.html

Internet Pharmacies

Lawful online pharmacies require a prescription for any medication. Most well-known chain pharmacies in the United States have an online **patient portal** that allows healthcare consumers to order and renew prescriptions. The portals also provide patient education information about drugs. Other services include sending an email or text message when a prescription is ready. Examples of legitimate online pharmacies include CVS (http://www.CVS.com), Walgreens (http://www.walgreens.com/pharmacy/), and Rite Aid (http://www.riteaid.com/).

Unfortunately, the high cost of drugs has forced many people to search for less expensive alternatives on the web. Unlawful Internet pharmacies allow consumers to purchase medications without prescriptions or consultation with a healthcare provider. Additionally, because their only interest is in making a sale, they may sell counterfeit or out-of-date medications, provide the wrong dosage, or sell medications that can create drug reactions. Furthermore, they do not warn purchasers of side effects or the appropriate method of taking a drug.

To help your clients avoid the pitfalls of these suspect pharmacies, assess their sources for drugs and assist them to find a legitimate online pharmacy (see Box 13-2). Warn your clients that any online site that does not require a prescription operates outside the law and may send questionable drugs. In 2010, the search engines Google, Bing, and Yahoo all agreed to a policy to allow only Verified Internet Pharmacy Practice Sites (National Association of Boards of Pharmacy, 2014) to advertise on the search engine web pages. The U.S. Department of Justice Drug Enforcement Administration maintains a website that allows the public to report unlawful Internet pharmacies at https://www.deadiversion.usdoj.gov/webforms/jsp/umpire/umpireForm.jsp.

Providing Supportive Systems

According to Pew Internet research conducted in 2012 (noted earlier), 42% of US adults went online to find others or to read about others with similar health conditions as a support system (Fox & Duggan, 2013b). The survey did not ask specific questions about use of online support groups, but online resources for people with health problems are located in online support groups. The idea of **support groups** is not new; they date back to the early 1900s as a method of working with persons suffering from psychological disorders (Klemm et al., 2003). Today, many support groups are online. Support groups use a variety of online forums, for example, patient portals, social networking websites, message boards, email lists, chat rooms, or any combination of these. Help given is similar to that in face-to-face groups.

There are hundreds of online support groups. Support group sites with the HONcode include Daily Strength.org (http://www.dailystrength.org/) and Mayo Clinic (http://www.mayoclinic.com/health/support-groups/MH00002). CaringBridge (http://www.caringbridge.org/) is an online support group that allows those with "significant health challenges" to stay in touch with their loved ones. PatientsLikeMe.com is especially popular for individuals with neuromuscular disorders. To learn more about PatientsLikeMe, view a YouTube video at http://www.youtube.com/watch?v=nqm-3nHJdGw&feature=related. A survey of 1,323 patients by Wicks et al. (2010) revealed that majority (74%) of the participants felt that the PatientsLikeMe.com site was moderately or very helpful. Participants also noted that sharing with others helped them when starting a new medication or changing a treatment plan.

The GriefNet Support (http://www.griefnet.org/) offers support to persons suffering from the loss of a loved one. The GriefNet Support discussion groups are varied and are oriented to the type of loss. They include, but are not limited to, support groups for those affected by terrorist attacks, widows or widowers, parents who have lost children, children who have suffered a loss, and those who are grieving from the loss of a pet. Trained counselors moderate many of their lists.

Support groups vary in sponsorship and the quality of the information. Healthcare providers who will answer questions sponsor some. Other support sites have a moderator who vets postings before publishing online. In groups sponsored by laypersons or organizations, the moderator may not be a healthcare provider. Most groups allow open discussion and permit members to answer each other's questions. Although there may be erroneous information posted, especially in nonmoderated groups, other members often quickly correct the misinformation.

For those groups that allow open discussion, membership is usually free and the discussion open for anyone to read, but one must join to post questions or replies. As a nurse, you may want to find one or two such groups in your specialty so that you can refer your patients to them. Before referring a patient, assess the group carefully. If referring a client to a moderated group, check the qualifications of the moderator. For a nonmoderated group, look at the archives, and follow the list for a while before recommending it.

You may even wish to join the group. A search by a web search tool for the name of the disease or condition followed by "forum" or "support group" will yield many groups for that condition. For all support groups, you should remind clients that the information they receive may be only an opinion; it may be an informed opinion, or it may not be. If information posted is a new treatment, the client needs to do further research by using qualified medical sites such as those sponsored by the government or formal organizations with known reputations in the field. Just as with web information, it may be necessary to teach clients how to evaluate the information they find in these groups. Additionally, unless users are very familiar with the reputation of the site sponsor and the provider, they should be careful about giving their names, email addresses, and especially their credit card numbers.

Online Support Groups

There are many advantages to online groups over face-to-face groups. They are asynchronous, members can participate at any time of day or night, and there is no restriction of membership by time, geography, or space. Group participants can create and edit a message before posting online. Group participants come from diverse perspectives, which provide varied experiences, opinions, and information sources. Lastly, the ability to post anonymously is helpful in discussing sensitive or potentially embarrassing situations.

Provider-Sponsored Groups

Healthcare providers, particularly hospitals or healthcare organizations, may provide online support for those for whom they provide care. These sites generally require passwords to enter and sometimes require specialized software. One of the earliest groups of this type was the ComputerLink project that supports caregivers of those with Alzheimer disease (Brennan & Moore, 1994; Brennan & Smyth, 1994).

PROVIDING WEB-BASED PATIENT INFORMATION

Most healthcare agencies have websites. The exact contents vary, but generally, they provide information about the organization, a map and directions to the agency, a list of the services offered, and other organizational information aimed at marketing. Some hospitals with obstetric services feature a web page that posts pictures of newborns that new parents can share access information with others. Other healthcare agencies post healthcare information related to their specialties.

Healthcare agencies may even develop a site that functions more like an **extranet** where access is restricted to only their clients, but the site has no ties to the clients' EHRs. Healthcare agencies should have written guidelines for use of the information provided on agency-developed web health sites. Agency guidelines are pertinent for extranets that deliver information designed for specific patients. Agency websites must address privacy and security issues, as well as adhere to criteria for all healthcare websites.

Creating a Web Page

Although you may not be the designer of a page posted on your agencies' website, you might use your expertise to evaluate the information it contains. Just as for all written communication, you need to think carefully about the target audience. Use web design principles to achieve your goal. Health Literacy Online: A Guide to Writing and Designing Easy-to-use Health Web Sites is a comprehensive resource online at http://www.health.gov/health-literacyonline/Web_Guide_Health_Lit_Online.pdf. It includes strategies, actions, testing methods, and resources. Two important factors you must consider when designing a website are verifying that the information is compliant with the American Disability Act and addressing usability principles.

Accessibility Factors in Web Design

Whether you are creating a healthcare website or evaluating one, you need to consider that the visitors may have disabilities. It is imperative, therefore, that the healthcare website is accessible. A 2008 to 2009 survey lists over 27 million (11.4%) US citizens with one or more disabilities (Center for Personal Assistance Service, 2014). It is likely that the percentage of those who are disabled is even higher in the population of those who access healthcare websites.

The website design should allow for use of a **screen reader** for persons with limited eyesight. Elementary screen readers are bundled with operating systems; for example, Microsoft Windows and Apple Mac operating systems both have **accessibility** features with speech recognition. However,

full-function screen readers are best for those with limited vision. The bundled screen readers, however, can help a visually challenged person install a screen reader. Besides translating text to speech, some screen readers can send information to a **Braille reader** placed near or under the keyboard (American Foundation for the Blind, 2013). Users then use their fingers to "read" the information.

Screen readers have vastly improved from earlier times when they could not interpret tables; however, considerations for alternatives to using the mouse, such as keyboard commands for navigation, are still necessary. Use text alternatives (called **Alt tags**) for graphics because screen readers cannot "read" a graphic. The tag should provide either textual information used by a screen reader in place of the illustration or a link to a site that explains the illustration in text. If there are clickable spots on a graphic (known as an **image map**), make provisions for finding these links using a screen reader. **Navigation bars** or graphical bars across the top of a page that provide multiple choices also need alternative methods of access.

Color blindness, which affects 12% of males of European descent and about 0.5% of females, can interfere with reading a web page, whereas the hearing disabled will miss any audio. Blinking items on a web page or quick changes from dark to light can cause seizures in people with photosensitive epilepsy (BC Epilepsy Society, 2008).

Usability

When health websites were evaluated by both **usability** experts and older adults, they agreed on many problem areas such as difficulty finding dropdown menus, too much information on the screen, too small a font size, lack of instructions for playing video, and navigation problems (Nahm et al., 2004). To avoid usability issues, a sampling of the intended audience should review the website; their feedback will allow you to identify and correct any problems. Although healthcare providers can evaluate the web content, the intended audience should conduct the usability testing. The National Institute on Aging and the National Institutes of Health have published guidelines on how to make a website senior friendly (National Institute on Aging, 2014). Furthermore, the U.S. Department of Health and

Human Services has a website dedicated to assist web designers to address usability issues (U.S. Department of Health & Human Services, 2014).

SUMMARY

The field of consumer informatics has developed along with the empowerment of the healthcare consumer. Consumers now have access to information that was previously unavailable such as the quality of care provided by hospitals and disease conditions. As consumers use the web more and more to find information, their relationship with healthcare providers will change. As this continues, healthcare providers must pay greater attention to how health literacy and health numeracy affect the teaching of clients.

Nurses must direct clients to high-quality websites with healthcare information and provide guidance for selecting support groups as ways to improve healthcare. By using patient portals, healthcare agencies provide more consumer education, some of it restricted to and individualized for their clients. These portals also serve as a marketing device.

Whether you design a website or a patient portal, you should use the design principles, as well as those in health literacy and health numeracy, to evaluate the appropriateness for clients. Websites with health information should be accessible to clients with disabilities. The intent of sites with healthcare information is to empower consumers to take an active part in their care to improve outcomes and quality of life.

APPLICATIONS AND COMPETENCIES

1. The fact that only slightly more than half the people who have found health information on the web discussed the information with their healthcare provider is somewhat disturbing. Discuss the following statements:

   a. Patients are leery of discussing information with their healthcare providers versus just listening to advice.

   b. Patients are afraid to take a more participatory approach to their healthcare.

   c. Reluctance to discuss information found on the web affects an individual's decision to follow the provider's treatment plan.

2. You are the nurse in a surgical center. A patient arrives with a printout of the complications of the surgery for which he or she is scheduled. Additionally, the information advocates alternative treatments. Discuss how you can work with this patient.

3. Find a high-quality web-based support group for a client with a condition of your choice and outline how you would teach the client about this site.

4. You are a nurse practitioner. The clinic where you are working wants to institute providing an online support group. What things would you want to consider?

5. Evaluate two health websites using a rubric you created or found with a search engine. Score the website using the rubric. What were the strengths and limitations? Discuss your findings.

REFERENCES

Ad Hoc Committee on Health Literacy for the Council on Scientific Affairs & American Medical Association. (1999). Health literacy: Report of the Council on Scientific Affairs. *Journal of the American Medical Association, 281*(6), 552–557. doi: 10.1001/jama.281.6.552

Agency for Healthcare Research and Quality. (2013a). *Health literacy universal precautions toolkit*. Retrieved from http://www.ahrq.gov/professionals/quality-patient-safety/quality-resources/tools/literacy-toolkit/index.html

Agency for Healthcare Research and Quality. (2013b). *The Patient Education Materials Assessment Tool (PEMAT) and user's guide: An instrument to assess the understandability and actionability of print and audiovisual patient education materials*. Retrieved from http://www.ahrq.gov/professionals/prevention-chronic-care/improve/self-mgmt/pemat/index.html

American Foundation for the Blind. (2013). *Refreshable Braille display*. Retrieved from http://www.afb.org/info/living-with-vision-loss/for-job-seekers/careerconnect-virtual-worksites/retail-worksite-for-blind-users/refreshable-braille-display-3652/12345

American Medical Informatics Association. (2014). *Consumer health informatics*. Retrieved from http://www.amia.org/applications-informatics/consumer-health-informatics

BC Epilepsy Society. (2008). *Epilepsy fact sheet*. Retrieved from http://www.bcepilepsy.com/files/PDF/Epilepsy_Fact_Sheet.pdf

Berkman, N. D., Sheridan, S. L., Donahue, K. E., et al. (2011, March). *Health literacy interventions and outcomes: An updated systematic review*. Rockville, (MD): Agency for

Healthcare Research and Quality (US); (Evidence Reports/Technology Assessments, No. 199.) Retrieved from http://www.ncbi.nlm.nih.gov/books/NBK82434/

Brennan, P. F., & Moore, S. M. (1994). Networks for home care support: the ComputerLink project. *Caring, 13*(8), 64-66, 68-70.

Brennan, P. F., & Smyth, K. (1994). Elders' attitudes and behavior regarding ComputerLink. *Proceedings of the Annual Symposium on Computer Applications in Medical Care*, 1011.

Center for Personal Assistance Service. (2014). *Disability prevalence data from the current population survey (2008–2009)*. Retrieved from http://www.pascenter.org/state_based_stats/disability_stats/index.php?state=us

Centers for Medicare and Medicaid Services. (2012, March 13). *Toolkit for making written material clear and effective*. Retrieved from http://www.cms.gov/Outreach-and-Education/Outreach/WrittenMaterialsToolkit/index.html

Chew, L. D., Bradley, K. A., & Boyko, E. J. (2004). Brief questions to identify patients with inadequate health literacy. *Family Medicine, 36*(8), 588–594. Retrieved from http://www.stfm.org/NewsJournals/FamilyMedicine

Chew, L. D., Griffin, J. M., Partin, M. R. et al. (2008). Validation of screening questions for limited health literacy in a large VA outpatient population. *Journal of General Internal Medicine, 23*(5), 561–566. doi: 10.1007/s11606-008-0520-5.

Cohen, E. (2007, December 20). *Are you a 'cyberchondriac'?* Retrieved from http://www.cnn.com/2007/HEALTH/12/20/ep.cyberchondriacs/index.html

Communicating with patients who have limited literacy skills. Report of the National Work Group on Literacy and Health. (1998). *Journal of Family Practice, 46*(2), 168–176. Retrieved from http://www.jfoonline.com

Crenshaw, J. T. (2011). Preoperative fasting: Will the evidence ever be put into practice? *American Journal of Nursing, 111*(10), 38–43. doi: 10.1097/1001.NAJ.0000406412.000 0457062.0000406424.

Dickens, C., & Piano, M. R. (2013). Health literacy and nursing: An update. *American Journal of Nursing, 113*(6), 52–57. doi:10.1097/01.NAJ.0000431271.83277.2f.

Exec. Order No. 12,866, 1 C.F.R. 2 (1993). Retrieved from http://www.reginfo.gov/public/jsp/Utilities/EO_12866.pdf

Exec. Order No. 12,988, 3 C.R.F. 4731 (1996). Retrieved from http://www.gpo.gov/fdsys/pkg/FR-1996-02-07/pdf/96-2755.pdf

Fergus, T. A. (2014). The Cyberchondria Severity Scale (CSS): An examination of structure and relations with health anxiety in a community sample. *Journal of Anxiety Disorders, 28*(6), 504–510. doi:10.1016/j.janxdis.2014.05.006

Fox, S., & Duggan, M. (2013a). *The diagnosis difference*. Retrieved from http://www.pewinternet.org/2013/11/26/the-diagnosis-difference/

Fox, S., & Duggan, M. (2013b). *Health online 2013*. Retrieved from http://www.pewinternet.org/files/old-media/Files/Reports/PIP_HealthOnline.pdf

Health on the Net Foundation. (2014, May 15. HONcode site evaluation form Health on the Net Foundation. Retrieved from http://www.hon.ch/cgi-bin/HONcode/Inscription/site_evaluation.pl?language=en&userCategory=providers

Hyde, S. S. (2004). Dialogues with Socrates. In R. E. Herzlinger (Ed.), *Consumer-driven healthcare* (pp. 262–269). San Francisco, CA: Jossey-Bass.

Kandula, S., Ancker, J. S., Kaufman, D. R., et al. (2011). A new adaptive testing algorithm for shortening health literacy assessments. *BMC Medical Informatics and Decision Making, 11*, 52–52. doi: 10.1186/1472-6947-11-52.

Kirsch, I. S., Jungeblut, A. Jenkins, L., et al. (1993, August). *Adult literacy in America: A first look at the findings of the National Adult Literacy Survey*. Retrieved from http://nces.ed.gov/pubsearch/pubsinfo.asp?pubid=93275

Klemm, P., Bunnell, D., Cullen, M., et al. (2003). Online cancer support groups: A review of the research literature. *Computers, Informatics, Nursing, 21*(3), 136–142.

Kutner, M., Greenberg, E., Jin, Y., et al. (2006, September). *The health literacy of America's adults: Results from the 2003 National Assessment of Adult Literacy*. Retrieved from http://nces.ed.gov/pubs2006/2006483.pdf

Medical Library Association. (2014). *Find and evaluate health information on the web*. Retrieved from http://www.mlanet.org/resources/userguide.html

Microsoft. (2014). *Test your document's readability*. Retrieved from http://office.microsoft.com/en-us/word-help/test-your-document-s-readability-HP010148506.aspx

Nahm, E. S., Preece, J., Resnick, B., et al. (2004). Usability of health web sites for older adults: A preliminary study. *Computers, Informatics, Nursing, 22*(6), 326–334; quiz 335–326.

National Association of Boards of Pharmacy. (2014, March 3). *Verified Internet pharmacy practice sites*. Retrieved from https://vipps.nabp.net/

National Center for Education Statistics. (n.d.a). National Assessment of Adult Literacy (NAAL): 1992 NALS products. Retrieved from http://nces.ed.gov/naal/nals_products.asp

National Center for Education Statistics. (n.d.b). National Assessment of Adult Literacy (NAAL): What is NAAL? Retrieved from http://nces.ed.gov/NAAL/

National Institute on Aging. (2014, March 20). *Making your website senior friendly: Tips from the National Institute on Aging and the National Library of Medicine*. Retrieved from http://www.nia.nih.gov/health/publication/making-your-website-senior-friendly

National Literacy Act of 1991, Pub. L. No. 102–3, 105 Stat. 7. Retrieved from http://www.gpo.gov/fdsys/pkg/STATUTE-105/pdf/STATUTE-105-Pg7.pdf

National Patient Safety Foundation. (2014). *Health literacy: Statistics as a glance*. Retrieved from http://www.npsf.org/wp-content/uploads/2011/12/AskMe3_Stats_English.pdf

Nielsen-Bohlman, L., & Institute of Medicine (U.S.), Committee on Health Literacy. (2004). *Health literacy: A prescription to end confusion*. Washington, DC: National Academies Press. Retrieved from http://www.nap.edu/openbook.php?record_id=10883&page=1

Open Education Database. (2014). *The ultimate guide to the invisible web.* Retrieved from http://oedb.org/ilibrarian/invisible-web/

Plain Writing Act of 2010, Pub. L. No. 111–274, 124–2861. Retrieved from http://www.gpo.gov/fdsys/pkg/PLAW-111publ274/pdf/PLAW-111publ274.pdf

Rothman, R. L., Montori, V. M., Cherrington, A., et al. (2008). Perspective: The role of numeracy in health care. *Journal of Health Communication, 13*(6), 583–595. doi: 10.1080/10810730802281791

Stagliano, V., & Wallace, L. S. (2013). Brief health literacy screening items predict newest vital sign scores. *Journal of the American Board of Family Medicine, 26*(5), 558–565. doi:10.3122/jabfm.2013.05.130096.

Starcevic, V., & Berle, D. (2013). Cyberchondria: Towards a better understanding of excessive health-related Internet use. *Expert Review of Neurotherapeutics, 13*(2), 205–213. doi: 10.1586/ern.12.162

U.S. Department of Education, & Office of Educational Research and Improvement. (2002, April). *Adult literacy in America: A first look at the findings of the National Adult Literacy Survey.* NCES 1993–275. Retrieved from http://nces.ed.gov/pubs93/93275.pdf

U.S. Department of Health & Human Services. (2008). America's health literacy: Why we need accessible health information. Retrieved from http://www.health.gov/communication/literacy/issuebrief/

U.S. Department of Health & Human Services. (2014, February 22). *Usability.gov home.* Retrieved from http://www.usability.gov/

van der Heide, I., Wang, J., Droomers, M., et al. (2013). The relationship between health, education, and health literacy: Results from the Dutch Adult Literacy and Life Skills Survey. *Journal of Health Communication, 18* (Suppl 1), 172–184. doi: 10.1080/10810730.2013.825668.

Webconfs.com. (2013). *Dynamic URLs vs. static URLs.* Retrieved from http://www.webconfs.com/dynamic-urls-vs-static-urls-article-3.php

Weiss, B. D., Mays, M. Z., Martz, W., et al. (2005). Quick assessment of literacy in primary care: The newest vital sign. *Annals of Family Medicine, 3*(6), 514–522. doi:10.1370/afm.405.

Wicks, P., Massagli, M., Frost, J., et al. (2010). Sharing health data for better outcomes on Patients Like Me. *Journal of Medical Internet Research, 12*(2), e19.

Wilson, M. (2009). Readability and patient education materials used for low-income populations. *Clinical Nurse Specialist CNS, 23*(1), 33–40; quiz 41–32. doi: 10.1097/01.NUR.0000343079.50214.31.

Woloshin, S., Schwartz, L. M., & Welch, H. G. (2005). Patients and medical statistics. Interest, confidence, and ability. *Journal of General Internal Medicine, 20*(11), 996–1000. doi:10.1111/j.1525-1497.2005.00179.x.

CHAPTER 14

Interoperability at the National and the International Levels

OBJECTIVES

After studying this chapter, you will be able to:

1. Define the three types of interoperability: foundational, structural, and semantic.

2. Describe a general pattern for developing standards.

3. Explain how standards affect the adoption of an interoperable electronic health record.

4. Interpret the effects on nursing of standards at all levels of healthcare.

5. Identify organizations involved in setting standards at the national and international levels.

KEY TERMS

Health Information Exchange (HIE)

Interoperability

Mapping

Nationwide Health Information Network (NwHIN)

Protocol

Reference Terminology Model

Regional Extension Centers (RECs)

Semantic interoperability

Standards

Unified Medical Language System (UMLS)

Without knowing he has been infected with a very contagious stage of a new type of flu, an individual walks into the international airport in Houston on his way to Seattle. While standing in the baggage check line, he starts up a conversation with the woman behind him, who will be in New Delhi in 24 hours. After checking his bag, he goes to the security line and there strikes up a conversation with a man who will be in San Diego in 4 hours. He is early for his plane, so he goes into one of the airport bars and begins talking to a woman who will be in Tokyo in 8 hours and then in Shanghai in 48 hours.

Today jet travel makes all points on the globe vulnerable to any communicable disease. Thus, health is an international concern. To protect us, countries must be able to exchange information pertaining to contagious diseases with other countries and within their own frontiers. This demands that healthcare systems be interoperable between communities, regionally and internationally. To achieve this goal, data transfer and reception must be interoperable.

The purpose of this chapter is to describe the many national and international efforts to make data exchange interoperable. It begins with an overview of **interoperability** and **standards**, which serves as a foundation for discussion of U.S.'s efforts for promoting an interoperable electronic health record (EHR). Information that follows provides perspectives on interoperability at the international level.

INTEROPERABILITY DEFINED

Simply stated, **interoperability** is the ability of two or more systems to pass information between them and to use the exchanged information. In healthcare, interoperability means that healthcare information systems can transmit and receive information within and across organizational boundaries to provide the delivery of optimum healthcare to individuals and communities (Healthcare Information and Management Systems Society [HIMSS], 2013). Interoperability is achieved either by adhering to accepted interface and terminology standards or by using a third system that seamlessly integrates the two systems. An example of the first option is the **protocols** that make the Internet possible, plus the use of a standardized terminology. The use of an rtf file to "translate" a file from one word processor to another is a case in which the second option, seamless integration, is used.

TYPES OF INTEROPERABILITY

The three types of interoperability are foundational, structural, and semantic (HIMSS, 2013).

Foundational interoperability refers to the transmission and reception of information so

that it is useful, but with no need for interpretation. Foundational interoperable systems are able to send and receive usable data from different systems.

Structural interoperability is a concept intended to coordinate work processes. It refers to the uniform format or structure of the exchanged messages. It is necessary to preserve the meaning and purpose of the information. With structural interoperability, data exchanged between information systems allow for interpretation at the data field level.

Semantic interoperability takes this one step further. In semantic interoperability, not only is the information transmitted so that it is understandable but, at its highest level, the interpretation and action on messages exchanged by two computers occur without human intervention. The effectiveness of semantic interoperability depends on the interaction between algorithms (rules), the data used in the message, and the terminology used to designate those data. Semantic operability allows authorized users to receive information from different EHRs to plan and provide safe and effective care. This type of functionality enables exchange of data from a laboratory system with the pharmacy system. It also enables exchange of data from one healthcare provider with another.

STANDARDS

Interoperability is not possible without standards. Imagine a situation in which each community sets its own time. In one city, it would be 1:00 PM, whereas in another 30 miles east, it would be 1:30 PM, and in still another 40 miles northwest, it would be 12:30 PM. This is similar to the situation that existed until the mid-19th century. Of course, the time was not so important then and the population was not as mobile. When the railroads arrived, it became necessary to standardize the time (WebExhibits, 2008). In 1883, the railroads set the first time zones in the United States and Canada. Britain had already established standard time 37 years earlier, in 1840, because of the rail system.

As the industrial revolution progressed, it was necessary to have more and more standards for the economy to prosper. Some may remember the Beta versus VHS videotape standards conflicts. A more recent standards conflict involved DVD formats—the Blu-ray disc versus HD DVD. Of course, the marketplace decided those standards. However, in healthcare, the marketplace's disparate decisions about standards create great inefficiencies.

A standard is an agreement to use a given protocol, term, or other criterion formally approved by a nationally or internationally recognized professional trade association or governmental body. Standards are vital to communication as well as in other areas. Even in casual communication, differences in language can result in miscommunication. For example, consider the following real-life example. The word "stroller" has several meanings depending on one's cultural background. Two meanings are a type of baby carriage or someone who is walking slowly. Hence, one person reading a sign reading "No strollers" in a museum might think one should not meander through the museum, and another person might interpret the sign to mean that baby carriages are not allowed. Although the results in casual life are not serious—in healthcare they can be—they can lead to serious communication errors or even outright lack of communication, which can be just as dangerous.

Standards influence nursing. They affect the use of equipment and documentation in EHRs. Standards setting organizations make decisions about what healthcare data to record; how to record it; what terminology to use; and what data to report to organizations. Because of the effect on nursing, nurses must have some understanding not only of the process but also of the groups involved in setting standards. Box 14-1

BOX 14-1   Acronyms for Standards and Standards Setting Organizations

AMA	American Medical Association
ANA	American Nurses Association
ANSI	American National Standards Institute
APR-DRG	All Patient Refined Diagnosis-Related Groups
ASTM International	American Society for Testing and Materials
CAP	College of American Pathologists
CEN	Comité Européen de Normalisation (or European Committee for Standardization)
CPT	Current Procedural Terminology
DICOM	Digital Imaging and Communications in Medicine
FHA	Federal Health Architecture
HCPCS	Healthcare Common Procedure Coding System
HIE	Health Information Exchange
HIO	Health Information Exchange Organization
HISPC	Health Information Security and Privacy Collaboration
HITSP	Health Information Technology Standards Panel
HL7	Health Level Seven
ICD-#	International Classification of Disease Version #
ICD-#-CM	ICD "number" Clinical Modifications
ICD-#-PCS	ICD "number" Procedural Codes
ICF	International Classification of Functioning, Disability, and Health
IEC	International Electrotechnical Commission
IHTSDO	International Health Terminology Standards Development Organisation

BOX 14-1   Acronyms for Standards and Standards Setting Organizations (*continued*)

ISI	International Statistical Institute
ISO	International Organization for Standardization
MS-DRG	Medicare Severity Diagnosis-Related Groups
NCHS	National Center for Health Statistics
NEDSS	National Electronic Disease Surveillance System
NEMA	National Electrical Manufacturers Association
NwHIN	Nationwide Health Information Network
NHS	National Health Service (UK)
NIST	National Institute of Standards and Technology
NLM	National Library of Medicine
OASIS	Outcome and Assessment Information Set
OBQI	Outcome-Based Quality Improvement
OMB	U.S. Office of Management and Budget
ONC	Office of the National Coordinator for Health Information Technology
OSI	Open Systems Interconnect
PHIN	Public Health Information Network
SNOMED CT	Systematized Nomenclature of Medicine: Clinical Terms
TC 215	ISO Technical Committee 215 (the group that set the nursing reference terminology model)
UHDDS	Uniform Hospital Discharge Data Set
UMLS	Universal Medical Language System
WHO	World Health Organization

displays some of the groups involved in setting standards, along with their acronyms. You could probably play a game of Scrabble by using just these acronyms.

U.S. EFFORTS FOR PROMOTING INTEROPERABLE ELECTRONIC HEALTH RECORDS

The Institute of Medicine's report *To Err is Human* (Kohn et al., 2000) resulted in the open realization for the need of efforts toward improving the delivery of healthcare in the United States. Creating EHRs became one of the pillars of these endeavors. The complexity of the endeavor was daunting.

Office of the National Coordinator for Health Information Technology

In May 2004, President Bush called for an EHR for Americans by 2014. To further this aim, he established the position of National Coordinator for Health Information Technology who heads the Office of the National Coordinator for Health Information Technology (ONC) (HealthIT.gov, n.d.a). The ONC is working to facilitate the adoption of health information technology (IT), as well as to promote nationwide **health information exchange** (HIE) (HealthIT.gov, n.d.e).

The Health Information Technology for Economic and Clinical Health (HITECH) Act, passed in 2009, provided funding opportunities to advance health IT. The ONC created six programs that serve as a foundation to assure the

BOX 14-2   Consumer eHealth Program Aims

Objective	Examples
Access	Increase access to health information for consumers and patients who have the right to obtain copies of health information from healthcare providers, healthcare agencies, and their health plans.
Action	Allow consumers to take action on their health information and use tools and resources that make the information meaningful to them.
Attitudes	Change attitudes so that consumers become active participants in their care with the support of eHealth tools.

Adapted from HealthIT.gov. (n.d.d). *Consumer eHealth Program overview.* Available at: http://www.healthit.gov/policy-researchers-implementers/consumer-ehealth-program

success of HITECH and to achieve IT adoption (HealthIT.gov, n.d.b; HealthIT.gov, n.d.g), all of which require interoperability and standards to have successful outcomes:

- Beacon Community Programs
- Consumer eHealth Program
- State Health Information Exchange Cooperative Agreement Program
- Health Information Technology Extension Program
- Strategic Health Information Technology Advanced Research Projects (SHARP) Program
- Workforce Development Program

Beacon Community Programs

The Beacon Community Program includes 17 demonstration projects funded by the ONC over 3 years (HealthIT.gov, n.d.c). The demonstration projects exemplify best practices for safe, secure, and cost-effective exchange of health information. You can learn more by watching the video, Beacon Community Program: Improving Health through Health Technology, at https://www.youtube.com/watch?v=DAQ2CnjL7tQ.

Consumer eHealth Program

The Consumer eHealth Program is a multifaceted initiative designed to improve consumer access to their health information, allow consumers to take action based on their health information,

and change the consumer attitudes so that they become partners in their own care. The Consumer eHealth Program summarizes the objectives as the "Three A's": Access, Action, and Attitudes. Box 14-2 provides examples of initiatives to address the Three A's. You can learn more about consumer eHealth by watching the video, ePatient Dave (Dave DeBronkart) recorded at the 2013 Consumer Health IT Summit, at http://www.youtube.com/watch?v=7aiTTwnvjWU.

State Health Information Exchange Cooperative Agreement Program

ONC developed two programs to facilitate the development of state HIEs. In 2010, the ONC developed the State HIE Cooperative Agreement Program. The program provided funding for states to build HIEs within the states and across state lines. In 2011, the ONC initiated the Challenge Grants program that provided monetary award to support state HIE efforts and interoperability. Grant recipients had to address privacy and security, use and integrated approach with Medicaid and state public health programs, monitor meaningful use, and comply with national standards.

The complexity of the effort to achieve interoperable IT adoption cannot be overstated. There are three main types of HIE: directed exchange, query-based exchange, and consumer mediated exchange (HealthIT.gov, 2014d). The directed exchange allows for sending and receiving of health information to care providers for coordinated care. Query-based exchange allows providers to find health information. Consumer-mediated exchange provides a way for consumers to collect and control their health information.

Health Information Technology Extension Program

The ONC's **Regional Extension Centers** (RECs) are components of the Health Information Technology Extension Program (HealthIT.gov, n.d.f). There are RECs located throughout the U.S. Trained REC staff members assist healthcare providers to understand and implement the EHR adoption. Educational components include vendor selection, workflow analysis necessary to decide on a vendor, and how to meet meaningful use requirements.

Strategic Health IT Advanced Research Projects Program

The ONC funded five research centers across the United States to develop innovations that speed up the processes for meeting meaningful use and adoption of Health IT. University of Texas at Houston, University of Illinois at Urbana-Champaign, Harvard University, Mayo Clinic of Medicine, and Massachusetts General Hospital each received a $15 million grant to conduct research over a 4-year period. The University of Texas research is on patient-centered cognitive support. The research addresses assisting the healthcare providers and patients to understand and adopt use of EHRs. The University of Illinois at Urbana-Champaign research addresses privacy and security of health IT in the areas of EHRs, HIEs, and telemedicine. Harvard University research addresses software applications and network designs using SMArt (Substitutable Medical Apps, reusable technology) architecture where healthcare providers, patients, and forward-thinking vendors drive innovations. Mayo Clinic of Medicine research addresses secondary use of health information with a unified EHR that provides for sharing health information on a large-scale among authorized users and services. Finally, Massachusetts General Hospital research addresses resources that medical device manufacturers can use to create interoperable products.

Workforce Development Program

The transition to using electronic communications and EHRs created a brick wall with a steep learning curve for busy healthcare providers, educators, and others working in the healthcare discipline. The knowledge deficit was especially challenging to those who grew up without computer technology before they were adults. The ONC workforce initiative addressed the deficit by sponsoring grants initiatives for creating curricula and educational opportunities for members of the healthcare workforce. Resources resulting from the Workforce Development Program and the final report can be found at http://www.healthit.gov/providers-professionals/workforce-development-programs.

Nationwide Health Information Network

The **Nationwide Health Information Network** (NwHIN) consists of standards, policies, and services necessary to allow for secure HIE (HealthIT.gov, n.d.i). Federal agencies and state-level, regional, and local HIE organizations, as well as integrated delivery networks (formerly known as NHIN Cooperative) conduct the work. Direct Project is an example of outcomes of the information network. Direct Project workgroups are developing standards and procedures to allow for secure information exchange at the local level so that a primary care provider can electronically exchange information with another provider.

> ### QSEN Scenario
> You are learning about the U.S. Office of the Nation Coordinator (ONC) and the HealthIT.gov SAFER Guides (http://www.healthit.gov/safer/guide/sg005), which are used by healthcare organizations to self-assess the safety and safe use of EHRs. Discuss the safety issues associated with interoperability and systems interfaces.

Health IT Adoption Surveys

The ONC conducts health IT adoption surveys of physician offices and hospitals in order to monitor the outcomes of the use of electronic HIE efforts. The surveys, conducted annually, monitor basic and full levels of EHR use. Results of the National Ambulatory Medical Care Survey showed that in

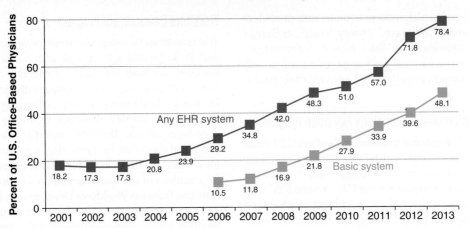

Figure 14-1. Growth in percentage of EHR systems use by U.S. office-based physicians, 2001–2013. Source: CDC/NCHS, National Ambulatory Medical Care Survey and Electronic Health Records Survey.

2013, 78% office physicians used some type of EHR, an increase from 18% in 2001 (Figure 14-1) (Hsiao & Hing, 2014). Basic system (includes the patient history, demographics, patient problem list, physician clinical note, computerized prescription orders, laboratory and imaging results) were in use by 48% of office physicians (p. 5). The adoption rate varies widely by state. As an example, North Dakota had the highest adoption rate of basic systems (83%), whereas New Jersey had the lowest rate (21%). The national average was 48%. In all cases, the state adoption rates were higher than the national average of 11% in 2006.

Survey respondents reported several benefits from using EHRs. More than half of the physicians reports that electronic records provided alerts to critical values (62%) and potential medical records (65%) (Jamoom et al., 2013; King et al., 2013). Eighty-one percent noted benefits from the ability to access the electronic records remotely. Finally, physicians who met meaningful use with 2 or more years' experience using EHRs were more likely to report clinical benefits from use. Experts anticipate the users will continue to see benefits after resolving issues.

U.S. Public Health Information Network

Although not part of the EHR efforts, the Public Health Information Network (PHIN) benefits from that work. The PHIN is a part of the Centers for Disease Control and Prevention (CDC), which is a national effort to increase the ability of public health agencies to electronically use and exchange information by promoting the use of standards (Centers for Disease Control and Prevention, 2014). The National Electronic Disease Surveillance System (NEDSS) is a major component of these efforts (Centers for Disease Control and Prevention, 2013d). The objective of the NEDSS is to develop and support integrated surveillance systems that can transfer appropriate public health, laboratory, and clinical data efficiently and securely over the Internet to allow quick identification and tracking of disease outbreaks, whether natural or from bioterrorism.

Unified Medical Language System

As you have seen, there are many standardized efforts and terminologies. Although some of these express concepts particular to a specific discipline (note: discussion of nursing terminologies is in the next chapter), many are interdisciplinary. It is essential, however, for users to be able to find all the information related to a given concept in all machine-readable sources such as clinical records, databases, biomedical literature, and various directories of information sources. "The **Unified Medical Language System** (UMLS) integrates and distributes key terminology, classification and coding standards, and associated resources to promote creation of more effective interoperable biomedical information services, including EHRs" (National Library of Medicine, 2014a).

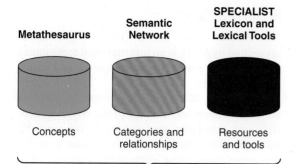

The Knowledge Sources
(delivered as machine-readable files)

Figure 14-2. Relationship of UMLS Knowledge Sources. (Courtesy of the National Library of Medicine. (2014b). UMLS Quick Start Guide. Available at: http://www.nlm.nih.gov/research/umls/new_users/online_learning/OVR_001.html)

The UMLS consists of three different but related types of knowledge sources: the Metathesaurus, Semantic Network, and the SPECIALIST Lexicon and Lexical Programs (Figure 14-2). The Metathesaurus is a large vocabulary database that has over 1 million health-related concepts (National Library of Medicine, 2014b), their names, and the linkages between them. The Semantic Network provides consistent categorization and relationships of the Metathesaurus concepts, including possible assignment of the categories to the concepts, and defines relationships between the semantic types. The SPECIALIST Lexicon provides resources and tools needed for the SPECIALIST Natural Language Processing (NLP) System. It contains many biomedical terms along with the information needed by the SPECIALIST NLP System. UMLS can potentially link information from EHRs with the biomedical literature. For additional information on the UMLS, use the online Quick Start Guide at http://www.nlm.nih.gov/research/umls/quickstart.html.

Effect of U.S. Efforts on Nursing and Patient Care

The decisions from the different health IT initiatives and the associated standards affect nursing practice. The standards used for health IT determine what and how nurses document patient care. These decisions determine the information that meaningful use (secondary analysis of the data) provides, which shapes national healthcare policy. Without nursing participation, the data will be unlikely to represent the contribution of nursing to patient care or provide national healthcare policy that is in the best interest of the patient and client.

INTERNATIONAL STANDARDS ORGANIZATIONS

Many organizations are involved in developing the standards demanded by the global nature of today's commerce. The two international groups that oversee much of the work involved in developing standards are the International Organization for Standardization (ISO, 2014a) and the International Electrotechnical Commission (IEC, 2014). As you might suspect, the IEC is concerned with electrical standards. It sets the standards for the equipment used in hospitals. The ISO sets standards in all other areas including health.

An international group has member national groups that perform work at the national level. There is often collaboration between these groups, as well as crossovers. For example, the U.S. National Committee of the IEC is an integral member of the American National Standards Institute (ANSI), which is the U.S. member of the ISO.

International Organization for Standardization

The ISO is a nonprofit group, established in 1947, that oversees many international standardization efforts. It has member national groups from more than 150 countries. There is a Central Secretariat in Geneva, Switzerland, that coordinates the system (ISO, 2010a). Some of its member institutions are part of the governmental structure of their countries, whereas others are from the private sector. Their purpose is to expedite standardization to facilitate international commerce and to promote cooperation in intellectual, technological, scientific, and economic activity.

ISO has technical committees in many fields. The committee for health informatics is technical committee number 215 (TC 215). Each technical committee has working groups with volunteers who do the work. Under TC 215, a working group of volunteers from many nations established a nursing **Reference Terminology Model**, known as ISO 18104:2014 (ISO, 2014b). A reference terminology model refers to a set of terms based upon evidence-based research. Some of the potential uses for this model include facilitating the documentation of nursing problems (diagnosis) and actions (interventions) in electronic information systems. The model also allows for the creation of nursing terminologies in a form that will make **mapping** (a form of matching concepts from one standardized terminology with those having similar meaning from another) among them easier.

International Electrical Commission

The IEC creates and publishes international standards for all electrical-related technologies (IEC, 2014). These standards serve as the basis for national standards in international contracts. The objectives include efficiently meeting the goals of a global market, assessing and improving the quality of products covered by its standards, and contributing to the improvement of human health and safety. In the healthcare field, their standards include medical electrical equipment and magnetically induced currents in the human body.

ASTM International

The original purpose of the ASTM International, created in 1898, as the American Society for Testing and Materials, was to address the frequent rail breaks in the evergrowing railroad industry. Today, it is an international organization; however, it still exerts a dominant influence among standards developers in the United States (ASTM International, 2014). Membership is by request, not by appointment or invitation, and anyone interested in its activities may join. Although there is no enforcement policy, in 1995 the United States passed the National Technology Transfer and Advancement Act, which requires the federal government to comply with privately developed standards when possible. Other governments—both local and worldwide—as well as corporations doing international business also reference ASTM standards.

Health Level Seven

The Health Level Seven (HL7) organization, accredited by ANSI, is an international community of healthcare subject matter experts and information scientists (Health Level 7, 2014b). Based in Ann Arbor, Michigan, HL7 began in 1987. It is an all-volunteer, not-for-profit organization, that sets standards for functional and semantic interoperability for electronic healthcare data. Its mission is to provide a "comprehensive framework and related standards for the exchange, integration, sharing, and retrieval of electronic healthcare information" (Health Level 7, 2014b).

Derivation of the term HL7 is from the position of these standards in the seven-level Open Systems Interconnect model, a framework for implementing protocols that pass control from the bottom layer up the hierarchy to the top level (Health Level 7, 2014a). The number seven in the name means that the standards being set are at the seventh, or the highest, messaging level of this model. At this level, the standards include those that address the terminology used; and at the functional level, identification of participants, electronic data exchange negotiations, and data exchange structuring. The lower six levels focus on the physical and logical connections between machines, systems, and applications. In very basic terms, HL7 standards are concerned with what data to transmit, for example, vital signs and demographic information, and what terminology and protocols to use for transmission of the data. There are many HL7 standards, each addressing a different portion of this process. The HL7 organization is very involved in setting standards for the EHR; several nurses are involved in these efforts.

Both the modern world with jet airplanes, which created a need for the quick dissemination of health data concerning disease outbreaks, and a new focus on healthcare outcomes made the need for the collection of healthcare data more visible. Healthcare data collection is not new; the first healthcare data collections occurred during the 16th century in England. Parish clerics recorded and published weekly the number of burials in the London Bills of Mortality. The publications served as early warning systems against the Bubonic Plague epidemics that decimated the European population several times in the 16th and 17th centuries.

You can view examples of records from the Bills of Mortality at http://www.history.ac.uk/ihr/Focus/Medical/epichamp.html.

In 1570, the parish clerics added baptisms to the statistics. In 1629, the London government took over responsibility for collecting these data because of the great value. In the last half of the 17th century, John Gaunt used these data to make some insightful observations on the patterns of mortality (Chute, 2000; WHO, 2014a). These efforts led to the modern concepts of epidemic and endemic disease patterns, and the beginning of the disciplines of population-based epidemiology, and the modern study of data terminologies and classifications.

International Classification of Disease

Developing the standards needed to implement data terminologies and classifications, however, was slow. The usefulness of classifying causes of death was discussed at the first International Statistical Congress in 1853 (WHO, 2010a). Later, Jacques Bertillon chaired a committee charged with creating uniform causes of death classification system. American Public Health Association recommended the use of the Bertillon Classification by Canada, the United States, and Mexico, at a meeting in Ottawa, Canada.

It was 1900 before there was any agreement in medicine on standardizing the causes of death. The first international classification of disease (ICD) standardization was the Bertillion Classification List of the Causes of Death. After acceptance in 1900, the Bertillon Classification became the ICD Version 1 (ICD-1). At that time, the recommendation was for revising the classification every 10 years to ensure that the system remained current with medical practice advances. The Mixed Commission, a group composed of representatives from the International Statistical Institute and the Health Organization of the League of Nations, had responsibility for the updates through ICD-5, a version that added morbidity and mortality conditions. The World Health Organization [WHO] (2014a, 2014b) took on the responsibility to review and prepare the ICD-6 edition in 1946. ICD-6 was approved in 1948 and WHO has published revisions ever since. Twenty years later, in 1968, the United States adopted the use of ICD codes.

The ICD classification of codes, whose full name is the International Statistical Classification of Diseases and Related Health Problems, is a detailed listing of known diseases and injuries (WHO, 2010b). Today, nations worldwide use ICD to record mortality and morbidity statistics. Every known disease (or a group of related diseases) has a description, classification, and a unique code. In the United States, the ICD codes are part of the standards required for use by the Health Insurance Portability and Accountability Act (HIPAA).

The 43rd World Health Assembly endorsed ICD-10 version for international use in 1990. Almost immediately, WHO began discussions and initiated the workgroup to address development of ICD-11. WHO projected the use of ICD-11 to be in place by 2017 (WHO, 2010b).

The United States, however, continued to use ICD-9-CM for another 24 years despite the fact that most of the rest of the world used ICD-10 (Centers for Disease Control and Prevention, 2013a, 2013b, 2013c; CMS.gov, 2013a). The National Committee on Vital and Health Statistics (NCVHS, 2013) forwarded several recommendations to the Office of the Secretary of Health and Human Services (HHS) to move to ICD-10. In 2009, HHS proposed that the United States adopt ICD-10 by October 1, 2011. A delay in the implementation moved the date to 2015. You will see the terms ICD-9 or ICD-10 used interchangeably with ICD-9 or ICD-10-CM in the United States. The CM is an abbreviation for clinical modification, the system used by care providers to classify and code diagnoses, symptoms, and procedures.

The ICD codes now used worldwide for morbidity and mortality statistics, and in the United States for billing, were the first efforts to standardize healthcare data for both national and international use. Unless you are a nurse practitioner or a certified nurse midwife, it is unlikely that you need to code a diagnosis, yet you need to be aware of these classifications. Nursing quality improvement efforts to identify aggregate groups of patients by disease type use the ICD codes. Although useful for statistical purposes, the ICD-9-CM codes are not **granular** enough, that is, they do not capture enough data, to be used to document patient care in electronic medical records (EMRs) or EHRs.

ICD-10-CM provides additional granularity for diagnosis codes. For example, ICD-9-CM uses three to five digits and ICD-10-CM uses seven digits. ICD-9-CM has 14,000 codes, but ICD-10-CM has 69,000 codes and also provides for extensive severity parameters (CMS.gov, 2014). For additional information about the differences between ICD-9-CM and ICD-10-CM, read the ICD-10 Overview online at http://www.roadto10.org/whats-different/.

International Classification of Functioning, Disability, and Health

The International Classification of Functioning, Disability, and Health (ICF) also fall under the auspices of the WHO. Measurement of health and disability for both individuals and populations use ICF codes (WHO, 2014c). ICF codes focus on the impact of disease on the human experience including social and environmental factors (Figure 14-3). The 54th World Health Assembly endorsed the ICF in 2001. The ICF classification acts to complement ICD-10 to provide information regarding functional status. Organization of the codes is around body structure, functions, activities of living, and participation in life situations. They also contain information on severity and environmental factors. Although not intended as a measurement tool, IDF codes place

emphasis on function rather than disease. The design of ICF codes was for relevance across all cultures, age groups, and genders, making them useful with heterogeneous populations.

Digital Imaging and Communications in Medicine

Another standards development group that has ties to both national (National Electrical Manufacturers Association) and international groups (IEC) is the Digital Imaging and Communications in Medicine (DICOM) organization. DICOM sets and maintains standards that allow electrical transmission of digital images (DICOM, 2014). Their work makes it possible to exchange medical digital images worldwide. Thus, if you have a magnetic resonance imaging done in London, England, and your doctor is in Chicago, IL, the DICOM standard makes it possible for doctor to see the image in Chicago just as if it had been done in the local radiology department.

Comité Européen de Normalisation

The European Committee for Standardization, or Comité Européen de Normalisation (CEN), is a collaboration of standards bodies in Europe. CEN

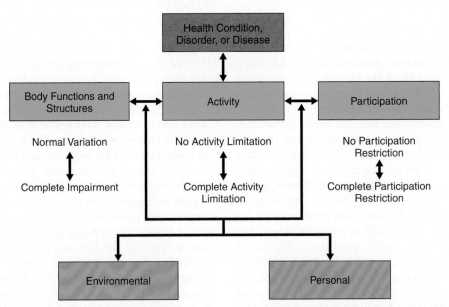

Figure 14-3. ICF codes focus on the impact of disease and the human experience. Source: World Health Organization. (2014c). *International classification of functioning, disability and health (ICF)*. Available at: http://www.who.int/classifications/icf/en/

has strong ties to the European Union politics, and common European legislation makes approved CEN standards the national standards (CEN, 2014). The standardization of healthcare informatics is the province of the CEN/TC 251. There are several standards relevant to nursing including the PrENV 14032, health informatics systems of concepts for nursing. This standard focuses on the application of nursing terminology within electronic messages and healthcare information systems.

International Health Terminology Standards Development Organisation

The International Health Terminology Standards Development Organisation (IHTSDO), a standards development organization created in 2007, is the outgrowth of the joint development of the Systematized Nomenclature of Medicine—Clinical Terms between the National Health Service in the United Kingdom and the College of American Pathologists in the United States (IHTSDO, 2014). Working with representatives of countries worldwide, this organization was created to promote more rapid development and worldwide adoption of standard clinical terminology for EHRs.

Development of International Standards

Group members of standard setting organizations are experts in their field who become members of a working or technical group of an organization, which has been delegated to set a specific standard. Anyone (including you) who is an expert in an area and has the time to devote to this endeavor can be a member of a working or technical standard setting group.

There are four main steps for developing standards. The first step in setting a standard is identification of a need. In the second step, the group designated to define the standard must state in operational terms what the standard will accomplish and how to accomplish it. The third step, defining terms and specifications for the standard is the longest, and one revised many times. Standards development involves a lengthy period of discussion, study of the literature, communication with those outside the group affected by the standard, and research. After definitions of terms and specifications, the fourth step is testing the standard.

If the number of parties affected by the new standard is large, the proposed standard is open for public comment. If the comments indicate problems, the group will return to the third step to refine the standard. If there are many changes from the original, the new proposal is open for public comment again. Eventually, members of the group vote on the standard. If they vote in favor, the standard goes to the parent organization for endorsement. If accepted by the parent organization, it then becomes a standard with a prefix indicating the group that set the standard and a number specific to that standard. When the standard needs updates, the approval process repeats itself.

BILLING TERMINOLOGY STANDARDIZATION

In the United States, there is agreement on the part of healthcare providers and patients that administrative or healthcare costs are too high. The National Health Expenditures Accounts reported that the administrative costs for 2008 were about 160 billion dollars (American Medical Association [AMA], 2014). Healthcare providers hope that the Patient Protection and Affordable Care Act, which went into effect in 2010, will address the cost concerns. Initiation of efforts to standardize government payments for hospital care in the 1980s was use of the diagnosis-related groups and modifications to the ICD codes. Following the lead of the government, many private insurers have also adopted them. Efforts to standardize billing for alternative healthcare providers, such as nurse practitioners, led to the Alternative Billing Coding (ABC) Set.

International Classification of Disease—Clinical Modification

The ICD codes discussed above, although useful for statistical and billing purposes, present a one-dimensional view of disease, because they focus only on etiology. The addition of CMs made the codes useful in billing. Development of CM codes allowed for capture of morbidity data from inpatient and outpatient records, physician office records, and National Center for Health Statistics surveys (CDC, 2013b). In the United States, healthcare providers transitioned from using ICD-9-CM to ICD-10-CM for billing purposes in 2014. Use of the ICD-10-PCS for procedure codes is also for billing purposes (CDC, 2013c).

Medicare Severity Diagnosis-Related Groups

The Medicare severity diagnosis-related groups (MS-DRG) are sometimes referred as the "daily rate guide," or simply MS-DRGs. The Health Care Financing Administration, now called the CMS, developed DRGs as a standardized patient classification system in the early 1980s. Originally intended as a review of the use of hospital resources, DRGs became a system for prospective payment. Under this system, categories of patients groups, determined the average consumption of hospital resources. The patient classification category served as the basis for hospital payment. The criteria used for assigning categories included medical diagnosis, surgery, complications, and usually age. In 2007, CMS began to use MS-DRG codes to reflect comorbidities (CDC, 2013b). Every patient receives a single MS-DRG, a process that done by a computer program called a "Grouper," based on information from the Uniform Hospital Discharge Data Set (CDC, 2010).

There are other DRG systems in use beyond the one used by CMS for Medicare patients. For example, the all patient-refined DRG (APR-DRG) represents non-Medicare patients. Other countries, such as England, France, Germany, the Netherlands, and Sweden, developed their own DRG systems based on the United States system (Quentin et al., 2013). In some countries with nationalized health systems, DRG codes determine hospital funding.

The Healthcare Common Procedure Coding System

The Healthcare Common Procedure Coding System (HCPCS) provides for a uniform billing systems for Medicare and other insurers (CMS.gov, 2013b). It consists of two levels: Level I and Level II. Level I uses the CPT (current procedural terminology) numeric coding developed and maintained by the AMA. Level II uses codes and descriptors for services, supplies, and products not includes in CPT codes. Examples of Level II codes include medical equipment, prosthetics, and orthotics. The intent of Level II is to supplement the CPT codes developed by the AMA and updated annually.

Outcome and Assessment Information Set

The DRGs are not the only government attempts to contain healthcare costs. Medicare-certified home care agencies must submit Outcome and Assessment Information Set (OASIS) data set to CMS as a part of the reimbursement procedure. OASIS is a group of data elements that represent a comprehensive assessment for an adult home care patient and the basis for measuring outcomes for Outcome-Based Quality Improvement (OBQI) (CMS.gov, 2012). Federal regulations require home healthcare agencies to collect, code, and transmit these data to their state center, which uploads them to CMS. OASIS standardizes what items are collected, and, by the use of a checklist, the terms used.

CMS provides the home health agencies feedback reports, OBQI Report, and the Patient Tally Report based upon the OASIS data (CMS.gov, 2013a, 2013b, 2013c). Currently, four reports are generated:

- Agency Patient-Related Characteristics Report
- Potentially Avoidable Event Report
- Outcome-Based Quality Improvement Report
- Process Quality Measurement Report

Derivation of the items in OASIS was from a study to develop a system of home care outcome measures. The Robert Wood Johnson Foundation and CMS funded development of OASIS (CMS.gov, 2012). The items include sociodemographic and environmental data, support systems, health status, and functional status attributes of adult (nonmaternity) patients. Individual agencies use OASIS data for care planning, demographics, and case mix reports of such patient characteristics as health and functional status at the start of care.

SUMMARY

Standards make commerce possible. From the light bulb you buy to the railroads, there are national and international standards both nationally and internationally. Technology used to care for patients has also met standards. Healthcare information standards are still in their infancy, particularly electronic information standards. Currently, interoperability continues to exist among many systems. This situation prevents early identification of epidemics and serious drug side effects as well as contribution to errors in patient care.

Data input into computers will become the healthcare records of the future; if these data are to be useful, it must meet standards. Professional organizations at the international and the national level, as well as governments, have recognized this problem, and are working to overcome it. Healthcare, however, is very complex and composed of many different stakeholders and disciplines, which further complicates this problem. The standards that are developed and adopted will determine important information for healthcare and will have a great effect on nursing and healthcare policy.

Analysis of standardized data warned of the Bubonic plague epidemic. Cooperation of the international community allows collection of data on the various outbreaks of flu at the time and place of origin and preventative measures be undertaken.

Because the tie of standards to the politics of healthcare, they are in continuous flux. Changes in technology compound the issues of standards and interoperability. The author attempted to make this chapter current at the time of its going to press.

APPLICATIONS AND COMPETENCIES

1. In your own words, describe interoperability and its three subtypes.

2. Working with two or three others, arrive at some standards for something simple such as entering a classroom or opening a book that a computer might interpret.

3. Using a drawing tool, such illustrations in Word or PowerPoint, diagram the use of standards used in a patient record for a patient's travel through:

   ■ An admission to the hospital from the emergency department
   ■ A home visit

   Consider the standards used for sharing laboratory or radiology testing, diagnosis and procedure coding, and billing. Summarize your analysis for use of standards.

4. Use the Internet to investigate further the activities of one of the standards setting groups. Employ the principles for evaluating websites described in Chapter 9.

5. Use a digital library to find an article that extends your understanding about interoperability and HIE. Make a list of "talking points" noted from the article to share with others.

6. Describe the function of the UMLS.

REFERENCES

American Medical Association. (2014). *Getting the most for our health care dollars.* Retrieved from https://www.ama-assn.org/ama/pub/advocacy/topics/health-care-costs.page

ASTM International. (2014). *The history of ASTM International—1898–1998: A century of progress. Chapter one: A broader view.* Retrieved from http://www.astm.org/HISTORY/hist_chapter1.html

Centers for Disease Control and Prevention (CDC). (2013a, June 19). *Classification of diseases, functioning, and disability.* Retrieved from http://www.cdc.gov/nchs/icd.htm

Centers for Disease Control and Prevention (CDC). (2013b). *International classification of diseases, tenth revision, clinical modification (ICD-10-CM).* Retrieved from http://www.cdc.gov/nchs/icd/icd10cm.htm

Centers for Disease Control and Prevention (CDC). (2013c). *Public health transition to ICD-10 CM/ PCS.* Retrieved from http://www.cdc.gov/nchs/icd/icd10cm_pcs.htm

Centers for Disease Control and Prevention (CDC). (2013d, December 10). *National Electronic Disease Surveillance System (NEDSS).* Retrieved from http://wwwn.cdc.gov/nndss/script/nedss.aspx

Centers for Disease Control and Prevention (CDC). (2014, February 24). *Public Health Information Network (PHIN).* Retrieved from http://www.cdc.gov/phin/

Chute, C. G. (2000). Clinical classification and terminology: Some history and current observations. *Journal of the American Medical Informatics Association, 7*(3), 298–303. Retrieved from http://www.ncbi.nlm.nih.gov/pmc/articles/PMC61433/?tool=pubmed

CMS.gov. (2012, April 5). *OASIS overview.* Retrieved from https://www.cms.gov/oasis/

CMS.gov. (2013a, June 26). *OASIS OBQI.* Retrieved from http://www.cms.gov/Medicare/Quality-Initiatives-Patient-Assessment-Instruments/HomeHealthQualityInits/HHQIOASISOBQI.html

CMS.gov. (2013b, September 9). *2011 ICD-10.* Retrieved from http://www.cms.gov/Medicare/Coding/ICD10/

CMS.gov. (2013c, December 5). *HCPCS—General information.* Retrieved from http://www.cms.gov/Medicare/Coding/MedHCPCSGenInfo/index.html

CMS.gov. (2014). Road to 10: The small physician route to ICD-10. Retrieved from http://www.roadto10.org/whats-different/

Comité Européen de Normalisation. (2014). *European Committee for standardization.* Retrieved from http://www.cen.eu/cen/pages/default.aspx

Digital Imaging and Communications in Medicine (DICOM). (2014, June). *DICOM homepage.* Retrieved from http://medical.nema.org/

Health Level 7. (2014a). *HL7 FAQs.* Retrieved from http://www.hl7.org/about/FAQs/

Health Level 7. (2014b). *What is HL7?* Retrieved from http://www.hl7.org/about/

Healthcare Information and Management Systems Society. (2013). *What is interoperability.* Retrieved from http://www.himss.org/library/interoperability-standards/what-is

HealthIT.gov. (n.d.a). *About ONC.* Retrieved from http://www.healthit.gov/newsroom/about-onc

HealthIT.gov. (n.d.b). *HITECH programs for health IT adoption.* Retrieved from http://www.healthit.gov/policy-researchers-implementers/health-it-adoption-programs

HealthIT.gov. (n.d.c). *Beacon Community Program.* Retrieved from http://www.healthit.gov/policy-researchers-implementers/beacon-community-program

HealthIT.gov. (n.d.d). *Consumer eHealth Program overview.* Retrieved from http://www.healthit.gov/policy-researchers-implementers/consumer-ehealth-program

HealthIT.gov. (n.d.e). *State health information (State HIE) resources.* Retrieved from http://www.healthit.gov/policy-researchers-implementers/state-health-information-exchange

HealthIT.gov. (n.d.f). *Regional extension centers (RECs).* Retrieved from http://www.healthit.gov/providers-professionals/regional-extension-centers-recs

HealthIT.gov. (n.d.g). *About the strategic healthcare IT advanced research projects (SHARP).* Retrieved from http://www.healthit.gov/policy-researchers-implementers/strategic-health-it-advanced-research-projects-sharp

HealthIT.gov. (n.d.h). *Workforce development programs.* Retrieved from http://www.healthit.gov/providers-professionals/workforce-development-programs

HealthIT.gov. (n.d.i). *Nationwide Health Information Network (NwHIN).* Retrieved from http://www.healthit.gov/policy-researchers-implementers/nationwide-health-information-network-nwhin

Hsiao, C.-J., & Hing, E. (2014). Use and characteristics of electronic health record systems among office-based physician practices: United States, 2001–2003. *NCHS Data Brief* (143), 1–8. Retrieved from http://www.cdc.gov/nchs/data/databriefs/db143.pdf

International Electrotechnical Commission. (2014). *What we do.* Retrieved from http://www.iec.ch/conformity/what/

International Health Terminology Standards Development Organisation. (2014). *Welcome to IHTSDO.* Retrieved from http://www.ihtsdo.org/

International Organization for Standardization (ISO). (2014a). *About ISO—ISO.* Retrieved from http://www.iso.org/iso/about

International Organization for Standardization (ISO). (2014b). *ISO 18104 L2003—health informatics—integration of a reference terminology model for nursing.* Retrieved from http://www.iso.org/iso/catalogue_detail.htm?csnumber=33309

Jamoom, E., Patel, V., King, J., et al. (2013). Physician experience with electronic health record systems that meet meaningful use criteria: NAMCS physician workflow survey, 2011. *NCHS Data Brief* (129), 1–8. Retrieved from http://www.cdc.gov/nchs/data/databriefs/db129.htm

King, J., Patel, V., Jamoom, E. W., et al. (2013). Clinical benefits of electronic health record use: National findings. *Health Services Research*, 49(1 Pt 2), 392–404. doi: 10.1111/1475-6773.12135. Retrieved from http://onlinelibrary.wiley.com/doi/10.1111/1475-6773.12135/pdf

Kohn, L. T., Corrigan, J., & Donaldson, M. S. (2000). *To err is human: Building a safer health system.* Washington, D.C.: National Academy Press. Retrieved from http://www.nap.edu/openbook.php?record_id=9728

National Committee of Vital Health Statistics. (2013, September 13). *NCVHS: Homepage.* Retrieved from http://www.ncvhs.hhs.gov/

National Library of Medicine. (2014a). *UMLS®.* Retrieved from http://www.nlm.nih.gov/research/umls/

National Library of Medicine. (2014b). UMLS Quick Start Guide. Retrieved from http://www.nlm.nih.gov/research/umls/new_users/online_learning/OVR_001.html

Quentin, W., Scheller-Kreinsen, D., Blumel, M., et al. (2013). Hospital payment based on diagnosis-related groups differs in Europe and holds lessons for the United States. *Health Affairs*, 32(4), 713–723. doi: 10.1377/hlthaff.2012.0876

WebExhibits. (2008). *History & info—Standard time.* Retrieved from http://www.webexhibits.org/daylightsaving/d.html

World Health Organization (WHO). (2014a). *History of the development of ICD.* Retrieved from http://www.who.int/classifications/icd/en/HistoryOfICD.pdf

World Health Organization (WHO). (2014b). *International classifications of disease.* Retrieved from http://www.who.int/classifications/icd/en/

World Health Organization (WHO). (2014c). *International classification of functioning, disability and health (ICF).* Retrieved from http://www.who.int/classifications/icf/en/

CHAPTER 15

Nursing Documentation in the Age of the Electronic Health Record

OBJECTIVES

After studying this chapter, you will be able to:

1. Analyze the opportunities that electronic documentation brings to nursing.
2. Define vocabulary associated with standardized terminologies.
3. Differentiate between the nursing minimum data set and nursing-focused terminologies.
4. Describe the benefits of using a standardized terminology in healthcare documentation.
5. Analyze issues surrounding the use of standardized terminologies.

KEY TERMS

Axes	Lexical	Ontology
Classify	Linked	Postcoordinated term
Combinatorial vocabulary	Linear list	Precoordinated term
Disjunctive	Mapping	Reference terminology
Granularity	Metathesaurus	Semantic
Harmonization	Minimum data set	Subset
Integrated	Monoaxial	Taxonomic vocabularies
Interdisciplinary terminology	Multiaxial taxonomy	
Interface terminology	Natural language	

ealthcare in the United States is undergoing a transformation. Additionally, fee for service is slowly giving way to a demand that reimbursement be based on outcomes not procedures (Topol, 2015). Given that nursing care greatly influences many patient outcomes, if nursing is to be valued, hence allowed to bill for its care, it needs evidence that this care positively affects outcomes (Moss & Saba, 2011; Dykes et al., 2013). This requires nursing data, which is only possible with electronic health records (EHRs) and standardized terminology. This fact has been acknowledged by the US government, which is supporting the use of clinical electronic records to provide this evidence (Boyd et al., 2010). Furthermore, the data that provide evidence of nursing's effect on outcomes must not only exist in EHRs, but must be presented in a readily identifiable and measurable way (Boyd et al., 2010; Moss & Saba, 2011; Harman et al., 2012).

NURSING AND DOCUMENTATION

The practice of documentation in healthcare is over 100 years old. In the 19th century and first half of the 20th century, most healthcare was delivered by the family physician who knew the patient, family, and all their maladies. He or she kept records, but they were simple by today's standards. Given the relative simplicity of healthcare at that time, detailed records were not necessary. Nursing's documentation, too, was relatively simple. It was designed for paper-based systems, generally used natural language, and focused on the care of one patient. Electronic documentation is slowly changing this scenario for nurses and all healthcare professionals. Although a record that details the care of one patient is still the number one reason for documentation, the data recorded are increasingly being used in many areas beyond the care of one patient, for example as a basis to make healthcare decisions and set healthcare policy.

To meet this need, nurses as well as others need to move beyond regarding conscientiously documented nursing notes as only a means of communication between nurses, or between physicians and nurses. The aforementioned perspective disregards these records' potential value for billing, research, and evidence-based practice. Before the age of litigation, nursing notes were often purged from patient records, leaving no lasting documentation of nursing's contributions to healthcare; hence, there was no way to retrieve these data (Thede, 2008), leading to the phenomenon of the invisibility of nursing. Due to a lack of nursing care documentation useful for billing, nursing care is

too often included as part of room cost, regardless of the level of care provided to an individual patient (Schwirian, 2013).

Too often, the focus in nursing documentation has been solely to record compliance with the medical regimen, or other Joint Commission reporting requirements. Although today nursing notes may be a permanent part of the record, nursing documentation is still not included in patient discharge abstracts that are prepared by hospital medical records departments. These abstracts, which include no indication that nursing care is a part of hospital care, are used by different agencies for various funding and statistical purposes, making nurses' contributions to healthcare virtually invisible. This situation will continue until we make nursing documentation both easily retrievable and standardized (Aslan & Emiroglu, 2013).

In community health, one state public health nursing group found that there was a "mystique" about nursing's contribution to public health and that nursing care was invisible to partners and stakeholders (Correll & Martin, 2009). In exploring this situation, they discovered that in addition to not being easily accessible or measurable, their documentation contained little that demonstrated nursing's value. Hannah et al. (2009) report that when the focus in EHRs is on physicians, there is no visibility for "...nurses' clinical judgments and decision making that are within the scope of nursing practice" (p. 524). These situations lead to erroneous perceptions of nurses and nursing care.

One has only to look at television medical dramas to realize the perception of nurses as handmaidens to physicians with no discernable cognitive skills. This perception is too often held by potential students (Weaver et al., 2013; Schwirian, 2013), the general public, and the physicians who provide advice to the screenwriters. To fully change the perception, we need to make nursing care visible not just to our patients but to other healthcare disciplines, regulatory agencies, and the general public. The best way to accomplish this is through nursing documentation. The documentation must contain data that are readily identifiable, accessible, and measurable and demonstrate the value of nursing. Nurses used to say that if it is documented, it was done; today, any nursing care that is not in electronic documentation in a way that it can be retrieved and used beyond the care of one patient is not going to be valued.

Making this transition is going to require a change in thinking about our documentation as well as changes in how we document. It involves being willing to learn new ways of thinking about and labeling our nursing problems, interventions, and outcomes. If we document interventions electronically with accurate, easily understood labels and relate them to specific problems and outcomes, electronic documentation can provide evidence that supports the value of nursing care. These data will improve nursing practice, make nursing care reimbursable, and be useful in allocating funding for healthcare (Jones et al., 2011).

TYPES OF STANDARDIZED TERMINOLOGIES

To change the perception of nursing through its documentation, we need to be familiar with standardized terminology and use it where appropriate. Figure 15-1 indicates changes in documentation uses as we move from paper records to electronic records and how the language used in documentation needs to change accordingly. If nursing care is to be valued beyond handmaiden to physicians or others, we need to be sure that nursing

> **QSEN Scenario**
>
> You are assisting an informatics nurse specialist to build data entry screens for a medical clinical area. She asks your assistance in getting the nurses to document using the standardized terminology that she is building into the system. How will you convince the rest of the staff of the value of using a standardized nursing terminology for documentation?

problems, interventions, and outcomes are part of the documentation.

Unfortunately, today, nursing data are seldom integrated into an EHR or a clinical data repository (Westra et al., 2015). Changing this situation requires that nurses champion, learn, and use a standardized terminology. A **standardized terminology** is one whose terms have agreed-upon definitions. It can be natural language, linear lists, taxonomic vocabularies, combinatorial vocabularies, or combinational vocabularies.

Natural Language

Although we may not be accustomed to thinking that the language we use every day is standardized, anyone who has tried to understand a foreign language quickly realizes this. Not only are different words in different languages used to communicate concepts, words also express

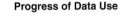

Progress of Data Use

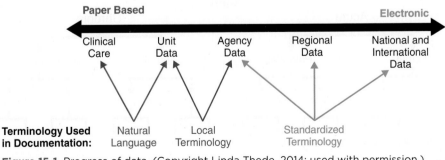

Figure 15-1. Progress of data. (Copyright Linda Thede, 2014; used with permission.)

the culture behind the language in ways that can make exact translations very difficult. There is no denying that your native **natural language**, or your everyday speaking tongue, is very expressive and that using it in documentation requires no change in how you think. However, it is notoriously difficult to analyze; hence, although it was suitable when we used paper records and focused on the care of one patient, it is not suited for the purposes for which documentation is used today.

Linear Lists or Vocabularies

You are probably familiar with these—think of a drop-down menu with choices that can be clicked to fill a blank. Some types of data, such as gender or physician, lend themselves well to a **linear list**, or what is often referred to as a **vocabulary**. An alphabetical list such as a dictionary is a linear list. Your agency may have a problem list from which you can select nursing problems to enter into the documentation. Many of the words in this list are terms, or linguistic labels used to represent a concept. If you have ever tried to construct such a list, you have no doubt realized two problems. One, the number of terms needed is unmanageable, and two, different nurses assign different meanings to the terms.

Lists such as these present an additional problem: There is no way to **classify** or group the terms so that they can be analyzed beyond the individual term. For example, the terms postoperative pain, chronic pain, and acute pain may each be on the list as well as other terms describing pain, but if one is searching for all situations where pain is a symptom, these separate entries make this cumbersome because every term that describes pain is needed in the query.

Taxonomic Vocabularies

A solution to the situation of looking for all pain conditions is to organize the list of terms into a taxonomy, or a grouping of terms with conceptual similarities into groups that share a common concept such as pain. Taxonomies are hierarchical; that is, they show different levels with each higher level being a broader concept or more general term for the concept below it. The terms with the most **granularity**, or the most specific terms, are on the lowest level of a taxonomy. Figure 15-2 is an example of a taxonomy. Notice that the terms higher up in taxonomy can all be used to describe any of the terms below it. For example, "acute" can describe either actual or potential pain. The terms at the lower levels in a taxonomy differ from the other items at that level, although they share a common train represented by the term at the level above it, called the parent. In a taxonomy, a trait can be analyzed at any level. For example, if you wished to analyze the characteristic of all cases of chronic pain, whether actual or potential, together with a given intervention, a taxonomy like that in Figure 15-2 (which has one axis and is **monoaxial**) would permit that use. Or, using the next lower level, one could just query for the interventions or outcomes for actual pain in the abdomen.

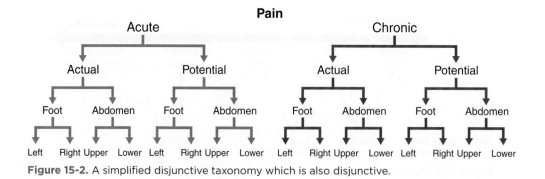

Figure 15-2. A simplified disjunctive taxonomy which is also disjunctive.

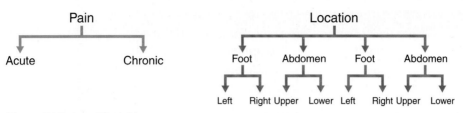

Figure 15-3. A multiaxial taxonomy.

The clinician generally uses the most granular, or most descriptive, term in documentation. The computer, which has the taxonomic structure programmed into it, provides the ability for clinicians to analyze data at any level in the taxonomy. Examples of taxonomic vocabularies are the North American Nursing Diagnosis Association International (NANDA-I) and the Nursing Interventions Classification (NIC). This arrangement lends itself well to statistical evaluation by allowing the data to be analyzed using either the most granular term or a higher-level term.

As you can see in Figure 15-2, **taxonomic vocabularies** share the problem with lists that they are difficult to expand without becoming repetitive. They do, however, help to reduce the number of terms and to organize terms so that searching can be done more easily. The repeating of the terms "actual" and "potential" at the second level of each branch, as well as the terms at the third and fourth levels, illustrates these difficulties. Figure 15-2 has only one axis and is monoaxial. It is also **disjunctive** because each term has only one parent.

You can easily see that in a monoaxial taxonomy, adding descriptors such as the length of pain would require a fifth level of repeated terms, a situation that quickly becomes unmanageable. Imagine trying to document the care of an ulcer on the left foot with this type of taxonomy. To solve these problems, **multiaxial taxonomies** are used, which have two or more axes such as is seen in Figure 15-3. Clinicians can then create terms from more than one axis. Multiaxial taxonomies, however, require an infinite number of taxonomies, and using all these taxonomies for documentation would be very involved.

Combinational Vocabularies

Solving these problems can be accomplished by creating what is called a **combinatorial vocabulary**, in which a term is created by combining terms from lists in different axes or categories. The International Classification of Nursing Practice (ICNP) is an example. Figure 15-4 illustrates the ICNP axes. Under each of these axes is a list of terms with agreed-upon definitions that can be used to describe that area. For example, under the client category are terms such as patient, significant other, family, or community. In the focus category, one finds terms such as pain and wound. The judgment category list contains terms such as slight, moderate, or severe, whereas the list for the duration category includes terms for the time the "focus" or area of concern existed. Not all descriptions needed in documentation require a term from each list; however, the rules of combination

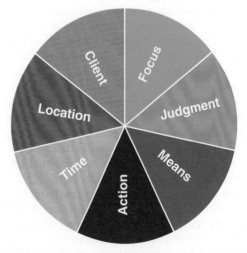

Figure 15-4. ICNP axes. (Reprinted with permission of the International Council of Nurses, 2014.)

TABLE 15-1	Example of an ICNP Combinatorial Term			
Client	Focus	Judgment	Location	Duration
Patient	Pain	Moderate	Lower Back	Three months

require that a created term includes a term from both the client and focus categories. Terms used in documentation that are created this way are called **postcoordinated terms**. An example can be seen in Table 15-1, which describes a patient with moderate lower back pain that has existed for 3 months.

The Systematized Nomenclature of Medicine (SNOMED) and the International Classification of Nursing Practice (ICNP) are examples of this type of standardized vocabulary. In the ICNP terminology, the divisions seen in Figure 15-4 are overall categories of terms deemed needed to document. The divisions are often called **axes**. To create a term, users select terms from lists in the axes. Rules of combination require users to select terms from specified axes, such as client and focus. Terms used in documentation that are created this way are called **postcoordinated terms**. One difficulty with combinatorial vocabularies is that it is possible to create terms that make no sense.

In specific areas such as obstetrics, it is known that specific terms will be used in documentation. In these cases, clinicians often have access to a list of **precoordinated terms**, or terms that are prepared by experts in a field by combining the terms from the various axes. These terms then are easily used in documentation, avoiding the need to create one's own term. The International Council of Nurses, which owns and maintains the ICNP, works with groups in various specialty areas to create what are called **subsets** of precoordinated terms that can be easily used with the terminology. (A subset is a smaller set of terms from a larger group of terms.) SNOMED has created a subset of nursing diagnoses that are precoordinated terms useful in nursing documentation. In the ICNP, the model in Figure 15-4 is used to create terms for not only nursing diagnoses but also nursing interventions and outcomes. Fortunately, these two groups are now working together and have created an equivalency table between the International Classification for Nursing Practice (ICNP) concepts and SNOMED CT concepts (Matney, 2014).

Ontologies

Does a combinatorial vocabulary solve all the problems associated with standardized terminologies? Given the breadth of healthcare and nursing, there will never be a perfect solution. However, attempts are being made to develop what are called **ontologies**. An ontology is the highest level of organization of a terminology. Complex and powerful, it provides the ability for concepts to be represented and linked to more than one concept. They are compositional, show relationships within a domain, and are a resource for building local terminologies, or nomenclatures (Hardiker, 2011a, 2011b).

OVERVIEW OF STANDARDIZED HEALTHCARE TERMINOLOGIES

Standardizing terminology in healthcare is not new. During the very early 20th century, medical professionals adopted standardized terminology that described patient mortality and morbidity. The International Classification of Diseases (ICD) formalized these terms (Levy, 2004) (ICD). The first version of the ICD, ICD-1, focused on mortality, but with the adoption of new versions, the ICD's breadth has been increased to include many other foci of healthcare such as etiology and diseases. The primary purpose of the ICD is statistical analysis of data regionally, nationally, and internationally. At times, it has been used for billing, although in the United States, the Current Procedural Terminology (CPT) codes are more appropriate for billing. Today, there are many standardized healthcare-focused terminologies such as:

- Current Procedural Terminology (CPT), a medical code set maintained by the American Medical Association that describes medical, surgical, and diagnostic services
- Digital Imaging and Communications in Medicine (DICOM), which is a standard for

handling, storing, printing, and transmitting medical images

- International Classification of Functioning, Disability and Health (ICF), which is a classification of functioning and disability
- Outcome and Assessment Information Set (OASIS), which is a set of data that represents core items used in assessing adult home care patients

NURSING-RELATED STANDARDIZED TERMINOLOGIES

The data needs for analyzing mortality, etiology, and billing are different from the data needs in clinical documentation. Standardizing the terminology used to describe the majority of clinical problems, interventions, and outcomes is relatively new. A few with which you are probably familiar are the staging numbers used to describe pressure ulcers, the Glasgow Coma Scale, and the APGAR (appearance, pulse, grimace, activity, respiration) rating of newborns. These are all standardizations useful in clinical care; however, each is limited to a very small area of patient care.

A few pioneers in the American Nurses Association (ANA) as early as the 1960s saw that nursing documentation was valuable and, if its value was to be recognized it, needed to be standardized. However, it took several decades and the push toward electronic records for more nurses to recognize the idea that our documentation is valuable. Today, as the use of an electronic medical record (EMR) becomes more prevalent along with a move toward interoperability of healthcare data, the need for standardized data that represent nursing care is even more imperative (Jones et al., 2010).

In 1989, the ANA created a committee to evaluate terminologies useful in nursing practice (Matney et al., 2012). This committee identified definitive criteria to evaluate the terminologies. These criteria required that the data set, classification, or nomenclature provides a rationale for its development and that the terminology support the nursing process by providing clinically useful terminology. The group asking for recognition also had to provide documentation of utility of the terminology in practice as well as its validity and reliability. A final requirement was identification of a specific group that would be responsible for maintaining and revising the system. Not only did the ANA recognize nursing-focused clinically useful terminologies, it also recognized three **interdisciplinary terminologies** (useful in all many healthcare disciplines) and two minimum data sets. Reflecting that since 2002 there have been no new requests for recognition for nursing terminologies, and in acknowledgment of the work currently underway to harmonize the various terminologies, on March 13, 2013, the ANA ceased work in this area.

Minimum Data Sets

A **minimum data set** is a list of categories of data, each of which has an agreed definition as to what it includes. They specify the type of data that will meet the essential needs of data users for a specific purpose, such as billing. They may or may not specify the terms to use for each category. The ANA-recognized U.S. Nursing Minimum Data Set (US-NMDS) specifies only the categories, not the terminology, to be used in each category. Other nations have also seen a need to define categories of information that are needed to provide adequate information about nursing care. Table 15-2, which compares the US-NMDS and the International Nursing Minimum Data Set (i-NMDS), illustrates the nursing care similarities between nations. (For additional information on the i-NMDS, see www.nursing.umn.edu/prod/groups/nurs/@pub/@nurs/documents/content/nurs_content_451375.pdf.)

Also recognized by the ANA is a Nursing Management Minimum Data Set (NMMDS). Developed to provide essential data elements useful to nurse managers and administrators (Kunkel et al., 2012), it allows administrators to pull together information that otherwise resides in many different places such as human resources, scheduling, or billing. It also adds information about staff mix and other items of interest to managers. The terms in the NMMDS "... describe contextual factors necessary to plan, conduct, and evaluate nursing services for any setting in which nurses work" (Kunkel et al., 2012, p. 134) and are coded into LOINC (Westra, 2015). By providing uniform terms with definitions and coding

TABLE 15-2	Comparison of the USA-NMDS and the i-NMDS	
Data Category	**USA-NMDS**	**i-NMDS**
Setting	Unique facility or service agency number Unique number of principal registered nurse provider[a] Unique patient number[a] Discharge or termination date Disposition of patient Expected payer for this bill	Agency location Ownership of facility Country system of payment Care personnel (number, gender, training and education, full-time equivalent for types of personnel) Ratio of patients to personnel
Patient Demographics	Personal identification[a]	Clinical service type Discharge status Reason for admission Dates for the start and end of a care episode
	Date of birth	Year of birth
	Sex	Gender
	Race and Ethnicity	
	Residence	Country of residence
Nursing Care	Nursing diagnosis[a]	
	Nursing intervention[a]	
	Nursing outcomes[a]	
	Nursing intensity[a]	

[a]Elements in the US-NMDS that are not in the US Uniform Hospital Discharge Data Set.

Source: University of Minnesota Center for Nursing Informatics. i-NMDS retrieved from www.nursing.umn.edu/prod/groups/nurs/@pub/@nurs/documents/content/nurs_content_451375.pdf

specifications, the NMMDS allows data to be collected and analyzed to provide information about nursing services at local, regional, national, and international levels.

Nursing-Focused Standardized Terminologies

In addition to recognizing two minimum data sets, the ANA recognized two terminologies that are interdisciplinary—that is, useful by all healthcare practitioners—one that is useful for nurse practitioners in billing for their practice, and eight nursing-focused terminologies, one of which the Patient Care Data Set, was retired in 2006. The Canadians have developed a standardized nursing terminology, which, although not ANA recognized, is a valuable addition to nursing.

ANA-Recognized Nursing-Focused Terminologies

In the United States, the most familiar terminology is the North American Nursing Diagnosis Association International (NANDA-I) (Schwirian &

Thede, 2011). NANDA-I provides the basis for nursing problems in most of the other ANA-recognized nursing-focused terminologies. This terminology, however, identifies and describes only those terms that are useful to document nursing diagnoses. The Nursing Interventions Classification (NIC) and Nursing Outcomes Classification (NOC) provide the terminology for nursing interventions and outcomes to fulfill all but the nursing intensity category of nursing specific data in the US-NMDS. The letters NNN are an acronym that refers to all three of these terminologies. All the other ANA-recognized nursing-specific terminologies contain terms for all three of these categories. Table 15-3 provides a brief description of each of the ANA-recognized data sets and terminologies. For more information about each of these terminologies, see the Web addresses in Table 15-3. For more in-depth information about each of these standardized terminologies, see dlthede.net/SNL/SNL.html.

With the exception of the International Classification of Nursing Practice (ICNP), all the nursing-specific ANA-recognized standardized terminologies are US developed. Additionally, with the same exception, they were designed as **interface terminologies**. An interface terminology is one that "interfaces" with the user—that is, the terms are used in documentation. The ICNP was originally designed as a **reference terminology**, but with the subsets of precoordinated terms described above, it is also useful as an interface terminology. A reference terminology is one that works behind the scenes. It takes a documentation term and gives it a code related to concepts at a higher level to allow a broader analysis. For example, in the figure of a simplified terminology in Figure 15-2, the documentation term acute pain of the left foot would be "coded" as the concept of pain, which is what would be used statistically. However, the ability to do analysis at lower levels is still preserved.

Canadian Health Outcomes for Better Information and Care (C-HOBIC)

To make visible the contributions of Canadian nurses, the Canadian Health Outcomes for Better Information and Care (C-HOBIC) (VanDeVelde-Coke et al., 2012; Hannah et al., 2012) was developed. C-HOBIC focuses on the collection of a set of nursing-sensitive outcomes in acute, long-term, home, and chronic care settings to support the sharing of clinical information among clinical disciplines and care settings (Hannah et al., 2009). These clinical outcomes have a concept definition, a valid and reliable measure, and empirical evidence linking them to nursing inputs or interventions (C-HOBIC, 2013).

Interdisciplinary Standardized Terminologies

The ANA recognized three interdisciplinary terminologies: the Systematized Nomenclature of Medicine—Clinical Terminology (SNOMED—CT); Logical Observations Identifiers Names and Codes (LOINC); and the Alternative Billing Codes (ABC). The ABC are used by nurse practitioners and other nonphysician practitioners for billing, but they are not used in documentation, so they are not discussed here.

SNOMED CT

Because of its international stature and its availability, comprehensiveness, and ability to capture data from all healthcare disciplines, SNOMED—CT (Systematized Nomenclature of Medicine—Clinical Terminology) is becoming an important standard in the EHR. The final rule for the initial set of standards from the Health Information Technology (HIT) Committee includes SNOMED CT as one of the options to electronically record, modify, and retrieve a patient's problem list for longitudinal care (Elhanan et al., 2011).

SNOMED is basically a reference terminology; however, with appropriate subsets, it can be used as an interface terminology. The SNOMED CT Nursing Work Group and the nursing terminology developers have integrated the diagnostic concepts of the CCC, Omaha System, North American Nursing Diagnosis Association International (NANDA-I), and Perioperative Nursing Data Set (PNDS) into SNOMED as a nursing problem list subset containing 369 unique coded concepts for documenting nursing diagnoses (Matney et al., 2012). Additionally, the International Council of Nursing (ICN) and the International Health Terminology Standards Development Organization (IHTSDO), which is now responsible for SNOMED CT, have an agreement to foster

TABLE 15-3 ANA-Recognized Standardize Nursing Terminologies

Terminology	Elements Contained	Year Recognized by ANA	Description/Comments
Nursing Minimum Data Sets			
U.S. Nursing Minimum Data Set (US-NMDS) www.nursing.umn.edu/prod/groups/nurs/@pub/@nurs/documents/content/nurs_content_451376.pdf	Delineates and defines categories of data needed to describe clinical nursing practice	1999	Designed for all healthcare settings. The categories have remained the same since their first release in 1988. Contains no terms for any category. Three of the 16 categories, nursing diagnosis, interventions, and outcomes are basis of all nursing standardized terminologies.
Nursing Management Minimum Data Set (NMMDS) www.nursing.umn.edu/prod/groups/nurs/@pub/@nurs/documents/content/nurs_content_451377.pdf	Categories and terms for environment nursing care, financial resources	2000	A standardized data set, contains categories and standardized terms for each category. Permits nursing managers to have more and better information about their nursing services as well as provide comparable data for benchmarking with other organizations
Nursing-Specific ANA-Recognized Standardized Terminology			
Clinical Care Classification (CCC) http://www.sabacare.com/	ND, NI, NO	1992	Originally developed to estimate home care expenditures for Medicare patients as the HHCC (Home Health Care Classification). Now expanded to all areas of healthcare. Used by permission, no royalty. Maintained by Sabacare
International Classification of Nursing Practice (ICNP) http://www.icn.ch/what-we-do/international-classification-for-nursing-practice-icnpr/	ND, NI, NO	2000	Designed as a reference terminology, terms are combinational, with the parts of a term selected from specific axes. Subsets, or a list of precoordinated terms, exist in specific areas and are being developed in other areas so that it can be used as an interface terminology. Developed and maintained by the International Council of Nursing (ICN). With SNOMED is part of the International Health Terminology Standards Development Organization (IHTSDO). Requires license fee to use

Name		Year	Description	Notes
North American Nursing Diagnosis Association International (NANDA-I) http://www.nanda.org/	ND	1992	Categorizes and defines nursing problems for documentation for all settings. Is a basis for many nursing terminologies' nursing problems. Requires license fee to use. Maintained by NANDA International	NANDA-I, NIC, and NOC are intended to be used together. Requires three separate licenses. When referencing all three, often referred to as NNN.
Nursing Interventions Classification (NIC) http://www.nursing.uiowa.edu/cncce/nursing-interventions-classification-overview	NI	1992	Categorizes and defines nursing interventions for documentation in all settings. Requires license fee to use. Developed and maintained by the University of Iowa Center for Nursing Classification & Clinical Effectiveness	
Nursing Outcomes Classification (NOC) http://www.nursing.uiowa.edu/cncce/nursing-outcomes-classification-overview	NO	1997	Categorizes and defines nursing outcomes for documentation. Requires license fee to use. Developed and maintained by the University of Iowa Center for Nursing Classification & Clinical Effectiveness	
Omaha System http://www.omahasystem.org/	ND, NI, NO	1992	Allows users to collect, classify, document, and analyze data for patients, families, and communities in home care, public health, and community nursing. Used with permission, no fee. Developed by the Omaha Visiting Nurse Association in conjunction with seven other community health agencies. Maintained by the Omaha System Organization	
Patient Care Data Set (Retired) http://www.nlm.nih.gov/research/umls/sourcereleasedocs/current/PCDS/	ND, NI, NO	1998–2006	Originally developed for acute care setting by Judy Ozbolt at the University of Virginia, in collaboration with member institutions of the University Health System consortium. Intended for nurses and nonphysician healthcare providers. Retired in 2006	

(continued)

TABLE 15-3 ANA-Recognized Standardize Nursing Terminologies (*continued*)

Terminology	Elements Contained	Year Recognized by ANA	Description/Comments
Perioperative Nursing Data Set (PNDS) http://www.aornjournal.org/article/S0001-2092(10)00993-2/fulltext	ND, NI, NO	1999	Provides data around the complete perioperative experience from preadmission to discharge. Developed as a means to validate nursing in an operative setting. Developed and maintained by the American Operating Room Nurses Association. Requires license fee to use
Interdisciplinary ANA-Recognized Standardized Terminology			
Logical Observation Identifiers Names and Codes (LOINC) http://loinc.org/		2002	Originally focused on standardization of names of laboratory tests. Now includes assessment measures for vital signs, obstetric measurements, and some clinical assessment scales. Developed by the Regenstrief Institute. Free to all users
Systematized Nomenclature of Medicine—Clinical Terminology (SNOMED—CT) http://www.ihtsdo.org/snomed-ct/		1999	Comprehensive, multilingual, clinical healthcare terminology. Basically a reference terminology, but has nursing subsets for documenting nursing problems. Free to all US users through the National Library of Medicine. Originally developed by the American College of Pathology, now owned and maintained by the International Health Terminology Standards Development Organization (IHTSDO)
Interdisciplinary ANA-Recognized Standardized Terminology for Billing			
Alternative Billing Codes (ABC) http://www.abccodes.com/ali/ARTpertinent_link/ARTMy_Health97.asp	Approximately 800 nursing procedures gathered from NIC[a]	2000	"...developed to process claims and alternative health care services not routinely included in traditional medical billing codes."[a] Useful for nurse practitioners

[a]Beintema, H., Isaacson, E., Lovinaria, D., et al. (2007). *Alternative billing concept coding system.* Retrieved from https://www.google.com/url?sa=t&rct=j&q=&esrc=s&source=web&cd=5&cad=rja&ved=0CFQQFjAE&url=https%3A%2F%2Fwiki.umn.edu%2F2Fpub%2F2FHealthInformatics%2F2FGroup1-VocabFall07%2FAssignment2final.docx&ei=JmWrUo6KleewyQHoqIGgAw&usg=AFQjCNH_Emr3flIbIFVqOHdAhmBgLtuuLQ&bvm=bv.57967247,d.aWc

ND, nursing diagnosis (phenomena, problems); NI, nursing interventions; NO, nursing outcomes.

interoperability in health information systems. This accord has resulted in an Equivalence Table between SNOMED CT and ICNP nursing diagnoses and outcomes (*e-Health Bulletin*, 2013, December), thus furthering the goal of a true interdisciplinary terminology that encompasses nursing.

LOINC

The Logical Observations Identifiers Names and Codes (LOINC) in its original form standardized the names and reporting of laboratory tests. It was created by, is maintained by, and is freely distributed by the Regenstrief Institute. Since its beginnings, it has expanded to include terms useful in assessment as well as clinical care, outcomes management, and research. Parts of the Clinical Care Classification and Omaha System are integrated into LOINC as is the UMMDS. The National Committee on Vital and Health Statistics (NCVHS) has recognized LOINC as a standard for laboratory test names.

ATTEMPTS TO MAKE TERMINOLOGIES INTEROPERABLE

With the plethora of standardized nursing terminologies, let alone other specialized healthcare and interdisciplinary terminologies, there is a hope that the use of any recognized standardized terminology will allow interoperability with other terminologies. In reality, this is not simple and never 100% successful. Remember from our discussion of natural language that in addition to standardizing meanings of words, a language expresses a culture. The same is true of a terminology; each is based on a philosophy. For example, the classification of NANDA-I is loosely based on Gordon's 11 health patterns, and the Omaha System focuses on terms specific to home health and public health needs. It is difficult to correlate these philosophies.

Mapping

Matching a term or concept in one standardized terminology with that in another has been referred to as **mapping**. There are two concepts involved in mapping one terminology with another: a lexical match and a semantic match. An exact **lexical** match is a word-for-word match (e.g., *pain* and *pain*). An exact **semantic** match is a match on the same meaning or a synonym (e.g., *convulsion* and *seizure*). The complete mapping of one terminology to another does not happen. There may be a match for some terms and concepts, but never for the entire terminology. In short, interchanging terminologies is fraught with difficulties.

Harmonization

One of the difficulties when mapping a term or concept in one terminology to another is that terminologies can differ in the granularity of terms—that is, one terminology might use concepts that are broader (less granular) than the other. Additionally, one terminology may contain concepts that are not available in the other terminology. Given that the nursing terminologies were developed with different aims, it is not surprising that they are not exactly equivalent. Terminologists today use the term **harmonization** to cover all the degrees of making standardized terminologies partially interoperable. It does not imply a complete matching.

Linking

Concepts may also be **linked** in a clinically relevant way. The term linked means that one term is related, or often used, with another. For example, a specific nursing intervention may often be associated or linked with a specific nursing diagnosis. Linked terms may be presented together for documentation purposes. For example, the nursing diagnosis "Comfort, Alteration in: Pain" is often linked to the nursing intervention "Assess/evaluate effectiveness of pain medication."

Integration

When terms in a terminology have been wholly absorbed into another entity as separate terms, those terms are said to be **integrated**. For example, the Unified Medical Language System (UMLS) has integrated into its metathesaurus the terms from all the ANA-recognized standardized terminologies. The UMLS **metathesaurus** is a list of concepts and terms from health-related standardized vocabularies that is used by the UMLS to index the literature. It is possible to search PubMed or Medline bibliographic indexes using terms from the ANA-recognized terminologies.

BENEFITS OF USING STANDARDIZED TERMINOLOGIES

With the increased use of electronic medical and healthcare records, the ease of uncovering information hidden in healthcare documentation is becoming far easier than in the past. Whether nursing documentation will provide this information is dependent on nursing's ability to use standardized terminologies. To quote Clark and Lang (1992), "If we cannot name it, we cannot control it, finance it, research it, or put it into public policy" (Clark & Lang, 1992, p. 128), and one might add, be reimbursed for it. When nursing documentation uses a standardized terminology in the EHR, it will generate quantitative data (Erdogan et al., 2013) that can be used to for these purposes.

Increasing Quality of Care

The first nursing informaticist, Florence Nightingale, saw documentation as a method for evaluating and enhancing patient care to further the profession. She would have recognized the value of standardized terminologies to support efficiencies in retrieving, linking, and exchanging data (Giannangelo & Fenton, 2008), a practice that reveals the impact of specific interventions on outcomes (Kripps, 2008) as well as informs best practice and research (Rutherford, 2008; Lundberg et al., 2008; Westra et al., 2008).

When nursing uses standardized terminologies, our data will be available for healthcare planning, giving nursing a voice in this process and improving policies related to patient care. These terminologies also facilitate developing care plans (Müller-Staub et al., 2007; Nunes et al., 2014). Additionally, standardized documentation meets many accreditation efforts as well as supporting decision-making (Correll & Martin, 2009). Standardized terminologies can provide clinical data to support current and new nursing practices, thus contributing to evidence-based practice.

Decreasing Costs of Care

Financial pressures in healthcare alone make it imperative that the nursing care in documentation be identifiable and measurable (Müller-Staub et al., 2007). Healthcare is facing a period of decreasing revenues as well as cuts in reimbursement when pay for performance, instead of services, becomes the norm. Standardized data that demonstrate outcomes will be necessary to justify reimbursement (Moss & Saba, 2011). Because nursing care is vital to healthcare outcomes, when an organization can accurately measure nursing care through queries of patient care data rather than by costly manual audits (Lundberg et al., 2008; Dykes et al., 2013), these data can be used to bill the nursing care provided to each patient rather than hiding nursing costs in room costs. If nursing can be viewed as revenue generating rather than as an expense, nurses will be more valued and adequate staffing will be realized as necessary to meet financial goals, with the end result that patient care will improve.

Contributing to Evidence-Based Practice and Clinical Decision Systems

The knowledge base of nursing is not static. When our documentation is able to be analyzed, it can contribute to the knowledge base of nursing, providing a strong background for evidence-based practice. Clinical nurses have a wealth of knowledge that is often not even documented, let alone in a way in which it can be analyzed and made part of the evidence for nursing actions. Too often, clinical nurses do not recognize the depth and breadth of their knowledge. When this knowledge is made visible in documentation and analyzed, the evidence for various practices can be supported by data, leading to those practices being more widely implemented and taught to nursing students.

Communication in Healthcare

Lack of communication in healthcare contributes to almost 59,000 errors in healthcare today (Keenan et al., 2013). Part of this problem is a lack of interdisciplinary communication. The use of standardized terminologies in transitions between care settings, documentation, and face-to-face communication can improve this situation.

STANDARDIZED TERMINOLOGIES ISSUES

Given the benefits of using a standardized terminology in documentation, it would seem that they would be universally adopted. However, there is a resistance to change in all of us and in the cultures of organizations. Additionally, the process of learning a new way of both thinking and documenting, together with a temporary decrease in productivity, is a barrier to implementation (Button et al., 1998). Another issue is that there is a higher level of accountability when documenting with standardized terminologies. Stating one's own diagnosis and actions using a standardized terminology makes one's judgments visible to all, which can be scary. When a standardized terminology is implemented, it is imperative that there be support not only from administration but also from colleagues.

Education for effectively using a nursing terminology can be costly and time consuming. A recent study of terminology users revealed that confidence in using a terminology is greatly affected by the quality of educational preparation (Thede & Schwirian, 2013a). This survey also revealed that follow-up education improves implementation and, when not offered, is desired by users. Education also affects the accuracy of use of the terminology as well as comfort in using the terminology (Thede & Schwirian, 2013b).

One of the biggest difficulties in implementing a nursing terminology is not outside forces, but the culture of nursing. Nursing's religious and military history, and the fact that nursing has been primarily a feminine occupation, has contributed to nurses' hesitancy in voicing opinions or making its contributions known. Old customs of communicating to physicians with comments such as "The patient appears to be bleeding" instead of stating it as a fact have also been a contributing factor. Fortunately, this type of communication is no longer prevalent, but the mind-set behind it lingers along with the historical legacies. If nursing is to become valued for its healthcare contributions, nurses need to take responsibility for their nursing actions, visibly label them, and support one another in decision-making and using the terminologies. Only we as nurses can accomplish this. If we wait for someone else to do it, it will never be done. We need to ask ourselves if improving patient care through our documentation is important enough for us to overcome the learning curve and achieve the cultural thought processes required to use a standardized terminology. Only you, as a nurse, can make this decision.

INTERDISCIPLINARY HEALTHCARE

Today, there is a big push for the various disciplines in healthcare to work together. This can be accomplished with standardized terminologies. For this reason, and the fact that these terminologies are freely available in the United States and many other countries, many agencies have elected to use SNOMED and LOINC. Not only can they improve documentation, but they also provide clinical care data that can be analyzed. The results of these analyses can support improvements in healthcare and provide true evidence-based practice. When all healthcare providers document their observations, problem identification, treatment, and outcomes, more effective—and more cost-effective—care will result. Because healthcare disciplines have different foci that are complementary, documentation becomes even more efficient if problems and interventions from all disciplines are documented in the same place.

Table 15-4 illustrates how patient outcomes improve when both medical and nursing data are considered. Unfortunately, too often, documentation reflects only medical foci and

TABLE 15-4	Comparison of Medical and Nursing Foci		
	If Focus is Only		
	Medical Data	**Nursing Problems and Interventions**	**Combination of Foci**
Diagnosis	Osteoporosis, Mild	Potential for physical injury due to throw rugs on hardwood floors, bathtub without handgrips, and inadequate lighting in bedroom	Medical diagnosis and nursing diagnosis identified
Treatment/ Intervention	Calcium 500 mg 3x a day Calcitonin— 200 U intranasally in alternate nostrils daily	Arrange for client to remove rugs, install handgrips in shower, and use higher wattage bulb in ceiling fixture in bedroom	Both medical diagnosis and nursing diagnosis treated
Outcome	Bone deterioration stopped or slowed, unsafe home	Bone deterioration continues, safe home	Bone deterioration stopped or slowed. Client's home is much safer.
	Fall and broken hip likely		**Healthy client, chance of fall greatly lessened**

lacks an agreed-upon way to express nursing interventions in a standardized, structured format. Consequently, nursing interventions are not valued, seen as important, or amenable to reimbursement, nor added to analysis used in healthcare planning. Worse, they often remain undone. Ideally, documentation would be expanded to include all healthcare disciplines such as physical and occupational therapy.

SUMMARY

Using a standardized nursing terminology for nursing care involves changes in thinking about documentation as well as learning to use the terminology accurately. Understanding the vocabulary pertaining to terminology—such as interface terminology, reference terminology, taxonomy, granularity, and precoordinated or postcoordinated terms—can help in understanding how a terminology is used. We need to recognize that the terminologies are not 100% interoperable because each is based on a somewhat different philosophy. Much knowledge currently concealed in nursing data could be uncovered with the use of standardized terminologies. The standardized terminologies provide data that can be used in linking assessments, interventions, and outcomes, as well as linking those outcomes to the literature, and making visible nursing's contributions to healthcare.

APPLICATIONS AND COMPETENCIES

1. Reflecting on your clinical practice, think of a clinical problem that you identified and the interventions that you planned and implemented.

   a. How did you communicate these to your colleagues and other healthcare professionals?

   b. Was it in a way that your knowledge base was identifiable?

   c. Could this communication be used to facilitate evidence-based practice?

   d. Could these actions be included in data analysis at the local, regional, national, and international level?

2. Why is it necessary for nursing documentation to contain comparable data?

3. Define what the following terms mean in the world of standardized terminology:

   a. Granular

   b. Harmonization

   c. Minimum data set

   d. Nomenclature

   e. Precoordinated term

   f. Postcoordinated term

   g. Lexical match

   h. Symantic match

4. Describe what is meant by a terminology used in the:

   a. Interface mode

   b. Reference mode

5. Relate the need for standardized data to creating accurate queries in a database.

6. Examine the pros and cons of using standardized terminologies.

REFERENCES

Aslan, G. K., & Emiroglu, O. N. (2013). Evaluation of the applicability of the clinical care classification system to the care of elderly nursing home residents. *Computers, Informatics, Nursing: CIN, 31*(4), 178–188. doi:10.1097/NXN.0b013e3182701028

Beintema, H., Isaacson, E., Lovinaria, D., et al. (2007). *Alternative billing concept coding system.* Retrieved from https://www.google.com/url?sa=t&rct=j&q=&esrc=s&source=web&cd=5&cad=rja&ved=0CFQQFjAE&url=https%3A%2F%2Fwiki.umn.edu%2Fpub%2FHealthInformatics%2FGroup1-VocabFall07%2FAssignment2final.docx&ei=JmWrUo6KIeewyQHoqIGgAw&usg=AFQjCNH_Emr3fIIblFVqOHdAhmBgLtuuLQ&bvm=bv.57967247,d.aWc

Boyd, A. D., Funk, E. A., Schwartz, S. M., et al. (2010). Top EHR challenges in light of the stimulus. Enabling effective interdisciplinary, intradisciplinary and cross-setting communication. *Journal of Healthcare Information Management, 24*(1), 18–24.

Button, P., Androwich, I., Hibben, L., et al. (1998). Challenges and issues related to implementation of nursing vocabularies in computer-based systems. *Journal of the American Medical Informatics Association, 5*(4), 332–334.

Canadian Outcomes for Better Information and Care (C-HOBIC). (2014). Retrieved October 31, 2013, from https://www.infoway-inforoute.ca/index.php/programs-services/standards-collaborative/pan-canadian-standards/canadian-outcomes-for-better-information-and-care-c-hobic

Clark, J., & Lang, N. (1992). Nursing's next advance: An international classification for nursing practice. *International Nursing Review, 39*, 109–112; 128.

Correll, P. J., & Martin, K. S. (2009). The Omaha System helps a public health nursing organization find its voice. *Computers, Informatics, Nursing: CIN, 27*(1), 12–15.

Dykes, P. C., Wantland, D., Whittenbur, L., et al. (2013). *A pilot study to explore the feasibility of using the Clinical Care Classification system for developing a reliable costing method for nursing services.* Paper presented at the American Medical Informatics Association, Washington, DC. Retrieved from http://www.ncbi.nlm.nih.gov/pmc/articles/PMC3900184/

International Council of Nurses. (2013, December). *e-Health Bulletin.* Retrieved from http://www.icn.ch/images/stories/documents/news/bulletins/eHealth/ICN_eHealth_Bulletin_Dec_2013.pdf

Elhanan, G., Perl, Y., & Geller, J. (2011). A survey of SNOMED CT direct users, 2010: Impressions and preferences regarding content and quality. *Journal of the American Medical Informatics Association, 18*(Suppl 1), i36–i44. doi:10.1136/amiajnl-2011-000341

Erdogan, S., Secginli, S., Cosansu, G., et al. (2013). Using the Omaha System to describe health problems, interventions, and outcomes in home care in Istanbul, Turkey: A student informatics research experience. *Computers, Informatics, Nursing: CIN, 31*(6), 290–298. doi:10.1097/NXN.0b013e318282eala.

Giannangelo, K., & Fenton, S. (2008). EHR's effect on the revenue cycle management coding function. *Journal of Healthcare Information Management, 22*(1), 26–30.

Hannah, K. J., White, P. A., Nagle, L. M., et al. (2009). Standardizing nursing information in Canada for inclusion in electronic health records: C-HOBIC. *Journal of the American Medical Informatics Association, 16*(4), 524–530. doi:10.1197/jamia.M2974

Hannah, K., White, P. A., Kennedy, M. A., et al. (2012). C-HOBIC—Standardized information to support clinical practice and quality patient care across Canada. *Nursing*

Informatics: Proceedings of the International Congress on Nursing Informatics, 2012, 142.

Hardiker, N. R. (2011a). Developing standardised terminologies to support nursing practice. In D. McGonigle & K. Mastrian (Eds.), *Nursing informatics and the foundation of knowledge* (2nd ed., pp. 111–120). Boston, MA: Jones and Bartlett Publishers.

Hardiker, N. R. (2011b). Developing standardised terminologies to support nursing practice [Electronic Version at usir.salford.ac.uk/17895/1/Mastrian_chapter_7_Hardiker_-_pre-print.pdf]. In D. McGonigle & K. Mastrian (Eds.), *Nursing informatics and the foundation of knowledge* (2nd ed., pp. 111–120). Boston, MA: Jones and Bartlett Publishers.

Harman, T. L., Seeley, R. A., Oliveira, I. N., et al. (2012). *Standardized mapping of nursing assessments across 59 U.S. military treatment facilities*. Paper presented at the AMIA Annual Symposium.

Jones, D., Lunney, M., Keenan, G., et al. (2011). Standardized nursing languages: Essential for the nursing workforce [Review]. *Annual Review of Nursing Research*, 28, 253–294.

Keenan, G., Yakel, E., Dunn Lopez, K., et al. (2013). Challenges to nurses' efforts of retrieving, documenting, and communicating patient care information. [Multicenter Study Research Support, U.S. Gov't, P.H.S.]. *Journal of the American Medical Association*, 20(2), 245–251. doi:10.1136/amiajnl-2012-000894.

Kripps, B. J. (2008). Toward standardized nursing terminology: The next steps. *CARING Newsletter*, 23(3), 4–8.

Kunkel, D. E., Westra, B. L., Hart, C. M., et al. (2012). Updating and normalization of the Nursing Management Minimum Data Set element 6: Patient/client accessibility. *Computers, Informatics, Nursing: CIN*, 30(3), 134–141. doi:10.1097/NCN.0b013e31823eb913.

Levy, B. (2004). Evolving to clinical terminology. *Journal of Healthcare Informatics Management*, 18(3), 37–43.

Lundberg, C., Warren, J., Brokel, J., et al. (2008). Terminology for the electronic health record that reveals the impact of nursing on patient care. *Online Journal of Nursing Informatics*, 12(2), 1–20. Retrieved from http://ojni.org/12_2/lundberg.pdf

Matney, S. (2014, April 7). *ICNP/SNOMED CT nursing terminology collaboration*. Retrieved from https://3mhealthinformation.wordpress.com/2014/04/07/icnpsnomed-ct-nursing-terminology-collaboration/

Matney, S. A., Warren, J. J., Evans, J. L., et al. (2012). Development of the nursing problem list subset of SNOMED CT®. *Journal of Biomedical Informatics*, 45(4), 683–688. doi:10.1016/j.jbi.2011.12.003.

Moss, J., & Saba, V. (2011). Costing nursing care: Using the Clinical Care Classification System to value nursing intervention in an acute-care setting. *Computers, Informatics, Nursing: CIN*, 29(8), 455–460. doi:10.1097/NCN.0b013e3181fcbe55.

Müller-Staub, M., Needham, I., Odenbreit, M., et al. (2007). Improved quality of nursing documentation: Results of a nursing diagnoses, interventions, and outcomes implementation study. *International Journal Nursing Terminology Classification*, 18(1), 5–16.

Nunes, S. T., Rego, G., & Nunes R. (2014). The experience of an information system for nursing practice: The importance of nursing records in the management of a care plan. *Computers, Informatics, Nursing: CIN*, 32(7), 322–332. doi:10.1097/CIN.0000000000000060.

Rutherford, M. (2008). Standardized nursing language: What does it mean for nursing practice? *Online Journal of Issues in Nursing*, 13(1). Retrieved from http://www.nursingworld.org/MainMenuCategories/ThePracticeofProfessionalNursing/Health-IT/StandardizedNursingLanguage.html

Schwirian, P. (2013). Informatics and the future of nursing: Harnessing the power of standardized nursing terminology. *Bulletin of the American Society for Information Science & Technology*, 39(5), 20–24.

Schwirian, P., & Thede, L. Q. (2011). The standardized nursing terminologies: A national survey of nurses' experiences and attitudes. *Online Journal of Issues in Nursing*, 16(2). doi:10.3912/OJIN.Vol16No02InfoCol01. Retrieved from http://www.nursingworld.org/MainMenuCategories/ANAMarketplace/ANAPeriodicals/OJIN/TableofContents/Vol-16-2011/No2-May-2011/Standardized-Nursing-Terminologies.html

Thede, L. (2008, August 18). The electronic health record: Will nursing be on board when the ship leaves?. *Online Journal of Issues in Nursing*, 3(3). Retrieved from http://www.nursingworld.org/MainMenuCategories/ANAMarketplace/ANAPeriodicals/OJIN/Columns/Informatics/ElectronicHealthRecord.aspx

Thede, L. Q., & Schwirian, P. M. (2013a). Informatics: The standardized nursing terminologies: A national survey of nurses' experience and attitudes—SURVEY II: Participants' education for the use of standardized nursing terminology "labels". *Online Journal of Issues in Nursing*, 18(2). doi:10.3912/OJIN.Vol18No02InfoCol01 Retrieved from http://www.nursingworld.org/MainMenuCategories/ANAMarketplace/ANAPeriodicals/OJIN/TableofContents/Vol-18-2013/No2-May-2013/Education-for-the-Use-of-Standardized-Nursing-Terminology-Col-1.html

Thede, L. Q., & Schwirian, P. (2013b). Informatics: The standardized nursing terminologies: A national survey of nurses' experience and attitudes—SURVEY II: Participants' perception of comfort in the use of standardized nursing terminology "labels". *Online Journal of Issues in Nursing*, 18(2). doi:10.3912/OJIN.Vol18No02InfoCol02. Retrieved from http://www.nursingworld.org/MainMenuCategories/ANAMarketplace/ANAPeriodicals/OJIN/Columns/Informatics/Informatics-Participants-Perception-of-Comfort-in-the-Use.html

Topol, E. (2015). *The patient will see you now: The future of medicine is in your hands*. New York, NY: Basic Books.

VanDeVelde-Coke, S., Doran, D., Grinspun, D., et al. (2012). Measuring outcomes of nursing care, improving the health of Canadians: NNQR (C), C-HOBIC and NQuiRE. *Nursing Leadership*, 25(2), 26–37.

Weaver, R., Salamonson, Y., Koch, J., et al. (2013). Nursing on television: Student perceptions of television's role in public image, recruitment and education. *Journal of Advanced Nursing*, 69(12), 2635–2643. doi:10.1111/jan.12148

Westra, B. L., Delaney, C. W., Konicek, D., et al. (2008). Nursing standards to support the electronic health record. *Nursing Outlook*, 56(5), 258–266 e251. doi:10.1016/j.outlook.2008.06.005.

Westra, B. L., Latimer, G. E., Matney, S. A., et al. (2015). A national action plan for sharable and comparable nursing data to support practice and translational research for transforming health care. *Journal of the American Medical Informatics Association*. doi:10.1093/jamia/ocu011

Healthcare Informatics

Change is a constant in healthcare. Informatics is becoming more and more important in the quest for patient safety, a factor put into focus by the Institute of Medicine's reports. Other demands on this maturing field are created by requirements of third-party payers for data that provide outcomes for healthcare. These demands illustrate the reality of the interdisciplinary nature of healthcare; no single specialty can provide the needed data if these goals are to be met.

Chapter 16 begins this unit by exploring nursing informatics as a specialty—the theories it is based on, its educational programs, and associated roles and organizations. Chapter 17 examines the basics of healthcare information systems with an overview of the process for system selection and implementation by using the systems life cycle. Chapter 18 explores healthcare information systems as enterprise-wide systems designed to improve the quality and efficiency of patient care delivery. The advent of informatics opportunities is associated with new challenges. Chapter 19 discusses some of the unresolved issues associated with clinical information systems. Finally, Chapter 20 discusses some of the cutting-edge telehealth developments in which care is provided or monitored by healthcare professionals in another location.

16

Nursing Informatics: Theoretical Basis, Education Program, and Profession

OBJECTIVES

After studying this chapter, you will be able to:

1. Describe the theory base for nursing informatics.

2. Evaluate whether a specific nursing informatics educational program is appropriate for your career goals.

3. Differentiate between the roles of informatics nurses and informatics nurse specialists.

4. Analyze nursing informatics roles for all nurses.

5. Identify professional health informatics groups.

KEY TERMS

Alliance for Nursing Informatics (ANI)

American Health Information Management Association (AHIMA)

American Medical Informatics Association (AMIA)

American Nursing Informatics Association (ANIA)

British Computer Society (BCS)

Chaos theory

Cognitive science

Data

European Federation for Medical Informatics (EFMI)

General systems theory

Healthcare informatics

Healthcare Information and Management Systems Society (HIMSS)

Informatics nurse

Informatics theory

Information

International Medical Informatics Association (IMIA)

Knowledge

Learning theories

Informatics nurse specialist

Nursing informatics theory

Nursing Informatics Working Group (NIWG)

Rogers' Diffusion of Innovations theory

Social informatics

Sociotechnical theory

Tacit Knowledge

Usability theory

User liaison

Wisdom

Although the term "informatics" is relatively new, the management of information started when the first caveman drew pictures to communicate and convey knowledge. Society has long since passed the time when pictures on a cave wall provided information. Although information is ultimately managed by people, the term informatics has come to denote the use of computers and information technology to manage healthcare information. The TIGER (Technology Informatics Guiding Education Reform) Initiative Report states that information technology is "the stethoscope of the 21st century" (Technology Informatics Guiding Education Reform, 2009, p. 24). **Healthcare informatics** is a broad multidisciplinary field with many specialties such as nursing informatics, medical informatics, dental informatics, and pharmaceutical informatics. The theoretical basis for nursing informatics includes nursing informatics theory, sociotechnical theory, change theories, general systems theory, chaos theory, cognitive science theory, usability theory, as well as learning theories. This chapter discusses educational preparation certification and roles for the informatics nurse specialist.

Generally, those who practice in their discipline's subspecialty are also licensed in their own profession such as nursing or dentistry. Health informatics is also broad enough to include subspecialties that are multidisciplinary—for example, social and consumer informatics. Despite all the subspecialties in healthcare informatics, a primary goal is interdisciplinary data management that facilitates holistic health and community health. There are a number of professional organizations pertinent to nursing informatics and informatics nurse specialists. Several organizations are interdisciplinary, reflecting the diversity of others who work in the field. This chapter also includes information on the national and international informatics organizations.

THEORIES THAT LEND SUPPORT TO INFORMATICS

Although information has been managed in one way or another since the beginning of time, as society became more complex in the early 1900s, theories about managing information developed. Information theory itself is a mathematical theory about communication, with the goal of finding the limits on reliably compressing, storing, and communicating data (Gray, 2013; Schneider, 2013). Informatics theory, which is a branch of applied probability theory, builds on information theory and uses concepts from change theories, systems theory, chaos theory, cognitive theory, and sociotechnical theory.

Nursing Informatics Theory

Nursing informatics theory is concerned with the representation of nursing data, information, and knowledge to facilitate the management and communication of nursing information within the healthcare milieu. It focuses on nursing phenomena and provides a nursing perspective, clarifies nursing values and beliefs, produces new knowledge, and develops standardized nursing terminology for use in electronic records. Graves and Cocoran (1989), in their seminal article on nursing informatics, devised an information model for nursing informatics based on Bloom's taxonomy. This model identified data, information, and knowledge as the key components of nursing informatics. Wisdom was first added to this structure by Nelson and Joos (as cited in Joos et al., 1992) shortly thereafter, but it was the 2008 ANA *Nursing Informatics: Scope and Standards of Practice* that officially incorporated wisdom into the nursing informatics model.

Data

Data are discrete, objective facts that have not been interpreted (Clark, 2010) or are out of context; they are at the atomic level. Data are described objectively without interpretation. They are the building blocks of meaning but lack context and hence are meaningless.

Information

Information is data that have some type of interpretation or structure; that is, it has a context. It is derived from combining different pieces of data (Clark, 2010). A set of data, such as vital signs, when interpreted over a period of time is information.

Knowledge

Knowledge is a synthesis of information with relationships identified and formalized. It changes something or somebody by creating the setting for formulating possible effective actions, evaluating their effects, and deciding on the required action (Clark, 2010). For example, interpreting a set of vital signs over a period of time and deciding on an action based on this information combined with nursing knowledge and experience is an example of knowledge.

Wisdom

Wisdom is achieved through evaluating knowledge with reflection. It involves seeing patterns and metapatterns and using them in different ways (Clark, 2010) and knowing when and how to apply knowledge to a situation (ANA, 2015, p. 3). For example, wisdom would be interpreting vital signs in a postsurgical patient as indicative of an infection and taking the appropriate action.

The Continuum

The informatics theory concepts are constructs, not absolutes, and are a continuum of an analog process. The simplified examples earlier in this section are used to make the process of converting data into wisdom easier to understand. Where

something falls on the continuum depends on the person or situation. A nurse with 10 years of experience may possess a great deal of **tacit knowledge**. This is the knowledge that has been earned with experience and reflection, but the knowledge is so ingrained that it is difficult for the nurse to verbalize or acknowledge. Nonetheless, this tacit knowledge provides a higher level of wisdom than that possessed by a new graduate.

The general idea of informatics theory is that the move from data to knowledge is a progressive process that follows a given path. As one moves up the continuum, each level becomes more complex and requires intellect that is more human. In practice, the lines between each of these entities are blurred and the process is iterative. The processes of converting data into knowledge include capturing, sorting, organizing, storing, retrieving, and presenting the data to give it meaning and produce information.

Figure 16-1 is a simplification of this continuum, one that might apply to a nursing student or a new graduate. In this figure, data are combined to produce information, and information is combined to produce knowledge. As another example, let's say we have as a datum (i.e., the smallest unit that can be processed) the number 37. If we combine the number 37 with the datum that this is a Celsius temperature for a person, we now have

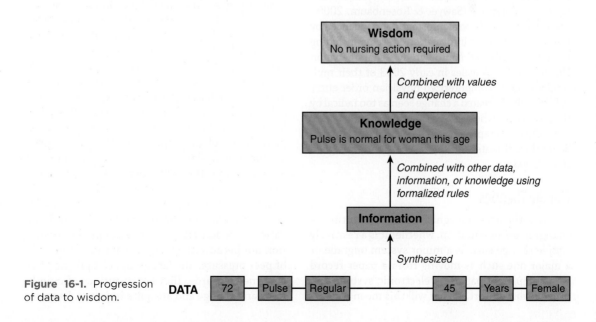

Figure 16-1. Progression of data to wisdom.

some information. Combining this still further with the fact that this is the normal body temperature, we have a small piece of knowledge. The individual adds wisdom by deciding on the action, if any, to take because of this knowledge.

Sociotechnical Theory and Social Informatics

Sociotechnical theory originated in the middle of the last century when it became evident that not all implementations of technology were increasing productivity. The overall focus of this theory is the impact of technology's implementation on an organization. Sociotechnical theory focuses on the interactions within an organization among information management tools and techniques and the knowledge, skills, attitudes, values, and needs of its employees as well as the rewards and authority structures of the employer (Akbari & Land, 2011). Its precepts can increase the understanding of how information systems should be developed.).

Introducing an information system is a social process that deeply affects an organization. Research based on sociotechnical theory is aimed at maximizing performance by designing or redesigning systems that fit the organizational system into which they are implanted. The sociotechnical point of view, which is the basis of **social informatics**, holds that a good design is based on an understanding of how people work and the context of the work, not just technologic considerations (Sawyer & Rosenbaum, 2000). The importance of social informatics is evidenced by the failure of many information systems including the much publicized shutdown by Cedars Lebanon Hospital in Los Angeles in early 2003 of their multimillion dollar computerized physician order entry (CPOE). CPOE created a change seen as too radical by the physicians, who believed that their interests were not sufficiently represented, the system was jammed down their throats, and that it was poorly designed (Bass, 2003).

Change Theories

Change theories recognize that instituting a change in documentation, whether it is a relatively simple change such as a minor system upgrade or a major one such as moving from a paper record to a completely paperless electronic system, can provoke discomfort. "What will this mean to me?" is always uppermost in the mind of a person faced with change. Whether affected individuals perceive the change as minor or major differs from individual to individual. Ignoring the psychosocial nature of changing information management is too often a one-way ticket to failure of the system. Two change theories that address the effects of change on people and organizations are discussed in the following subsections.

Rogers' Diffusion of Innovations Theory

Rogers' theory, diffusion of innovations, was first published in his 1962 book of the same name. This theory examines the pattern of acceptance that innovations follow as they spread across the population and the process of decision making that occurs in individuals when deciding whether to adopt an innovation. Although the theory was based on depression-era rural research that studied how Midwestern farmers adopted hardier corn (Rogers, 2003), this theory is still applicable in North America and other parts of the world. As an example for when this theory is helpful, when making decisions on how to implement changes, such as computerized provider order entry (CPOE), it is best to assess the nursing units that might best adopt the changes.

Societal Changes

Rogers classifies people into five categories (Figure 16-2) to view how innovations are accepted by the general population (Rogers, 2003). Innovators, the first category, readily adopt the innovation. They constitute a very small percentage, about 2.5% of the population. These persons are often seen as disruptive by those who are averse to risk taking, so innovators are usually not able to sell others on the innovation. This job is left to the next category, early adopters, who comprise 13.5% of the population. They are respectable opinion leaders who function as promoters of an innovation. The next group, the early majority (34%), is averse to risks but will make safe investments. The late majority, who make up another 34% of the adopters, need to be sure that the innovation is beneficial. They may adopt the innovation not because they see a use for it, but because of peer pressure. The last group, comprising 16%, is termed laggards. They are suspicious of innovations and change and are quite resistant. Laggards

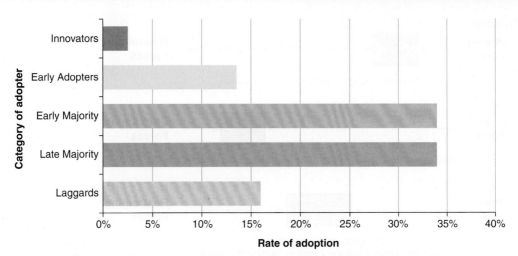

Figure 16-2. How individuals adopt innovation: Innovators to Laggards. (Data from Rogers' Diffusion of Innovation Theory, 1995. Reprinted from Melnyk, B. M., & Fineout-Overholt, E. (2015). *Evidence-based practice in nursing and healthcare: A guide to best practice* (3rd ed.). Philadelphia, PA: Wolters Kluwer with permission.)

must be certain that the innovation will not fail before they will adopt it. Instead of discounting this group, we should be listening to them. They may grasp weaknesses that others fail to see.

Individual Changes

In Rogers' theory, individuals go through five stages in deciding to adopt an innovation. Like all stage theories, progress is not uniform, and adopters can show behaviors from more than one stage at a time or revert completely to an earlier stage. In the first stage, knowledge of an innovation, the potential adopter gains an understanding of how the innovation operates (Rogers, 2003). This can occur passively, through either education or advertisements, or actively in response to a felt need or incentives. The second stage, persuasion, is based on the perception of the relative advantage of the innovation, compatibility with existing norms, and its observability. At this stage, an individual forms an opinion about the innovation—negative, neutral, or positive. In the third stage, the individual uses personal opinions to make a decision. A potential adopter may try the innovation or base an opinion on the experience and opinion of a respected peer who has tried the innovation. The individual then decides to either adopt or reject the innovation. If the decision is positive, the fourth stage, or implementation, follows. At this

stage, the adopter wants knowledge, such as how to use the innovation and how to overcome problems with its use. Confirmation, the fifth stage, may occur when reinforcement of the decision is sought. Conflicting information about the innovation may cause the adopter to reverse a decision.

Lewin's Field Theory

Whereas Rogers' theory identified the stages that individuals go through in making a change, **Lewin's field theory** provides a guide to helping individuals achieve a positive decision in relation to an innovation. This theory holds that human behavior is related to both personal characteristics and the social milieu in which the individual exists (Smith, 2009). It focuses on the variables that need to be recognized and observed in a situation of change and uses these variables to create a model of the stages that occur during change. Lewin divides these changes into three stages or force fields: unfreezing, moving, and refreezing. Ways of moving a group from the first to the last stage need to be part of a plan for implementation of a system. The three stages are illustrated in Figure 16-3.

Unfreezing

The unfreezing stage is based on the idea that a balance of driving and restraining forces that creates equilibrium supports human behavior. To institute

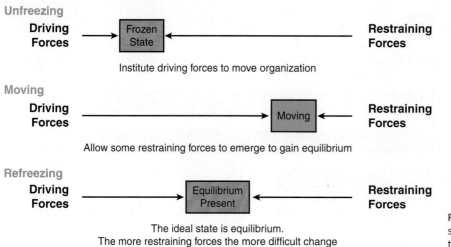

Figure 16-3. The three stages of Lewin's field theory.

change, the driving and restraining forces that are part of the maintenance of equilibrium in the organizational culture and individual have to be changed. To unfreeze, one must identify and change the balance so that the driving forces are stronger than the restraining forces. Driving forces can be involvement in the process, respect of one's opinion, and continuous communication during the process. Unfortunately, restraining forces are harder to identify and treat because they are often personal psychological defenses or group norms embedded in the organizational or community culture.

Moving

In the moving stage, the planned change is implemented. Its success depends on how situations were handled in the first stage. This is not a comfortable period. Anxieties are high, and if they are not successfully dealt with, the change may be unsuccessful. Additionally, it is important to recognize that in this stage, movement may occur in the wrong direction. This is especially likely to happen if the new system has many problems, if it is not supported by administration, or if it has had no end-user involvement. Thus, it is important to have the support of administration in the planning process, involve users so that the system serves them instead of creating more work, thoroughly test the system before implementation for both bugs and usability, provide adequate training, and deal with any implementation problems immediately. In the Cedars Lebanon case, the new

CPOE system created more work and resulted in a movement in the wrong direction despite a decree that all people must use the system (Bass, 2003). Decrees do not "move" people.

Refreezing

In the **refreezing** stage, equilibrium returns as the planned change becomes the norm and it is surrounded by the usual driving and restraining forces. For this state to occur, individuals need to feel confident with the change and feel in control of the procedures involved in the new methods. One way to assist this process would be to provide a well-designed help system that can provide answers to frequent procedures as well as those that a user may use only occasionally. Another approach to help cement the change would be to have the organization recognize new skills. However, keep in mind that if the change is too strongly reinforced, it might be difficult to enact subsequent changes.

General Systems Theory

General systems theory is a method of thinking about complex structures such as an information system or an organization. A simplified description of systems theory holds that any change in one part of a system will be reflected in other parts of the system. Von Bertalanffy (1973), a biologist, introduced the original theory. It was developed in part as a reaction against reductionism, or the reducing of phenomena to small parts, studying each, and ignoring the actions that each part creates in other parts. In systems theory, the focus is on the interaction among the various parts of the system instead of regarding each individual part as standing alone. It is based on the premise that the whole is greater than the sum of its parts and is the basis for holistic nursing.

To be part of a system, a phenomenon must be able to be isolated from its surrounding area for analysis yet be part of the functioning of the whole system. Systems are open or closed. Whereas, an open system continually exchanges information with the environment outside the system, a closed system receives no input from the outside. This classification is more of a continuum than an absolute. Few, if any systems, are 100% closed or 100% open.

The objective of any system is to be in equilibrium, which is maintained by the correction forces from a feedback loop. Negative feedback results when there is a lack of something. The action it produces is to add the missing item to restore a variable to its state of equilibrium. Positive feedback results when there is too much of something. The action in positive feedback is to take away the excess. These two concepts can be confusing until one remembers that positive feedback results when the system finds too much of something and negative feedback when it finds something missing. Whether feedback is positive or negative is based on what the system finds, not its action.

The feedback loop operates using input, process (throughput), and output (Figure 16-4). Input involves adding information or matter to a system. Process is the throughput, or evaluation of the input, that the system performs using the input information; output is the information or action that results from what the processing finds. This output may produce no action, or the action needed from either negative or positive feedback. A simple example is inputting a patient's temperature into a computer system, the computer processing that data by combining it with the order that if this patient's temperature is more than 101°F, a specific medication should be given, and presenting the information to the nurse along with the action that needs to be taken. This is positive feedback—there was too much of something, body heat. The action it produced was to tell the nurse to give a medication. Another example

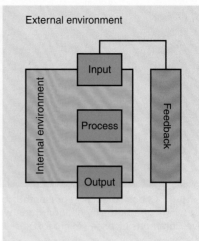

Figure 16-4. General systems theory.

is the physiologic body processes governed by hormones, as well as the entire human body.

You interact with systems all your life. Families, communities, and most inanimate objects are systems. The more complex the system, the more chaotic it is. A perfect example of a system is a computerized information system. Making a change in one area invariably affects other sections in ways that were never envisioned, which explains why it is often not a simple matter to make desired changes in systems. Adding an information system to a healthcare agency produces an even more complicated system. Systems theory provides a way of studying both the information system itself and its interaction with the environment. These interactions are also the focus of sociotechnical theory, but that theory would frame the problem in a different way.

Chaos Theory

Chaos theory was first encountered by a meteorologist, Edward Lorenz, in 1963 (Dizikes, 2011) when attempting to predict the weather with a set of 12 equations. This theory is often associated with the so-called butterfly effect, or the result on worldwide atmospheric conditions caused by the flapping of one butterfly's wings. Yet, chaos theory has a true mathematical basis. The analogy comes from the small differences in the starting points of a butterfly flapping its wings (Figure 16-5), which produce different effects and which over time

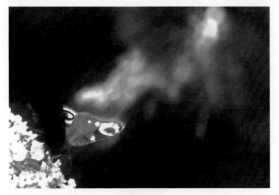

Figure 16-5. Chaos theory represented by the flapping wings of a butterfly changing the weather (Creative Commons License—Microsoft).

produce changes. Chaos theory deals with the differences in outcomes depending on conditions at the starting point. For example, the conditions where an information system is first envisioned will affect the overall design.

Chaos theory, like general systems theory, addresses an entire structure without reducing it to the elemental parts. This makes it useful with complex systems such as information systems. The idea behind this theory is that what may appear to be chaotic actually has an order. It is based on the recognized fact that events and phenomena depend on initial conditions. Chaos theory is nonlinear. It allows us to question assumptions that we normally might reach using linear thought. Seeing things reframed as a whole can stimulate new thinking and new approaches.

Cognitive Science

Cognitive science is gaining more importance in informatics. It is the study of the mind and intelligence (Thagard, 2010) and how this information can be applied. It is interdisciplinary; includes philosophy, psychology, artificial intelligence, neuroscience, linguistics, and anthropology; and is a part of social informatics. It adds to informatics concepts that focus on how the brain perceives and interprets a screen (Turley, 1996). These factors are important in all aspects of information systems. When designing input screens, the screen locations where information is entered must be organized to facilitate data entry.

Cognitive science is also a factor when presenting information; for example, characteristics such as color, font, and screen display affect clinical judgment because they are processed along with onscreen text and data. Additionally, cognitive science addresses the amount of information that an individual can absorb and use constructively. Principles from these theories provide a guide to developing systems that allow users to concentrate on the task, rather than requiring cognitive tasks to deal with the computer interface. Cognitive theory can also aid a informatics nurse specialist in understanding the information processing done by a nurse in decision making, thus facilitating the design of tools to support these processes (Staggers & Thompson, 2002).

Usability Theory

Although usability was a problem long before computers, it gained significance with the advent of computers and the Web and is an integral part of informatics. **Usability theory** represents a multidimensional concept and involves users' evaluation of several measures, each one representative of their effectiveness in performing a task. It involves the ease of use, users' satisfaction that they have achieved their goals, and the aesthetics of the technology. It uses information from both the cognitive science and sociotechnical theories. Box 16-1 outlines the five goals of usability.

BOX 16-1 The Five Goals of Usability

1. It is easy for users to accomplish basic tasks the first time they use the product.
2. Once learned, the design permits users to quickly and easily perform the needed tasks.
3. If it is not used for a period of time, it is easy to reestablish one's proficiency in using the product.
4. Users make very few errors, but any that they do make are easily remedied.
5. The design is pleasant to use.

Source: Nielsen, J. (2012). *Usability 101: Introduction to usability*. Retrieved from http://www.nngroup.com/articles/usability-101-introduction-to-usability/

TABLE 16-1 Contributions of Theories to Informatics	
Theory	**Contributions to Informatics**
Change	Increase the chance of success in implementing a system by attending to the reactions to the change
Chaos	Improve the design of an information system
Cognitive science	Improve the ability of user to gain knowledge from an information system
General systems	Contribute to the understanding of the complexity of an information system
Learning theory	Teach the use of a system and design or select computer-aided instruction
Nursing informatics	Convert data into information and information to knowledge; nurse adds wisdom
Sociotechnical theory and social informatics	Improve interaction between an information system and the organizational culture
Usability	Improve ease of use and satisfaction with an information system

Learning Theories

Learning theories are important in informatics as well as in all nursing endeavors. Users must be taught to use a system, and use of these theories can decrease the time for training as well as the time for learning. For more information on learning theories, see Chapter 21.

Summary of Theories

See Table 16-1 for a summary of what the various theories contribute to informatics.

INFORMATICS IN EDUCATIONAL PREPARATION

Both the National League for Nursing and the American Association of Colleges for Nursing, which are accrediting bodies for nursing programs, have recommendations for including informatics in nursing education preparation (American

Association of Colleges of Nursing, 2008; National League for Nursing, 2008). Basic informatics knowledge is essential for safe and effective nursing practice at the generalist level and all advanced practice levels. Understanding the possibilities and limitations of information management and technology assists the nurse to have realistic expectations of information systems.

The overall discipline of informatics has a core curriculum that is supplemented by informatics principles and knowledge specific to each healthcare discipline. A course at the master's level of education should include content integrating technology in practice and on improving healthcare delivery. It should also include analyzing strategies for using information communication technologies to reduce risk. Although formal educational programs provide an excellent foundation for jobs in informatics, as with all healthcare providers, there must be a commitment to lifelong learning.

Today, many nurses practicing in the field of nursing informatics gained their knowledge through self-learning and continuing education; nevertheless, there is a move toward requiring advanced formal academic preparation in the field, especially for the high-end jobs. Before commencing on a career in informatics, it is helpful to have a thorough, in-depth, understanding of clinical practice in one's discipline, which can only be gained through at least 5 years of experience in the field (ANA, 2015, p. 47). Computer competency alone, although helpful, is insufficient for a career in informatics. Computers are only a tool in informatics; information management is the focus. This knowledge requires clinical experience.

All informatics careers require continuing education that is often obtained at professional conferences. The American Medical Informatics Association (AMIA), Healthcare Information and Management Systems Society (HIMSS), and American Health Information Management Association (AHIMA) have large educational and research meetings including tutorials for novice practitioners. Additionally, some universities sponsor 1- or 2-week intensive informatics courses. Three annual conferences, one sponsored by Rutgers College of Nursing, a second one by the University of Maryland School of Nursing, and a third by ANIA (American Nursing Informatics Association), are all excellent places for continuing education.

The four categories for nursing informatics education are (1) online courses, (2) graduate programs with a specialty in nursing informatics, (3) graduate and undergraduate programs with minors or majors in nursing informatics, and (4) individual courses in nursing informatics within graduate/undergraduate programs. Online courses may be standalones that provide just continuing education, may be part of a program that leads to a certificate in nursing informatics, or may belong to a formal degree-granting program that may or may not be 100% online.

Many educational institutions have informatics programs. Given the many foci of informatics, it follows that each educational program will have a different focus. Some concentrate on applied informatics, others on informatics research. At present, there is no accrediting body that examines informatics education, such as there is for nurse practitioner education programs. Thus, prospective students need to ask many questions

---

BOX 16-2   Questions Prospective Students Should Ask of an Informatics Program[a]

1. What is the focus of the informatics program? For example:
   a. Clinical systems
   b. Knowledge generation/research
   c. Decision support
   d. Healthcare specialty
2. What types of jobs do graduates of the program obtain?
3. Who are the faculty in informatics?
   a. What is their informatics experience?
   b. What are their qualifications to teach informatics?
   c. What are their interests in informatics?
4. Is there a preceptorship or internship?
   a. If so, for how long?
   b. How are these assignments found?
5. How long has the program been operating?
6. What courses are currently available versus those being planned but not yet offered?
7. If the program is online, how much on-campus time is required?

[a]These questions are in addition to those normally asked of any educational program.

---

when examining programs. Questions specific to an informatics program are listed in Box 16-2.

Informatics for All Nurses

Informatics nurse specialists cannot work in a vacuum. The best systems are developed by collaboration between informatics nurse specialists and practicing clinicians. This avoids one of the common reasons for system failure: neglecting the expertise and needs of end users. To foster a productive relationship, practicing clinicians need to have a basic understanding of informatics (see Box 16-3). If a system is to assist the clinician in providing quality care, it is imperative that the

BOX 16-3   Some Informatics Facts for All Nurses

- **Data should be entered only once**.
- One piece of data can be presented in many different ways and contexts.
- Data from monitors of physiologic processes can be integrated into an electronic record.
- Computers can transform data by calculating either numbers or words.
- Computers require standardization of data if they are to permit learning from aggregated data.
- Decision support can be part of an informatics system.
- Output is only as good as input.
- Only a clinician understands how information flows through the clinical area; it is imperative that this information be communicated to informatics personnel.
- An information system will not solve organizational problems.
- Aggregated, unidentified data about patient care can, and should, be available to all practicing clinicians for the purpose of improving patient care.

clinician have an understanding of the role of data in not only providing but also tracking and trending individual patient care. As data are synthesized and converted to information and knowledge, all nurses need to use this information/knowledge wisely. Everyone needs to realize that a computer can work with only the data that it has. The principle "garbage in, garbage out" should have as a corollary "data lacking, output defective." When evaluating an outcome, be it a research result or output from a computer, examine the data categories (fields) on which it was based.

There is often an unrealistic expectation that a new information system will solve all problems, some of which may be organizational problems. An information system is apt to magnify organizational problems such as poor communication between departments, lack of accountability, and lack of administration support for the planned information system. It is important to be able to separate organizational problems from informational system problems and solve the former before the new system is implemented.

NURSING INFORMATICS AS A SPECIALTY

Nursing is a subspecialty in informatics, with roles and tasks in both disciplines. It is important to differentiate the terms informatics nurses and informatics nurse specialists. According to the *Nursing Informatics Scope & Standards of Practice*, those who enter the nursing informatics field because of an interest or experience are **informatics nurses**. Nurses with either a graduate education degree in nursing informatics or a field relating to informatics are **informatics nurse specialists** (American Nurses Association [ANA], 2015, p. 17). The roles of informatics nurses vary with their job and specialty in healthcare, but the general foci of nursing informatics are the following seven areas, as set out in seminal work by the National Institutes of Health, National Center for Nursing Research (NCNR) Priority Expert Panel on Nursing Informatics (Pillar & Golumbic, 1993):

1. Using data, information, and knowledge for patient care
2. Defining data in patient care
3. Acquiring and delivering patient care knowledge
4. Creating new tools for patient care from new technologies
5. Applying ergonomics to nurse–computer interfaces
6. Integrating systems
7. Evaluating the effects of nursing systems

Practice in each of these areas requires different knowledge and skills on the part of the informatics nurse.

One of the main objectives of nursing informatics in the clinical area is to integrate data from all areas pertinent to nursing care and present it in a manner that enables the clinical nurse to provide quality care. Many sources of information are needed for patient care. The overall goal in nursing informatics is to optimize information management and communication to improve individual healthcare and the health of populations (ANA, 2015).

Florence Nightingale's Role in Nursing Informatics

Some might say that Florence Nightingale was the first informatics nurse specialist, given that the fundamental building block in informatics is data, despite her lack of a formal educational program. Recognizing the value of data in affecting healthcare, she collected data and systematized recordkeeping practices in Crimea (Nightingale & Goldie, 1997). Using these data, she developed the first version of the pie graph known as a "polar area diagram" or "coxcombs" to dramatize the need for reform to stop the needless deaths caused by the unsanitary conditions in military hospitals (School of Mathematics and Statistics, St. Andrews University Scotland, 2003). With the advent of the computer, the use of data has become far easier and more widespread than it was in Ms. Nightingale's time.

When decisions are based on the data available, collection and analysis of nursing data become very important. Without nursing data, the value of nursing will continue to be hidden to those in policymaking positions. Through nursing informatics, the healthcare information systems that are being developed can include the nursing data needed to improve patient care and show the value that nurses add to healthcare.

Informatics Nurse Specialist Certification

In 1992, the ANA recognized nursing informatics as a specialty. The second edition of the *ANA Nursing Informatics: The Scope and Standards Practice* outlines the characteristics of the specialty, defines the specialty, and describes how it differs from other health and nursing specialties (ANA, 2015). It also explains in detail the basic theories behind nursing informatics, presents a discussion of the sciences that provide a foundation for informatics, and discusses standardized nursing terminologies and the importance of interoperability. The publication is a necessary basic reference for anyone interested in the field.

Certification validates the nurse's education and experience in the specialty. It provides evidence of competence and quality of knowledge. Initial administration of the informatics nurse specialist certification examination was in 1995. The informatics

nurse specialist exam is updated on a regular basis to reflect current informatics practice. The prerequisites for writing the certification examination include a bachelor's degree in nursing (or relevant field), an active registered nurse (RN) license, 2 years of practice full-time equivalent as an RN, and 30 hours of continuing education in informatics within the last 3 years. The applicant must also meet *one* of the following three practice requirements (American Nurses Credentialing Center, 2014):

1. 2,000 hours practice in informatics nursing within the last 3 years
2. A minimum of 1,000 practice hours in informatics nursing in the last 3 years plus completion of a minimum of 12 hours of academic credit in informatics courses as part of a graduate-level informatics nursing program
3. Completion of a graduate program in nursing informatics with a minimum of 200 hours of a faculty-supervised practicum in informatics

Passing the examination provides certification for 5 years, at which time the certification can be renewed if specified educational and practice requirements are fulfilled. To renew the certification, the nurse can apply twelve months prior to the expiration date. Renewal requirements are:

1. Current licensure as an RN
2. ANCC certification as a informatics nurse specialist
3. Completion of 75 professional development hours, of which 51% (38.25 hours) relate to the specialty. The other half of professional development hours can be from academic credit, presentations, publication or research, preceptor hours, and professional service.
4. Completion of a minimum of 1,000 practice hours

ROLES FOR NURSES IN THE INFORMATICS SPECIALTY

As can be seen from the broad areas that informatics and its specialty nursing encompass, and considering the evolving nature of this specialty, nurses in this realm have a variety of roles and work areas. Whereas some informatics nurses have only on-the-job training, certified informatics nurse specialists work in settings where there is increased complexity and expectations for systems. Keep in mind that although the roles of informatics nurses and informatics nurse specialists may differ (Table 16-2), there is often much overlap, and job descriptions vary from agency to agency. Understanding the role of the informatics nurses and informatics nurse specialists assists clinical nurses working with them to improve clinical systems. The following subsections more closely examine each of these positions.

Informatics Nurse

Informatics nurses, regardless of their role or area of practice, interact with a variety of individuals at many organizational levels, from anyone who uses the system to the chief executive officer. These interactions are important in gaining collaboration with clinicians, making decisions about how to interpret data, and obtaining administrative support for new practices. They also permit the informatics nurse to identify how information flows through an organization, assess for real and potential communication problems, and, when necessary, devise alternative methods of communication.

Informatics nurses serve in a variety of roles. In **user liaison** role, the informatics nurse is the communications link between nurses and others involved in computer-related matters. Other job functions can be managing nursing applications or chairing the nursing computer coordinating committee. Informatics nurses may also act as data systems managers for a specialty such as oncology.

TABLE 16-2   Example Roles of an Informatics Nurse versus a Informatics Nurse Specialist

Roles	Responsibilities
Informatics Nurse	
Systems educator	Plans, coordinates, and facilitates education for all computer applications and computer software for all user groups. Develops and trains all user groups on clinical computer applications and online documentation processes. If employed by a vendor, systems educator may be responsible for documenting a new system and providing "train the trainer" education to healthcare agency personnel.
Information technology nursing advocate	Assesses the needs and opportunities for nurses with the technology. Looks at both the functional and operational needs of clinical users when using the system and translates these needs into information technology–specific solutions
Superuser	Supports the system in a given unit. Assists users with functionality, procedural issues, and basic troubleshooting. Often holds a clinical position in the assigned unit
System specialist	May work at many different levels from the unit to the full agency. Acts as a link between nursing and information services and is both a nursing resource and a representative
Clinical systems coordinator/ analyst	Responsible for coordinating aspects of planning, design, development, implementation, maintenance, and evaluation of the clinical information system. Troubleshoots issues with systems. Supports a clinical system

(continues)

TABLE 16-2   Example Roles of an Informatics Nurse versus a Informatics Nurse Specialist (*continued*)

Roles	Responsibilities
Informatics Nurse Specialist	
Project manager	Plans and implements an informatics project. Must be able to communicate effectively with all levels of management, users, and system developers. Must also be cognizant of all factors involved in the project including, but not limited to, managing change, assessing the need for the new project, and planning for its implementation
Consultant	Provides expert advice, opinions, and recommendations from consultant's area of expertise. Must be able to analyze what the client wants, as well as what is needed, and integrate these to create what is possible, technologically and politically. May be employed within an organization, by a vendor, or self-employed
Director of clinical informatics	Facilitates the development, implementation, and integration for an agency information system. Assists in developing the strategic and tactical plans of the system. Develops plans for implementation and gaining acceptance of systems
Researcher	Uses informatics to create new knowledge. Encompasses research in any area of nursing informatics. May be involved in basic research on the symbolic representation of nursing phenomena, clinical decision-making, or applied research of information systems. Could be involved in developing decision support tools for nursing or models of representation for nursing phenomena
Product developer	Participates in the development of new information systems including designing, developing, and marketing of informatics solutions for nursing problems. Must understand the needs of both business and nursing
Policy developer	Contributes to health policy development by identifying nursing data, its availability, structure, and content, which are used to determine health policy. These policies encompass not only information management but also health infrastructure development and economics
Entrepreneur	Analyzes nursing information needs in clinical areas, education, administration, and research; develops and markets solutions

Informatics Nurse Specialist

Informatics nurse specialists working for either a healthcare agency or a vendor may be project directors for the installation of an information system. They may also be involved in product management or product definition. In this position, the nurse may also be responsible for seeing that the product is updated. This involves being aware of new developments in the field as well as the current and future needs of clients both inside and outside the organization. Some nurse informatics specialists who work for vendors are involved in marketing. Marketing requires skills in listening and anticipating needs as well as the ability to identify the real decision maker.

Informatics Nurse Specialists also act as consultants, either working independently or working for an organization. Consulting is a high-pressure field in which individuals often must make instant decisions based on personal knowledge and an analysis of only the known facts. This involves the role of a liaison and an expert. Many consulting jobs involve a heavy travel schedule. Nurses in academia who are involved in nursing

informatics are usually involved in teaching nursing informatics, research, or both. Box 16-4 describes a typical day for a informatics nurse specialist.

QSEN Scenario

You are a member of a multidisciplinary team that is selecting a new clinical information system that meets the requirements of "meaningful use" identified by the HITECH Act. How do the roles of the informatics nurse specialist, clinical nurse, and nursing administration team member contribute to the system selection process?

BOX 16-4   A Day in the Life of a Informatics Nurse Specialist: Healthcare System Implementation/Support Stage

My name is Omega R. Finney, and I am an informatics nurse. I work for a five-hospital healthcare system with an extensive network of ambulatory offices. We are in the process of implementing our new electronic health record (EHR) in one of our five hospitals and providing ongoing support to the remaining four hospital locations.

My years of clinical experience as a nurse prepared me for my career in informatics. My experience helps me directly relate to my end users, empathize with them, and address their concerns. My clinical experience also helps with the documentation that is needed for service request tickets.

A typical day for me as an informatics nurse during a Go-Live involves several tasks, responsibilities, and duties. During a 12-hour day, I may use many of the skills I learned from my nursing career such as the nursing process, prioritization, critical thinking, clinical experience, and multitasking. Below is a timeline of a typical 12-hour day for me supporting one hospital during a Go-Live onsite, while simultaneously remotely supporting four hospitals.

6:00 AM to 9:00 AM: The morning begins in the Command Center with shift report from night-shift team member. We discuss any outstanding issues, service request tickets to follow up on during day shift, and build awaiting approval in our internal Change Control.

I then follow up on any outstanding service request tickets placed by end users that work night shift. In between placing calls, I answer "How-To" calls about everything from placing orders to medication reconciliation to discharging a patient.

10:00 AM to 10:45 AM: Internal Change Control is held in the Command Center at this time. Everyone from all teams stops to listen to proposed changes; because our EHR is integrated, changes can affect other modules and downstream systems.

11:00 AM to 12:00 PM: During this time, end users begin to place service request calls to our help desk, and a ticket is created for each. Once I receive a ticket, I call the end user and attempt to resolve the issue over the phone for the Go-Live site. If it is a remote site, I have the following options: remote into their computer, assist over the phone, email information, or refer to an on-site educator.

BOX 16-4 A Day in the Life of a Informatics Nurse Specialist: Healthcare System Implementation/Support Stage (*continued*)

12:00 PM to 1:30 PM: It's time to round on inpatient units and assist end users where needed. Before leaving the Command Center, the manager on duty has assessed which inpatient units are requiring the most help or have requested assistance. Rounding on the floors allows me to interact with end users, answer their questions, provide shoulder-to-shoulder support, and address their concerns.

Example of a typical physician support situation I assist with during rounding:

• A physician is attempting to discharge a patient for the first time in our new EHR and has general questions about where to document. I introduce myself, direct the physician where to document, and answer any questions all at the same time. I direct the physician through the workflow in a manner that works for a physician and wait until the physician has completed the documentation. I then ask if there are any final questions. I then follow up with the nurse of the patient discharged to see if the nurse has any questions regarding the discharge.

1:30 PM to 2:15 PM: It's time for Lunch! It is very important to take time to eat and take a mental break.

2:15 PM to 3:30 PM: Return to Command Center for a meeting with other team members to resolve an issue. My colleagues and I assess the problem, diagnose the issue, test for a possible solution, and then evaluate.

In order to test the solution, my colleagues and I perform integrated testing. Each one of us has a specific role to perform during testing. We admit patients in our test environment, take them through the workflow, and then evaluate if the solution solves the issue. If the solution works, the changes are then documented for next internal Change Control.

3:30 PM to 6:00 PM: Typically, I spend the remainder of my day in the Command Center following up on service request tickets, answering phone calls, and answering emails.

During this time, Hospital Leadership may come by to ask workflow questions. This gives me a chance to answer their questions, address concerns, or escalate issues to my manager or director.

6:00 PM to 6:15 PM: The evening ends with shift report to my night-shift team member. We discuss any outstanding issues and service request tickets to follow up on during night shift.

An implementation can be very exciting, an adrenaline rush and a lot of work, but it is worth the effort. Tomorrow will bring more meetings, new end users, new service request tickets, and new issues to solve.

Omega R. Finney, RN-BC, MSN,CPOE
Application Coordinator

INFORMATICS ORGANIZATIONS

Worldwide, multidisciplinary and nursing informatics specialty groups focus on using informatics to improve healthcare. In the United States, the largest nursing informatics professional association is the **American Nursing Informatics Association (ANIA)**. ANIA has annual educational conferences, provides continuing education forums, and disseminates informatics updates with an organization newsletter (ANIA, 2014). ANIA members also receive a discounted subscription rate for *Computers, Informatics Nursing: CIN* journal.

Multidisciplinary Groups

Given the interdisciplinary nature of informatics, many of the formal organizations involve practitioners from all areas.

International Medical Informatics Association (IMIA)

The **International Medical Informatics Association (IMIA)** was established in 1967 as TC4, a Technical Committee within the International Federation for Information Processing. IMIA is a non-political, international, scientific organization whose goals include promoting informatics in healthcare, promoting biomedical research, advancing international cooperation, stimulating informatics research and education, and exchanging information.

Many countries belong to IMIA through national organizations such as the AMIA, which represents the United States and the **European Federation for Medical Informatics (EFMI)**, which represents Europe. The members have national meetings to focus on issues pertaining to their nation, which allow members to establish a national network where ideas can be shared, and provide a place to gain information for specific national problems. These organizations also provide journals and are a source of up-to-date information for their country. The members of IMIA also take part in MedINFO, a feature of IMIA, which is held every 3 years. A list of member countries' organizations is present on the IMIA Web page (http://www.imia.org/).

Healthcare Information and Management Systems Society (HIMSS)

Another international organization, **Healthcare Information and Management Systems Society (HIMSS)**, has offices in Chicago, Washington, DC, Brussels, and other locations across the United States and Europe (HIMSS, 2014a). Founded in 1961, HIMSS is a not-for-profit organization dedicated to promoting a better understanding of healthcare information and management systems. In 2003, HIMSS formed a Nursing Informatics Community to provide support to the nursing role in informatics. HIMSS meets annually and publishes a quarterly journal and several guides to the field. They offer accreditation as a Certified Professional in Healthcare Information and Management Systems.

American Health Information Management Association (AHIMA)

The American College of Surgeons formed the **American Health Information Management Association (AHIMA)** in 1928 to improve clinical records (AHIMA, 2014). The name, AHIMA, reflects today's situation in which clinical data have expanded beyond either a single hospital or a provider. AHIMA offers credentialing programs in health information management, coding, and healthcare privacy and security.

Nursing Informatics Profession Associations

The multidisciplinary groups sometimes have smaller working groups, some of which are nursing focused. The IMIA Nursing Working Group has sponsored an International Nursing Informatics Conference every 3 years since 1982. The themes of these conferences provide a look into how the concerns of nursing informatics have broadened from a concern in 1982 with computers in nursing through integrating caring and technology in nursing, a realization of the impact of informatics on nursing knowledge, to the recognition of the importance of the consumer or human in healthcare.

Nursing Working Groups of Larger Organizations

AMIA and EFMI both have nursing working groups. AMIA's nursing working group, the **Nursing Informatics Working Group (NIWG)**, is responsible for promoting the integration of nursing informatics into the broader context of healthcare. NIWG also works to influence US policymakers regarding the use of nursing information. EFMI's nursing working group was formed to support European nurses and nursing informatics as well as to build informatics contact networks (EFMI, 2012).

British Computer Society Nursing Specialist Group

A very active group is the **British Computer Society (BCS)** Health Nursing Group. One of its aims is to disseminate information about current nursing informatics applications and to encourage the publication of research and development material in this area (BCS, 2014). This is accomplished by interacting with other groups such as the Royal College of Nursing, the Clinical Professions and Health Visitor's Association (CPHVA/Amicus), and the NHS Connecting for Health's National Advisory Group for the National Programme.

Alliance for Nursing Informatics

In 2004, the **Alliance for Nursing Informatics (ANI)** united many of the local, smaller, nursing informatics groups. The organization is sponsored by

AMIA and HIMSS (Alliance for Nursing Informatics, 2014; HIMSS, 2014b). Membership is through affiliation with a nursing-focused informatics group, a nursing working group or a local or national group. These groups retain their dues, programs, publications, and organizational structures, but are united through ANI to create a unified voice for nursing informatics. Representatives of each of the organizational groups make up the governing directors group that guides the strategic goals and activities of ANI (2014). Their website (http://www.allianceni.org/) features link to all the member groups. ANI membership includes the nursing working groups of AMIA, HIMSS, and ANIA.

SUMMARY

Nursing informatics is a subspecialty in both nursing and health informatics. Nursing informatics focuses on helping clinicians acquire and integrate patient care data from many sources. The theory basis for nursing informatics includes sociotechnical, change, general systems, cognitive science, usability, chaos theories, and learning theories.

Many nurses working in informatics learned on the job as informatics nurses, but the trend today is for a more formal education in the field to prepare nurses for the role of informatics nurse specialists. Many types of programs exist for those who wish to specialize in nursing informatics. They range from programs granting graduate degrees to continuing education offerings. There is no accrediting body yet for informatics nurse specialist education as there is for nurse practitioners; therefore, the wise prospective student should investigate any academic program before enrolling.

Within nursing informatics, there are many different areas of concentration and roles including project manager, systems manager, and independent contractor. Nursing informatics, however, is not solely the province of informatics nurse specialists; all nurses must be involved if successful information systems are to be developed and implemented. There are many areas where informatics nurses work, as well as various job foci.

Health informatics organizations at the international and national level are mostly multidisciplinary. Besides nursing working groups in the multidisciplinary groups, there are organizations that focus only on nursing informatics interests.

APPLICATIONS AND COMPETENCIES

1. Using one episode in a recent clinical experience, describe how you mentally move data through information and knowledge to wisdom. Keep it small, such as giving a medication or assessing a patient for lung congestion.

   a. How did you evaluate and combine the different pieces of data?

   b. What was the outcome of this process?

   c. Reflect on how an information system could assist this process.

2. The theories supporting informatics come from many different areas.

   a. By using the sociotechnical theory, make a plan to assess the readiness of an organization for either a new information system or an update to the current plan.

   b. In adopting a spreadsheet, in which category of Rogers' diffusion theory would you place yourself?

   c. Think of planning a change for an organization with which you are familiar. What are some of the restraining forces and the driving forces? How would you proceed?

   d. Think of some of the various organizations with which you are familiar. Where would you classify them on the open–closed continuum of systems theory?

   e. Relate the cognitive theory to the design of a Web page.

3. Interview an informatics nurse to discover her or his responsibilities. Into which of the role(s) discussed in this chapter would you place this individual?

4. Conduct an Internet search to identify two formal educational programs in nursing informatics that would most interest you. Identify three key factors about the programs that you found to be most interesting and explain why.

5. Investigate the activities of one of the informatics professional organizations. Some methods for accomplishing this include checking their home page, attending a meeting, or interviewing a member/officer in one of the groups.

REFERENCES

Akbari, H., & Land, F. (2011, November 16). *Socio-technical theory*. Retrieved from http://istheory.byu.edu/wiki/Socio-technical_theory

Alliance for Nursing Informatics. (2014). *About ANI*. Retrieved from http://www.allianceni.org/about.asp

American Association of Colleges of Nursing. (2008). *The essentials of baccalaureate education for professional nursing practice*. Retrieved from http://www.aacn.nche.edu/Education/pdf/BaccEssentials08.pdf

American Health Information Management Association. (2014). *AHIMA facts*. Retrieved from http://www.ahima.org/about

American Nurses Association. (2015). *Nursing informatics: Scope and standards of practice* (2nd ed.). Washington, DC: American Nurses Publishing.

American Nurses Credentialing Center. (2014). *Informatics nursing certification eligibility criteria*. Retrieved from http://www.nursecredentialing.org/informatics-eligibility.aspx

American Nursing Informatics Association (ANIA). (2014). *American Nursing Informatics Association main menu*. Retrieved from https://www.ania.org/

Bass, A. (2003, June 1). *Health-care IT: A big rollout bust. CIO*. Retrieved from http://www.cio.com/article/29736/Health_Care_IT_A_Big_Rollout_Bust

British Computer Society (BCS). (2014). *About BCS—The Chartered Institute for IT*. Retrieved from http://www.bcs.org/

Clark, D. (2010, November 15). *Understanding and performance*. Retrieved from http://www.nwlink.com/~donclark/performance/understanding.html

Dizikes, P. (2011, February 22). When the butterfly effect took flight. *MIT News Magazine*. Retrieved from http://www.technologyreview.com/article/422809/when-the-butterfly-effect-took-flight/

European Federation for Medical Informatics (EFMI). (2012, July). *EFMI WG NURSIE nursing informatics in Europe*. Retrieved from http://www.helmholtz-muenchen.de/ibmi/efmi/index.php?option=com_content&task=view&id=25&Itemid=121

Graves, J. R., & Cocoran, S. (1989). The study of nursing informatics. *Image: Journal of Nursing Scholarship, 21*, 227–231.

Gray, R. M. (2013, March 3). *Entropy and information theory*. New York, NY: Springer Verlag. Retrieved from http://ee.stanford.edu/~gray/it.html

Healthcare Information and Management Systems Society (HIMSS). (2014a). *About HIMSS*. Retrieved from http://www.himss.org/ASP/aboutHimssHome.asp

HIMSS. (2014b). *Alliance for Nursing Informatics*. Retrieved from http://www.allianceni.org/

Heylighen, F., & Joslyn, C. (1992, November 1). What is systems theory? In F. Heylighen, C. Joslyn, & V. Turchin (Eds.), *Principia Cybernetica Web (Principia Cybernetica, Brussels)*. Brussels: Principia Cybernetica. Retrieved from http://pespmc1.vub.ac.be/SYSTHEOR.html

Joos, I., Whitman, N. I., Smith, M. J., et al. (1992). *Computer in small bytes*. New York, NY: National League for Nursing Press.

National League for Nursing. (2008, May 29). *NLN Board of Governors urges better preparation of nursing workforce to practice in 21st century, technology-rich health care environment*. Retrieved from http://www.nln.org/newsreleases/informatics_release_052908.htm

NCNR Priority Expert Panel on Nursing Informatics. (1993). *Nursing informatics. Enhancing patient care: A report of the NCNR priority expert panel on nursing informatics*. Bethesda, MD: U.S. Department of Health and Human Services, U.S. Public Health Service, National Institutes of Health, National Center for Nursing Research.

Nightingale, F., & Goldie, S. M. (1997). *Letters from the Crimea, 1854–1856*. Retrieved from http://preview.tinyurl.com/2auahra

Rogers, E. M. (2003). *Diffusion of innovations* (5th ed.). New York, NY: Free Press.

Sawyer, S., & Rosenbaum, H. (2000). Social informatics in the information sciences: Current activities and emerging directions. *Informing Science, 3*(2), 89–95. Retrieved from http://inform.nu/Articles/Vol3/v3n2p89-96r.pdf

Schneider, T. D. (2013, July 31). *Information theory primer*. Retrieved from http://www.ccrnp.ncifcrf.gov/~toms/paper/primer/primer.pdf

School of Mathematics and Statistics, St. Andrews University Scotland. (2003, October). *Florence Nightingale*. Retrieved from http://www-history.mcs.st-andrews.ac.uk/Biographies/Nightingale.html

Smith, M. K. (2009, November 4). *Kurt Lewin: Groups, experiential learning and action research*. Retrieved August 1, 2010, from http://www.infed.org/thinkers/et-lewin.htm

Staggers, N., & Thompson, C. B. (2002). The evolution of definitions for nursing informatics: A critical analysis and revised definition. *Journal of the American Medical Association, 9*(3), 255–261.

Technology Informatics Guiding Education Reform. (2009). *The TIGER initiative: Collaborating to integrate evidence and informatics into nursing practice and education: An executive summary*. Retrieved January 24, 2011, from http://www.tigersummit.com/uploads/TIGER_Collaborative_Exec_Summary_040509.pdf

Thagard, P. (2010, June 9). *Cognitive science—The Stanford encyclopedia of philosophy*. Retrieved August 22, 2011, from http://plato.stanford.edu/entries/cognitive-science/

Turley, J. (1996). Toward a model for nursing informatics. *Image: Journal of Nursing Scholarship, 28*(4), 309–313.

von Bertalanffy, L. (1973). *General system theory: Foundations, development, applications*. Harmondsworth: Penguin.

Warner, H. R. (1995). Medical informatics: A real discipline? *Journal of the American Medical Association, 2*(4), 207–214.

CHAPTER 17

Electronic Healthcare Information Systems, Electronic Health Records, and Meaningful Use

OBJECTIVES

After studying this chapter, you will be able to:

1. Describe how the electronic medical record (EMR), electronic health record (EHR), and the electronic personal health record (ePHR) relate to emerging clinical information systems.

2. Discuss the importance for use of data standards for EHRs.

3. Discuss the progress toward adoption of the EHR and information exchange.

4. Discuss the relationship between "meaningful use" and best practices for healthcare delivery.

5. Describe efforts to assure health information privacy and security for EHRs and health information exchange.

KEY TERMS

American Recovery and Reinvestment Act (ARRA)

Audit trail

Clinical Document Architecture (CDA)

Continuity of Care Document (CCD)

Healthcare information system (HIS)

Health Information Technology for Economic and Clinical Health (HITECH) Act

Meaningful use

The **healthcare information system (HIS)** is a composite made up of all the information management systems that serve an organization's needs. The complexity of HIS is largely independent of the size of the organization because healthcare provides a common core of patient care services. At the very minimum, most healthcare providers have electronic systems for billing patient care services. Facilities using advanced technologies have numerous systems that manage every service provided to the patient. This chapter focuses on a few basic components and processes common to HISs that are essential for all nurses to understand. The relationship between the HIS and the US government initiative for meaningful use is also discussed.

Every nurse needs to appreciate the individual's role as it relates to HISs. As nurses, we need to understand what systems can do to help us efficiently manage information that relates to patient care. We need to appreciate how to improve the healthcare delivery system using the exchange of deidentified data from the US HealthIT.gov meaningful use initiative. We must recognize how electronic documentation underpins the discovery of evidence-based practice for improved patient outcomes. We should expect the HIS to support the nursing care delivery process and the documentation of care; the HIS must not negatively impact our practice. That being said, we should not expect a technology solution to mimic the paper chart world.

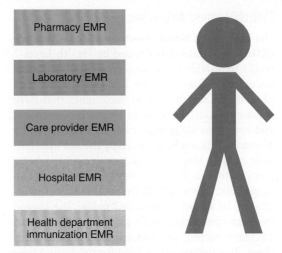

Figure 17-1. Patient data in virtual database silos. (nicubunu_Stick_figure. Creative Commons License, Retrieved from openclipart at https://openclipart. org/tags/stick%20man)

EMR, EHR, EPHR, AND THEIR RELATIONSHIPS TO EMERGING CLINICAL INFORMATION SYSTEMS

The patient's health information is at the forefront of clinical information systems. A brief review of the different types of patient records should help set the scene for emerging clinical information systems. The EMR (electronic medical record), EHR (electronic health record), and ePHR (electronic personal health record) are now being integrated into the design of clinical information systems.

As noted in Chapter 12, the EMR is an electronic version of the traditional record used by the healthcare provider. It is a legal record that describes the care that a patient received during an encounter with the healthcare agency. Instead of hospital visit information being located in one or more manila folders in medical records, the EMR is a searchable database. For example, providers could search for all admissions for treatment of congestive heart failure or all surgeries. A patient can have many EMRs: one at the health department for immunizations, one at each hospital where care has been provided, and one at each healthcare provider's office.

When the EMRs reside in the individual provider information silos, there is no standard for recording data, which leads to data redundancy (repeated entries of the same information) and subsequent entry discrepancies. As an example, the hospital where the care was originally provided may have accurate dates for the admission or surgery; however, on readmission when asked about previous surgeries, the patient's memory of those dates or types of surgeries may vary from the actual information. The information belongs to the patient, but the healthcare provider owns the data in the EMR. Where no EHRs and health information exchange (HIE) programs exist, EMR data reside in virtual silos, which are different databases that do not communicate among all the providers (Figure 17-1).

The EHR is a transportable subset of the EMR designed for use by healthcare organizations and physician practices and other providers. It provides a bridge connecting the EMR and the ePHR. "The EHR is a longitudinal record of patient health information generated by one or more encounters in any care delivery setting" (Health Information and Management Systems Society [HIMSS], 2014, para. 1). The patient owns the data.

Data Standards

The EHR uses two types of data standards for data communication: the Clinical Document Architecture and the Continuity of Care Document.

Clinical Document Architecture

The EHR uses **Clinical Document Architecture (CDA)** data standards devised by Health Level 7 (HL7) to provide a common structure for clinical documents. The structure has three levels that provide the ability to send documents that have sufficient "code" in them to be machine-readable and yet are easily interpretable as a document by a human. This can be achieved by the use of extensible markup language tags that designate what a piece of text is. For example, a first name will be tagged just like in HTML (hypertext markup language), as will other required fields. The tagged items can be automatically placed as data into an electronic record, and humans can read the document. This format is intended for use by any type of clinical document such as demographics, vital signs, medications, progress notes, history and physical, consults, nursing documents, laboratory and radiology reports, and discharge summaries.

Continuity of Care Document

The **Continuity of Care Document (CCD)** uses the CDA architecture to provide a "snapshot" of a patient's health information, including insurance information, medical diagnoses and problems, medications, and allergies (American Academy of Family Physicians [AAFP], 2014), which is to be integrated with EHRs to provide the sharing of data with multiple providers. It is a result of the harmonization of the CCD developed jointly by the American Society for Testing and Materials (ASTM) International, Massachusetts Medical Society, HIMSS, AAFP, and the American Academy of Pediatrics ASTMs with HL7's CDA specifications. The CCD has defined what data are shared, and the CDA defines how data are shared with the EHR. In this manner, the CDA is used for other clinical documents that need sharing.

The terminology for an electronic record can be confusing because the terms EMR and EHR may be used as if the meanings are identical. However, it is important to know that the terms refer to two different types of records. Not only can healthcare providers extract pertinent information from electronic records that enhance the effectiveness of care, but the information also has the potential for use in quality and evidence-based care knowledge management. Both the EMR and EHR electronic clinical databases allow healthcare providers to review and analyze changes over time. Liang (2007) lists five ways (see Box 17-1) the EHR can fill gaps in knowledge between evidence and practice. The information continues to be valid today.

The effort to improve patient care outcomes resulted in a chaotic effort when healthcare providers transitioned from a paper record to an electronic record. Without any "mental models" about how to extract information from electronic systems, the adoption process is tainted by "paper chart thinking" (Baron, 2007, p. 549). There is still inconsistent communication between those who are involved in the universal design of the electronic record, those attempting to implement it, and those who are considering implementation. Agencies that are adopting or want to adopt electronic documentation may not understand the advantages of an interconnected record and the importance of interoperability for sharing

---

BOX 17-1 Ways the EHR Can Address the Gaps in Clinical Knowledge

The EHR can address the gaps in knowledge in evidence and clinical practice in the following ways:

- By detecting information and knowledge from current records that can efficiently affect clinical outcomes
- By shortening the time from knowledge discovery to implementation
- By monitoring quality improvement outcomes that result from knowledge-driven changes in providers' practices
- By empowering the patient to become a partner in care with the healthcare provider(s)
- By providing real-world knowledge versus controlled clinical trials about treatment effectiveness and outcomes

Source: Liang, L. (2007). The gap between evidence and practice. *Health Affairs, 26*(2), w119–w121.

information pertinent to improvement of patient outcomes. In the ideal world, the EHR summary data are owned by the patient, have patient input, and are used by multiple healthcare organizations.

THE NEED FOR EHRS

Why is there a need for healthcare records to be electronic? As clearly outlined in the seminal IOM reports (see the "Benefits of Electronic Records" section later in this chapter), it is to make patient care safer (Committee on Quality of Health Care in America & Institute of Medicine, 2001; Page, A., & Institute of Medicine [U.S.], 2004; Kohn et al., 2000). The paper record and the associated information silos are not good enough anymore. The need for an electronic record is recognized worldwide, not just in the United States. The following subsections examine the strengths and weaknesses of paper records versus EHRs and culminate in an explanation of meaningful use.

Paper Records

Strengths of Paper Records

The wonderful thing about paper is that it is very transportable. The paper record can be used as soon as we find it (assuming it has not been misfiled; see next section) and pick up a pen to write. We do not have to wait in line for a computer terminal, log in, click to drill down to menus, or wait for a window to open. The paper record requires no electricity, no maintenance, and no downtime. In an ideal paper chart world, we can chart very quickly. In fact, when the health information system "goes down" (is not working), we use paper records as a backup method for charting until the system starts working again.

Weaknesses of Paper Records

Potential to be Incomplete

A nursing student completing her senior internship in a hospital that used the paper record system stated that documenting on paper "made her think." When asked what she meant, she said that she was used to a computer documentation system that provided checkboxes and data entry screen prompts, which, she felt, guided her in electronic

documentation. She said that when there was a blank nursing progress note, she had to "think" about what to chart. It was clear that she realized that without those prompts, her entries might be incomplete.

Logistical Issues

Unlike the electronic record, paper records do not have a backup system. They also can be easily damaged or destroyed. Parts of the paper record can be destroyed accidentally or, rarely, purposely. A part of the drudgery, particularly for night staff, includes stamping new forms and deleting duplicate updated patient information such as laboratory and x-ray reports. In the paper record world, it is easy to stamp a chart form with the wrong stamp plate. Stamp machines are heavy and cumbersome and require maintenance. Filing copies of testing reports in paper records is very time consuming and prone to human error, such as misfiling a report.

Paper records for patients who require a lengthy hospital stay can become very large, heavy, and difficult to store on a nursing unit. Retrieving old records for a new admission is often challenging. If the paper record is misfiled, there may be a significant time delay before the paper record is delivered to the nursing unit. Finding information for a patient with multiple readmissions is often overwhelming and may require searches through stacks of manila folders.

Illegibility and Medical Errors

Lack of legibility is another criticism of the paper record. It is often very difficult to read handwriting of others. Script versions of certain terms have led to serious and sometimes fatal medical errors. As a result, the National Coordinating Council for Medication Error Reporting and Prevention (2014) and the Joint Commission (2013) made recommendations to stop using certain dangerous abbreviations. The Joint Commission issued a Sentinel Event Alert on the use of dangerous abbreviations in 2001, and healthcare agencies have worked fervently ever since to correct the problems. It was later incorporated into standards for information management. Examples of abbreviations commonly misinterpreted include the abbreviations for cubic centimeter, every day, and morphine sulfate. Healthcare workers often misinterpret cubic centimeter (c.c.) as units, every day (q.d.) as four times per day (q.i.d.), and morphine sulfate (MSO_4) as magnesium sulfate ($MgSO_4$).

Difficulty in Trending Data

Trending data in the paper record world is tedious and prone to error. The user has to graph vital signs data and draw connecting lines to portray a trend on a vital signs flow sheet. Information such as intake and output (I&O) is initially charted on a clipboard in the patient's room and then transferred to the paper record at the end of the shift. If the patient got behind or ahead of his or her fluid volume needs, it usually is not discovered until the nurse charts the date—when it is too late to make an efficient correction. Totaling the I&O for complex care patients can be extremely time consuming and prone to error. A calculator is often required to add and subtract numbers for an I&O total. Use of the EMR can avoid all of the errors; the data can be entered as they are generated, and the total is automatically calculated. Further, it can provide an up-to-date record for the healthcare provider who wants this information before the end of the shift.

Electronic Records

Disadvantages of Electronic Records

If health information is stored electronically, what are the ramifications of a disaster, such as a tornado, fire, or hurricane destroying the HIS location? What about major equipment failures?

Benefits of Electronic Records

Using the electronic record in documenting patient care has many benefits, which outweigh the risks noted previously.

Continuity of Care

For example, consider what happened to paper versus EHRs when Hurricane Katrina hit the US gulf coast in 2005. The inherent weaknesses of the paper health records were realized: thousands of Americans were affected when physicians' offices, healthcare agencies, and hospitals were under water. Paper health records were destroyed, and the continuity of care was breached. In contrast, the Veterans Administration (VA) patients experienced a relatively minor continuity of care issue because the VA uses EHRs with a health information infrastructure. The VA patient care issues were associated with the initial isolation of patients and the lack of communication and electricity, not the permanent loss of medical care information.

Uses of the EMR, EHR, and ePHR all minimize the "decentralized and fragmented nature of the healthcare delivery system" that we were warned about in the Institute of Medicine (IOM) report *To Err is Human: Building a Safer Health System* (Kohn et al., 2000, p. 3). The report was the first of several, all of which outlined the inherent weaknesses in our healthcare delivery system. The report challenged us to make healthcare safe. The electronic record provides ways to make healthcare safer with the use of real-time documentation and instant communication with all providers who need access to the information wherever they are—in another department or in a remote office. In addition, decision support systems with just-in-time alerts can guide providers when delivering patient care.

The IOM report, *Crossing the Quality Chasm: A New Health System for the 21st Century* (Committee on Quality of Health Care in America & Institute of Medicine, 2001), outlined the critical need for restructuring healthcare to improve patient outcomes. The report identified six areas of focus, stating that healthcare should be safe, effective, patient centered, timely, efficient, and equitable. It provided a scenario of a working mother's plight with healthcare before, during, and after her diagnosis of breast cancer. Many of the problems she experienced could have been mitigated with the EHR, beginning with the failure of her past mammograms to be mailed, the failure of the physician to notify the patient of an abnormal finding on a previous mammogram, and the time spent locating her x-ray information in preparation for surgery. The scenario is not new to those of us who work in the paper record world; we see it happen every day.

Private and Secure Information

Information privacy and security is a benefit of the electronic record. The electronic record includes an **audit trail** that details information about when the record was accessed, the original point of access, what particular components were accessed, the date, and times. Access to the electronic record is controlled by delineation of user privileges. In contrast, there is no means of knowing who picked up a paper chart or what information was reviewed.

Searchable and Analyzable Information

The ability to search and extract information and to trend the information to create knowledge to inform practice is another benefit of the electronic record. If the electronic record is a well-designed database with a standardized healthcare vocabulary, it can be searched quickly and efficiently. For example, if a patient presented with a wound infection that was not responding to therapy, the patient's temperatures could be viewed in a graph output to visualize the patterns of temperature elevation spikes. Information from patients with chronic diseases, such as readmission patterns for those with diabetes or heart failure, could be analyzed for proactive intervention.

Real-Time Information

The electronic record provides the opportunity for real-time information that can be collected and communicated in an effective and efficient manner. As soon as a medication or vital sign is done, it can be entered into the record and viewed by other care providers who have access to the record. As another example, consider the patient who is referred from a provider's office to a facility for an outpatient test, such as a magnetic resonance imaging. If the referring office is connected to the same information system as the provider's office, the staff will be able to view the available appointments and schedule the test before the patient leaves the office. When the tests are completed, the test results can be communicated to the referring provider in an efficient manner, and the test results can be added to the patient's record electronically.

Data entry can be automated by using synchronization with monitoring devices, or the user can key it in. Multiple users can easily view and document on different parts of the electronic record simultaneously, unlike the paper record. When providing care in the paper world, the chart is not usually with the patient, so the first step is to locate it. The paper chart may be in a stack of charts with doctor's orders, with a physician writing orders or progress notes, or being reviewed by another care provider.

The electronic record is simply a tool for the clinician to use when telling the story about patient care and making pertinent decisions. If we do not take advantage of the real-time documentation, we miss opportunities to share just-in-time information with other care providers. Real-time documentation provides a window of opportunity for early interventions and improved patient outcomes. Nurses must embrace the potential values of the electronic record, demonstrate real-time documentation that can facilitate communication, and use the record to extract information to improve patient outcomes. Real-time documentation requires a culture change for nurses who practiced in a paper chart world. It also requires a workflow redesign, which includes ready access to computers for charting at the point of care.

Improved Quality

One of the most important benefits of the electronic record is improved patient care outcomes. In noncomputerized systems, test results can be easily lost or misplaced, requiring repeated testing. Ordered treatments can be overlooked or not documented. An electronic information system can improve the quality of care by preventing these all-too-common difficulties. Physicians entering orders into the system eliminates transcription errors. The HIS can compare the electronic order with recommended dosages in the database and provide the physician with information about the drug prescribed using clinical reminders (decision support system). When the order is integrated with the patient's information about the drugs that the patient is concurrently receiving, as well as drug allergies, drug mismatches can be better avoided. The HIS can generate clinical reminders to ensure that the patient receives the correct drug.

THE ELECTRONIC RECORD AND MEANINGFUL USE

The number of EHR adopters continues to grow, which is necessary to meet care new outcome knowledge spurred by meaningful use, an initiative that uses EHRs to improve patient care. Meaningful use originated with the **American Recovery and Reinvestment Act (ARRA)**

(Recovery.gov, 2014), signed into law by President Obama on February 17, 2009. ARRA and the **Health Information Technology for Economic and Clinical Health (HITECH) Act**, a part of ARRA, were milestones in the history of HIT. The HITECH Act outlined four purposes:

- Define meaningful use
- Use incentives and grant programs to foster the adoption of EHRs
- Gain the trust of the public regarding the privacy and security of electronic healthcare data
- Promote IT innovation

The HITECH Act provided monetary incentives to hospitals and eligible providers that met "meaningful use" requirements. The term **meaningful use** refers to the use of information from EHRs to make improvements in the delivery of healthcare (Blumenthal & Tavenner, 2010). Meaningful use requires an interoperable HIS for data exchange. A full-text summary of the meaningful use objectives and measures is online in a *New England Journal of Medicine* article, "The 'Meaningful Use' Regulation for Electronic Health Records" (http://www.nejm.org/doi/full/10.1056/NEJMp1006114).

According to research done by Mathematica Policy Research, Harvard School of Public Health, and Robert Woods Johnson Foundation (2013), 44% of hospitals in the United States had adopted a basic EHR as of 2012. The adoption rate by smaller and rural hospitals was slower than larger, private, and urban hospitals. The meaningful use definition, finalized in July 2010, allowed hospitals and providers to qualify for incentive payments beginning in 2011. It provided a two-tiered implementation plan. The CMS website at http://www.cms.gov/Regulations-and-Guidance/Legislation/EHRIncentivePrograms/Meaningful_Use.html has additional information about meaningful use.

Meaningful use has three stages. Stage 1 focuses on data capturing and sharing. Stage 2 focuses on advanced clinical processes. Finally, Stage 3 focuses on improved clinical outcomes. Eligible providers, hospital, and critical access hospitals must meet the thresholds for the first stage prior to meeting ones for the second stage. Meaningful use requires that all EHRs be certified to verify the interoperability for sending and receiving health data. An overview of Stages 1 and

2 meaningful use objectives for eligible providers is displayed in Table 17-1.

In 2014, as a part of meaningful use Stages 1 and 2, eligible providers were required to select and report 9 of 64 clinical quality measures in three of the following six domains: patient and family engagement, patient safety, care coordination, population and public health, efficient use of healthcare resources, and clinical processes/effectiveness. Note that the ability to report electronic syndromic surveillance data to public health agencies could assist with identifying and containing disease outbreaks, such as the Ebola hemorrhagic fever virus that erupted in 2014 across the world. Additional information about the clinical quality measures is online at http://www.cms.gov/Regulations-and-Guidance/Legislation/EHRIncentivePrograms/ClinicalQualityMeasures.html.

The HITECH Act provided $27 billion in incentives for healthcare agencies and authorized providers to adopt EHRs over 10 years (The Commonwealth Fund, 2011). The dollar amount was adjusted to be $35 billion (Thune et al., 2013). CMS (Centers for Medicare and Medicaid) was responsible for the distribution of the incentive payments for providers. The incentives occurred between 2011 and 2014. Comprehensive information about the HITECH Act is available online at http://healthit.hhs.gov/. Information about the CMS incentive programs is available online at http://www.cms.gov/ehrincentiveprograms/.

The HITECH Act continues be hotly debated in the political arena. A report by Senators Thune et al. (2013) to Kathleen Sebelius, who was the Secretary of Health and Human Services at that time, identified deficiencies in the effort to obtain meaningful use: lack of clear plan for interoperability, increased healthcare costs related to EHRs, lack of oversight, placing patient privacy at risk, and concerns about program sustainability. The nonprofit organization HIMSS responded to the Senators' report using supporting evidence. Using the HIMSS EMR Analytics Adoption Model at http://www.himssanalytics.org/stagesGraph.asp (discussed in Chapter 20), HIMSS (2013) noted the EHR Incentive Program increased adoption for EHRs by 80% for Stages 5 and 6, where Stage 6 indicates full adoption of all components, including the EMR, CCD to share data, data warehousing, and

TABLE 17-1 Stages 1 and 2 Meaningful Use Core and Menu Objectives for Eligible Providers

Core objectives to enable EHRs to support healthcare	**Stage 1** 1. Use computerized provider order entry (CPOE). 2. Use drug–drug and drug–allergy interaction checks. 3. Maintain an up-to-date list of diagnoses. 4. Create and transmit prescriptions electronically. 5. Maintain an active medication list. 6. Maintain an allergy list. 7. Record demographics. 8. Record vital signs. 9. Record smoking status for patients 13 years and older. 10. Use one clinical decision support rule. 11. Provide patients the ability to view online, and transmit information within 4 days after information is available to the provider. 12. Provide clinical summaries for each office visit. 13. Protect electronic health information. **Stage 2**—Meet all 13 objectives above plus 4 additional ones. 1. Include clinical lab test results in the EHR. 2. Perform medication reconciliation. 3. Submit electronic data to immunization registries. 4. Use secure electronic messaging to communicate with patients on relevant health information.
Menu objectives that provide flexibility for providers to choose	**Stage 1**—Select 5 of the following menu objectives; at least 1 is a public health measure. 1. Implement drug formulary checks. 2. Use clinical lab test results in the EHR as structured data. 3. Create patient lists by condition for quality improvement, reduction of disparities, research, or outreach. 4. Send patient reminders for preventive and follow-up care. 5. Use certified EHR technology to provide patient education resources. 6. Perform medication reconciliation for patients received from another setting/provider. 7. Provide a summary of care for patients referred to another setting/provider. 8. Able to submit electronic immunization information. 9. Able to submit electronic syndromic surveillance data to public health agencies. **Stage 2**—Select 3 of the following menu objectives. 1. Submit electronic syndromic surveillance data to public health agencies. 2. Record patient notes electronically. 3. Have imaging results accessible in the EHR. 4. Record family history data. 5. Report cancer cases to public health cancer registry. 6. Report specific cases to a specialized registry.

Source: The Eligible Professional Meaningful Use Table of Contents Core and Menu Set Objectives at http://www.cms.gov/Regulations-and-Guidance/Legislation/EHRIncentivePrograms/Downloads/Stage2_MeaningfulUseSpecSheet_TableContents_EPs.pdf; the Eligible Professional's Guide to Stage of the EHR Incentive Program at http://www.cms.gov/Regulations-and-Guidance/Legislation/EHRIncentivePrograms/Downloads/Stage2_Guide_EPs_9_23_13.pdf

data continuity with the emergency, ambulatory, and outpatient departments (HIMSS Analytics, 2014). Adoption at Stage 7 increased 63%. HIMSS recognized the potential for fraudulent billing and abuse but noted that the organization is actively involved with mitigating these problems. HIMSS noted that CMS and the Office of the National Coordinator for Health Information Technology (ONC) provide oversight using periodic reviews and that privacy and security is at the heart of all EHR interoperability efforts.

The ONC submits an annual report on the adoption of electronic records in the United States to the US Congress. In October 2014, the ONC reported that as of 2013, 59% of hospitals and 48% of physicians "had at least a basic EHR system" (ONC, 2014, p. 9). The report noted that the vast majority of the states in the United States had the ability for secure sharing of electronic health information by "trusted parties" and the ability to find and request patient information from other providers (ONC, 2014, p. 33). The most current information on HIE, which is necessary for EHR data exchange, is available from the HealthIT.gov Program Measures Dashboard at http://healthit.gov/policy-researchers-implementers/state-hie-implementation-status.

> ### QSEN Scenario
> A friend asks you to explain the rationale for meaningful use. How should you respond?

THE ELECTRONIC RECORDS PRIVACY AND SECURITY: HIPAA REVISITED

As noted with the concerns about EHR adoption, assurance of patient privacy and security is a significant concern. In the United States, the Health Insurance Portability and Accountability Act (HIPAA) of 1996 has had a tremendous impact on the policies and procedures for clinical information systems. The law initiated a new standard for protecting information for individuals who have health records that are stored or transferred by using clinical information systems. Under HIPAA, health information for individuals has federal protection. Efforts to strengthen privacy and security under HIPAA continue. For example, changes in 2013 addressed improved patient privacy protection and provided healthcare consumers new rights to their health information (HHS.gov, 2013).

Although there is a tremendous amount of education and news about HIPAA and HIPAA breaches, the law is too often misunderstood. To complicate things, the law has been constantly amended. Moreover, HIPAA is frequently *misspelled as HIPPA*. The acronym is also misquoted as "health information," instead of "health insurance."

HIPAA law has two components: one is privacy and the other is security. The law reaches further than the origin of the clinical HIS and extends to consultants, agencies, and businesses that contract with the owner of the HIS. Nurses generally have an exceptional understanding of the privacy (confidentiality) part of the law. However, the data security part of the law may not be as clear to nurses and other healthcare providers. The Department of Health and Human Services (http://www.hhs.gov/ocr/privacy/hipaa/understanding/index.html) has easy-to-read information on HIPAA privacy and security.

Security of protected health information is more than logging in and out of the electronic record or assuring that the computer screen is not viewed by those who do not have the need to know. All users must attest to using a certified EHR technology, conduct a risk analysis, and make any necessary updates to correct problems (EHR Incentive Program, 2014). For additional information on the requirements for EHR certification, go to http://www.cms.gov/Regulations-and-Guidance/Legislation/EHRIncentivePrograms/downloads/15_Core_ProtectElectronicHealthInformation.pdf. It relates to transfer, removal, disposal, and reuse of the electronic information. Every healthcare worker who works with patient information data must be familiar with the agency's policies and procedures for storage of data that are extracted from the EHR, such as for quality improvement studies. Storage of data pertains to remote shared agency servers, hard drives, flash drives, and any other optical media.

The agency's HIPAA security officer is responsible for the policies and procedures that address data security issues.

SUMMARY

The rapid emergence of electronic records in healthcare is driving change for the way we record care and how it is communicated to clinical information systems. The CDA data standard allows the EHR data machine to be readable, and the CCD data standard provides a snapshot of the patient's health information.

The most rapid changes for adoption of electronic records are with the EMR and EHR. Within the next five to ten years, the ePHR should be adopted by healthcare consumers because it allows them to access their personal health information. To make health communication possible, states are creating HIE programs, and most states have the systems in place.

Meaningful use, a component of the HITECH Act, provides a means for eligible providers, hospitals, and critical access hospitals to use and communicate data to improve patient outcomes. There are three stages for meaningful use. The purpose of Stage 1 is to verify that the EHR could capture and share data. In Stage 2, users utilize advanced clinical processes to analyze data and make care improvements. As a result of the first two stages, improved outcomes are expected with Stage 3 of meaningful use. The ultimate goal of electronic data exchange is for meaningful use of deidentified data. There is a great potential for learning best practices of data from large groups of individuals.

The CMS and ONC are conducting ongoing reviews to ensure that progress is made to facilitate data communication exchange between EMRs, EHR, and the clinical information systems. Use of ePHRs is still in its infancy but should gain popularity within the next decade.

Because patient's health information privacy and security are critical for the success of data exchange, HIPAA regulations continue to be strengthened. Everyone who uses EHRs is required to attest that they are using certified EHR technology.

APPLICATIONS AND COMPETENCIES

1. Use a drawing tool, such as the Illustrations menu in Microsoft Word or PowerPoint, to depict the relationships of the EMR, EHR, and the ePHR to emerging clinical information systems.

2. Conduct a literature or Web search on the CDA and CCD data standards that extends your understanding of the terminology. Cite the resource and summarize your findings.

3. Review the most recent update for HIE adoption on the HealthIT.gov Program Measures Dashboard at http://healthit.gov/policy-researchers-implementers/state-hie-implementation-status. Summarize your findings.

4. Do a literature search for the terms meaningful use and best practice to extend your understanding of the topics. Summarize your findings for current development issues. Cite your sources.

5. Examine the policies and procedures to assure health information privacy and security for your college/university student health services or the healthcare agency where you work. Summarize your findings and describe efforts to assure health information privacy and security for EHRs and HIE.

REFERENCES

American Academy of Family Physicians (AAFP). (2014). *ASTM Continuity of Care (CCR)*. Retrieved from http://www.aafp.org/practice-management/health-it/astm.html

Baron, R. J. (2007). Improving patient care. Quality improvement with an electronic health record: Achievable, but not automatic. *Annals of Internal Medicine, 147*(8), 549–552.

Blumenthal, D., & Tavenner, M. (2010). The "meaningful use" regulation for electronic health records. *New England Journal of Medicine, 363*(6), 501–504. Retrieved from http://www.nejm.org/doi/abs/10.1056/NEJMp1006114. doi:10.1056/NEJMp1006114

Committee on Quality of Health Care in America & Institute of Medicine. (2001). *Crossing the quality chasm: A new health system for the 21st century*. Retrieved from http://books.nap.edu/catalog.php?record_id=10027#toc

EHR Incentive Program. (2014, May). *Eligible professional meaningful use core measure, measure 13 of 13*. Retrieved from http://www.cms.gov/Regulations-and-Guidance/Legislation/EHRIncentivePrograms/downloads/15_Core_ProtectElectronicHealthInformation.pdf

Health Information and Management Systems Society. (2013, May 17). *HIMSS response to Senators' reboot*. Retrieved from http://www.himss.org/files/HIMSSorg/Content/files/20130517_HIMSS_Response_Senate_Reboot.pdf

Health Information and Management Systems Society (HIMSS). (2014). *Electronic health record (EHR)*. Retrieved from http://www.himss.org/library/ehr/

HHS.gov. (2013, January 17). *New rule protect patient privacy, secures health information*. Retrieved from http://www.hhs.gov/news/press/2013pres/01/20130117b.html

HHS.gov. (n.d.). *Summary of the HIPAA security rule*. Retrieved September 18, 2010, http://www.hhs.gov/ocr/privacy/hipaa/understanding/srsummary.html

HIMSS Analytics. (2014). *EMR Adoption Model*. Retrieved from http://www.himssanalytics.org/hc_providers/emr_adoption.asp

Kohn L. T., Corrigan J. M., & Donaldson M. S. (Eds.), *To err is human: Building a safer health system*. (2000). Retrieved http://www.nap.edu/catalog/9728.html#toc

Liang, L. (2007). The gap between evidence and practice. *Health Affairs*, *26*(2), w119–w121.

Mathematica Policy Research, Harvard School of Public Health & Robert Woods Johnson Foundation. (2013). *Health information technology in the United States: Better information systems for better care, 2013*. Retrieved http://www.rwjf.org/en/research-publications/find-rwjf-research/2013/07/health-information-technology-in-the-united-states-2013.html

National Coordinating Council for Medication Error Reporting and Prevention. (2014). *National coordinating council for medication error reporting and prevention*. Retrieved from http://www.nccmerp.org/

Recovery.gov. (2014). *The recovery act*. Retrieved from http://www.recovery.gov/

The Commonwealth Fund. (2011, June 23). *Quality matters: Innovations in health care quality improvement*. Retrieved from http://www.commonwealthfund.org/publications/newsletters/quality-matters/2011/june-july-2011/in-focus

The Joint Commission. (2013, June 18). *The official "do not use" list of abbreviations*. Retrieved from http://www.jointcommission.org/facts_about_the_official_/

The Office of the National Coordinator for Health Information Technology (ONC). (2014, October). *Update on the adoption of health information technology and related efforts to facilitate the electronic use and exchange of health information*. Retrieved from http://www.healthit.gov/sites/default/files/rtc_adoption_and_exchange9302014.pdf

Thune, J., Alexander, L., Roberts, P., et al. (2013, April 16). *Rebook: Re-examining the strategies needed to successfully adopt Health IT*. Retrieved from http://www.amia.org/sites/amia.org/files/EHR-White-Paper.pdf

CHAPTER 18

Design Considerations for Healthcare Information Systems

OBJECTIVES

After studying this chapter, you will be able to:

1. Compare the systems life cycle with the nursing process.
2. Discuss the role of the superuser in the systems life cycle.
3. Discuss how a business continuity plan mitigates risk.

KEY TERMS

Big-bang conversion	Initiating	Return on investment (ROI)
Bugs	Needs assessment	Rollback
Business continuity plan	Parallel conversion	Rollout
Context-sensitive help	Phased conversion	Scope creep
Contingency plan	Pilot conversion	Superuser
Controlling	Project goal	Systems life cycle
Debugging	Project requirements	Test scripts
Disaster recovery	Project scope	Vanilla product
Executing	Regression testing	Vaporware
Go-live	Request for information (RFI)	Workflow analysis
Implementation	Request for proposal (RFP)	

Healthcare information system existence began with formalized healthcare. As the complexity of healthcare has grown, so has the complexity of information. Patients see many providers and have records in many places. The electronic health record (EHR) incentive program and meaningful use requirements of the Health Information Technology for Economic and Clinical Health (HITECH) Act prompted care providers, hospitals, and critical access hospitals to either change from a paper record or change from an older electronic system to a new HIS that is certified for data exchange (meaningful use and EHR certification are discussed in Chapter 17). This chapter focuses on design concepts that must be considered when implementing a new electronic system including workflow redesign, technical competencies of the users, project management principles, the systems life cycle, and a business continuity plan.

WORKFLOW REDESIGN

The need for workflow redesign when making a change from the paper record or from an older system to a newer clinical information system (CIS) cannot be emphasized enough. In contrast to the paper record environment where forms were often designed for the care providers, the electronic system focuses on the *patient* with collaborative information sharing patient data among the care providers. This means that workflow redesign has to consider the patient, the work done by all the care providers, and organizational needs, not just nursing needs. All participants in the design and implementation process must carefully listen to users' perceptions about the impact of a system implementation, recognize barriers to change, and identify strategies to work through the barriers. Lack of a thoughtful and focused redesign process will be inevitably result in a new system that is plagued with problems.

One approach for workflow redesign is to use the same method as we do for patient problems: identify the purpose, goals, and expected outcomes. The workflow redesign should be orchestrated by a multidisciplinary committee, which first identifies what an automated system is expected to accomplish. The committee should also establish broad goals and maintain compliance with standard setting organization requirements and rules and laws of regulatory agencies. The design of an efficient workflow process must include documentation of patient care, creation of reports, electronic prescribing of medications, and computerized provider order entry (CPOE).

Workflow redesign is not for the faint-hearted. It requires a tremendous amount of work and collaboration between the various discipline members. Without that communication, the work could easily be compared to the Chinese parable about the blind men and the elephant. According to the parable, each blind man touched a different part of the elephant and came away believing that the part he touched represented the big picture. If the blind men had communicated what part of the elephant they were describing, they would have had a much richer picture of the true representation of an elephant. An example of a complex process in healthcare is the redesign of the paper medication administration record (MAR) to create the electronic version (eMAR).

In the paper record world, the MAR is used primarily by the nurse or medical secretary to record medication information and by the nurse when administering medications. In contrast, the eMAR is used by multiple disciplines. The physician uses it to order medications, the pharmacists use it to review/verify the orders and dispense the medications, and the nurses use it to organize their care for a group of patients and to document medication administration. Staggers et al. (2007), in their study to identify critical online medication tasks for acute care, described some of the challenging issues associated with medication administration. For example, nurses often chart data associated with a medication, such as a pulse when administering digoxin and a blood sugar when administering insulin. In addition, nurses chart sites where injections were given. When carefully designed, the eMAR can guide the nurse in organizing medication administration and facilitate documentation of this complex process.

Workflow design must also address inconsistencies within the organization. For example, Detwiller and Petillion (2014) found inconsistencies for the Interior Health CIS. The Interior Health is a health authority in British Columbia, Canada. Inconsistencies included naming differences for radiology and laboratory tests, as well as diet types and textures. There were also process variances for programs and support services. Some programs used paper processes and others used electronic processes. The experience shared for the Interior Health CIS demonstrates the importance of workflow design addressing the details. Healthcare has a tremendous number of details that must be addressed to assure patient safety.

CISs allow for the construction of critical pathways. Critical pathways provide a foundation for multidisciplinary documentation that focuses on the attainment of a specific clinical outcome within a defined length of time, which is a concept that should be under consideration when redesigning workflow. The pathway identifies the patient-desired outcomes. The criteria required for their achievement are predetermined by representatives of the multidisciplinary groups involved in the care of patients with a particular diagnosis. The development of the critical path is based on a review of the literature and a synthesis of findings. The structure of the path allows for the documentation of assessment elements, interventions, patient response to interventions, and coordination of documentation by all disciplines. The Agency for Healthcare Research and Quality (AHRQ, 2013) has resources online for developing critical paths (see Critical Path Method, at http://healthit.ahrq.gov/health-it-tools-and-resources/workflow-assessment-health-it-toolkit/all-workflow-tools/critical-path-method).

TECHNOLOGY COMPETENCIES

All users of computerized CISs must have effective technology competencies. Examples of computer competencies for clinicians include basic desktop software, documentation, and communication: the types of competencies discussed in this textbook. Nurses must understand that they must invest the time to learn how to use the technology (Kellermann & Jones, 2013). Leadership should address technology competencies, computer literacy, and keyboarding skills long before implementing a computerized system from a paper system. It may take a couple of years to plan and install a system; during that time, the staff should attend workshops and classes to gain the necessary skills. In a hospital setting, leadership should foster skill-learning activities by encouraging the nursing units to develop intranet web pages and to use e-mail for communication.

In a provider office setting, all providers and staff should assist with planning and training for a new system. An example of what not to do is from the following experience shared by a family nurse practitioner (FNP). The FNP stated that the physician owner in an office where she worked independently selected an electronic medical record (EMR) for the practice. The physician completed the training in <1 week. The FNP and staff received no training. After the system was installed, the learning curve was so steep when making the transition that the FNP quit the job.

Many healthcare agencies administer computer competency tests to assess learning needs of employees. The types of competency tests vary widely from self-assessments to timed, proctored quizzes. The 2009 TIGER (Technology Informatics Guiding Education Reform) report includes numerous informatics competencies educational resources (TIGER, 2009). A nursing informatics website, Nursing-Informatics.com, contains links to a variety of tutorials and skills self-assessments.

Because employees with low skill levels may feel intimidated by testing environments, it is very important to communicate that the purpose for the use of competency assessment tools is supportive rather than punitive. Computer games might be a strategy for the development of hand–eye motor skills necessary for using a mouse. See Table 18-1 for a listing of resources that can assist

TABLE 18-1 Resources for Technology Skills Development	
Name	Where to Locate
Solitaire or Spider Solitaire	Type "Solitaire" or "Spider Solitaire" into a search engine
Typing Game	http://www.freetypinggame.net/
GCFLearnFree	http://www.gcflearnfree.org/
Nursing-Informatics.com	http://www.nursing-informatics.com/
Others	Type "free typing practice" or "using mouse skills" into a search engine

users in developing technology skills. There are free websites with online lessons that allow users to learn about computers and to gain competency with how to use a computer and software, such as the operating system, e-mail, word processing, and spreadsheets. GCFLearnFree.org sponsored by Goodwill Community Foundation International is free and includes online lessons that are enhanced with videos.

Leadership should support the nursing staff as they gain the computer-necessary competencies (Huryk, 2010, p. 610). Experienced nurses with little or no computer competencies may require significant support because they must revisit the role of a novice. Asking nurses to revisit the change theory concepts (see Chapter 16 for more information on change theories) may be a way to heal any feelings of inadequacy and discomfort. Although abuse of computer privileges is unlikely, if it occurs, it should be addressed the same way as other performance issues such as time and attendance are addressed—with enforcement of policies and procedures and with individual counseling.

NEED FOR INTEROPERABILITY

In healthcare, one or two services or departments may adopt a health information technology (HIT) solution long ahead of others. As an example, HIT was used by laboratory systems and admissions departments for several decades prior to use for care delivery and documentation. The EHR should be able to share data among healthcare agencies. HIT problems do not begin to surface until the systems "bump into each other" because the systems cannot talk to one another; that is, they are not interoperable. Today, EHRs should be able to share data with other systems in order to realize the cost–benefits for use (Apfield et al., 2014). Interoperability (the ability to share data, as noted above) is a goal of the HITECH Act for EHRs. (For a full discussion of interoperability, see Chapter 14.)

Consider the following possible scenario: The facility where you work is thinking about buying a new documentation system (let's call it System A). System A is currently in use in outpatient areas, but inpatient areas are on another system (System B), and ER and surgery use other products (Systems C and D). In such a case, because inpatient and outpatient information needs are vastly different, the two types of systems may not to "talk" with each other. As a result, nurses may need to use different passwords and learn to use two or more systems while also delivering complex patient care. When looking up patient visits, nurses may need to query the systems independently. An example of a common problem is that the patient is seen in the emergency department (ED) and data are entered into the ED information system. When the patient is admitted to the hospital using a different CIS, the information has to be summarized or documented again by using the acute care documentation system. Another example is that when the hospital-discharged patient is followed up in an outpatient clinic, the outpatient clinic might not be able to access the inpatient data from the outpatient information system.

In another scenario, as of 2013, the immunization registry for the state of Colorado was not compatible with the computer systems used by care providers (Whitney, 2013). As a result, providers were not updating the registry, and documentation required a double entry—once in the provider's computer system and another in the state's immunization registry. Therefore, the registry was not a reliable source of information to make decisions about whether a vaccine was missed. This problem should be ameliorated once the state HIE, provider computer, and immunization systems can share data as a part of meaningful use Stage 2, discussed in Chapter 17.

HEALTH IT SYSTEM COST–BENEFITS

This next section discusses cost–benefit as a component of the systems life cycle. However, given the recent changes in adoption of health IT as a result of the HITECH Act, background on the subject is important. A research report by Hillestad et al. (2005) estimated that health IT adoption could save more than 81 billion annually. That savings has not yet occurred. According to Kellermann and Jones (2013), annual expenditures on healthcare grew from $2 trillion in 2005 to $2.8 trillion in 2013.

Because the incentives for EHR adoption affect eligible physicians, hospitals, and critical access hospitals, it is important to understand the cost issues for providers as well as others who are adopting EHRs. Many providers who adopted systems found soon afterward that they needed to replace the EHR because of mergers, acquisitions, and/or lack of support or organizational relationships to groups/hospitals (Kosiorek, 2014). Furthermore, physicians state the systems cost too much and negatively impact patient care (McBride, 2014). A survey conducted by Medical Economics reported that 70% of physicians stated that purchase of the EHR was not worth the costs (Verdon, 2014). It is possible that the physicians did not have clear expectations when selecting an EHR, did not receive appropriate training, or did not have the knowledge and experience to make purchase choices for computers and equipment. The take home point is that cost is an extremely important factor that must be considered when making an initial purchase or a change to a new system.

PROJECT MANAGEMENT AND THE SYSTEMS LIFE CYCLE

Project Management

Project management is an essential skill of the informatics nurse specialist. The term refers to the management of a project from start to finish. It requires excellent communication and team-building skills, organizational planning, and time and resource management. To identify project management software solutions, go to Project-Management.com at http://project-management.com/ or conduct a Web search.

Some healthcare agencies contract out or hire professional certified project managers to assure project success. The systems life cycle is the backbone for project management. The Project Management Institute (http://www.pmi.org) publishes the Project Management Body of Knowledge (PMBK), an excellent resource for learning more about project management and the systems life cycle.

Systems Life Cycle

The term **systems life cycle** refers to the process that begins with the conception of a system until the system is implemented. According to Bernard (2009, p. 70), "the purpose of IT systems

life cycle is to optimize technology deployments for performance, efficiency and cost containment, including the costs of maintaining the networks and systems and even user training." The systems life cycle is analogous to the nursing process because it begins with assessment, has multiple places for iteration, and ends with evaluation (Figure 18-1). Like the nursing process, it never really ends because changes can be made as a result of evaluation findings; thus, a new cycle begins. Unlike the nursing process, the wording and number of steps involved differ according to the agency or author. To provide consistency in the use of terminology across an organization, healthcare agencies often provide glossaries and templates for users. One example is the Duke University Project Management website (http://oit.duke.edu/enterprise/project-mgt/) that includes a glossary, templates, and flow charts (Duke Office of Information Technology, n.d.).

Step 1: Initiating

Every system begins with an idea. In the **initiating** phase, project planners identify and analyze the project goals and needs (requirements). This first phase is a critical step. Many system implementation failures can be attributed to a poor needs assessment. All system stakeholders must be a part of this process, not just the information systems personnel. A **stakeholder** is anyone who has something to gain or lose from a project. Examples of stakeholders include the healthcare agency's top executives, nursing executives, financial personnel, nursing clinicians, and any other personnel who may need to use the system.

Project Goals and Scope

The first task in initiating the process is to identify the project goal. The **project goal** is a succinct statement that describes the project. Goals should be specific and measurable. Instead of using the term project goal, some references use the term project definition (Box 18-1).

The next task is to define the **project scope**, which refers to all the elements that are entailed in the project. For example, a project scope may address the implementation of an electronic documentation in the emergency department or it may entail deployment of electronic documentation throughout the entire hospital. **Scope creep** is a term that describes unanticipated growth of the

Systems Life Cycle

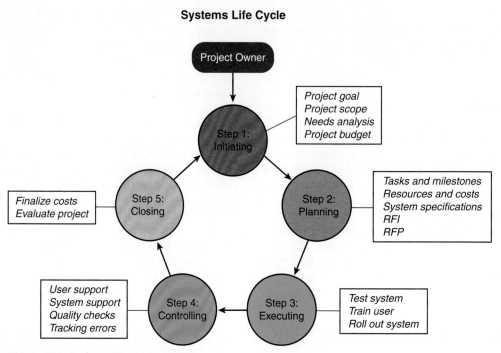

Figure 18-1. Systems life cycle.

project. It can develop because of "we don't miss what we never had" situations. Once the users understand that a database or new system can manage information more effectively, they often specify new requirements, causing the scope of the project to creep (get larger). The problem with scope creep is that time and resources add up to money. Scope creep can cause project budget overruns.

Project Requirements

The **project requirements** stage involves using a needs assessment to identify the expectations or requirements of the system. In this part of the cycle, data and information pertinent to the project goal and scope are put together and translated to the needs for the system. The team identifies which features are essential to the new system and which are nice to have. At this point, a team member may go back to the clinicians and ask them to differentiate their needs from their wants. Some teams use a rating scale to determine the necessity of a feature, with patient safety features being given a higher priority.

The **needs assessment** is comparable to a brainstorming session. Questions that should be addressed include the following:

- Why do we want an information system?
- What do we want the system to do?
- Do we need to communicate with another department?
- Are system-generated alerts required?
- What information do we record in the patient record?
- Do we need to print reports?
- Of all the system "wants," which are essential needs and which are nice to have?

As a comparison, think about your needs assessment process when purchasing an automotive vehicle. Considerations for making a purchase

---

BOX 18-1 Example Project Goal Statements

- Implement computerized patient order entry, CPOE, by December 1, 2015.
- Implement computerized documentation in the ED by April 1, 2016.

would include the amount of money you have to spend, the expected number of passengers, and when and why you want to use the vehicle. Gas consumption may be another consideration—whether there is a cost–benefit in purchasing a hybrid. Service should be important. You would want to consider the reputation and reliability of the service department, the cost of oil changes, and routine maintenance. In the process of making a purchase decision, the buyer usually reads news reports and compares auto manufacturers, vehicle types, and auto dealers.

Likewise, project management team members must consider all the factors considered for the purchase of a vehicle when selecting an information system: the reason for the purchase, what the system needs to accomplish, and the alternatives available. When reviewing the alternatives, decision makers must consider the alternatives that best meet their requirements, the experiences of other users, and the type and reliability of service. This detailed analysis is done to determine the **return on investment (ROI)** and cost–benefit analysis. ROI is the cost savings that are realized. (ROI is discussed in more detail in Chapter 19.) **Cost–benefit** analysis is an examination of the difference between the projected revenues and expenses (Investopedia, 2015).

The needs assessment for an HIS is similar to a vehicle purchase. All participants in the needs assessment process must do their homework. A list of possible vendor products should be determined. This is often done by using word of mouth, reading news reports, reading journal article reports, and Listserv communication. A **request for information (RFI)** with a summary of the information is sent to vendors. Information from the return of the RFI is used to determine which vendors should be considered. Vendor products should be compared by using a tool such as a matrix. In doing so, participants must understand the IT terminology.

The time and quality of a needs assessment can make or break the success of system implementation. A **request for proposal (RFP)** is a detailed document sent to potential vendors asking for information on how their product will meet the users' needs. The document should be a list that that the vendor can answer using yes/no including

information about customization and future releases (Hunt et al., 2004). A well-written RFP allows the users to compare products effectively. It has three parts—one that describes the method and deadline for responses, one that describes the organization, and one with a listing of details of expectations such as requirements, training, and support.

HIS project requirements refer to needs, such as the following:

- Schedule, design, and budget constraints
- The number of system users
- The department(s) that will use the system
- The type of application, for example, desktop application or enterprise application
- Where the software and data will reside
- How and where the data are backed up
- Requirements for system redundancy (if one system fails, another system takes over seamlessly)
- The type and availability of system support

Every project involves risks; the project development team should always carefully explore risks and never minimize them when identifying project requirements. Risks are all those things that could interfere with the success of the project. They include personnel, finances, equipment, interoperability issues, training, security, and time issues.

Step 2: Planning

Planning is the second step in the systems life cycle. This critical phase requires a detailed assessment of the current processes including workflow analyses, timelines, and the implied changes of the new processes. Effective planning can breed trust and confidence among the users and team members.

Analysis of Workflow

Workflow analyses are critical components of the planning phase. A **workflow analysis** analyzes and depicts how work is accomplished. Each nursing task has a distinct workflow. It is important to analyze workflow in the paper record system (or legacy electronic system), and then, project work might best be accomplished using the new electronic system. As an example, consider the workflow that begins with:

- A physician's medication order and ends with the medication administration of digoxin
- Administering intravenous Lasix and ends with the documentation of the drug
- Checking a blood glucose level, subsequently administering a combination of NPH and regular insulin, and ends with the documentation of the procedures

The process for "who" does what, when, and how differs for each example. The "it depends" has to be considered. In the first example, it depends on how the physician's order was written. Was it written by the physician or was it a verbal or phone order? If the order was written on the paper chart, did a medical secretary or a nurse transcribe the order?

An effective way to visualize what happens is to diagram the activity. Project planners can diagram the activity using drawing tools in any program that includes the use of drawing shapes such as OpenOffice.org Draw, Microsoft PowerPoint, or specialized software, such as Microsoft Visio. A process flow diagram uses special symbols to convey a certain meaning. For example, the oval shape is used to convey the start and stop processes, the rectangle shape indicates a process, and the diamond shape indicates a decision (Figure 18-2).

Selecting a System

Selecting a system is one of the most daunting decisions for the stakeholder committee members. Healthcare organization enterprise solutions have the potential of improving or disrupting the complex care delivery process. There are significant financial investments ranging from thousands of dollars to multiple millions of dollars. Project

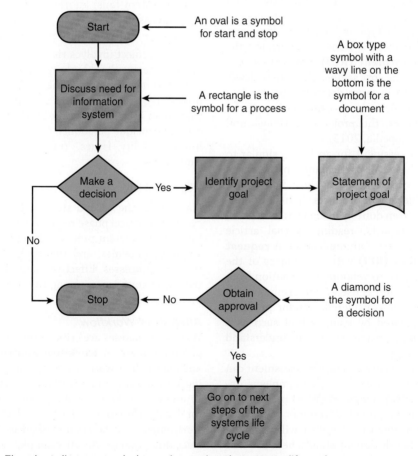

Figure 18-2. Flowchart diagram symbol meanings using the systems life cycle.

planners can mitigate the risks of making a mistake using a structured process, effective risk and needs analyses, and careful product investigation.

The selection member participants must educate themselves to be able to make an informed decision. Participants should investigate pertinent literature. Journals with comprehensive pertinent articles include *CIN* (*Computers Informatics Nursing*), *JAMIA* (*Journal of the American Medical Informatics Association*), the *Journal of Healthcare Information Management*, and the *International Journal of Medical Informatics*.

Nursing participants should consider membership in nursing informatics professional organization and stay abreast of common issues and concerns using informatics Listservs. Nurses should network with other system users and attend professional informatics education sessions, such as HIMSS and American Medical Informatics Association. It is important for the selection committee not to be overly dependent on the vendor's advice. Vendors are in the business of making money, and they are trained to market their product to make sales. They have been known to minimize system weaknesses.

Be cautious about vendors' promises of upcoming new features or product releases. Broken promises of computer system products are known as **vaporware**. The selection committee members should also make site visits to interview others. Before selecting sites to visit, it is important to talk with several agencies and listen to both good and bad features. No system is perfect, and the success of a system may have as much to do with the agency as the vendor. Although the vendors often arrange the visits, users should make sure that they candidly speak with other users without the vendor's presence. During a site visit, talking with clinical users as well as with information system personnel and those in leadership positions will provide the most knowledge.

The site visitation team should include several potential users, not just IT services or administrative personnel. Using a list of prepared questions for all visits allows users to make comparisons between the different sites. Visitors should see the system in operation. The staff nurse may be a part of the visitation team or may be demonstrating

the system from the host site. In either position, the selection team must be open-minded and both listen carefully to what is said and be attuned to what is not said. The nurse demonstrating the system at the host site should be honest and fair in discussing the system.

Step 3: Executing

The third stage of the systems life cycle is **executing** the system. This phase involves customizing the system to meet the needs of the organization. The system is tested to make sure that it works as planned. Once there is agreement that the system meets the user requirements, the staff members are trained and the system is implemented (called a **rollout**).

System Design and Testing

Once the system is selected, the next step is to customize the system design so that it is compatible with the user requirements. Typically, the vendor will provide the user with a standard product, sometimes known as a **vanilla product**. It is similar to the standard desktop computer that the buyer can customize with additional features such as additional memory or an extra monitor. Just as in the customization of a desktop computer, extra features come at an additional fee.

During the system design phase, system documentation must be developed. It is an important feature started in the planning phase and continued with each change made in the system. Some vendors provide "canned" or standardized data entry objects and output boxes, while others allow unlimited customization by the customer. The decision to build your own or take what you get should be made in the very early stages of the vendor selection and discovery process. The need for up-to-date and complete system documentation that flows with the user processes cannot be overemphasized.

The testing phase is just one of many critical phases that must be addressed intently before the system is implemented. System errors and issues, commonly called **bugs**, must be identified and addressed. The process of correcting the errors is called **debugging**. The testing of the new system is ongoing, during, and after the system build. The testing needs to include features and expected functionality of the system, hardware, backups, downtime, restarts, data capture and storage, and network communication.

Application functionality is often referred to as **regression testing** and interfaces, and communication/network functionality is usually called integration testing. A set of situations commonly called scenarios or **test scripts** are devised to depict normal and abnormal events that could occur. Clinicians may be involved in devising the features and functionality scenarios and in the actual testing. Several test scripts should be written for each functional part of the software and for the integration of data across interfaces to ensure consistent quality of output. A test script may not catch everything that does not work as expected, but each time a new issue is discovered, it should be added to the set of scripts. Over the years, a collection of test scripts can become extremely accurate and reduce the issues discovered during implementation. This will improve user acceptance of the system or changes to an existing system and the user's trust and confidence in the IT department. The trust and confidence for IT are imperative for moving the institution forward with an electronic information system.

System **superusers** are identified to assist in the system building and testing. Superusers should be clinical nurses and staff who are recruited from each of the areas where the system will be deployed. Superusers can help sell the other clinicians and assist in later implementation and training. They are invaluable to the success of the implementation phase. The participation of end users in initial testing provides the design team with valuable developmental information. Observation of users during testing highlights training needs. Many times, something that is considered intuitive by the design team may prove confusing for the user.

QSEN Scenario

You volunteered to be a superuser for a new CIS. What are the nurse superuser's unique attributes that contribute to the process of system building and testing?

Training

The need for basic computer training that is uncovered in the needs assessment phase should be met before training for the actual system occurs. Computer literacy issues can be dealt with in separate learning sessions and target only those who need to know instead of planning training with the lowest common denominator of learner in mind. User training is another essential step leading to a successful **go-live** or rollout. Both terms refer to the implementation of a new system. The training sessions should use effective pedagogical teaching/learning theory and methods. (See Chapter 21 for more information about teaching/learning theory.) Training should be done within a few weeks of the system implementation for "just-in-time" learning. If completed too early, without reinforcement, the learning will be forgotten.

Training should be done with the user needs in mind. Many facilities use superusers to assist with the training sessions. A needs assessment may be helpful to identify training resources. An analysis of needs can assist the training developers to create modules that meet the needs of novices to expert computer users. It can also be helpful to identify availability of the staff. Training should also include instructions on how to obtain help for the system. An ideal system will contain **context-sensitive help** or help that is modified based on where in the system help was accessed. Providing online tutorials and video clips on the computer can also assist clinicians to use the system successfully.

During training sessions, end users should take responsibility for learning to use the new system by asking questions and providing feedback on the functionality and features for the system to serve their needs best. Training activities should be viewed as multipurpose activities. The trainer not only teaches intended users how to use a system but also makes determinations about specific support that will be required during the rollout. During the training sessions, security and data accuracy must be addressed. By discussing these issues in the context of system use, the user responsibilities related to security become more meaningful.

A common training mistake is to simply show the user where system features are located and explain how they are used. A better approach is to develop several scenarios or simulation case studies that the clinician experiences on a daily basis so that the user can apply learning. After a brief introduction to the system, the user is allowed to work through the learning modules. Some agencies develop self-learning modules, place them on the nursing unit PCs, and use them in addition to classroom training.

Another mistake is to provide too much information in a single training period. Rather than planning a 4- to 5-hour class, it is better to break the training session down into shorter 1- to 2-hour classes. Learning to use a new computer system can be overwhelming to many. After a short period, the mind can become saturated, evident by restlessness and inattention of the learners.

Implementation

The **implementation** or go-live is a significant milestone. Many agencies build the momentum to that milestone with preparatory "count down the days ..." presentations, memos, and posters. The implementation team may choose to order T-shirts—one color for the trainers and super-users and another for the staff. The celebration often includes a media release to the local newspapers. The implementation is yet another key phase in the systems life cycle. It needs to be carefully planned and implemented. If not done well, the users might be tempted to bypass essential features that were put in place to make patients safer.

Success of the go-live is dependent on the support system. Adequate system and user support are crucial. It may be necessary to schedule additional staff for the first few days or weeks, depending on the number of users affected and the workflow impact. Initially, 24-hour on-site support may be required, with later support provided from a help desk. Vendor support is important in the initial stages of implementation to troubleshoot unforeseen issues and to resolve any issues quickly. The goals should be to have as little disruption in patient care delivery as possible.

Each system implementation plan should have a **contingency plan** for a **rollback**. A rollback refers to backing out of the implementation—the cancellation of the system implementation. The contingency plan should be detailed and address risks of significant implementation problems. Clinicians should not be expected to use a CIS that jeopardizes patient care. If the system is carefully tested prior to implementation and the users are trained and ready, rollback issues are minimized.

There are four main approaches used to implement health information systems: the big-bang approach, pilot conversion, phased conversion, and parallel conversion. There are strengths and weaknesses of each approach. All approaches involve change by very busy health practitioners, and change involving care of patients should never be considered lightly. To optimize the success of any new health information system, nursing leadership and clinical nurses should be involved in the selection, planning, training, and implementation planning processes.

Big-Bang Conversion. The **big-bang conversion** is used when switching from one computer system to another. The entire institution implements the system at the same time. This method can be most disruptive to the clinical setting. It is used most frequently when there is no initial system, the system in use is old, or there is a requirement for implementation on a specific date, such as the beginning of a new fiscal year. As a nonclinical example, many universities are switching from university-run old and failing email systems to a free one provided by Microsoft or Google. When making a switch, the universities use the big-bang approach and migrate all the email accounts at one time. Likewise, healthcare agencies may use the approach when switching CISs. The associated risk and required support for this major transition are dependent on the size of the agency.

Pilot Conversion. The **pilot conversion** is done to "test the waters" to see what issues might occur when making a transition to a new CIS. This approach enables the testing of a system on a smaller scale. For instance, a new documentation system or point-of-care device may be implemented on one care unit for a period of time for the purpose of evaluation. For the overall evaluation to be successful, project planners should establish specific evaluation criteria. The pilot testing should be completed within a defined time period. Project planners might use the pilot conversion when transitioning from the paper chart to an electronic charting system or when switching charting system vendors. Usually, use of pilot implementation helps to determine operational or training needs for future implementation of the system. It involves the least risk.

Phased Conversion. The **phased conversion** is used to bring up a new system gradually in a controlled environment. The phased conversion is done incrementally with several alternative approaches. One is to implement one component of the system to a group of departments throughout the organization. New systems can be phased in on one nursing unit or department at a time. The choice of the initial phased roll area is usually done with the staff members who are most likely to champion the system. The personnel who are implementing the system can learn from training sessions and go-lives and implement that learning in the next phase.

Parallel Conversion. The **parallel conversion** requires the operation and support of the new and the old system for a period of time. The implementation plan normally addresses the specific operational needs and defines the timing of the implementation. Project planners may target certain departments or care units with specific dates for a switchover to the new system. This method allows an organization to allocate resources in an efficient manner. It involves the least risks but increased workload for the users. Training can be done with just those who need to know.

Step 4: Controlling

Controlling is the fourth phase of the systems life cycle. Even the best systems have bugs and issues. System maintenance is an ongoing process. The information system staff members who work on the help desk are key personnel for keeping the system running smoothly. They need to have customer service communication skills and be able to talk using words that the user who is experiencing problems can understand, appreciate the complex role of the clinician, and be able to recognize potential patient safety issues. All issues should be documented, prioritized, and tracked by using a database.

Step 5: Closing

Although evaluation should be a part of every phase of the systems life cycle, there should be a planned evaluation at least 6 months after implementation. Before that, improvements may be difficult to identify because of issues related to adjusting to new methods of working. If a pre-evaluation was done before implementation, comparisons can be made. Clinicians may find changes that would make the system easier to use. In such cases, clinicians should provide a thorough explanation of the needed change and the rationale behind it. In addition to clinician recommendations, issue tracking at the help desk about common problems will lead to the establishment of effective adjustments and system improvements. Established teams and analysts must continually evaluate and deal with identified issues.

BUSINESS CONTINUITY PLAN

Business continuity plan is the term used by IT for **disaster recovery**. Some resources differentiate the two terms, indicating that "business continuity" refers to how to continue IT services in the case of a disruption (Public Safety Canada, 2014) and "disaster recovery" refers to the recovery of IT services after a disaster. Although electronic systems are safer than paper systems, there is still an element of risk that must be addressed with planning. If health information is stored electronically, what are the ramifications of a disaster, such as a tornado, fire, or hurricane destroying an HIS location? Is there off-site storage of the HIS data? What are the ramifications of a pandemic where a significant number of the IT staff are ill and unable to work? What about major equipment failures?

IT, just like nursing services, must have a written plan, equipment, and services that outline actions to manage potential disasters. It includes precautions taken to minimize the loss of data due to a disaster. In the case of a major power outage, it might be use of the backup power supply. In the case of a fire, it might be an automated shutdown of the HIS system before the sprinklers turn on. Other precautions include mirroring the major servers to a remote site. The plan would include procedure to restore mission critical processes as quickly as possible. It would also include how to address data entry after the system is restored.

The Federal Emergency Management Agency (FEMA) provides direction for business continuity planning at Ready.gov (Ready.gov, 2012). The Ready.gov website includes rationale and an overview of the business continuity impact analysis. It also includes worksheets and requirements necessary to complete the process.

SUMMARY

The HITECH Act spurred rapid adoption of healthcare information systems. The importance of design, selection, and implementation of healthcare information systems cannot be overemphasized. The process is complicated because the usability of the systems depends upon many factors. Examples discussed include the details of workflow design, the technology competence of the users, the ability to share data with other systems, and the cost–benefits. Project management guides the process for identifying, selecting, and implementing a system. Project management skills are important for the informatics nurse specialist. Project management addresses the people, equipment, and timeline necessary for successful implementation of a system.

Healthcare agencies need a strategic plan to guide in selecting and implementing necessary information systems. The implementation process for information systems uses a process known as the systems life cycle, which parallels the nursing process. The involvement of end users, such as practicing nurses, in all stages of the systems life cycle is crucial to a successful system implementation. A well-planned and well-implemented system can provide many patient care benefits, including improved efficiency in both documentation and communication. Electronic information systems can also provide aggregated data for use in improving clinical practices. When standardized nursing languages (discussed in Chapter 15) are included in the documentation system, nursing data will be available for unit, institution, and regional uses. Aggregated nursing data have the capacity to demonstrate the values that nursing brings to healthcare.

The business continuity plan is an essential component for maintaining the integrity of patient data in the event of a disaster. It usually includes redundancy of data in an off-site storage center. It also addresses system maintenance in the event of a shortage of personnel. FEMA provides the necessary resources for providers and hospitals to use to create a business continuity plan.

APPLICATIONS AND COMPETENCIES

1. Use drawing word processing or presentation software to draw the process of medication administration, beginning either with the physician's order in the paper record environment or with an electronic information system.

2. Compare the systems life cycle with the nursing process. How are they alike or different?

3. Discuss how the role of the nurse clinician superuser is helpful in the design and implementation of life cycles.

4. Create a lesson plan to use when implementing a clinical documentation system on a nursing unit. Be sure to incorporate concepts of change theory and teaching learning theories.

5. Conduct a search on the topic of business continuity plan for a resource that extends your understanding of the topic. Summarize your findings and cite your source.

REFERENCES

AHRQ. (2013, May). *Critical path method.* Retrieved from http://healthit.ahrq.gov/health-it-tools-and-resources/workflow-assessment-health-it-toolkit/all-workflow-tools/critical-path-method

Apfield, J. C., Jahangir, A., & Sethi, M. K. (2014, October). The lowdown on EMRs. *AAOS Now.* http://www.aaos.org/news/aaosnow/mar13/advocacy1.asp

Bernard, R. (2009). System life cycle planning. *Security Technology Executive, 19*, 68, 70, 72.

Detwiller, M., & Petillion, W. (2014). Change management and clinical engagement: Critical elements for a successful clinical information system implementation. *Computers, Informatics, Nursing, 32*(6), 267–273; quiz 274–265. doi:10.1097/CIN.0000000000000055.

Hillestad, R., Bigelow, J., Bower, A., et al. (2005). Can electronic medical record systems transform health care? Potential health benefits, savings, and costs. *Health Affairs (Millwood)*, *24*(5), 1103–1117. doi:10.1377/hlthaff.24.5.1103.

Hunt, E. C., Sproat, S. B., & Kitzmiller, R. R. (2004). *The nursing informatics implementation guide*. New York, NY: Springer.

Huryk, L. A. (2010). Factors influencing nurses' attitudes towards healthcare information technology. *Journal of Nursing Management*, *18*(5), 606–612. doi:10.1111/j.1365-2834.2010.01084.x.

Investopedia. (2015). Definition of 'cost-benefit analysis'. Retrieved from http://www.investopedia.com/terms/c/cost-benefitanalysis.asp

Kellermann, A. L., & Jones, S. S. (2013). What it will take to achieve the as-yet-unfulfilled promises of health information technology. *Health Affairs*, *32*(1), 63–68.

Kosiorek, D. (2014). Analyze cost, usability features carefully when considering EHR switch. Use the experience your practice gained during its first EHR implementation to make your new system work for you. *Medical Economics*, *91*(3), 39–40, 42–33. Retrieved from http://medicaleconomics.modernmedicine.com/medical-economics/content/tags/cloud-computing/analyze-cost-usability-features-carefully-when-consid

McBride, M. (2014). Measuring EHR pain points: High cost, poor functionality outweigh benefits, ease of access. *Medical Economics*, *91*(3), 28, 30. Retrieved from http://medicaleconomics.modernmedicine.com/medical-economics/content/tags/ehr/measuring-ehr-pain-points-high-cost-poor-functionality-outweigh-b

Public Safety Canada. (2014). A guide to public safety planning. Retrieved from http://www.publicsafety.gc.ca/cnt/rsrcs/pblctns/bsnss-cntnt-plnnng/index-eng.aspx

Ready.gov. (2012). Business continuity plan. Retrieved from http://www.ready.gov/business/implementation/continuity

Staggers, N., Kobus, D., & Brown, C. (2007). Nurses' evaluations of a novel design for an electronic medication administration record. *Computers, Informatics, Nursing: CIN, 25*(2), 67–75. doi: 10.1097/01.NCN.0000263981.38801.be.

Technology Informatics Guiding Education Reform (TIGER). (2014). Informatics competencies for every practicing nurse: Recommendations for the TIGER Collaborative. Retrieved from http://www.thetigerinitiative.org/docs/tigerreport_informaticscompetencies.pdf

Verdon, D. R. (2014). EHRs: The real story. Why a national outcry from physicians will shake the health information technology sector. *Medical Economics*, *91*(3), 18–20, 27. Retrieved from http://medicaleconomics.modernmedicine.com/medical-economics/content/tags/ehr/physician-outcry-ehr-functionality-cost-will-shake-health-informa

Whitney, E. (2013, January 22). *Growing pains as doctors adopt electronic records*. NPR. Retrieved from http://www.npr.org/blogs/health/2013/01/22/169984966/growing-pains-as-doctors-offices-adopt-electronic-records?ft=1&f=1128&sc=tw

CHAPTER 19

Quality Measures and Specialized Electronic Healthcare Information Systems

OBJECTIVES

After studying this chapter you will be able to:

1. Discuss the current trends for clinical information systems meaningful use. Summarize your findings and cite the sources you used.

2. Discuss the pros and cons for the use of best-of-breed versus integrated health information technology solutions.

3. Identify two quality measures that would benefit the nurse who has a voice in the selection of an electronic clinical system.

4. Describe the advantages for the integration of data from pharmacy, laboratory, and radiology information systems with the electronic patient record.

5. Explain why the Leapfrog Group recommends the use of computerized provider order entry.

6. Discuss the factors that impact the management of patient flow in hospitals.

7. Identify at least three factors that would promote the adoption of clinical information systems by nurses.

KEY TERMS

Active RFID

Aggregated data

Best-of-breed

Certification Commission for Healthcare Information Technology (CCHIT)

Clinical decision support system (CDSS)

Closed-loop safe medication administration

Electronic medication administration record (eMAR)

Health information technology (HIT)

Integrated enterprise system

Integrated interface

Mission critical

Passive RFID

Physician Quality Reporting System (PQRS)

Positive patient identifier (PPID)

Radiofrequency identifier (RFID)

The healthcare industry uses a variety of information systems to support and communicate for the delivery of patient care and to manage business operations. As discussed in Chapter 18, healthcare information systems (HISs) are a composite made up of all the information management systems that serve an organization's needs. These include applications that track patients, those that manage financial data associated with the staff payroll and billing for services rendered, and patient care services including nursing, pharmacy, radiology, and laboratory services. In a well-designed system, there is an interface between systems to support the sharing of data so that the data do not have to be reentered. An interface allows for the sharing of data between systems.

Two approaches are used when selecting a vendor system: best-of-breed or integrated solutions. The **best-of-breed** approach refers to the selection of systems that best meet the needs of particular services or departments from different vendors, and it requires building an integrated interface at the institutional level. The **integrated interface** approach refers to the selection of a collection of HISs that are already interfaced; however, the systems may not all be best of breed. An **integrated enterprise system** is an information system designed to meet the needs of the organization at large, which may include multiple geographically separated hospitals and clinics. The purpose of this chapter is to provide some background for quality initiatives and to explore some specific HIS applications.

QUALITY MEASURES FOR HEALTH INFORMATION TECHNOLOGY

Healthcare organizations and care providers who make decisions to purchase **health information technology (HIT)** have several resources available. Clinical nurses and nurse leaders should be familiar with nationally recognized quality measures for HIT. Nurses must also be knowledgeable about innovative reimbursement incentive efforts to reward quality care, such as the Physician Quality Reporting System (PQRS) by the Centers for Medicare and Medicaid Services

(CMS). Nurses, especially if involved in the system selection process, must also understand organizational efforts to address quality care and have the necessary knowledge to judge vendor systems. As an example, vendor system analysis reports might show software components for two different vendor systems to be very similar and equally robust, but the vendor support for planning and implementing the system differs. One vendor may have a better track record of successful implementation of computerized provider order entry (CPOE) than the other.

Physician Quality Reporting System

The President authorized the **Physician Quality Reporting System (PQRS)** in December 2006 when he signed the Tax Relief and Health Care Act of 2006 (CMS.gov, 2014a). The purpose of the CMS initiative was to provide financial incentives to eligible providers for cost-effective high-quality care. PQRS uses incentive payments for quality reporting and payment adjustments for unsatisfactory reporting. Detailed information about PQRS is available online at CMS website.

Historically, our healthcare delivery system paid for the number of patients served and the number of resources consumed. There were no financial incentives to improve care—just moral and ethical ones. Hospitals that worked on decreasing patient care costs by decreasing the length of stay and reducing the number of unnecessary tests and medications lost revenue. In other words, the healthcare system rewarded poor care.

The PQRS is voluntary for all fee-for-service providers who bill Medicare Part B, including nurse practitioners, clinical nurse specialists, and certified nurse midwives. As an incentive, qualified participants receive a bonus of approximately 2% (may vary by year) of the revenue, subject to a cap. A collaborative effort of the Physician Consortium for Performance Improvement, convened by the American Medical Association, the National Committee for Quality Assurance, and specialty medical associations, identified the evidence-based quality measures used for reporting. The quality measures address care classifications such as advanced care planning, perioperative care, medication reconciliation, imaging, and screening for fall risk. Participants are asked to include information on the use of electronic health records (EHRs) and electronic subscribing.

EHR Certification

The original purpose of certification was to standardize EHR systems to allow extraction of data for meaningful use. Certification is a quality measure to ensure interoperability and healthcare data communication. Certification programs were developed specifically to meet the requirements of ONC-ACB (the Office of the National Coordinator-Authorized Certification Bodies), set forth by the Health Information Technology for Economic and Clinical Health (HITECH) Act. The National Institute of Standards and Technology (NIST) must recognize certification programs used for EHRs. NIST developed the testing tools, test cases, procedures, and test data for interoperability required to meet meaningful use objectives.

The **Certification Commission for Healthcare Information Technology (CCHIT)** pioneered the certification process for the US government. In 2014, CCHIT took a strategic direction to provide assistance to healthcare providers and vendors attempting to meet the HIT regulations. There was a mass volume of vendor EHRs (CCHIT, 2014) that required certification. CCHIT made the strategic direction change to assist many vendor EHRs to meet meaningful use objectives.

HIT Research and Analysis Reports

Many companies specialize in researching HIT solutions to assist healthcare providers and institutions making purchase solutions. The research reports also serve to assist vendors make decisions for modifying their systems to meet market needs. Considering the millions of dollars involved in adopting new systems, the use of research findings to select a solution makes great sense. Examples of vendor research companies include HIMSS Analytics (http://www.himss-analytics.org/) and KLAS (http://klasresearch.com/). HIMSS Analytics, a nonprofit organization associated with HIMSS, provides benchmarking reports based on provider information. (HIMSS Analytics is discussed in more detail in Chapter 20.) KLAS provides reports based on information

from providers who rate the systems. Both HIMSS Analytics and KLAS offer provider participants the results of their reports at no charge.

SPECIALTY HEALTHCARE INFORMATION SYSTEMS

Take a moment to think about all the different services that are necessary to deliver patient care. Even within the nursing department, there are various services including nursing administration, intensive care units, surgery, and postanesthesia care. It is no different for any other discipline service in a hospital, such as the laboratory and radiology. Each of those smaller services has a specialized information need, but most or all share two common needs: access to the patient electronic record and the ability to send charges to the financial management department. When healthcare providers select a system, they weigh the options for best-of-breed solutions, which serve as the best solution for a specialized service or they choose a vendor package that provides an integrated enterprise solution to meet the needs of many or all the services. This section addresses just a few of the many specialty HISs.

Admission, Discharge, and Transfer

The admission, discharge, and transfer (ADT) system was one of the first information systems used in healthcare. It is the backbone of the clinical and business portion of most hospital systems. In the early years, ADT systems were standalone best-of-breed systems with an interface to financial systems; however, ADT is now also a common part of integrated enterprise solutions. This application provides and tracks patient details, such as demographics and insurance information, medical record numbers, care providers, and next of kin. All patient interactions are tracked or linked to this basic information. Laboratory results find their way to the appropriate provider or care area based on the important information contained in this portion of the information system. It is important, therefore, that the data in this system should be updated and verified on a regular basis.

Financial Systems

Financial systems are another distinct application in the HIS. They are considered by some as the second backbone of the system because they track financial interactions and provide the fiscal reporting necessary to manage an institution. Financial systems are **mission critical**, which means that the services are vital to the existence of the organization. A few functions of financial systems are to ensure a higher collection rate from payers, to expedite payments for accounts receivable, to minimize third-party payer denials of care, and to prevent underpayment for care.

The problem that many healthcare organizations are facing today is how to get their legacy financial system to communicate with the clinical information system (CIS). Some of the systems in use date back several decades and are not able to meet the demands of regulators and consumers. To avoid building costly interfaces at the institutional level, some healthcare organizations choose to purchase systems that include financial systems, but it is an expensive proposition that costs in the hundreds of millions of dollars range. The integration of the two systems is necessary for efficient billing and to allow for process improvement analysis.

Providers and healthcare agencies recognize the challenges of being able to stay in business and meeting the requirements of regulators and payers. Besides the billing and reimbursement from third-party payers, consumers want to know their out-of-pocket expenses prior to checking into the hospital. Providers and hospitals want to be able to bill Medicare without being accused of fraud. Unfortunately, EHR technology does make it easier to commit fraud (Levinson, 2014). Two examples of EHR features that make fraud easier are the copy/paste function and the ability to over-document. Copy/paste-type frauds occur when the provider does not verify information for accuracy. Overdocumentation fraud occurs when there is incorrect or irrelevant documentation that suggests services were rendered but they were not.

Unfortunately, fraud accusations—true or not—are in the news daily. As an example, a New Jersey physician received fraudulent reimbursement from Medicaid by billing personal services performed by three people with no medical licenses (Bowman, 2010). An Illinois cardiologist went to prison for fraud after receiving $13 million from Medicare and 30 other private and public insurance programs for services he never rendered (Yin, 2010). He accessed insurance information on patients without their knowledge and hired others to bill for fake services. To place the gravity of the fraud matter in perspective, the costs for Medicare and Medicaid in 2009 were $54 billion. In 2010, CMS initiated a program that uses auditors and high-tech computer software to scan Medicare and Medicaid records for bogus claims (Versel, 2010). The anticipated savings are 2 billion dollars over a 3-year period.

The initiative is clearly only a dent in the rampant fraud problem. In 2013, 74% of Medicaid criminal convictions were cases of fraud. There were 1,197 criminal indictments and 991 criminal convictions (CMS.gov, 2014b). Medicaid Fraud Control Unit (MFCU) was able to recover almost $1 billion for all fraud. An example of a criminal case occurred in New York where the owner of several pharmacies submitted false claims totaling $7.7 million (CMS.gov, 2014b; MFCU, 2013). His sentence included a 3-year prison term with a requirement to pay back to the New York Medicaid Program the money he stole.

CLINICAL INFORMATION SYSTEMS

CISs are a conglomerate of integrated and interoperable information systems and technologies that provide information about patient care. The core information systems are the ancillaries: laboratory, radiology, and pharmacy. The build of the clinical documentation system uses data from the core ancillary systems. Other components of the CIS are the CPOE, the **electronic medication administration record (eMAR)**, and positive patient identifier (PPID) systems, such as the barcoded medication administration system.

CIS vendors, like other software companies, continuously work to improve the quality of their products. They make the improvements available as version releases and as major upgrades. Major upgrades are usually associated with a fee and may require equipment upgrades. Major software upgrades could also introduce new software bugs. For these reasons and others, healthcare institutions may choose not to make software changes. On the other hand, nurses who are critical of a certain CIS need to be aware that their concerns may be related to the version of software, not the manufacturer.

Ancillary Systems

The laboratory and radiology systems provide a means of storing and viewing clinical testing and diagnostic patient information. Laboratory systems, one of the earliest clinical systems, have been in use by small and large hospitals for several decades. Laboratory systems integrate data from all the standard laboratory departments including hematology, chemistry, microbiology, blood bank, and pathology. Radiology systems integrate data from patient diagnostic and therapeutic services, including the picture archiving and communication system (PACS). The PACS allows for digital versions of all diagnostic images, such as x-rays and magnetic resonance images, to be stored in the electronic patient record. The pharmacy system provides a means for stocking and recording medications dispensed by the pharmacy. The three ancillary information systems provide a foundation for other clinical systems.

Clinical Documentation

Clinical documentation applications are available in various formats. A good documentation system, whether for nursing or another discipline, is part of the clinical workflow and supports the communication of real-time information. Clinical documentation software is designed by using rules so that when the assessment data with abnormal values, such as a pulse rate or blood pressure, are entered, the abnormal values stand out because they are displayed in a different color. A patient list report can help the nurse to manage assignments and workload (Figure 19-1). These systems remove the need to find the paper chart and allow all who use the electronic chart to access information whenever and wherever it is needed.

The design of screens can support assessment documentation by listing systems, or practitioners can be alerted by the system with a pop-up box to complete or verify essential information, such as allergies. Numerical laboratory data, such as a white blood count, hemoglobin, and platelet count, can be displayed in a graph format to visualize trends. Nurses can document medication administration on the eMAR as well as view overdue medications, which are highlighted in red (Figure 19-2). In a well-planned documentation system, there is little need for the entry of free text, although the ability to do so should be maintained for those occasions when there is no place to document the information and a comment is necessary. Many CIS allow use of tablet technology

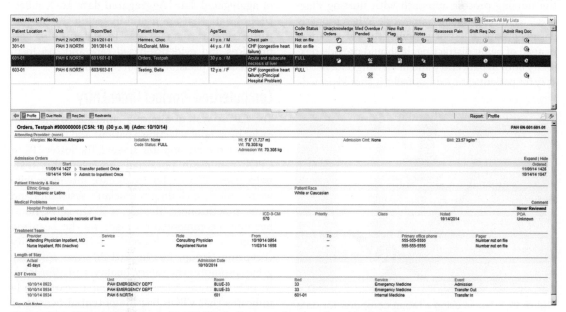

Figure 19-1. Patient list report. (© 2014 Epic Systems Corporation. Used with permission.)

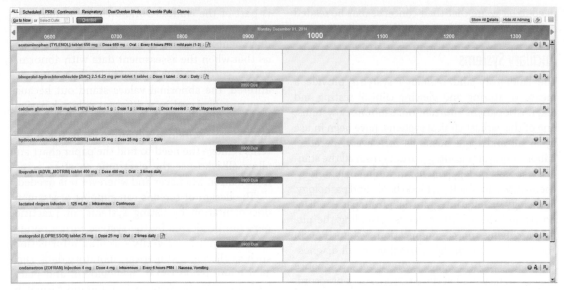

Figure 19-2. eMAR displaying overdue medications. (© 2014 Epic Systems Corporation. Used with permission.)

for data entry at the point of care (Figure 19-3). When these systems work well, it is because the healthcare professionals who use the system were involved in the planning, designing, implementation, and evaluation of the system.

Nursing information systems sometimes use the nursing process approach with nursing diagnoses as the organizing framework. When properly designed, data collection supports clinical workflow instead of being distracting. It should provide flexibility both in data entry and in viewing data necessary for patient care. Additionally, it should provide

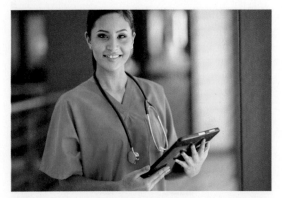

Figure 19-3. Nurse using a tablet computer for data entry (shutterstock.com/michaeljung).

easy access to reference information such as policies and procedures as well as online literature.

Clinical documentation systems should provide for the retrieval of data used in long-range planning and research. The use of clinical data by practicing nurses can be facilitated by easy availability of aggregated data. **Aggregated data** are a collection of data that are useful in seeing the big picture. Aggregate data is useful for determining best practices and evidence-based care and can form the basis for decision support systems.

Computerized Provider Order Entry

The CPOE system allows a clinician to place an order by simply selecting a patient and the needed service from a computer screen. The letter "P" in CPOE can mean physician; however, this textbook uses "P" to refer to all care providers who write orders, including physician's assistants and nurse practitioners. The use of CPOE is the number one recommendation made by the Leapfrog Group to improve patient safety and quality (Leapfrog Group, 2014a, 2014b). The advocacy group promotes the safety, quality, and affordability of healthcare. A Leapfrog Group research study indicates that CPOE has the potential benefit of averting approximately 3 million preventable adverse medication errors (ADEs)—an annual benefit of $7.5 billion dollars per year. According to the Leapfrog Group, one ADE adds an average of $2000 to hospitalization costs, excluding liability insurance claims and lost productivity.

When a provider writes an order by using CPOE, the order is immediately sent to the appropriate department. This saves time, and it prevents transcription errors. Additionally, order entry systems facilitate the capture of financial information for restocking and billing purposes. The advantages attributed to CPOE are electronic prescribing (e-prescribing) and quality improvement (Agency for Healthcare Research Quality, 2012). The use of e-prescribing can reduce errors and improve the quality of care because the medication order is checked against a set of rules, such as allergies, drug dosage, administration routes, frequency of administration, and drug-to-drug interaction, by using **clinical decision support system (CDSS)** information. CDSS is a computer application that uses a complex system of rules to analyze data and presents information to support the decision-making process of the knowledge worker. That is, if a medication order is entered and the dosage exceeds normal limits for that medication, the provider will be given this information. The system should also provide information about any potential drug incompatibilities and patient allergies.

Medication Administration

The use of HIT for medication administration is a process that goes hand-in-hand with CPOE with the purpose of making patient care safer by reducing potential and actual errors. In the paper record world, the medication administration process resided in three record silos—the doctor's order, the pharmacist's verification/dispensing records, and the nurse's administration/paper documentation record. In reality, electronic medication administration is a medication use process addressed with the use of the eMAR.

> ### QSEN Scenario
> The healthcare agency where you are a nurse uses the eMAR and a PPID for closed-loop medication administration. What is your role as a nurse in preventing medication errors?

eMAR

The eMAR, discussed in Chapter 18, is a multidisciplinary record that communicates the complex process of medication use. The implementation of CPOE and CDSS requires the use of the eMAR. The eMAR guides the nurse to use the six rights when administering medications: the right drug, the right dose, the right time, the right route, the right patient, and the right documentation. If well designed, it includes all the pertinent documentation appropriate for the medication that is administered. Because the eMAR can provide a view of information in the database, the nurse can query it to display scheduled medications and medications that are pending, past due, and/or previously administered. The eMAR provides a mechanism for efficient nurse time utilization as well as facilitates the delivery of safe care.

Positive Patient Identifier

A **positive patient identifier (PPID)** uses a bracelet with a barcode to verify the patient's identification. The PPID with bar-coded or **radiofrequency identifier (RFID)**-tagged bracelets is used with the eMAR for **closed-loop safe medication administration**. The term "closed loop" means that the right patient received the right medication, and it is an essential component of patient safety improvements. The Joint Commission first issued a recommendation for accurately identifying patients in 2003. The following year, the U.S. Food and Drug Administration recommended the use of barcodes on patient identification bracelets. Leung et al. (2014) reported that use of barcode technology does improve patient safety associated with medication administration.

The medication administration procedures when using barcoding or **passive RFID** are similar. Both procedures require the use of a barcode or RFID scanner that is either handheld or built into a laptop or tablet computer. The nurses first scan their barcode or RFID tag on their ID badge to identify themselves in the system. Next, the nurses scan the barcode on the medication and finally scan the patient's armband prior to administering the medication (Figure 19-4). If the tag uses **active RFID**, which means that the RFID tag is battery powered and constantly transmitting signals, the use of a scanning device is not necessary,

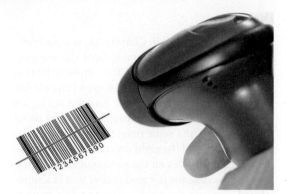

Figure 19-4. Scanning a barcode, which is located on the patient's armband (shutterstock.com/florin oprea).

because the identifier will be recognized by the computer (Thrasher, 2013). The use of active RFID would allow PPIDs without disturbing the patient (e.g., when hanging an intravenous [IV] line while a patient is sleeping). The drawback to active RFID is that it is more expensive than passive RFID.

The outcomes of research on the use of barcoded medication administration (BCMA) with the eMAR are promising. Research at St. Joseph/Candler Health System in Georgia compared medication errors matching nursing units at two tertiary care hospitals that used BCMA with the eMAR (Seibert et al., 2014). The findings of the study indicated that medication error accuracy, when eliminating wrong-time errors, improved at hospital 1 from 92% to 96%, and at hospital 2, accuracy improved from 93% to 96%. Another study researched the use of BCMA and the eMAR in a variety of settings (Leung et al., 2014). The researchers found that use of BCMA and the eMAR essentially eliminated transcription errors. Barcode-assisted dispensing systems reduce dispensing errors by 93% to 96%, as well as reducing potential dispensing errors by 85%.

The complexity of the medication process cannot be overemphasized. CPOE and BCMA are not magic bullets. Examples of factors that facilitate or impede the safe administration of medications include the quality of the workflow analysis, physician verification of current medications, CPOE and BCMA hardware and software, the medication barcode, the barcode on the patient armband, and the process for medication administration. Nurses who find the BCMA impeding the ability to administer medications have been known to use work-arounds

in order to administer medications. However, they may not understand the possible negative consequences and threats to the patient's safety. The results of a study conducted in two large hospitals located in the Midwest and the East coast of the United States revealed 31 types of potential medication errors and 7 types of process work-arounds (Kaplan, 2008; Koppel et al., 2008). The classifications for potential errors were related to technology, tasks, organization, patients, and the environment. The types of workarounds were as follows:

- Scanning the medication without verifying the medication list, drug name, and dose
- Physicians not verifying the eMAR current medication list, resulting in additional medication given to the patient
- Administering the medication without reviewing the parameters for administration
- Bypassing the policy for a check by a second provider or the second nurse confirms without verifying the medication
- Administering medications without reviewing new medication orders
- Administering medications without scanning the patient barcode to confirm the patient's identification
- Administering the medication without scanning the medication barcode to confirm the correct medication, dose, and time

The researchers noted that when patient armband barcodes did not work, nurses often used nonstandard procedure and printed extra copies of the barcode (Kaplan, 2008). Consequently, information management services take efforts to thwart the nonstandard procedures. When workarounds are observed, there must also be an investigation and correction of the issues that impede the safe medication administration process.

MANAGING PATIENT FLOW

Patient flow is a long-standing hospital issue that must be addressed to provide safe and efficient patient care. The problems associated with patient flow are multifactorial and are based on the principle of supply (staffing, hospital beds, and resources) and demand (patients). Hospitals have to operate with nearly full bed capacity for economic efficiency purposes. Staffing, supplies, and resources are budgeted according to the average occupancy. Most hospital budgets have very little flexibility.

The demand for hospital care resources is affected by the aging population, many of whom have chronic diseases such as congestive heart failure, diabetics, and chronic renal disease. This medically fragile population often has acute episodic needs because of their disease processes. As a result, the population is negatively impacted during the annual flu season. Patients expect to be treated at the time of need. If they are unable to see a care provider during office hours, they use emergency services where patient flow problems begin. Emergency beds fill quickly because of the lack of available hospital beds for patients who need to be admitted, causing a patient traffic jam.

The Joint Commission issued a recommendation requiring hospitals to discover and minimize barriers to well-organized patient flow in 2004 and the scoring went into effect on January 1, 2005 (The Joint Commission, 2012). Beginning January 1, 2014, the Joint Commission recommended that emergency department (ED) times not exceed 4 hours to assure patient safety and care quality. The original recommendation resulted from a root cause analyses for sentinel events, which reported that ED overcapacity was a contributing factor in 31% of sentinel event cases (McBeth, 2005). Hospital leaders quickly recognized the difficulty in planning, tracking, and managing patient flow, and as a result, many, especially the large facilities, turned to informatics bed management systems. According to the American Hospital Association (2007, p. 29),

"The goal of bed management is to accurately place the patient in the right unit with the right level of staff and right level of care the first time."

Tracking Systems Solutions

Tracking systems solutions allow hospitals the ability to improve the flow of a patient through the system. The new tracking systems provide for real-time information for patients and staff (Drazen & Rhoads, 2011). A variety of informatics solutions provide real-time location services (RTLS) for patient flow, staffing, and equipment and also provide documentation of time lapses, which is used in the analysis of data and planning.

Of course, like any software solution, leadership must do an analysis of the issues prior to selecting a solution. Software solutions make bad systems worse, not better. MEDHOST, Radianse, Reveal RTLS, McKesson Horizon Enterprise Visibility, and the Versus RTLS all use RFID tags to monitor patient locations (MEDHOST, 2014; McKesson, 2014; Radianse, 2014; Versus Technology, 2014). Features common to many of the popular patient-tracking systems include the visual display of beds, which indicates the patient status (e.g., discharge, fall risk, methicillin-resistant *Staphylococcus aureus* [MRSA]), bed availability display, instant transport notification, and equipment (e.g., wheelchairs and intravenous pumps) locators.

Tracking systems are often used to facilitate patient flow in settings such as the emergency department and clinic settings (Figure 19-5).

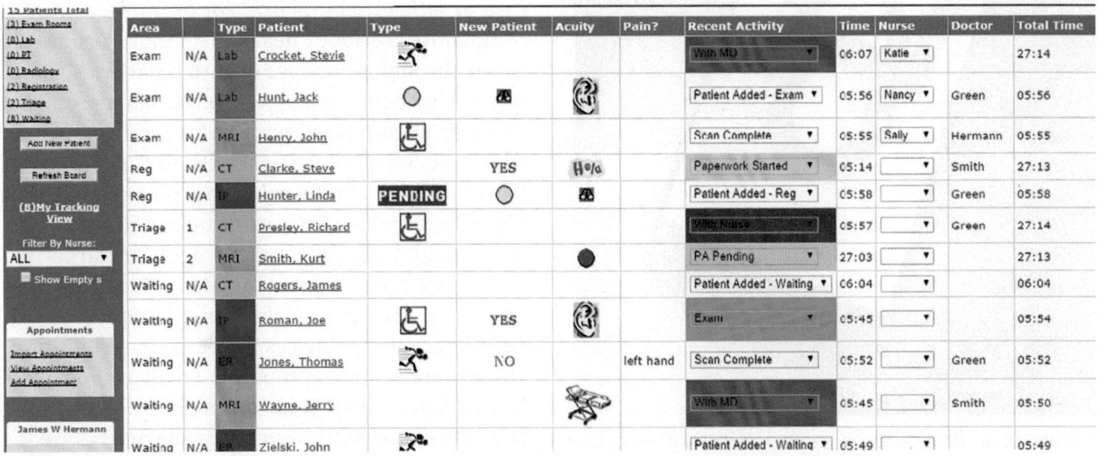

Figure 19-5. PatientTrak.net—a cloud-based service from Lumin Medical LLC. (Used with permission.)

The demand for use of location service technology will continue to increase because as of 2014, CMS core measures included reporting data for the emergency department admission decision time to departure time for admitted patients (National Quality Measures Clearinghouse, 2013; AHRQ, 2011).

In some fast-paced settings, such as perioperative, it is beneficial to track members of the perioperative team to understand workflow. Huynh et al. (2011) developed a Web-based application, POS Trac, for the iPhone/iPod Touch devices. The Web-based application worked on other smartphones, as well. The mobile app allowed team members to record the type of providers, tasks, and interruptions associated with moving the patient through the perioperative system.

Voice Communication Systems

Communication systems facilitate the exchange of information needed by the various healthcare disciplines. Examples include the use of e-mail, Internet, and intranet systems. Although these systems may not be integrated with clinical systems, they enhance information flow within the organization and workflow patterns. They have an indirect impact on clinical practice.

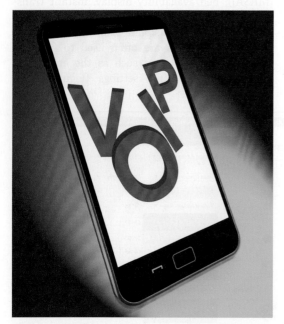

Figure 19-6. Smartphone using VoIP (shutterstock.com/Stuart Miles).

Some suggest that voice-over internet protocol (VoIP) is a technology of the past in the healthcare arena. Hospitals and healthcare providers are gravitating toward the use of smartphones for voice communication (Figure 19-6). Smartphones allow for voice communication, text messaging, and applications that facilitate the delivery of healthcare. It is clear that there is no "one size fits all" solution for healthcare providers. The promise is that the popularity of the smartphone with the benefits of multipurpose use will influence the adoption rate. By 2013, there were approximately 1 billion smartphones in use in the world and the number will top 3.3 billion in 2018 (Mobile Marketing Experts, 2014; Ericsson, 2014). Factors influencing the adoption include the ability to disinfect the device, data encryption and antitheft prevention, and the ability to integrate with EMR (electronic medical record) and EHR. There is little certainty for the direction that voice communication systems will take in the future. However, we can anticipate that overhead paging systems and pagers will become extinct and that smartphones will be at least one component in future systems.

POINT-OF-CARE SYSTEMS

Clinical systems should be accessible at both the point of care and quiet places where the nurse is able to sit down and reflect on patient care events to chart accurately. Nurses' attitudes about the use of clinical systems are often shaped by the ease or difficulty in its use. For example, common complaints are about heavy carts that are difficult to get through doorways or into a patient's room. Any rolling device is subject to the same problems as those encountered with poles for IVs, such as wheels sticking because of spills on the floor from IV solutions or other solutions, wheels that "fall off" of moveable carts, or difficulty in pushing a cart because of the cart's weight or carpeting. To answer nurses' concerns, some facilities have chosen to use lightweight tablet computers with built-in scanning devices for barcode recognition. Others are using laptops on small rolling platforms. With every solution, new problems arise (e.g., problems with battery life, device failure, or theft of portable devices).

SUMMARY

Today's complex healthcare delivery environment requires the use of numerous specialized electronic HISs. Nurses should be aware of the advantages and disadvantages of choosing best-of-breed systems versus integrated enterprise solutions. Quality initiatives such as the physician quality reporting initiative (PQRI) and CCHIT are driving forces for information technology adoption. CCHIT has an aggressive agenda for certifying vendor solutions for the electronic record, which includes ambulatory, inpatient, and specialty practice and specialty care EHRs. CCHIT is also certifying health networks that share data from the electronic record.

The two backbones for the clinical and business portion of most hospital systems are the ADT system and the financial system. Both have been in existence for several decades. Because many of the legacy systems have run their course, there is a growing trend to replace them by using integrated enterprise solutions to share data with the CIS.

The foundation for the CIS is made up of data from laboratory, radiology, and pharmacy information systems. Therapeutic and diagnostic data seamlessly interface with the clinical documentation system and allow the clinician visual alerts for abnormal values and data trends over time. CPOE is designed to reduce order errors and to expedite the delivery of safe patient care. Medication administration is a complex process involving the provider who orders the medication, the pharmacist who checks the order and dispenses the medication, and the nurse who administers the medication. The eMAR provides real-time communication among all who are involved in the process. The PPID is verified by using barcoding or RFID-tagged armbands. It provides for a closed-loop medication administration in which the right patient receives the right medication correctly and on time.

The Joint Commission 2004 recommendation requiring hospitals to discover and minimize barriers to patient flow spurred hospitals to look for informatics solutions. As a result, some hospitals have various electronic tracking systems for patient beds, personnel, and equipment such as wheelchairs. Data from the tracking systems can be analyzed to improve patient flow from admission to discharge, thereby improving the efficiency of the use of scarce resources such as ED and telemetry beds.

The nurse plays a key role in the adoption and use of information technology. The access and use of CISs should be designed to assist the nurse in the delivery of efficient, safe care. Consideration must be made for the selection and placement of equipment such as desktop computers, laptops, tablets, scanners, and medication storage devices. Although the workflow using electronic systems is different from paper record systems, the focus on quality patient outcomes remains the same.

APPLICATIONS AND COMPETENCIES

1. Search the Internet and current literature for clinical information systems meaningful use. Summarize your findings and cite the sources you used.

2. Review the PQRS website. Compare the incentive for a quality care concept with the traditional fee-for-service concept. Will the use of incentives impact the adoption of HIT on patient care? Why or why not?

3. Explore the use of best-of-breed versus integrated HIT solutions at a local hospital. Discuss the pros and cons for each approach.

4. Describe the advantages for the integration of data with the electronic patient record for each of the ancillary information systems listed below.

   a. Pharmacy

   b. Laboratory

   c. Radiology

5. Review the Leapfrog Group website and then explain why the Leapfrog Group recommends the use of CPOE.

6. Search the Internet for information about managing patient flow. Summarize your findings to explain how changing hospital processes can improve patient flow outcomes. Conduct an Internet search for HIS research and analysis services. On the basis of your findings, identify two quality measures that would benefit the nurse who has a voice in the selection of an electronic clinical system.

7. Explain at least three factors that would promote the adoption of clinical systems by nurses using findings from the literature.

REFERENCES

Agency for Healthcare Research Quality. (2011, October). *Section 3. Measuring emergency performance—Improving patient flow and reducing emergency department crowding: A guide for hospitals (No. 11(12)-0094)*. Retrieved from http://www.ahrq.gov/research/findings/final-reports/ptflow/section3.html

Agency for Healthcare Research Quality (AHRQ). (2012, October). *Patient safety primers: Computerized provider order entry*. Retrieved from http://psnet.ahrq.gov/primer.aspx?primerID=6

American Hospital Association. (2007). Improving patient flow patient satisfaction and patient safety. *Hospital and Health Networks*, 81(11), 28–29. Retrieved from http://www.hhnmag.com/

American Hospital Association. (2014, April 14). *The American Hospital Association exclusively endorses the patient flow management solution form MEDHOST*. Retrieved from http://www.medhost.com/news-and-events/press-releases/the-american-hospital-association-exclusively-endorses-medhost-patientflow-hd

Bowman, D. (2010, September 10). 'Fake doctors' treated patients in Medicaid fraud scheme. *FierceHealthcare: Daily News for Healthcare Executives*. Retrieved from http://www.fiercehealthcare.com/story/fake-doctors-used-medicaid-fraud-scheme/2010-09-10

Certification Commission for Healthcare Information Technology (CCHIT). (2014, January 1). *CCHIT announces new strategic direction with global focus: Plans to offer counsel and policy guidance to HIT stakeholder*. Retrieved from http://preview.tinyurl.com/ll6m78n

CMS.gov. (2014a). *Physician quality reporting system*. Retrieved from http://www.cms.gov/Medicare/Quality-Initiatives-Patient-Assessment-Instruments/pqrs/index.html

CMS.gov. (2014b). *Medicaid fraud control units fiscal year 2013 annual report*. Retrieved from http://oig.hhs.gov/oei/reports/oei-06-13-00340.pdf

Drazen, E., & Rhoads, J. (2011, April). Using tracking tools to improve patient flow in hospitals. *California HealthCare Foundation*. Retrieved from http://www.chcf.org/~/media/MEDIA%20LIBRARY%20Files/PDF/U/PDF%20UsingPatientTrackingToolsInHospitals.pdf

Ericsson. (2014). *Ericsson mobility report*. Retrieved from http://www.ericsson.com/mobility-report

Huynh, N., Taaffe, K., Fredendall, L., et al. (2011). The use of a mobile application to track process workflow in perioperative services. *Computers, Informatics, Nursing*, 29(6), 368–374. doi:10.1097/NCN.0b013e31820662ab

Kaplan, M. (2008, July 2). *Barcoded technology to reduce medication administration has flaws*. Retrieved from http://www.medicalnewstoday.com/printerfriendlynews.php?newsid=113498

Koppel, R., Wetterneck, T., Telles, J. L., et al. (2008). Workarounds to barcode medication administration systems: Their occurrences, causes, and threats to patient safety. *Journal of the American Medical Informatics Association*, 15(4), 408–423. doi:10.1197/jamia.M2616

Leapfrog Group. (2014a). *Computerized physician order entry*. Retrieved from http://www.leapfroggroup.org/56440/SurveyInfo/leapfrog_safety_practices/cpoe

Leapfrog Group. (2014b). *The Leapfrog Group fact sheet*. Retrieved from http://www.leapfroggroup.org/about_us/leapfrog-factsheet

Leung, A. A., Denham, C. R., Gandhi, T. K., et al. (2014). A safe practice standard for barcode technology. *Journal of Patient Safety*. doi:10.1097/PTS.0000000000000049. Retrieved from http://www.pubfacts.com/detail/24618650/A-Safe-Practice-Standard-for-Barcode-Technology

Levinson, D. R. (2014, January). *CMS and its contractors have adopted few program integrity practices to address vulnerabilities in EHRs*. Retrieved from https://oig.hhs.gov/oei/reports/oei-01-11-00571.asp

McBeth, S. (2005). Mitigate impediments to efficient patient flow. *Nursing Management*, 36(7), 16–17.

McKesson. (2014). *McKesson visibility solution manages hospital capacity*. Retrieved from http://www.mckesson.com/providers/health-systems/enterprise-intelligence/mckesson-performance-visibility/

MEDHOST. (2014). *MEDHOST*. Retrieved from http://www.medhost.com/

Medicaid Fraud Control Units (MFCU). (2013). *Fiscal year 2013 annual report*. Retrieved from http://oig.hhs.gov/fraud/medicaid-fraud-control-units-mfcu/index.asp

Mobile Marketing Experts. (2014). *Global mobile statistics 2104 part A: Mobile subscribers; handset market share; mobile operators*. Retrieved from http://mobithinking.com/mobile-marketing-tools/latest-mobile-stats/a#smartphonepenetration

National Quality Measures Clearinghouse. (2013). *Emergency department (ED): Admit decision to ED department time for admitted patients*. Retrieved from http://www.qualitymeasures.ahrq.gov/content.aspx?id=46482

Radianse. (2014). *Radianse reveal RTLS solutions for healthcare*. Retrieved, from http://www.radianse.com/reveal-how-it-works.html

Seibert, H. H., Maddox, R. R., Flynn, E. A., et al. (2014). Effect of barcode technology with electronic medication administration record on medication accuracy rates. *American Journal of Health-System Pharmacy*, 71(3), 209–218. doi:10.2146/ajhp130332

The Joint Commission. (2012). Standards revisions addressing patient flow through the emergency department. Joint Commission Perspectives. Retrieved from http://www.jointcommission.org/assets/1/6/Stds_Rev_Patient_Flow.pdf

Thrasher, J. (2013, June 20). *Active RFID vs. passive RFID: What's the difference?* Retrieved from http://blog.atlasrfidstore.com/active-rfid-vs-passive-rfid

Versel, N. (2010, March 29). CMS to fight Medicare, Medicaid fraud with high-text 'bounty hunters'. *FierceHealthcare: Daily News for Healthcare Executives*. Retrieved from http://www.fiercehealthit.com/story/cms-fight-medicare-medicaid-fraud-high-tech-bounty-hunters/2010-03-29

Versus Technology. (2014). *Versus technology: RTLS-RFID for patient flow and asset management*. Retrieved from http://www.versustech.com/

Yin, S. (2010, August 12). Fraud: Cardiologist billed Medicare, other insurers $13M for untreated patients. *FierceHealthcare: Daily news for healthcare executives*. Retrieved from http://www.fiercehealthcare.com/story/fraud-cardiologist-billed-medicare-other-insurers-13m-untreated-patients/2010-08-12

20

Quality Measures and Electronic Healthcare System Issues

OBJECTIVES

After studying this chapter, you will be able to:

1. Use the EMR Adoption model to analyze the level of adoption for a healthcare agency.
2. Discuss the risks and opportunities for sharing clinical data.
3. Discuss how the privacy and confidentiality of patient electronic information is currently addressed in healthcare.
4. Discuss how the issue of interoperability affects the sharing of patient health information.
5. Provide an example that demonstrates the significance of workflow redesign as it relates to a clinical documentation system.
6. Identify ways that healthcare is addressing The Joint Commission's patient safety goals with the use of health information technology.
7. Provide at least two examples of strong passwords, with an explanation about why the password is strong.

KEY TERMS

Accuracy of data	Data security	Strategic plan
Authentication	Intangibles	Tangibles
Biometrics	Single sign-on	Unintended consequences
Clinical Decision Support System (CDSS)	Spear phishing	Voice recognition
	Stark rules	Workflow redesign

The use of health information technology (HIT) is improving patient care outcomes. The rate of adoption of technology solutions is growing. Not all the issues associated with its use have been resolved. The transition from a paper record world to an automated one is a huge endeavor. Healthcare practitioners are slow to adopt new solutions that they believe could jeopardize patient care while they are "unlearning" legacy processes and "learning" new approaches. This chapter focuses on a few of the issues associated with the adoption of HIT.

THE ADOPTION MODEL FOR THE ELECTRONIC MEDICAL RECORD

Unraveling the complexity of healthcare delivery systems when planning the adoption of information technology can be a daunting process. HIMSS Analytics, a nonprofit subsidiary of Healthcare Information and Management Systems Society (HIMSS), defined an adoption model, as seen in Table 20-1, for the electronic medical record (EMR). The model serves as a guide for healthcare providers who are transitioning from the paper record to the electronic record. It should be useful for multidisciplinary information technology implementation committees involved with system procurement and budget planning.

At Stage 0, all the basic clinical systems (laboratory, pharmacy, or radiology) are not in place (HIMSS Analytics, 2014). At Stage 1, all three of the basic clinical systems exist. At Stage 2, there is physician access to obtain and view results from a clinical data repository (CDR) fed by the clinical systems. At this stage, there is also a "controlled medical vocabulary" (standardized healthcare vocabulary) and a **clinical decision support system (CDSS)** for conflict checking in place. At Stage 2, the system is capable of health information exchange.

At Stage 3, there is integration of the clinical documentation with the CDR with at least one other hospital service. There is error checking for order entry by using CDSS, and a picture archive and communication system available outside of radiology by using a secure network such as an intranet is in place. Clinical documentation includes nurses' notes, the electronic medication administration record (eMAR), flow sheets, and care plans. At Stage 4, computerized provider order entry (CPOE) and CDSS related to evidence-based

TABLE 20-1	EMR Adoption Model
Stage	Cumulative Capabilities
7	Complete EMR (electronic medical record); CCD (continuity of care document) transactions to share data; data warehousing; data continuity with ED (emergency department), ambulatory, OP (outpatient)
6	Physician documentation (structured templates), full CDSS (variance and compliance), full R-PACS (radiology—picture archiving and communication system)
5	Closed-loop medication administration
4	CPOE, CDSS (clinical protocols)
3	Nursing/clinical documentation (flow sheets), CDSS (error checking), PACS available outside radiology
2	CDR, controlled medical vocabulary, and CDSS may have document imaging; HIE–capable
1	Ancillaries—laboratory, radiology, pharmacy—all installed
0	All three ancillaries not installed

Source: HIMSS Analytics. (2014). *Healthcare providers: EMR Adoption model*. Retrieved from http://www.himssanalytics.org/home/index.aspx

care protocols are in place on at least one patient care area. This level is achieved with implementation of only one patient service.

At Stage 5, the closed-loop medication administration is achieved by using the eMAR and a method for autoidentifying the patient is integrated with the pharmacy system. At Stage 6, physician–patient documentation and the ability to view all radiology images is available on at least one patient care area. At the highest level of implementation, Stage 7, clinical information can be shared electronically with authorized providers, payers, patients, and others through a regional health network, creating a true electronic health record (EHR), as defined in this book. The healthcare provider no longer uses paper records to manage patient care. Furthermore, the healthcare provider uses a clinical data warehouse to analyze clinical data patterns for improving the quality of care.

The issues associated with the adoption of HIT become evident when viewing the percentage of adoption at each stage. According to HIMSS Analytics, as of 2008, 4.3% of 5,050 healthcare agencies were between Stages 4 and 7. Six years later, by the third quarter of 2014, 63.9% of 5,453 healthcare agencies were between 4 and 7, with the highest level of adoption achieved by 3.4% of providers (HIMSS Analytics, 2014) (Figure 20-1). The most current adoption data for the United States and Canada is on the HIMSS Analytics website at http://www.himssanalytics.org.

Adoption of the EHR places the patient as the first and foremost recipient of benefits. Providing the best possible patient care requires access to the data generated in patient care situations and systems, which can monitor for known problem areas and anticipate others (Box 20-1). Although we are making headway, there is still much work ahead before this goal becomes an everyday reality.

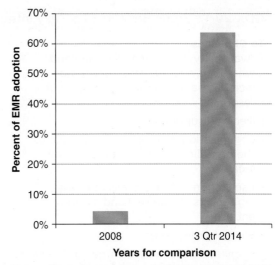

Figure 20-1. Comparison of HIMSS Analytics EMR Adoption model Stages 4 to 7 for 2008 and 2014. (Data from HIMSS Analytics. (2014). *Healthcare providers: EMR Adoption model.* Adapted from http://himssanalytics.org/)

period. It also guides the acquisition of resources and for budget priorities. It should be a living and breathing document that allows for flexibility. As an example, it should provide the ability to incorporate the use of new evolving technologies. The costs associated with the use of an HIT solution, such as CPOE, are often in the thousands to multi-millions of dollars range, depending on the size of the institution. As a result, the stakeholders must be able to see that the expenditures are offset by patient outcome benefits; they must see a return on investment (ROI). If the use of information technology is not supported by the institution's strategic plan, it will probably not be funded.

STRATEGIC PLANNING

Healthcare agency strategic planning lays the groundwork for the adoption of healthcare information technology; it is essential for successful system implementation (Gattadahalli, 2013). A **strategic plan** is a road map that guides the institution in meeting its mission. It directs decision-making practices over a 3- or 5- to 10-year

RETURN ON INVESTMENT

The ROI is an important issue serving as a barrier to the adoption of electronic systems. Improving patient care outcomes and managing costs should align with the strategic plans for healthcare agencies. The process of ROI requires scrutiny regarding risks and the associated values (Health Resources and Services Association [HRSA], n.d.). In other words, is the risk offset by the potential value? If so, what data are available to support the value?

BOX 20-1   Some Benefits of a Fully Integrated Electronic Health Record

To Clinicians
- Availability of information when and where it is needed. This information includes patient data and bibliographic resources.
- Decision support.
- Organization of information specific to the discipline so that it can be easily located.
- Facilitation of the process of preparing reports for internal and external entities.
- Ease of order entry.
- Elimination of multiple entries of the same data.

To Patients
- Knowledge of who has access to their data.
- Individualized treatment anywhere the computer-based patient record is available.
- Ability to check the accuracy of their record.
- One location for all healthcare data.
- Evidence-based healthcare.

To Researchers and Policymakers
- Time savings in obtaining data.
- Large databanks yielding more valid and precise research.
- Ability to answer questions at local, state, national, and possibly international levels.

Persons involved in budget-making decisions must identify goals and methods for measuring achievement for both tangible and intangible values and risks. A classic 2006 study indicated that although there are increased expenses associated with the use of information technology, there is an ROI in the acute care setting (Menachemi et al., 2006). Maviglia and colleagues (2007) researched the cost–benefit of barcode medication administration system for a large tertiary care hospital. They found that that costs totaled $2.24 million over 5 years. The ROI was a decrease in adverse drug events (ADEs) from medication dispensing errors for an annual savings of $2.2 million. The hospital was able to break even after 1 year.

Tangibles are those values that can be clearly measured, calculated, and quantified with numerical data. Examples of tangibles include a decrease in length of stay, a decrease in anti-infective medication costs, a decrease in the number of unnecessary medications and tests, and a decrease in charges per admission. There is not much variance in tangibles between healthcare settings.

Intangibles are those values that are not easily calculated or in which the results cannot be directly attributed to the investment. Examples of intangibles include improved decision-making, communication, and user satisfaction. Intangibles may vary between healthcare settings because

of the differences in factors, such as organizational culture, physical environments, population served, and staffing.

Fortunately, the results of a number of studies spurred efforts by individual healthcare organizations in larger geographical areas to initiate the adoption of CPOE to improve patient care outcomes. The results from the research studies have been used to benchmark data and to calculate ROIs. The impact of ROI by government regulatory requirements, incentive payments, and noncompliance fines must be accounted for as well.

REIMBURSEMENT

Reimbursement is a crucial issue for healthcare agencies, physicians, and other providers. The Centers for Medicare & Medicaid services passed the Physician Self-Referral Law in an effort to prevent Medicare fraud (CMS.gov, 2013c). The law is more commonly known as Stark law or **Stark rules** because Congressman Peter Stark introduced it. It has been criticized for interfering with collaborative innovations and limiting the ability of healthcare agencies and providers to design seamless solutions for sharing healthcare information using technology. The law was relaxed in August 2006 to provide an incentive for physicians to adopt a certified EHR. The amended law allowed hospitals to donate "certified" interoperable systems to physicians. On the other hand, the law was criticized for swaying physicians to use the hospital's choice of clinical information system vendor. In 2013, CMS, the Office of the Inspector General, and the U.S. Department of Health and Human Services published new rules that extended the date for protected donations through December 31, 2021 (Mohammed, 2014).

ISSUES RELATED TO ELECTRONIC HEALTH INFORMATION

There are five main issues associated with electronic health information: (1) interoperability standards, (2) user design, (3) workflow redesign, (4) quality measurement, and (5) **data security**. Theoretically, the certification requirement resolves issues associated with the EHR. However, they still apply to commercial vendor EMR products, which have to communicate with the EHR.

The terms EMR and EHR are often used interchangeably, but the differences are very important. The EMR belongs to the healthcare agency. Information associated with the EMR can be a composite of several different information systems that may or may not be integrated. The EHR includes certain information from healthcare agency EMRs as well as other healthcare providers (e.g., physicians, nurse practitioners, and pharmacies). The EHR allows health information to be shared with consumers, authorized providers, and public health personnel. Information embedded in the EHRs provides a strong foundation for new knowledge formation. Examples of information stored in the EHR include patient histories, medical tests, medications, and images (HealthIT.gov, 2013b).

Interoperability Standards

The lack of interoperability standards interferes with the ability to share information by authorized users, including the patient. Interoperability is especially a significant issue as it relates to clinical information system and the EMR. Clinical information systems refer to a group of technology-enabled systems, which may or may not be originally designed to share data with one another.

Purchasing from a single vendor does not assure the buyer that the system is seamlessly interoperable. Large well-known vendors commonly purchase smaller popular applications and then design interfaces with other vendor applications. The resulting lack of interoperability requires nurses to document the same data in more than one area or application because the data do not flow over to another application. Many times the deviations seem minor, but in reality, the deviation from system standard can become a huge issue when attempting to standardize, update, and maintain data or to integrate applications, develop interfaces, or aggregate data between systems. One of the significant rewards of a clinical information system is the ability to share data. The Office of the National Coordinator for Health Information Technology (ONC) certification program has ameliorated many of the issues associated with interoperability (HealthIT.gov, 2014).

User Design

User design of data entry screens is an issue because many healthcare providers involved in the design process have no background knowledge of or skills with database design. As a result, providers approach user design by thinking about using the paper chart. Until all healthcare providers have some kind of education on informatics and database design basics, the issue will not be resolved. Examples of screen design issues include lack of using uniform pain scales, terminology, pain documentation, pressure ulcer prevention programs, and falls prevention programs. These design issues affect the ability to analyze the data for evidence-based practice decisions. They also make documentation of care challenging for nurses who float to other units or who work for temporary assistance agencies. Finally, lack of uniformity introduces new opportunities for extending the time for documentation, user frustration, and documentation errors.

Workflow Redesign

Workflow redesign is one of the many difficult issues that healthcare providers face when planning and designing the application of electronic systems. As noted several times earlier, one of the problems is the lack of experience or lack of knowledge about other ways to accomplish work. Another problem relates to resistance to change. Workflow redesign also relates to the tedious processes involved in identifying how work changes with a technology solution. It involves creating process flow diagrams that paint "before" and "after" pictures of workflow. Finally, redesign involves the nuts-and-bolts questions about the presence of computers. Common questions faced by nurses are as follows:

- How many computers are needed?
- Where should the computers be located?
- Should the computers be placed on wheeled stands (computer on wheels) so that they can be moved or should they be at the bedside?
- What are the fire marshal regulations for storing moveable or wall-mounted computers in patient unit hallways?
- If laptops or tablets are used, can these be prevented from being stolen?
- How can unauthorized users be prevented from using the computer?
- When documenting care in public places, can unauthorized eyes be prevented from viewing the data?

A team of researchers at the University of Wisconsin studied the how HIT affected workflow in relationship to the healthcare staff, the patients, and between organizations (AHRQ, 2010). The researchers also developed an interactive tool for assessing workflow in outpatient settings that is available from the AHRQ website at http://healthit.ahrq.gov/health-it-tools-and-resources/workflow-assessment-health-it-toolkit. The toolkit provides a basis for understanding the complexity of workflow analysis (AHRQ, 2011).

Quality Measurement

A CDR has the potential to allow us to measure quality. The goal for the use of HIT is improved patient outcomes and quality of care, not the use of HIT. A quality measurement issue is to design data fields in a way that allows users to query the data for answers. Clinical application vendors need to work with providers to identify quality measures and design data entry windows to capture the data so that the computer can analyze it.

Data Security

Data security issues are the responsibility of the information systems team. Data security has three aspects. The first deals with ensuring the accuracy of the data, the second with protection of the data from unauthorized eyes inside or outside the agency, and the third with internal or external damage to the data.

Informatics nurses and clinical nurses are involved in building entry screens prior to a system implementation. Nurses, as well as the technical staff, need to understand the principles of data security. **Accuracy of data** can be improved with methods that check the data during input. For example, when a user chooses phrases for input from a list, the person needs to be sure that only recognized terms are entered. To check that the desired phrase was chosen before leaving the page, the user can be presented with a screen that shows the items that will be entered into the record. Another factor for consideration is how to handle incorrect entries. Generally, a provision is allowed for the entry to be corrected within a time period, but a record of all entries is kept in an audit trail. An audit trail provides a list of who accessed the system, the date, the time, and the activity.

Protection of the data from prying eyes involves the use of audit trails and making decisions about how much access individual users should have. Who has access to what information differs from agency to agency. For pure ease of use, all professional healthcare workers would have access to any patient record in the system. This is very helpful when patients are transferred from one department to another, and it is allowed in some institutions. Its use must be backed up by audit trails or by a record of which individual worker accessed which record at what time and where. Additionally, those audit trails must be routinely examined to determine if breaches of security are occurring. Audit trails are closely scrutinized after the admission of persons who are well known.

Audit trails can identify the user who accessed the record by username, the Internet Protocol (IP) address, the pages accessed, and the length of time of the access. A famous breach occurred in 2008 when UCLA Medical Center fired thirteen employees and suspended six others for looking at the medical record for celebrity Britney Spears

(Ornstein, 2008). Electronic access assisted in identifying the employees.

Making decisions about how much access users have varies from one institution to the next. Most institutions provide access only to records of those patients on the unit where the healthcare worker is stationed and index the employees by job description. Limiting access too severely will prohibit holistic care and can put patients in jeopardy.

Accuracy of the original data is also the responsibility of users. There have been situations in which clinicians have entered anything into a mandatory field just to continue in the system. Not only does this put patient care at risk, but it also compromises the integrity of the database. This cavalier attitude can be attributed to a multitude of factors: lack of awareness of what is done with the data, an unwieldy system for entering data, time pressures, and inadequate training on using the system. That said, system designers must understand nurse workflow and require only essential mandatory fields, not ones that may be impossible to complete. Regardless of the cause, attempts to bypass mandatory data entry fields must be addressed if data are to be valid.

Protection from System Intrusions

With the rise of the Internet and the actuality that most agencies are now connected to it, preventing outsiders from accessing institutional information has become a major responsibility of the information services department. One of the first lines of defense for protecting against unauthorized access is a firewall. A firewall operates in one of two ways. Either it examines all messages entering and leaving a system and blocks those that do not meet specific criteria or it allows or denies messages based on whether the destination port is acceptable. Firewalls require constant maintenance. To ensure that the system is safe from prying eyes, some agencies hire white hat hackers who attempt to penetrate their information systems. White hat hackers are persons who are ethically opposed to security abuse. Their job is to identify security weaknesses. This allows information services to devise protection for any security breaches that are found.

Systems also need protection from outsiders who gain physical entrance to the agency and from insiders who are intent on gaining unauthorized access. Security audits completed by independent consultants identify potential system security vulnerabilities. The first line of defense against this type of breach includes staff education on the importance of data security. Staff should be encouraged to expect identification from unfamiliar persons and to refuse access to anyone without recognized authorization.

Phishing and Spear Phishing Security Breaches

The concept of phishing was discussed in Chapter 5 on email, so you may be curious about why it is being discussed again in this chapter on healthcare system issues. To steal confidential patient information, criminal hackers use phishing email tactics to lure the care provider into revealing private information. **Spear phishing** tactics use what appears to be legitimate business email from a person well known to the email recipient. It is a scam that lures an employee into revealing private login information (SearchSecurity.com, 2011; Technopedia, 2014). For example, in a healthcare agency, the employees might receive what appears to be a legitimate employee email from within the agency, such as from human resources, nursing services, or information services. The scam is that the email will ask the recipients to update their login and password information or to verify it. When the recipients respond, the perpetrator steals their login and password and then uses the information for criminal purposes by hacking into the hospital's information system. All phishing scams should be reported to the Antiphishing Working Group at http://www.antiphishing.org.

Protection from Data Loss

Computer data need to be protected from being lost because of either a system problem or disaster, natural or otherwise. This latter element took on new importance after the fall of the World Trade Center on September 11, 2001, hurricanes Katrina and Rita in 2005, and the tornadoes that destroyed Mercy Medical Center in Joplin, Missouri, in 2011 and Moore Medical Center in Moore, Oklahoma, in 2013. To provide this protection, data must be backed up routinely and stored off-site in a secure place. These backups should be periodically examined to make sure that they are accurate and can be easily reinstalled on the system. Additionally, a disaster recovery plan needs to be devised and tested. This plan should be made in conjunction with key people in the agency to ensure adequate protection. The objective in disaster recovery is to allow work to resume by using the same standards as before the disaster with the least amount of effort. One of the first tasks in planning for disaster recovery is to do a risk analysis. This analysis will determine vulnerabilities and appropriate control measures. Identification of system weaknesses can prevent the actual occurrence of a disaster. A disaster plan should be tested at least twice a year. Healthcare accrediting bodies have standards to assure protection from data loss.

UNINTENDED CONSEQUENCES OF INTRODUCTION OF ELECTRONIC SYSTEM

The introduction of technology into a healthcare delivery system can result in unintended and unexpected consequences. An **unintended consequence** refers to an outcome, good or bad, that was not planned or deliberate. Researchers have reported on unintended consequences for the use of CPOE and CDSS. The findings from the research studies should assist nurses in avoiding these problems and recognizing the necessary compromises that must be made to ensure patient safety. Results of research conducted by Jones et al. (2011) provide a guide to reduce unintended consequences of medical records.

CPOE

Nurse–physician communication and workflow issues are unintended consequences from the use of CPOE (Cowan, 2013). Classic research investigating CPOE revealed nine types of unintended consequences (Ash et al., 2009). Two of the consequences related to the way work (more and new work) and workflow changed after CPOE. For example, the providers were responsible for entering orders instead of the nurses or secretaries. At least initially, work tasks took a longer time as the users learned to adjust to a new ordering system.

System demands were the third consequence. The CPOE system required unintended system design, support, and maintenance that involved personnel, software, and hardware requirements.

Communication and emotions were two other unintended consequences. Although patient information was readily available, some users used the computers to replace face-to-face communication when indeed communication never occurred; there was only the appearance of communication. The information was entered into the computer, but the person who needed it did not know. Computers should enhance, not replace, other types of communication.

Emotions ranged from love to hate. Personnel who were comfortable with automated systems acclimated to CPOE, but those who were uncomfortable experienced strong negative emotions. CPOE led to power shifts, and some believed the physician was perceived as losing power, but others felt that pharmacists lost power because the physician took responsibility for ordering medications. The dependence on technology was considered an unintended consequence of problems and productivity loss associated with computer downtimes.

The research on the effects of CPOE revealed new kinds of errors and problems with confusing user-screen designs, and order option presentations had the potential to result in new errors. Use of long drop-down menus had the potential for inadvertent selection of the wrong patient. Other potential errors were related to medication dosing errors and orders that overlapped.

Duplicate orders are another unintended consequence of CPOE. Magid et al. (2012) reported a problem with duplicate orders for "high-alert" medications, which occurred after implementing CPOE in a specialty hospital. They used the high-alert drugs identified by the Institute of Safe Medication Practice (ISMP) as noted on the website http://www.ismp.org. The research team identified 5,442 duplicate orders over an 84-week period. They devised interventions such as activating alerts, one-on-one training sessions, emails to prescribers, reminders at conferences, and training session. As a result, they were able to reduce the number of duplicate orders significantly.

Decision Support Systems

A research study that investigated CDSS also revealed unintended consequences (Ash et al., 2009). The research findings identified "patterns" of unintended consequences as (1) those related to content and (2) those related to the way information was presented on the computer screen. Consequences related to content included the possibility of continuing unnecessary daily orders, such as chest x-rays. Content also related to the way orders had to be entered, resulting in a lack of full information from other professionals. There were problems that related to difficulties in updating the clinical decision support rules and wrong or misleading alerts. There were also problems related to inadequate communication between systems, resulting in a lack of supplies or misinformation about the costs of laboratory testing. Consequences related to clinical decision support representation on the computer screen related to order information that was required but not available and alert fatigue from too many alerts.

As in the CPOE research, CDSS research revealed unintended potential errors. Examples include the accidental selection of an autocomplete word when typing and notifications that were delivered in an untimely manner. Finally, potential errors could occur when editing and correcting a clinical decision support rule.

RULES AND REGULATIONS: THE JOINT COMMISSION

The Joint Commission has challenged the healthcare organizations it surveys with annual national safety goals (The Joint Commission, 2014). HIT can augment three of the top patient safety goals for 2014. The first goal (2014) is to improve the accuracy of patient identification. Agencies using barcode identification assist in providing the patient two identifiers to meet the goal (Stage 5 of the EMR Adoption model in Table 20-1). The Joint Commission also recommends use of barcode identification when there is a one-person identification for starting a blood transfusion. The second safety goal is to improve communication. Goal 2.03.01 addresses communicating critical results for tests and procedures. The CDSS in clinical information systems facilitates alerting those who need to know of tests and procedures with critical values.

The sixth goal addresses alarm safety. With the increasing number of alarms used in healthcare

facilities, alarm fatigue is a huge issue. Alarm fatigue occurs when the clinician ignores or turns off alarms after becoming desensitized due to the constant noise (MacDonald, 2014). The result threatens patient safety. The Joint Commission made three recommendations to reduce alarm fatigue. The first is to filter alarms. In other words, make decisions for which alarms are necessary. The second is to develop policies and procedures on the use of alarms. Finally, educate the staff about the use of alarms.

DISEASE SURVEILLANCE SYSTEMS AND DISASTER PLANNING

When all health records are electronic, aggregated data from the records could be trended to detect infectious disease outbreaks and bioterrorism. In 2010, the Centers for Disease Control and Prevention realigned its divisions within the Public Health Information Network to form the Division of Preparedness and Emerging Infections (DPEI) (Centers for Disease Control and Prevention, 2011). The division incorporated the responsibilities of the former National Electronic Disease Surveillance System (NEDSS). The purpose of DPEI is to work with public partners to "prepare for, prevent, and respond to infectious diseases, including outbreaks, bioterrorism, and other public health emergencies, through cross-cutting and specialized programs, technical expertise, and public health leadership" (Centers for Disease Control, 2011). Early detection (or potential disease) or bioterrorism health problems can be accomplished by using syndromic surveillance systems.

Syndromic Surveillance

Syndromic surveillance is the collection of health indicators from individuals and populations that present before diagnoses are made and that provide information on the health of a community (Centers for Disease Control and Prevention, 2014a). The Health Information Technology for Economic and Clinical Health (HITECH) Act allowed for coordination of syndromic surveillance using data reporting with the EHR and Meaningful Use. The Centers for Disease Control and Prevention (CDC), with assistance of the

International Society for Disease Surveillance, provides messaging guides that support Meaningful Use at http://www.cdc.gov/phin/resources/PHINguides.html#ss. The messaging guides are continually updated on the CDC website.

Syndromic surveillance exists at the country and global levels. For example, the Public Health Information Network (PHIN) covers the entire United States with state data collected under the authority of state or local health departments. Data are exchanged using interoperable information systems for both routine and emergency purposes (Centers for Disease Control and Prevention, 2014b). The World Health Organization (WHO) (2014) also uses syndromic surveillance to detect and follow communicable diseases. The WHO Pacific surveillance system publishes reports weekly. The WHO November 16, 2014 report noted 15,145 cases of Ebola and 5,420 deaths. In 2014, the dangers of Ebola spreading to other countries made international news when infected patients were identified in the United States and Spain.

Disaster Response and Planning

Hurricane Katrina, the disastrous storm that struck the US Gulf Coast in August 2005, served as initial notice to inform HIT about disaster planning. After the storm, the KatrinaHealth website (http://www.katrinahealth.org) was almost immediately established in conjunction with local and state governments; Dr. David Brailer, the then National Coordinator for HIT; the Markle Foundation; and pharmaceutical companies (Markle Foundation, American Medical Association, & Gold Standard, 2006). The website served as a portal for authorized physicians and pharmacists to obtain electronic prescription medical records for victims of the storm. Reflective analysis for KatrinaHealth is available online at http://katrinahealth.org/katrinahealth.final.pdf. The report included seven recommendations that local, state, and national policymakers and governments must consider:

- Plan for disasters now.
- Use existing available resources such as the regional health information organizations (RHIOs).
- Create interoperable EHRs.
- Integrate emergency response systems into nonemergent systems.
- Establish systems that can be easily accessed.
- Establish effective communication channels.
- Overcome policy barriers.

Healthcare professionals, information technology specialists, and those in leadership positions continue to learn from disasters. The efforts serve as catalysts for improved communication channels and the development of improved informatics solutions to improve the lives of future victims.

The Regional Coordinating Center (RCC) for hurricane response was established in October 2005 (Kim et al., 2013). The mission for RCC was to use HIT with the National Institute of Health's Centers of Excellence in Partnerships for Community Outreach, Research on Health Disparities and Training to assist with the renewing and rebuilding of the healthcare systems that were affected by hurricanes Katrina and Rita. The RCC embarked on building partnerships with local healthcare systems among the different Gulf Shore states to assist in the rebuilding process. The goals for this project included the use of EHRs, telepsychiatry, and screening and surveillance systems. Project leaders for RCC recognized that the reconstruction process was very complicated and that it would take time to accomplish.

RCCs are now under the direction of FEMA (Federal Emergency Management Agency) and organized into regions of the United States as Regional Response Coordination Centers (RRCC). RRCCs coordinate the immediate emergency response to a disaster or catastrophic event for the federal government (FEMA, 2014).

PROTECTION OF HEALTHCARE DATA

Health Insurance Portability and Accountability Act

The 1996 Health Insurance Portability and Accountability Act (HIPAA) has affected the entire healthcare entity, including HIT. The law addressed several areas pertaining to healthcare information, including simplifying healthcare claims, providing standards for healthcare data transmission, and ensuring the security of healthcare information. The purpose of the law was to improve the effectiveness and efficiency of healthcare. It was also designed to prevent medical fraud by standardizing the electronic exchange of financial and administrative data. The HIPAA law applies only to (1) healthcare providers that "furnish, bill, or receive payment for healthcare in the normal business day" and who also transmit any transactions electronically; (2) healthcare clearinghouses; or (3) health plans (CMS.gov, 2013b).

The area that has generated the most public attention has been the privacy and security rules that address many of the privacy, confidentiality, and security issues already discussed in this chapter. There have been many areas of disagreement among the stakeholders about the rules, and legitimate concerns exist on both sides. One rule requires that in each agency, a specific person be assigned the responsibility for overseeing efforts to secure electronic data. As a result, each healthcare agency that has to abide by the rules has a person designated as the HIPAA officer. This person must be proficient in information technology, auditing, agency policies and practices, ethics, state and federal regulations, and consumer issues. The ONC provides a Privacy and Security Toolkit for providers to use as a guide when addressing privacy and security for electronic exchange of information (HealthIT.gov, 2013a).

Although data privacy issues generate the most media attention, HIPAA also maintains "technology neutral" methods for the transmission of data among healthcare organizations. Technology neutral means that any computer system can import and read the data. (This is similar to the rich text format (RTF) that permits most word processors to read documents created by other word processors.) To simplify and encourage electronic transfer of administrative and financial healthcare data among payers, plans, and providers, HIPAA requires the use of national code standards.

HIPAA also calls for the use of "national identifiers for providers, health plans, and employers" (CMS.gov, 2013a). Use of the national provider identifier went into effect in 2008 for Medicare fee-for-service providers. The original call for a unique patient identifier was put on hold permanently because of privacy issues.

Privacy

Protecting patient privacy is an important professional responsibility. Being sick does not make intrusions into one's personal life justifiable. In some instances, people have been denied employment because of known medical conditions. This can make patients hesitant to share their health history when they know that it will be entered into a record for anyone with access to read. Patient privacy also needs to be considered when interviewing a patient. The environment should be such that the interview cannot be overheard. Additionally, information routinely asked of patients should be scrutinized to ensure that it is pertinent to the care that can be rendered in the agency. Another item to consider is the placement of computers on which charting is done. Ideally, the computer screen should not be visible to anyone except the person charting. The nurse must log off before leaving the computer; otherwise, anyone who approaches the computer will be able to access private information.

Confidentiality

Confidentiality is a constant balancing act. The more confidential we make a record, the more difficult it becomes to use it. Before computerized records, we gave minimal concern to confidentiality. We believed that the record was safe. Yet, in most institutions, anyone with a white coat and a name badge that reads "Doctor or Nurse X" could pick up a record and read it. Additionally, when a patient was sent to another area, such as the operating room, the chart was tucked under a corner of the gurney from where anyone could easily remove it. Not only did this make it easy for the staff in another area to view the record, but it also raised questions about confidentiality that were seldom addressed.

Authentication

Computerized records have brought the issue of confidentiality to the forefront. Even with the flaws in paper records, it was difficult to obtain information from more than one or two records at a time. When records are computerized, if one gains unauthorized entrance to the system, it is easy to access many records. Hence, the first line of protection is to defend against unauthorized access or entrance to the system. This is achieved with a login process that authenticates that the person using the system is permitted access. **Authentication** simply means verifying the identification of the person logging into the system. It can be accomplished by using passwords, smartcards, **biometrics** (use of physiologic characteristics), or a combination of these.

Login Name and Passwords

Anyone who has ever used a network in a healthcare agency or a secure site on the World Wide Web has become familiar with login names (user ID) and passwords. Most systems today rely on a login name and a password for authentication. Various systems of designating login names are used, such as first initial and last name, most of which are easy to guess, and they generally remain the same as long as one is using the same network. Thus, the rules for passwords are much more stringent and vary from agency to agency.

The best passwords involve a combination of upper and lower case letters and numbers in a manner that will not form a word (e.g., "Sec9uR7ity"). This prevents someone with an electronic dictionary from trying various passwords until the right one is found. Additionally, making passwords case sensitive (i.e., one must use lower and upper case letters in the same way each time the password is used) also makes them more difficult to guess.

> ### QSEN Scenario
> The healthcare agency where you work requires you to use a strong password. How does a strong password help protect health information in electronic records?

Password Policies

Policies on how often to change passwords are based on the premise that after a given length of time, one's password has been compromised, either purposely or accidentally. The system administrator determines the length of time. Additionally, most systems prohibit users from reusing a password. Forcing a change too frequently can result in users writing the password down and pasting it either near the computer or on the back of an ID badge. Not changing frequently enough leaves users open to having the security of their account breached. One of the problems faced by network administrators is providing logins and passwords to temporary users, such as temporary staff and nursing students. Because an unused account is an invitation to hackers, there must be a network policy for closing the accounts of both temporary users and workers who leave their positions in the company or institution.

Network administrators require password access to clinical information systems to protect the privacy and security of patient records. They also have to deal with regulatory pressure, security threats, and the cost of help desks. Password problems are among the top day-to-day issues encountered at information technology help desks.

Automatic Logout

Automatic logout is another function used to preserve data confidentiality. Knowing emergencies often arise that involve calling a nurse away from the computer, most systems will time out after a given length of time with no input activity. If the time interval is too short, this can be annoying to users who have to go through the entire login process again. If it is too long, it could allow someone else to perform unauthorized activities by using the original user's login. If the clinician is at the computer and involved in a phone call, simply moving the mouse may be interpreted as activity and keep the system from logging the user out.

Single Sign-On

Use of a **single sign-on** is an issue for the use of clinical information systems. Single sign-on allows the user to access multiple clinical applications with only one login/password for authentication. Use of logins for every clinical application is problematic. Having multiple passwords that expire on a regular basis creates the same problem as having passwords expire too frequently—the users creatively use methods to write down the passwords by which they can easily be discovered. Each login requires authentication and forces the busy professional to wait before completing a transaction. It is more efficient for users to have a single sign-on for the use of clinical information systems, which improves workflow and prevents accidental breaches of security and confidentiality.

Professional Responsibility to Protect Confidentiality

Confidentiality of private information located in computerized records starts with the users. Users need to understand the need for protecting their account; they must tailor behaviors to guarantee this protection. Users need to understand that between the times they log in and out, they are responsible for anything that is done from their account. When a nurse leaves a computer screen unattended with patient data exposed, the patient's confidentiality is breached. To make matters worse, any other person who recognizes that the nurse is logged in has the opportunity to make entries into the system under the nurse's name. The computer would not be able to tell the difference. It is very important for nurses to learn to log off the computer before leaving. Logging off is a habit that can be learned as easily as locking the doors of the house or car.

The most secure method of authentication is biometrics—the use of physiological characteristics such as iris scan, fingerprint, or a voiceprint that is presumably unique to the particular person. For the iris scan, users stand approximately 3 to 10 inches away from a high-resolution camera to be authenticated (Wilson, 2005; Fontana, 2014). The authentication process uses 200 or more points from the iris. Verification takes only seconds. Airports and border control stations use iris scanning for international travelers to clear customs (U.S. Customs and Border Protection, n.d.). The iris scan is very accurate, but it is less beneficial in the busy healthcare environment because the users must remove their glasses and focus on the camera (Biometric Newsportal, n.d.).

The rich whorls, ridges, and patterns of fingerprints are useful for authentication. The users press their fingers against an optical or silicon surface reader for less than 5 seconds. The accuracy is improved with the use prints from more than one finger. One of the limitations of fingerprint biometrics is that the finger should be clean and dry and not smudged with grease, dirt, or ink, such as newspaper print. Fingerprint recognition is a common option used to authenticate access to smartphone, tablets, and laptops.

Palm vein technology is an authentication system used for the candidates who take the NCLEX exam (Pearson, 2014). The scanner uses an infrared light source to examine the veins in the hand. The resulting digital template is used for authentication when the candidate enters the testing center after breaks.

Voice recognition is another type of biometric used for security. Voice recognition creates voiceprints using a combination of two authentication factors: what is said and the way that it is said (Nuance, 2014). It can also be used at a distance with a telephone. Voice biometrics is more commonly used in the banking industry as much of banking business is done over telephone lines. Voice recognition has potential for increased use in healthcare because it is two to three times more accurate than fingerprinting and less expensive than other biometric systems.

RADIOFREQUENCY IDENTIFICATION

RFID refers to smart labels or intelligent bar codes that can communicate with a network. RFID is designed to take the place of the Universal Product Code that we see on almost any product we purchase, whether it is a package of CD-ROMs at the office supply store or a box of cereal at the grocery store. We may have seen or used RFID on a pass card attached to a vehicle windshield for access to toll roads. Another nonmedical use is to tag pet dogs and cats for easy identification in case they are lost. In 2007, the United States began to embed RFID chips in passports (Kelly, 2014).

RFID is of two types: passive and active (RFID 101.com, 2014). The passive tags are lighter, less expensive ($0.5 per tag) (RFID Journal, 2014), have read-only capability, and can be read at a distance of 1 to 10 feet. The passive, implantable (inserted under the skin) tag uses a U.S. Food and Drug Administration chip. The active tags are more expensive (several dollars), have read–write capability, and can be read at distances of 1 to 300 feet.

Currently, RFID is used in many healthcare agencies to track patients (Martinez-Pérez et al., 2012), including newborn babies. The "Hugs" Infant Protection System by Stanley Healthcare Solutions is an example of how RFID is used in healthcare. Each baby receives an ankle band with an embedded RFID chip. If there is an unauthorized removal of the baby, an alarm is sounded. An example of successful use was reported when a baby's abduction was thwarted from Garden Grove Medical Center (Wicklund, 2012). The perpetrator, posing as a care provider, tricked the mother into leaving the room and stole the baby using a tote bag. The RFID on the baby's ankle tripped the door locks out of the labor and delivery unit, thereby thwarting the baby abduction.

RFID is also used in healthcare agencies to track equipment such as wheelchairs and intravenous pumps and used to track the location of patients (Supply Insight, 2015). Another use of this technology is to track hospital personnel, such as doctors and nurses (Chen & Collins, 2012). Although the use of the technology with patients and personnel has been controversial in some settings, decisions have been made in favor of improved care delivery systems and patient safety.

RFID solutions have been used to facilitate identification. A unique identifier number can be used to identify "at-risk" patients who may need emergency medical treatment. These unique identifier numbers can also be used to locate patients with memory impairments who may wander away from their rooms or caregivers (Positive ID, n.d.). The RFID tag can be implanted under the patient's skin or worn as a bracelet. The only information contained in the chip is the patient's name, address, allergies, picture, and the unique identifier, which is used to obtain health record information. The healthcare provider uses a wall or handheld scanner to obtain the information.

SUMMARY

The issues associated with migration from a paper medical record to full implementation of the electronic record are extremely complex and arduous. The good news is that progress is being made one step at a time and, sometimes, one keystroke at a time. There is collaboration among the government, private and professional organizations, vendors, healthcare agencies, and healthcare professionals. The EMR Adoption model developed by HIMSS Analytics serves as a road map for those

who have undertaken or plan to undertake the electronic journey.

The healthcare organization's strategic plan serves as a foundation for the successful implementation of a system. Selection decisions for health information system solutions don't come easily. In this day of financial scrutiny, stakeholders need to see an ROI. Risks and opportunities for tangible and intangible payoffs must be explored.

The HIT steering committee should be a multidisciplinary team that includes the top leadership, clinicians, information technology personnel, and all others whose work might be influenced by the new system. The oversight committee must address hard issues such as interoperability standards, user design of data entry screens, workflow redesign, and quality measurement desired outcomes. All users must have a clear vision of the opportunities to improve nursing outcomes and save unnecessary, avoidable hospital costs, while at the same time meet The Joint Commission's and other accreditation body regulatory requirements. Everyone who is involved with the system design and implementation should be familiar with literature findings and research results to anticipate and avoid negative unintended consequences. No potential problem should be minimized; rather, it should be addressed proactively.

As the issues of interoperability and system integration are addressed, the United States will be able to take proactive interventions to recognize communicable disease outbreaks by using analysis of symptoms in a secure central database. Several initiatives addressing the creation of disease and syndromic surveillance systems can also be used for bioterrorism. As an example, the CDC NEDSS system is already in place. The EHR has the ability of expediting safe care and saving lives during a disaster if the data are stored in an RHIO's secure databases so that they are accessible wherever the victim receives care.

Issues regarding privacy, confidentiality, and data security still persist. Healthcare data privacy and security are of utmost importance to those who provide and receive care. The associated challenges are how to expedite the delivery of healthcare and communication among providers while at the same time protecting the health information system data. As new technology develops, new issues will surface. The more things change, the more they stay the same.

APPLICATIONS AND COMPETENCIES

1. Use the EMR Adoption model to analyze and describe the level of adoption for a local healthcare agency.

2. Discuss the opportunities for clinical data sharing in your city or region. Support the associated risks and opportunities with current literature.

3. Discuss the methods for ensuring privacy and confidentiality of patient electronic information in a local clinical setting. Identify the penalties the agency uses for employees that breach confidentiality and security policies.

4. Interview a leadership representative from information technology at a healthcare agency to assess interoperability issues within the different health information systems. Summarize the findings in a written report.

5. Create literature on workflow redesign, as it relates to a clinical documentation system. Afterward, interview a nurse on a unit that is using any method of HIT to assess any nurse workflow issues. Explain why workflow is or is not an issue for the nursing staff.

6. Analyze how a local healthcare agency is addressing The Joint Commission's patient safety goals. Is the agency using HIT to address the safety goals? Why or why not?

7. Search the Web for tools that measure the strength of a password. Use the tool to assist you to create two examples of strong passwords. Provide an explanation for how you were able to create a strong password.

REFERENCES

Agency for Healthcare Research and Quality. (2010). *Incorporating health information technology into workflow redesign (Wisconsin)*. Retrieved from http://healthit.ahrq.gov/ahrq-funded-projects/incorporating-health-information-technology-workflow-redesign

Agency for Healthcare Research and Quality. (2011). *Workflow assessment for Health IT toolkit*. Retrieved from http://healthit.ahrq.gov/health-it-tools-and-resources/workflow-assessment-health-it-toolkit

Ash, J. S., Sittig, D. F., Dykstra, R., et al. (2009). The unintended consequences of computerized provider order entry: Findings from a mixed methods exploration. *International Journal of Medical Informatics*, 78(Suppl 1), S69–S76. doi: 10.1016/j.ijmedinf.2008.07.015.

Biometric Newsportal. (n.d.). *Biometric systems and solutions*. Retrieved from http://www.biometricnewsportal.com/default.asp

Centers for Disease Control and Prevention. (2011, April 1). *Division of Preparedness and Emerging Infections (DPEI)*. Retrieved from http://www.cdc.gov/ncezid/dpei/

Centers for Disease Control and Prevention. (2014a). PHIN messaging guide for syndromic Emergency department, urgent care, inpatient and ambulatory care settings. Retrieved from http://www.cdc.gov/phin/library/guides/SyndrSurvMessageGuide2_MessagingGuide_PHN.pdf

Centers for Disease Control and Prevention. (2014b). *Public Health Information Network (PHIN)*. Retrieved from http://www.cdc.gov/phin/

Chen, J. C., & Collins, T. J. (2012). Creation of a RFID based real time tracking (R-RTT) system for small healthcare clinics. *Journal of Medical System*, 36(6), 3851–3860. doi:10.1007/s10916-012-9858-7.

CMS.gov. (2013a). *National provider identifier standard (NPI)*. Retrieved from http://www.cms.gov/Regulations-and-Guidance/HIPAA-Administrative-Simplification/NationalProvIdentStand/index.html

CMS.gov. (2013b). *Overview HIPAA—General information*. Retrieved from http://www.cms.gov/Regulations-and-Guidance/HIPAA-Administrative-Simplification/HIPAAGenInfo/index.html

CMS.gov. (2013c). *Physician self-referral*. Retrieved from http://www.cms.gov/Medicare/Fraud-and-Abuse/PhysicianSelfReferral/index.html

Cowan, L. (2013). Literature review and risk mitigation strategy for unintended consequences of computerized physician order entry. *Nursing Economics*, 31(1), 27. Retrieved from www.nursingeconomics.net

Federal Emergency Management Agency (FEMA). (2014). *Response & recovery*. Retrieved from http://www.fema.gov/response-recovery

Fontana, J. (2014, January 10). *Authentication pushing password out to pasture*. Retrieved from http://www.zdnet.com/authentication-pushing-password-out-to-pasture-7000025007/

Gattadahalli, S. (2013, January 1). Ten practices for Health IT strategic planning. *Journal of AHIMA*. Retrieved from http://journal.ahima.org/2013/01/01/ten-practices-for-health-it-strategic-planning/

HealthIT.gov. (2013a). *Nationwide privacy and security framework for electronic exchange*. Retrieved from http://www.healthit.gov/policy-researchers-implementers/nationwide-privacy-and-security-framework-electronic-exchange

HealthIT.gov. (2013b). *What is an electronic health record (EHR)*. Retrieved from http://www.healthit.gov/providers-professionals/faqs/what-electronic-health-record-ehr

HealthIT.gov. (2014, November 7). *About ONC HIT certification program*. Retrieved from http://www.healthit.gov/policy-researchers-implementers/about-onc-hit-certification-program

Health Resources and Services Administration (HRSA). (n.d.). *What return on investment (ROI) models can I use?*

Retrieved from http://www.hrsa.gov/healthit/toolbox/RuralHealthITtoolbox/Financing/roi.html

HIMSS Analytics. (2014). *HIMSS Analytics.* Retrieved from http://www.himssanalytics.org

Jones, S. S., Koppel, R., Ridgely, M. S., et al. (2011). *Guide to reducing unintended consequences of electronic health records.* Prepared by RAND Corporation under Contract No. HHSA290200600017I, Task Order #5. Rockville, MD: Agency for Healthcare Research and Quality (AHRQ). Retrieved from http://www.healthit.gov/unintended-consequences/

Kelly, K. (2014, May 2). *Keep your RFID passport data secure.* Retrieved from http://www.practicalhacks.com/2011/05/02/keep-your-rfid-passport-data-secure/

Kim, T. J., Arrieta, M. I., Eastburn, S. L., et al. (2013). Post-disaster Gulf Coast recovery using telehealth. *Telemedicine Journal and E-Health, 19*(3), 200–210. doi:10.1089/tmj.2012.0100.

MacDonald, I. (2014, January 22). Hospitals rank alarm fatigue as top patient safety concern. *FierceHealthcare.* Retrieved from http://www.fiercehealthcare.com/story/hospitals-rank-alarm-fatigue-top-patient-safety-concern/2014-01-22

Magid, S., Forrer, C., & Shaha, S. (2012). Duplicate orders: An unintended consequence of computerized provider/physician order entry (CPOE) implementation: Analysis and mitigation strategies. *Applied Clinical Informatics, 3*(4), 377–391. doi:10.4338/ACI-2012-01-RA-0002.

Markle Foundation, American Medical Association, & Gold Standard. (2006, June 13). Lessons from Katrina Health. Retrieved from http://www.markle.org/publications/894-lessons-katrinahealth

Maviglia, S. M., Yoo, J. Y., Franz, C., et al. (2007). Cost-benefit analysis of a hospital pharmacy bar code solution. *Archives of Internal Medicine, 167*(8), 788–794. doi:10.1001/archinte.167.8.788.

Menachemi, N., Burkhardt, J., Shewchuk, R., et al. (2006). Hospital information technology and positive financial performance: A different approach to finding an ROI. *Journal of Healthcare Management, 51*(1), 40–58; discussion 58–59.

Mohammed, A. S. (2014, January 10). Just in time—EHR Stark Law exception, anti-kickback safe harbor extended through December 31, 2021. Retrieved from http://blog.ecgmc.com/2014/01/10/just-in-time-ehr-stark-law-exception-anti-kickback-safe-harbor-extended-through-december-31-2021/

Nuance. (2014). *Voice biometrics.* Retrieved from www.nuance.com/for-business/customer-service-solutions/voice-biometrics/index.htm

Ornstein, C. (2008, March 15). *Hospital to punish snooping on Spears.* Retrieved from http://articles.latimes.com/2008/mar/15/local/me-britney15

Pearson. (2014). *State-of-the-art identification: Palm vein pattern recognition for the NCLEX®examination.* Retrieved from http://www.pearsonvue.com/nclex/NCLEX_PalmVeinFAQ.pdf

Martinez Pérez, M., Cabrero-Canosa, M., Vizoso Hermida, J., et al. (2012). Application of RFID technology in patient tracking and medication traceability in emergency care. *Journal of Medical Systems, 36*(6), 3983–3993. doi:10.1007/s10916-012-9871-x.

Positive ID. (n.d.). *PositiveID—Identity theft, credit monitoring, implantable microchip, electronic health records.* Retrieved from http://www.positiveidcorp.com/health-id.html

RFID 101.com. (2014, November 29). *RFID 101: Guide to radio-frequency identification (RFID) technology.* Retrieved from http://www.rfid-101.com/

RFID Journal. (2014). *Frequently asked questions.* Retrieved from http://www.rfidjournal.com/faq/

SearchSecurity.com. (2011, March). *Spear phishing.* Retrieved from http://searchsecurity.techtarget.com/sDefinition/0,sid14_gci1134829,00.html

Supply Insight. (2015). *Supply Insight sustainable RFID solutions.* Retrieved from http://supplyinsight.com

Technopedia. (2014). *What is spear phishing?* Retrieved from http://www.techopedia.com/definition/4121/spear-phishing

The Joint Commission. (2014). *2014 Joint Commission national patient safety goals.* Retrieved from http://www.jointcommission.org/hap_2014_npsgs/

U.S. Customs and Border Protection. (n.d.). *NEXUS program description.* Retrieved from http://www.cbp.gov/travel/trusted-traveler-programs/nexus/nexus-overview

Wicklund, E. (2012, August 12). Thanks to Hugs, an abduction is averted. *MHealthNews.* Retrieved from http://www.mhealthnews.com/news/thanks-hugs-abduction-averted

Wilson, T. V. (2005, November 11). *How biometrics works.* Retrieved from http://www.wpro.who.int/southpacific/programmes/communicable_diseases/disease_surveillance_response/PSS-16-November-2014/en/

World Health Organization. (2014, November). *Pacific syndromic surveillance report.* Retrieved from http://www.wpro.who.int/southpacific/programmes/communicable_diseases/disease_surveillance_response/PSS-16-November-2014/en/

CHAPTER 21

Evolving Trends in Telehealth

OBJECTIVES

After studying this chapter, you will be able to:

1. Define the two overall classifications of technology used in telehealth.
2. Discuss some of the ways that telehealth can deliver healthcare.
3. Illustrate the opportunities for autonomous nursing practice in telehealth.
4. Discuss the main issues in implementing telehealth.
5. Analyze the ways that telehealth could influence the present healthcare system.

KEY TERMS

Biometric garment	Store and forward (S&F)	Telenursing
E-intensive care	Telehealth	Telepresence
Portable monitoring devices	Telehomecare	Teletrauma
Real-time	Telemedicine	
Robotics	Telemental health	

During the 1998 Around the World Alone sailboat race, one of the racers, while in the South Atlantic, developed an abscess on his elbow that could have caused him to lose his arm. Using a wireless computer and satellite technology, he contacted a doctor in Boston who directed his treatment and saved the arm (Lynch, 1998). Not all telehealth applications are this dramatic, but the incident demonstrates the power of this emerging vehicle for delivering healthcare. Although much attention has been given to the aspect of telehealth that addresses the delivery of acute care or specialist consultations, telehealth is far more versatile. We can use telehealth to provide home nursing care **(telenursing)**, electronic referrals to specialists and hospitals, teleconsulting between specialists and general practitioners or nurse practitioners, minor injury consulting, and consulting through call centers.

Terms such as "telehealth" and "telemedicine" are often used interchangeably to refer to health services delivered using electronic technology to patients at a distance. According to the American Telemedicine Association (ATA) (2012), **telemedicine** refers to the electronic exchange of patient information between two sites for improving the patient's health status, and **telehealth**, a broader term, extends beyond the delivery of clinical services. The International Council of Nursing defines *telenursing* as telecommunications technology in nursing to enhance patient care (International Council of Nurses, 2010). This chapter focuses on emerging developments and applications using the term telehealth unless specified otherwise in the references used to support the information.

TELEHEALTH BASICS

Telemedicine technology does not have to be complex, as the sailor in the Around the World Alone sailboat race proved. Most cases would not involve self-treatment. Generally, technology can be used in two ways to deliver telehealth: **store and forward (S&F)** and two-way communication. The line between these two modes is becoming less and less distinct because many services use both types of communication. There is a wealth of information about telehealth on the Internet. A good place to begin is the American Telemedicine Association at http://www.americantelemed.org/home. Telehealth has emerging multidimensional aspects with advances in the Internet and mobile apps, which allow the consumer to take control of personal health.

Store and Forward Technology

In S&F technology, a digital camera, scanner, or technology (e.g., x-ray machine) that generates electronic images captures a still image electronically and then that image is sent to a specialist for interpretation later (American Telemedicine Association, 2013). Radiology, dermatology, pathology, and wound care specialties lend themselves very well to this technique. S&F also includes asynchronous transmission of clinical data, such as the results of an electrocardiogram, magnetic resonance imaging (MRI), or blood glucose levels, between two sites. This type of communication is often between healthcare providers. S&F offers the only affordable way for practice of medicine in remote communities, such as those in Alaska. An example for use of S&F is when a radiologist located at a different site from where the x-ray was done reads it. We use this method in healthcare frequently.

Real-Time Telehealth

Real-time telehealth involves the patient and the provider interacting at the same time by using interactive video/television. Real-time telehealth requires the use of telecommunications devices that permit two-way communication. The oldest of these is the telephone, but current telehealth technology generally includes videoconferencing using two-way video and audio. Although videoconferencing is possible with a modem and plain old telephone service, a higher quality of service is usually preferred. The required level of service depends on the type of services offered. Some services require at least a secure T1 fiberoptic line or a line on an integrated digital network, which must not only connect the sites but also extend to the rooms where both the patient and the distant consultant are located. Telehealth also may use large satellite systems that have a global audience. In short, any two-way communication technology offering both audio and video has, or will find, a use in telehealth.

Real-time telehealth also makes use of special instruments that can transmit an image to a clinician at a different location. These include an ear–nose–throat scope, a camera that captures skin observations, and a special stethoscope. They can be used either in real-time or in S&F mode. In addition, by using a combination of **robotics** (use of robots) and virtual reality, a surgeon with special gloves and the appropriate audio and video technology is able to perform surgery by manipulating surgical instruments at the remote site. This procedure uses **telepresence**. Telepresence is the use of technology to provide the appearance of a person's presence, although he or she is located at a remote site (Federation of American Scientists, n.d.). It is still in development and requires a 100% reliable system and a very high bandwidth.

TELENURSING

Telenursing, as part of telehealth, is not new. Telenursing in nondisaster settings is a nursing specialty. Telenursing offers nurses a chance to create more collaborative and autonomous roles and at the same time reduce the overall cost of healthcare.

Today, telenurses work in various settings. An international study completed between 2004 and 2005 revealed that 37% of telenurses reported working in hospital and college settings

(Grady & Schlachta-Fairchild, 2007). Telenursing was described as a nurse who works with telehealth technologies. The majority of the nurses indicated that they learned telenursing skills on the job. An interesting finding, given that majority of the nurses had no prior experience with telehealth before their telenursing positions, is that the majority (89.2%) of those surveyed indicated that telehealth should be included in basic nursing curriculum. Although the research is dated, telehealth is still not a standard component for entry-level registered nurse education in the United States, although faculty may introduce the concept in community nursing courses.

OTHER TELEHEALTH EXAMPLES

As healthcare shifts away from the hospital and into the home and community, the therapeutic uses for telehealth increase. A much broader range of healthcare professionals such as nurse practitioners, nutritionists, social workers, and home healthcare aides have roles in the provision of telehealth. One problem that has plagued the use of telehealth in the past is that payers have focused on acute medical care; however, reimbursement for telehealth services is slowly beginning to improve. Until the reimbursement issue is completely resolved, much of our population will remain underserved. As a result, instead of treating illnesses in the early stages, without the use of telehealth, the illnesses progress to a stage where they are very costly to treat.

Telehomecare

A trend in modern healthcare is to focus on the patient instead of the provider or agency. **Telehomecare** refers to the monitoring and delivery of healthcare in the patient's home rather than the provider's work setting. The greatest use of telehomecare is that it allows the patient the comforts of his or her own home, improves quality of life, and avoids time-consuming costly visits to office appointments or hospital admissions. Telehomecare uses the concepts from the "medical home," where there is coordinated care provided in a home that is "accessible, family-centered, continuous, comprehensive, coordinated, compassionate, and culturally effective" (HRSA, 2014, para. 2).

The ongoing monitoring allows identification of potential problems before they become significant problems. Because telehomecare can eliminate unnecessary emergency room visits and hospital visits, it is cost-effective.

Telehealth for Chronic Disease Care

For patients with chronic diseases, such as cardiac, pulmonary, diabetes, and chronic renal failure, telehealth can be a powerful self-management tool. Home health monitoring services provide patients with devices that can collect and transmit vital signs: cardiac rhythm, blood glucose, and weight (Table 21-1). The data sent by using a telephone line or broadband connection to the healthcare provider can be stored in the patient's electronic health record (EHR). The healthcare provider's central monitoring station can view data from all patients that they are monitoring and see any alerts indicating significant changes. The computer screen that the healthcare provider views looks very similar to the central monitoring station in an intensive care unit (ICU) or step-down unit. Various companies host home health monitoring services.

Research studies support the use of remote monitoring to reduce emergency department visits, reduce hospital readmission rates, improve care, and reduce costs. Blinkhorn (2012) did a meta-analysis of telehealth research for chronic kidney disease (CKD). He identified four classifications for use of telehealth in the care of CKD: teleconsultation, teleconferences, teledialysis (remote monitoring using communication with an automated peritoneal dialysis or hemodialysis

TABLE 21-1	Examples of Telehomecare Devices
Vendor	Device
ViTelCare Health	HomMed Health Monitoring System
Philips	Motiva remote care manager
MD2	Medication dispensing system

machine), and telemonitoring. His research revealed telehealth improved disease management and fewer hospital days for CKD with some of the studies. Guédon-Moreau et al. (2014) researched the outcomes of remote monitoring in 310 patients with implantable cardioverter defibrillators in France. Research results showed a decrease in nonhospital and hospital costs.

Other monitoring devices are growing in popularity with those who have chronic diseases. All of the devices provide a means for remote monitoring. For example, patients with heart problems might have pacemakers, insertable cardiac monitors, implantable cardiac defibrillators, and cardiac resynchronization therapy devices (Medtronic, 2014). Patients with diabetes might have an insulin pod or insulin pump. The insulin pod attaches has an adhesive side with a small needle that attaches to the patient's body and communicates wirelessly to a handheld remote control. The insulin pump attaches to a belt or waistband of clothing with tubing that connects to a subcutaneous covered needle that delivers insulin. Patients can customize the insulin delivery based upon their input about diet intake and blood sugar results. Although still under development, some diabetics might qualify for an implantable blood glucose monitor that simulates the functioning of a pancreas (GlySens, 2014).

The Centers for Medicare & Medicaid Services have traditionally not reimbursed for telehomecare, so the studies reported in the literature are prototypes funded with grant money. For example, home care agencies in New York began using telehomecare after receiving a York State Department of Health telemedicine grant (Wood, 2011). Home care service reported decreases in hospitalization rates ranging from 5% to 10% after implementing the service.

Telehomecare is also in use by major medical centers worldwide. Piedmont Healthcare (2014), a large medical center based in Atlanta, Georgia, uses telemonitoring. Piedmont Healthcare reported that telehomecare monitoring heart failure patient readmission rates were 75% lower than that for patients not in the program (Mattia, 2007).

The Veterans Administration (VA) also uses telehomecare. The researchers reported a separate 4-year longitudinal study with 774 veterans diagnosed with diabetes mellitus (Jia et al., 2009). The veterans were divided into a treatment group and a control group. All veterans had been an inpatient in the VA or used the emergency services within the previous 12 months. Patients in the treatment group received services from the VA Care Coordination Home Telehealth program. Patients in the control group did not have telehealth services. The study results showed an improved accessibility to healthcare, reduction of preventable hospitalizations, and decreased costs for care over time.

Portable Monitoring Devices

Portable monitoring devices, available from a number of vendors (see Table 21-1), have many similarities. For example, they include an input device and various types of peripheral monitoring equipment. Many of the input devices use a touch screen with text and audio to ask assessment questions about the patient's health. The patient can respond to questions by choosing answers such as true/false, none/better/worse, yes/no, and 0–10. Programming of some of the devices includes branching questions. Answers to some questions may result in the display of patient education information.

There are some differences for self-monitoring equipment. While most provide access to a central monitoring station using a telephone line, others allow access using high-speed and wireless connections. The peripheral monitoring accessories can vary among vendor products. Examples of monitoring accessories include a blood pressure cuff, electrocardiogram, blood glucose meter, weight scales, fluid status monitor, pulse oximeter, monitors for PT/INR (prothrombin time/international ratio), peak flow meter, and a spirometer.

What are the future trends for home monitoring devices? We can expect vendors to design the equipment so that the monitoring data will integrate with the EHR to share with authorized healthcare agencies and providers. For example, Honeywell HomMed health monitoring system integrates the patient monitoring data with an EHR. We can also expect the devices to provide patient decision support with context-sensitive health education information, reminders to take medication and doctor's appointments, feedback regarding vital sign monitoring results, and motivational messages. One example of a home monitoring system that uses a television monitor or a 3G-enabled tablet computer is Philips Motiva remote care manager (Philips Healthcare, 2013).

Consumer and Healthcare Provider Telehealth Devices

Healthcare consumer self-monitoring is growing in popularity with the release of low-cost or free health and wellness apps available without a prescription. There are thousands of health and wellness apps for smartphone and tablets available from the Apple and Google Play stores. A caveat to the availability of the apps is that Federal Drug Administration (FDA) has not approved many of them so they may have questionable value.

In addition to apps, there are wearable devices, for example, Fitbit and Google Glass. Depending on the specific device, the wearable Fitbit assists the user to monitor sleep quality, calories burned, and body activity (Fitbit, 2015). Fitbit also has a WiFi smart weight scale that allows the user to track their weight, body mass index, and percent body fat. The wearable Fitbit device and smart scales connect to the iOS or Android smartphone app. Users can also use to social aspect of Fitbit to share and compare progress with others.

Google Glass (Figure 21-1) incorporates a small computer with camera and video functions on the corner of eyeglass frames (Google, 2014). Google Glass connects with the iOS or Android smartphone Glass app using WiFi or Bluetooth. With Google Glass, the user can do several things, for example, take pictures and videos, make a phone call, and navigate, send a message, connect with Google Hangouts, and use the Google search engine. Google Glass technology is still in its infancy. Healthcare consumers will find how to use it to improve their health.

Google is working with healthcare providers to develop strategies that will improve delivery of care with Google Glass. For example, doctors at Beth Israel Deaconess Medical Center in Boston are beta testing Google Glass in the emergency department (Gaudin, 2014). The Google Glass devices they are testing are custom designed for use in the healthcare setting, for example, the doctors are able to view a patient's chart using the wearable computer.

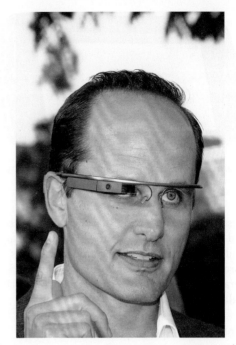

Figure 21-1. Google Glass (shutterstock.com/Joe Seer).

Telemetry self-monitoring devices are available. For example, AliveCor (http://www.alivecor.com) provides that ability to monitor one's heart rhythm using a case attachment for iPhone or Android smartphone for purchase without a prescription (AliveCor, 2014). The AliveCor monitoring device is FDA approved for use. To obtain a cardiac tracing, the user places their fingers on the metal plates of the smartphone attachment (Figure 21-2) or place the device on the person's

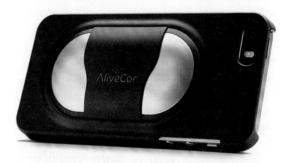

Figure 21-2. AliveCor heart smartphone case attachment. (Used with permission.)

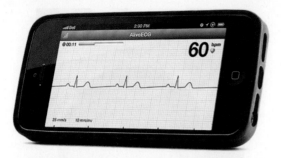

Figure 21-3. AliveCor heart monitor app on a smartphone. (Used with permission.)

chest. The cardiac tracing that displays on associated smartphone app (Figure 21-3) is similar to Lead I of the 12-lead electrocardiogram. Users can store their telemetry tracings in a secure cloud storage as well as share the tracing with their healthcare providers.

Automatic Pill Dispensers/Reminders

Automatic pill dispensers/reminders are another type of telehomecare device. The pill dispensers include auditory reminders to prompt patients to take their medications, even if the medication is not a pill. Some of the automatics pill dispensers provide patient reminders to take the medication with food or to take an insulin injection. One example, with the MD2 Plus MedSmart system, if the patient does not dispense the medications within a specified timeframe, the system notifies the caregiver by telephone. If the caregiver does not answer the telephone, the device phones the support center. The MD2 remote monitoring of compliance is through a secure website. In addition to the MD2 Plus MedSmart system, several other companies make automatic pill dispensers with reminders.

Wearable Monitoring Garments

Our current healthcare system remains disease focused; we seek care after something has gone wrong. Emerging wearable **biometric garment** technology allows for a proactive approach that allows for early identification of symptoms before problems develop. Early identification of symptoms has the potential for maintaining the patient's quality of life, reducing acute

exacerbations of disease processes, and avoiding unnecessary medical costs. The concept of wearable garments with built-in physiological monitoring devices uses nanotechnology and is fascinating.

Consider the concept of "smart underwear" where sensors printed on the waistband of underwear monitor biomarkers in sweat and tears (Kane, 2010). The underwear sensors make "autonomous" diagnoses and dispense appropriate drugs. Researchers are developing smart underwear for use by warriors who might be injured in battle. Of course, others who have an altered health status could also use them.

Wearable biometric garments can also be designed for use with portable home monitoring devices (Villalba et al., 2009). Consider a shirt for cardiac and respiration monitoring in addition to a portable blood pressure cuff and weight scale with Bluetooth capabilities for data transfer. The grouping of devices is a part of the Heart Failure Management System used in Europe.

Telemental Health

Telemental health is the use of telehealth to deliver psychiatric healthcare. The Telemental Health, a special interest group of the ATA, website at http://www.americantelemed.org/i4a/pages/index.cfm?pageID=3326 includes up-to-date educational presentations on current telemental health projects. Research on the use of telemental health reports that care provided with the use of telehealth technology is comparable to face-to-face care.

Healthcare providers use telehealth to deliver care for various mental health problems. Its use is more prevalent in rural areas, prisons, and other areas where access to a mental health professional is difficult or impossible. Telehealth is also used to care for veterans. A 2011 4-year study reported the use of telehealth to provide evidence-based psychotherapy for veterans with posttraumatic stress disorder (PTSD) (Stachan et al., 2012). Veterans with PTSD may have difficulties receiving care in busy medical centers. The travel time to receive care and symptom severity are also factors. Telehealth provides a means to delivery evidence-based care in convenient settings for the veterans.

Clinic Visits

Use of telehealth benefits rural areas where residents traditionally have few options for healthcare and few, if any, specialists. For example, Maine includes many barrier islands inhabited by residents, many of whom make their livelihood from lobster work. Travel to the mainland for these residents can be very inconvenient and result in loss of income. To address the healthcare delivery problem, Sunbeam Health Services provides virtual doctors' visits by using a ship staffed by nurses and equipped closed circuit television (Main Sea Coast Mission, 2014). Telehealth services are also provided from a renovated clinic on Swan's Island, one of the barrier islands.

E-Intensive Care Units

Remote monitoring of critical care patients is not new. Hospitals, such as Stormont-Vail in Topeka, Kansas, were doing remote telemetry monitoring for patients in small outlying communities of Kansas in the 1970s. The current use of telepresence of ICU intensivists in critical care is redefining the meaning of critical care remote monitoring. According to the Leapfrog Group, the mortality rate of ICU patients is 10% to 20%; however, the use of intensivists to manage or comanage patients can reduce hospital mortality by 30% and ICU mortality by 40% (Leapfrog Group, 2014). The Leapfrog Group recommends the use of ICU physician staffing and supports the use of telemedicine intensive services to meet that need. Telepresence in critical care is currently being delivered with the use of videoconferencing tools, such as eICU (VISICU, Baltimore, MD), and robotics, such as RP-7 (InTouch Health, Santa Barbara, CA).

QSEN Scenario

After sharing information about the e-intensive care unit concept with a nursing colleague, the colleague asks you how the system affects the quality and safety of patient care. How should you respond?

---

eICU

iCare Intensive Care at North Colorado Medical Center provides telepresence using a camera, microphone, and speaker in the patient rooms (Banner, 2014). The bedside team activates the camera during patient rounds when there is a need for the off-site intensivists and the expertise of critical care nurses located at the iCare Command Center in Banner Desert Medical Center.

The Banner Health system includes hospitals located across seven states: Alaska, Arizona, California, Colorado, Nebraska, Nevada, and Wyoming. The iCare Command Center located in Mesa, AZ, monitors Banner system critical care beds (Banner, 2014). The command center staff has access to patient monitoring information, laboratory values, and x-rays. The cameras and microphones make it possible for the off-site experts to speak with the patients and on-site care providers by using HIPAA-compliant transmissions. Patients receive information about the service upon admission to the hospital and are encouraged to ask questions or express concerns about the service.

Reports on the use of eICU provide promising results for the use of telehealth in critical care. Taylor (2013) reported implementing eICU in 2009 to improve ICU outcomes and to decrease costs for care. In 2005, the cost of taking care of a patient on the ventilator was $28,000 at High Point Regional Health in North Carolina. After implementation of eICU in 2012, the cost was $18,500 after investing in eICU services, which cost $800/patient. With iICU services, there was a reduction of the average length of stay by more than half, decreasing from 14.2 days to 7 days.

Kowitlawakul (2011) conducted a study with 117 critical care nurses working in two metropolitan healthcare systems where eICU technology was not used. She used the Technology Acceptance Model developed by Davis (1985). The model assessed five constructs: perceived usefulness, perceived ease of use, attitude toward using, intentions to use, and actual systems use to determine computer acceptance behavior. The study results showed that although all of constructs had some significance, perceived usefulness was a key determinant on the nurses' acceptance of eICU technology. The researcher recommended that nurses and physicians be involved at the beginning of the planning for adoption of eICU technology. A physician who supports the use of technology should be identified as the person responsible for patient care management before implantation. Finally, administrators should respect the autonomy of the nurses and physicians by providing the necessary education prior to system implementation.

Nurses agree that improved patient outcomes are extremely important, but implementing **e-intensive care** has implications for the entire ICU environment. The use of these eICU tools requires extensive planning and communications as well as workflow redesign. The most important factor is buy-in by all affected departments, including not only the ICU staff but also attending physicians, hospital leadership, information services, and respiratory therapy.

Robotics

Robotics is yet another way to provide telepresence of ICU intensivists. One example is the RP-7i robot; RP is short for remote presence (InTouch Health, 2014). The robot is the height of a person who is 5 feet 6 inches and has a large flat screen monitor where a person's head would be; a small camera with tilt, pan, and zoom features; and a couple of antennas on top of the monitor (Figure 21-4). The robot also has two-way audio that allows for conversations between the clinical site and the remote expert. It receives and sends data through a wireless network. It rolls about the floor on three spheres and has built-in infrared sensing devices to help guide it around obstacles. Other versions of the robot have a smaller base or a computer carried by a healthcare provider. The robots are FDA approved for use.

The remote teleintensivist expert controls the robot using RP software and a joystick. The software can be used with a laptop or a desktop computer. Dual monitors allow the physician to view a patient's electronic medical record on one monitor and to control the robot using the second monitor. The movement of the robot's camera tilt, pan, and zoom features allows the physician to examine the patient, read a chart, view x-rays mounted on a light board, or observe physiological monitor data. The robot's "head" (the monitor) is able to move 360 degrees, allowing it to "face" the ICU person. The

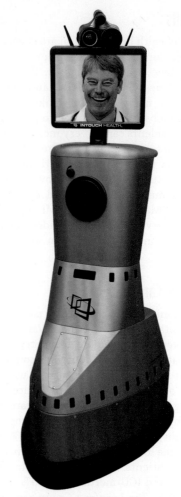

Figure 21-4. RP-7i robot. (Courtesy of InTouch Health.)

robot's audio and video features allow for real-time interaction between the physician at the remote site and the patient and care providers in the ICU.

Robotics are used in a variety of settings. Wake Forest Baptist Medical Center uses robots at its network remote hospitals to assist the physicians at the remote agencies to provide stroke care (Covington, 2014, April 9). The telehealth service provides the networked hospitals with 24-hour access to stroke specialist physicians.

Robotic telepresence is also used in the care of sick newborn infants at Longview Hospital in Washington (Tolandes, 2014). The hospital is in the network of Oregon Health and Science University, which also provides expertise in neonatology to rural and midsized community hospitals. It is also in use for neonatal care at New Albany Hospital in Tupelo, Mississippi (Byers, 2014). The expert care supports physicians and families where the infant was born and can prevent the necessity for the infant's transport to another care facility.

Early research on the use of remote telepresence using robotics in critical care demonstrated positive outcomes. Vespa et al. (2007) compared data for a period of time before and after using robot telepresence. They noted that the face-to-face response time for routine and urgent pages was reduced from 3.5 hours to less than 10 minutes. Because of the rapid response times, patient outcomes improved and the ICU length of stay was reduced. The researchers attributed a cost savings of $1.1 million to the use of robot telepresence.

Teletrauma Care

Rural hospitals and clinics have been able to use telehealth to augment trauma care **(teletrauma)** because they are able to obtain reimbursement for these services (CMS.gov, 2014a). Teletrauma is used to obtain second opinions and advice from trauma care experts. Teletrauma care has also been used to deliver care in parts of the world torn by violence and war.

Rural hospitals in places like Northern California and Eastern Maine are using telehealth equipment to connect with trauma experts. The rural physicians and staff want to provide the best possible care to the patients while keeping the inconvenience of care, travel, and expense of care as low as possible. As of 2007, University of California, Davis (UC Davis), pediatric intensivists had completed over 200 videoconferencing consultations with remote hospital emergency departments and ICUs (UC Davis Health System, 2007). Thirty percent of the consultations were related to trauma care for children. Eastern Maine Health System (EMHS, 2014) has reported the use of teleconferencing to improve emergency patient outcomes. The telemedicine hub site, located at Eastern Maine Medical Center, was designed to provide 24/7 support for the care of patients located in multiple rural care hospitals.

Research on the use of teletrauma care in rural settings has shown promising evidence-based outcomes and significance for use in rural health settings. Duchesne et al. (2008) reported a 5-year study of 814 trauma patients, comparing the outcomes before and after the implementation of telemedicine in rural Mississippi settings. The trauma patients who experienced teletrauma care had a decrease in the length of stay at the local community hospital (1.5 hours vs. 47 hours) and a decrease in transfer time to trauma centers (1.7 hours vs. 13 hours). The hospital costs for the trauma patients decreased from $7,632,624 to $1,126,683.

Disaster Healthcare

Telehealth has been used successfully in providing healthcare in disasters (Block, 2010; Markle Foundation, American Medical Association, & Gold Standard, 2006). Almost immediately after Hurricane Katrina hit the Gulf Shore states in the United States in 2005, the KatrinaHealth website was established to facilitate communication and to assist victims to access their electronic prescription medication records. As a result, many nurses were able to distribute medications in temporary living communities established across the United States where victims had been transported. One example of such a community was the Rock Eagle 4-H camp in Georgia. The home economics building was converted into a clinic and was open 24 hours to serve 240 to 500 victims. Volunteer physicians and nurse practitioners staffed part of the clinic. Another part was staffed by volunteer nurses. The local health department nursing leadership coordinated all the care. Nurses used desktop computers with access to the Internet and secure logins to access information to assist the victims. With the assistance of the electronic prescribing, a local pharmacy was able to make daily deliveries of prescribed medication. The clinic volunteer nurses provided care in traditional ways, and the patient records were all on paper; however, access to the Internet played a major role in access to supplies and the provision of care.

Telehealth was used in a number of disasters following Hurricane Katrina. Bon Secours Hospital in Baltimore, Maryland, used it during horrific blizzards when streets were impassible (Wood, 2012). It was also used after a tornado struck Lone Star, Oklahoma. Patients from the Lone Star area received care at Mercy Hospital in Ardmore, Oklahoma. TeleICU physicians and staff covered care for the 10-bed ICU, thereby freeing up Mercy staff to assist with disaster care.

EDUCATION COMPONENT OF TELEHEALTH PROJECTS

Most telehealth projects have a built-in patient educational component. In some, education is delivered during the "visits" and in others through Web pages. Telehealth is also useful in the educational needs of healthcare professionals, not only for continuing education but also for preparing practitioners. Telehealth education is especially useful in rural areas where it is difficult to recruit healthcare professionals and where costs and difficulty of travel and time away from the workplace are barriers.

Several successful education projects support the use of telehealth. For example, the Native People for Cancer Central Telehealth Network provides education for American Indians and Alaskan Natives who live in Washington and Alaska. During 2008 and 2009, the network provided monthly interactive educational meetings using videoconferencing equipment at 28 tribal clinics (Doorenbos et al., 2011). The educational sessions addressed the latest cancer updates and cultural issues related to cancer care. Evaluations of the educational sessions were very positive and supported the cost-effective use of telehealth education.

Fitzner and Moss (2013) reviewed the literature related to telehealth and "emerging technologic tools" that supported best practice for diabetes self-management. Findings of their research supported the use of telehealth for education and training when it provides benefit, when it does not negatively affect the provider's care, and when costs are reimbursed. The researchers identified ten areas for best practice for use of telehealth delivery of education and training, which are applicable to health education in all settings, not just diabetes (Box 21-1).

ISSUES WITH TELEHEALTH

Telehealth in its many forms can provide many benefits such as enhanced patient care, reduced travel time, increased productivity, access to specialists, and enlarged educational opportunities for all. Many issues, however, surround this mode of healthcare delivery. Four main issues relate to (1) reimbursement, (2) medicolegal issues, (3) technical issues, and (4) research.

Reimbursement Issues

Reimbursement remains a large barrier to the widespread adoption of telehealth (Center for Telehealth & e-Health Law (CTeL), 2014). CTeL conducted a survey of all states and found that 45 had some type of reimbursement for telehealth services. The 2009 American Recovery and Reinvestment Act (ARRA) stimulus money included telemedicine (LeRouge & Garfield, 2013). The Centers for Medicare & Medicaid Services maintains websites, updated annually, on telehealth services (CMS.gov, 2014b, 2014c). Information on Medicaid reimbursement is

---

BOX 21-1 Best Practices for Use of Telehealth for Education and Training

1. Use multiple approaches combining face-to-face with more than one technology.
2. Provide regularly scheduled meetings to motivate and engage users.
3. Use interactive communication.
4. Provide immediate feedback to questions.
5. Keep the patients' health information secure.
6. Provide accurate information.
7. Address the patient's personal and cultural needs.
8. Provide coordinated care.
9. Provide technology and information for use that addresses the need of the patient.
10. Provide convenient access, including the ability for the patient to receive information when at home.

Source: Fitzner and Moss (2013, p. 6).

available online at http://www.medicaid.gov/Medicaid-CHIP-Program-Information/By-Topics/Delivery-Systems/Telemedicine.html.

Of the examples in this chapter, the majority was supported with grants. Despite successes, the telehealth projects were discontinued when the grants expired. Our healthcare system today is shaped by third-party payers, both government and private. Currently, there continues to be no uniformity for the reimbursement of telehealth/telemedicine services (CTel, 2014). For telemedicine to survive/thrive, reimbursement must be a joint effort between states, the federal government, and private payers. Reimbursement considerations must be made with the best interests of the patients' healthcare needs and outcomes in mind.

A 2006 study, a follow-up study on the ATA and AMD Telemedicine Study, showed progress in reimbursement for telehealth. In 2008, the Centers for Medicare & Medicaid Services modified their reimbursement policy for telemedicine as a result of the 2006 Tax Relief and Healthcare Act (Naditz, 2008).

Medicolegal Issues

The medicolegal issues for telehealth relate to licensure, liability, and medical malpractice (LeRouge & Garfield, 2013; Wesson & Kupperschmidt, 2013). Licensure is an issue when the telehealth provider is located in another state or country. Certification and licensure requirements are state-level decisions. Liability and medical malpractice are issues when the licensing/credentialing laws do not specify the use of telehealth (LeRouge & Garfield, 2013). Additional information on medicolegal issues is discussed in Chapter 25.

Technical Issues

The safety of the patient is always a concern with developing uses of new technology. As stated earlier in the chapter, all the projects seen thus far have been of a very high quality, with no compromise in patient safety. In an endeavor to set standards in telenursing, the American Academy of Ambulatory Care Nursing (AAACN) established the telehealth nursing practice special interest group in 1995. The AAACN developed telehealth nursing practice administration and practice standards (American

Academy of Ambulatory Care Nursing, 2011a) that address standards for telenursing, including staffing, competency, ethics, patient rights, and the use of the nursing process in telehealth. They followed this with the publication of the Telehealth Nursing Practice Essentials (Espensen & American Academy of Ambulatory Care Nursing, 2009). The organization also published the Telehealth Nursing Practice Resource Directory (American Academy of Ambulatory Care Nursing, 2011b).

The directory includes resources and information to assist nurses to "improve the quality, efficiency, and effectiveness" of their practice. The AAACN offers certification for telehealth nursing. The application can be downloaded from the AAACN website at http://www.aaacn.org/.

The ATA has adopted core standards for telemedicine operations, which address three types of standards: administrative, clinical, and technical. Administrative standards cover issues related to human resource management, HIPAA, research protocols, telehealth equipment use, and fiscal management. Clinical standards uphold the individual discipline standards of professional practice and standards of care as they relate to telehealth. Technical standards relate to requirements for safety and the function of telehealth equipment, the requirements for policies and procedures, and the need for redundant systems to ensure network connectivity.

SUMMARY

As technology improves, the possibilities for telehealth are endless. Telehealth technologies can be classed as either S&F or real time. S&F is an asynchronous method in which images are sent to a distant location where the images are examined at the convenience of the specialist. Real-time telehealth, a synchronous mode, involves both the patient and the consultant interacting at the same time. Telepresence created with eICUs, two-way video teleconferencing, and robotics is used to augment care delivered in ICUs and emergency departments. Telehomecare monitoring devices are empowering patients to live independently and to be proactive in the early detection of healthcare problems before they happen.

Telehealth offers many opportunities for nurses. Telehealth is valuable in education, both professionally and for patient care and disaster care. As telehealth becomes more widespread, issues still need to be resolved. Access to care remains an issue. Although the Veterans Administration is using telehealth, it is not helping to meet the needs of all veterans. There are about 21.5 million veterans in the United States (CNN, 2014). However, there are only 151 medical centers and 827 clinics available. Breaking news reports in 2014 highlighted the backlog on veterans receiving timely care (Daley & Tang, 2014).

Medicare has finally begun to reimburse telehealth care in the United States; however, since Medicaid is controlled at the state level, variations in reimbursement still exist. The telecommunications infrastructure can also be a problem. As with many innovations, use of telehealth will change the way healthcare is delivered. These changes will create opportunities for many. Care that is more preventive reduces emergency room visits and hospital admissions. It has the potential to upset the financial base of the present acute care system.

APPLICATION AND COMPETENCIES

1. Define the two overall classifications of technology used in telehealth. Provide examples for how your healthcare work setting uses the classifications.

2. Search the digital library for examples of current uses for telehealth. Identify at least one journal article. Summarize the findings using bullet points. Cite the source(s) you used.

3. Write two or three paragraphs illustrating the essential competencies for telenursing.

4. Select one of the issues in implementing telehealth and discuss the different approaches for resolving the issue.

5. Analyze two research studies done with telehealth. Compare the findings for similarities and differences.

6. Explore the ways that telehealth could influence the healthcare system in your country.

REFERENCES

AliveCor. (2014). *AliveCor home.* Retrieved from http://www.alivecor.com

American Academy of Ambulatory Care Nursing. (2011a). *Telehealth nursing practice administration and practice standards* (5th ed.). Pitman, NJ: Author.

American Academy of Ambulatory Care Nursing. (2011b). *Telehealth nursing practice resource directory* (6th ed.). Pitman, NJ: Author.

American Telemedicine Association. (2012). *Telemedicine nomenclature.* Retrieved from http://www.americantelemed.org/resources/nomenclature#.U1QPgqLYMt9

American Telemedicine Association. (2013). *State Medicaid best practice: Store and forward best practice.* Retrieved from http://www.americantelemed.org/docs/default-source/policy/state-medicaid-best-practice---store-and-forward-telemedicine.pdf

Banner Health. (2014). *Banner iCare™ monitoring.* Retrieved from http://www.bannerhealth.com/Locations/Arizona/Banner+Baywood+Medical+Center/Programs+and+Services/Intensive+Care/iCare+monitoring.htm

Blinkhorn, T. M. (2012). Telehealth in nephrology health care: A review. *Renal Society of Australasia Journal, 8*(3), 132–139. Retrieved from http://www.renalsociety.org/RSAJ/about/about_main.html

Block, C. (2010, April 21). *UTMB responds to disasters.* Retrieved from http://telemedicinenews.blogspot.com/2010/04/utmb-responds-to-disasters.html

Byers, R. (2014, January 17). *Doctors use robot to help sick infants.* Retrieved from http://www.wtva.com/news/national/story/Doctors-use-robot-to-help-sick-infants/6Kq8vYHw-0-EGtRloBudAA.cspx

Center for Telehealth & e-Health Law (CTel). (2014). *Reimbursement.* Retrieved from http://ctel.org/expertise/reimbursement/

CMS.gov. (2014a). *Telehealth rural health fact sheet series.* Retrieved from http://www.cms.gov/Outreach-and-Education/Medicare-Learning-Network-MLN/MLNProducts/downloads/TelehealthSrvcsfctsht.pdf

CMS.gov. (2014b). *Telehealth.* Retrieved from http://www.cms.gov/Medicare/Medicare-General-Information/Telehealth/index.html?redirect=/telehealth/

CMS.gov. (2014c). *Telehealth services.* Retrieved from http://www.cms.gov/Outreach-and-Education/Medicare-Learning-Network-MLN/MLNProducts/downloads/TelehealthSrvcsfctsht.pdf

CNN. (2014, November 14). *Department of Veterans Affairs fast facts.* Retrieved from http://www.cnn.com/2014/05/30/us/department-of-veterans-affairs-fast-facts/

Covington, O. (2014, April 9). *Wake Forest Baptist adds 11th to telestroke network.* Retrieved from http://www.bizjournals.com/triad/news/2014/04/09/wake-forest-baptist-adds-11th-hospital-to.html

Daley, M. & Tang, T. (2014, June 6). *VA Chief: 18 vets off waiting list have died.* Retrieved from http://www.cnn.com/2014/05/30/us/department-of-veterans-affairs-fast-facts/

Davis, F. D. (1985). *A technology acceptance model for empirically testing new end-user information systems*. Retrieved from http://dspace.mit.edu/handle/1721.1/15192

Doorenbos, A. Z., Kundu, A., Eaton, L. H., et al. (2011). Enhancing access to cancer education for rural healthcare providers via telehealth. *Journal of Cancer Education, 26*(4), 682–686. doi:10.1007/s13187-011-0204-4.

Duchesne, J. C., Kyle, A., Simmons, J., et al. (2008). Impact of telemedicine upon rural trauma care. *The Journal of Trauma, 64*(1), 92–97; discussion 97–98.

EMHS. (2014). *EMHS telehealth: Improving access to healthcare in Maine's rural communities*. Retrieved from http://emh.com/dynamic.aspx?id=14710

Espensen, M., & American Academy of Ambulatory Care Nursing. (2009). *Telehealth nursing practice essentials*. Pitman, NJ: American Academy of Ambulatory Care Nursing.

Federation of American Scientists. (n.d.). *Glossary*. Retrieved from http://www.fas.org/spp/military/docops/usaf/2020/app-v.htm

Fitbit. (2015). *Fitbit site for activity trackers & more*. Retrieved from https://www.fitbit.com

Fitzner, K., & Moss, G. (2013). Telehealth—an effective delivery method for diabetes self-management education? *Population Health Management, 16*(3), 169–177. doi:10.1089/pop.2012.0054.

Gaudin, S. (2014, April 14). *With Google Glass, the doctor can see you now. Healthcare IT*. Retrieved from http://www.computerworld.com/s/article/9247720/With_Google_Glass_the_doctor_can_see_you_now?taxonomyId=132&pageNumber=1

GlySens. (2014). *GlySens—next generation glucose monitoring for better diabetes health*. Retrieved from http://glysens.com/

Google. (2014). *Google Glass*. Retrieved from http://www.google.com/glass/start/

Grady, J. L., & Schlachta-Fairchild, L. (2007). Report of the 2004–2005 International Telenursing Survey. *CIN: Computers, Informatics, Nursing, 25*(5), 266–272.

Guedon-Moreau, L., Lacroix, D., Sadoul, N., et al. (2014). Costs of remote monitoring vs. ambulatory follow-ups of implanted cardioverter defibrillators in the randomized ECOST study. *Europace: European Pacing, Arrhythmias, and Cardiac Electrophysiology, 16*(8), 1181–1188. doi:10.1093/europace/euu012.

Health Resources and Services Administration (HRSA). (2014). *What is a medical home? Why is it important?* Retrieved from http://www.hrsa.gov/healthit/toolbox/Childrenstoolbox/BuildingMedicalHome/whyimportant.html

International Council of Nurses. (2010, August 11). *Network history*. Retrieved from http://www.icn.ch/networks/tele-network-history/

InTouch Technologies. (2014). *InTouch telemedicine system*. Retrieved from http://www.intouchhealth.com/products-and-services/

Jia, H., Chuang, H.-C., Wu, S. S., et al. (2009). Long-term effect of home telehealth services on preventable hospitalization use. *The Journal of Rehabilitation Research and Development, 46*(5), 557–562.

Kane, D. (2010, June 17). *NanoEngineers print and test chemical sensors on elastic waistbands of underwear*. Retrieved from http://ucsdnews.ucsd.edu/newsrel/science/06-17Elastic-Waistbands.asp

Kowitlawakul, Y. (2011). The technology acceptance model: predicting nurses' intention to use telemedicine technology (eICU). *Computers Informatics Nursing: CIN, 29*(7), 411–418. doi:10.1097/NCN.0b013e3181f9dd4a.

Leapfrog Group. (2014). *ICU physician staffing*. Retrieved from http://www.leapfroggroup.org/56440/SurveyInfo/leapfrog_safety_practices/icu_physician_staffing

LeRouge, C., & Garfield, M. J. (2013). Crossing the telemedicine chasm: Have the U.S. barriers to widespread adoption of telemedicine been significantly reduced? *International Journal of Environmental Research and Public Health, 10*(12), 6472–6484. doi:10.3390/ijerph10126472.

Lynch, A. (1998). *Bleeding sailor performs self-surgery via e-mail/Boston doctor advises solo racer—SFGate*. Retrieved from http://articles.sfgate.com/1998-11-19/news/17737296_1_viktor-yazykov-sailor-e-mail

Maine Sea Coast Mission. (2014). *Sunbeam*. Retrieved from http://www.seacoastmission.org/sunbeam.html

Markle Foundation, American Medical Association, & Gold Standard. (2006, June 13). *Lessons from KatrinaHealth*. Retrieved from http://www.markle.org/publications/894-lessons-katrinahealth

Mattia, J. (2007, May 21). *How Piedmont Hospital cut heart failure patient readmissions by 75 percent*. Retrieved from http://www.healthleadersmedia.com/content/89750/topic/WS_HLM2_TEC/How-Piedmont-Hospital-Cut-Heart-Failure-Patient-Readmissions-by-75-Percent.html

Medtronic. (2014). *Medtronic for healthcare professionals*. Retrieved from http://www.medtronic.com/for-healthcare-professionals/

Naditz, A. (2008). Medicare's and Medicaid's new reimbursement policies for telemedicine. *Telemedicine Journal and e-Health, 14*(1), 21–24. doi:10.1089/tmj.2008.9996.

Philips Healthcare. (2013). *Taking care where it is needed: Philips Motiva Mobile—empowering patients*. Retrieved from http://www.healthcare.philips.com/pwc_hc/main/shared/Assets/Documents/Homehealthcare/Telehealth/Motiva_2Pager_09.pdf

Piedmont Healthcare. (2014). *Heart failure program*. Retrieved from http://www.piedmont.org/medical-care/Heart-Failure-Services.aspx

Strachan, M., Gros, D. F., Yuen, E., et al. (2012). Home-based telehealth to deliver evidence-based psychotherapy in veterans with PTSD. *Contemporary Clinical Trials, 33*(2), 402–409. doi:10.1016/j.cct.2011.11.007.

Taylor, G. (2013). Improving the patient experience with an eICU. Telehealth helps provide round-the-clock patient care. *Healthcare Executive, 28*(5), 50.

Tolandes, L. (2014, January 20). *Telemedicine network cuts emergency transport for ill babies*. Retrieved from http://tdn.com/news/local/telemedicine-network-cuts-emergency-transport-for-ill-babies/article_ec1336ae-824f-11e3-8bbe-001a4bcf887a.html

UC Davis Health System. (2007). *Telemedicine extends trauma care to rural areas*. Retrieved from http://www.ucdmc.ucdavis.edu/welcome/features/20070314_telemed_parsapour/

Villalba, E., Salvi, D., Ottaviano, M., et al. (2009). Wearable and mobile system to manage remotely heart failure. *IEEE Transactions on Information Technology in Biomedicine, 13*(6), 990–996. doi:10.1109/titb.2009.2026572.

Wesson, J. B., & Kupperschmidt, B. (2013). Rural trauma telemedicine. *Journal of Trauma Nursing, 20*(4), 199–202. doi:10.1097/JTN.0000000000000012.

Wood, D. (2012, June 4). *Disasters showcase the effectiveness of telehealth*. Retrieved from http://www.nursezone.com/nursing-news-events/more-news/Disasters-Showcase-the-Effectiveness-of-Telemedicine_40102.aspx

Wood, D. (2011). *Telehealth successes in patient health management*. Retrieved August 31, 2011, from http://www.amnhealthcare.com/News/news-details.aspx?Id=35158

Computer Uses in Healthcare Beyond Clinical Informatics

The information that we gain from healthcare informatics allows us to become knowledge workers so that we can improve the welfare of others. The process of transforming data into knowledge is the crux of informatics, but it does not end there. The combination of knowledge and critical thinking skills is empowering and provides rich opportunities to improve nursing decision making and practice settings. The theme for this unit is computer uses in healthcare beyond clinical informatics.

Chapter 22 explores the use of technology for online learning for nursing education or ongoing clinical education requirements. Chapter 23 looks at the nurse administrator's role in the use of computers and information systems to analyze data and make business decisions and the nurse's role as it relates to clinical information systems. Chapter 24 addresses basic competencies in data analysis and research that provide a foundation for decision making in nursing and healthcare. Finally, Chapter 25 addresses the legal and ethical responsibilities of the nurse as they relate to informatics. Topics that are discussed include the professional codes of ethics, Health Insurance Portability and Accountability Act of 1996 (HIPAA), Web 2.0/3.0, telehealth, the implantable patient identifier, and copyright issues.

CHAPTER 22

Educational Informatics: e-Learning

OBJECTIVES

After studying this chapter, you will be able to:

1. Describe how different online teaching methodologies contribute to learning using Bloom's taxonomy of learning.

2. Compare online quizzing and survey features with that of print versions.

3. Identify the strengths and weaknesses of e-learning.

4. Discuss the learning opportunities that simulations provide in nursing education.

5. Describe how online databases of teaching/learning resources such as the MERLOT project benefit learners.

6. Discuss emerging trends for e-learning.

KEY TERMS

Animations

Asynchronous learning

Augmented reality

Avatar

Blended courses

Bloom's Taxonomy of Learning

Drill and practice

E-learning

Flipped classroom

High-fidelity

Instructional games

Learning assessment

Learning content management system (LCMS)

Learning management system (LMS)

Learning style

Low-fidelity

Multimedia

Simulations

Sharable Content Object Reference Model (SCORM)

Streaming video

Synchronous learning

Tutorial

Virtual reality (VR)

You may have heard or read **e-learning** (electronic learning) advertisements—"Go to school in your pajamas" or "Earn a college degree without ever leaving your home." You may be taking a course that is offered completely online or with parts of the course online **(blended course)**. You may be earning an online degree. But then again, you may be taking classes at a traditional brick and mortar school where you have schoolwork that requires the use of a computer for learning activities and quizzing functions. If your learning falls into any of these situations, you have much personal experience on the topics presented in this chapter on e-learning.

E-LEARNING DEFINED

E-learning is another of the "e-words" that has crept into our language; it indicates a marriage between electronics—generally a computer—and educational software. It includes many different types of instruction using technology, from instruction using only the text portion of a computer to Internet-based distance learning using a multimedia-capable computer. The term "e-learning" places the emphasis on student learning and pedagogy. Older terms, such as computer-assisted instruction, computer-aided instruction (CAI), and computer-based learning, emphasized the technology.

E-learning is the use of computers/technologies to enhance and facilitate learning. This can include using the Internet to improve access to learning opportunities. With technologic advances and the Internet, we have experienced an explosion of resources to support e-learning. E-learning can occur anywhere the user has Internet access, including the traditional classroom setting. A combination of the traditional face-to-face classroom and online formats for learning is called a blended (or hybrid) course.

BENEFITS FOR THE LEARNER

Technology-enhanced instructional methodologies allow learners to take ownership of their learning. It provides mechanisms to allow the learner to interact with knowledge concepts and to practice

and evaluate learning gains. E-learning provides a foundation for nurses who want to advance their education and obtain college degrees when time, work, family, or distance makes it difficult to attend school in the traditional brick building setting. E-learning is used in healthcare facilities to provide continuing education (CE) programs to nurses at times when they are mentally and physically able to learn, rather than after a busy 12-hour work shift. E-learning provides a means for nurses to obtain CE hours to acquire and maintain their specialty certifications. In spite of the pains of occasional technology glitches, nurses who truly embrace e-learning would rather fight than give it up. E-learning is also used in primary care settings to assist with training the healthcare workforce.

HOW WE LEARN

The focus of educational activities is on achieving outcomes in the different domains of learning: knowledge, skills, and attitudes. Resources for such activities appear in many formats, including lectures, reading, and self-learning computer activities. To understand the benefits of e-learning, let's first examine how we learn. Education is the mental manipulation of data, information, and knowledge by learners to achieve outcomes. Learning can be facilitated by a teacher, whether face-to-face or mediated by learning resources ranging from paper to a video, an interactive simulation, or any combination of these. The job of an educator, whether a nurse providing patient education, a teacher in a formal class, a designer of educational aids, or a parent, is to facilitate this process.

No matter the format used for education, the primary focus must be on learning, not on the technology or lack of it. Informatics is about using the best methods to manage information, and e-learning focuses on the appropriate use of computerized technology to achieve educational aims. Factors such as learning goals, outcomes, and characteristics of the topic determine the best instructional methods needed. Simply moving a class or course to a computer format is not necessarily an improvement. Educators must pay attention to how the technology is used as well as to what it will add to the learning situation. Each technology method from simple computer-assisted learning to virtual reality (VR) possesses different attributes. An attribute such as color, movement, or music may or may not add to the learning process.

Learning theories are helpful to understand the concept of learning when combined with technology. This section examines several learning theories: Dale's Cone of Experience, **learning styles**, and **Bloom's Taxonomy of Learning**.

Dale's Cone of Experience

Dale's Cone of Experience, based on the work of Edgar Dale in 1946 (Figure 22-1), provides a visual about how people learn (Atherton, 2013; Thalheimer, 2006). Dale's original model did not include any percentages. This particular model is concept based but not evidence based and, as a result, remains very controversial. The model provides an intuitive explanation about the learning experience and helps to explain why student nurses learn best from clinical experiences with patients

and families and from simulation laboratories. Interactive teaching methodologies using e-learning open up opportunities for students to apply learning. How people learn is complex and individual.

Learning Styles

A person's learning style is the way he or she perceives, remembers, expresses, and solves problems. Learning style surveys, available online, provide excellent self-assessment tools. For example, the Solomon and Felder Index of Learning Styles Questionnaire at http://www.engr.ncsu.edu/learningstyles/ilsweb.html includes 44 items. After submitting the survey, the learner receives a report indicating where he or she scored on scales for the following types of learning: active (doing) or reflective (thinking), sensing (learning facts) or intuitive (discovery), visual (pictures) or verbal (words), and sequential (using linear steps) or global (seeing the big picture). An associated Web page suggests learning strategies that complement the various learning styles.

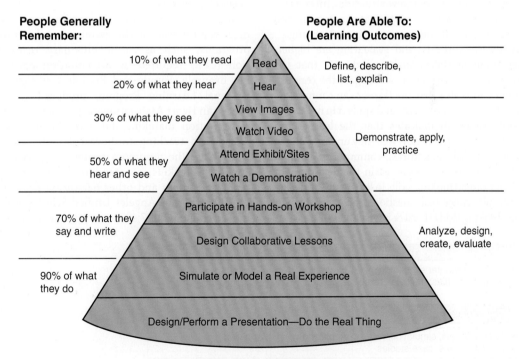

Dale's Cone of Experience

Figure 22-1. Dale's Cone of Experience. (Used with permission. From Pastore, R. S. (2005). *Principles of teaching*. Retrieved from http://teacherworld.com/potdale.html)

Bloom's Taxonomy and Learning Methods

Bloom's Taxonomy of Learning (Bloom, 1956) delineates progressively complex domains of learning to include knowledge, comprehension, application, analysis, synthesis, and evaluation. The taxonomy was later modified by Anderson and Krathwohl to make "creating" rather than "evaluating" the highest level of learning (Anderson et al., 2001).The design of e-learning addresses one or more of the domains (Figure 22-2).

When designing e-learning programs, educators need to keep in mind the level of learning necessary to meet the goal of the learning activity. Knowledge, comprehension, and application are lower-order thinking skills. Knowledge indicates the ability to recite discrete facts. Flash cards, games, and quizzes assist the learner to memorize terms. Comprehension indicates that the learner can explain the concept. Simulations, animations, and tutorials assist the learner to visualize and describe complex concepts. Application indicates that the learner can understand the concepts well enough to apply it to a new situation. Interactive tutorials, simulations, instructional games, and case studies assist the learner to apply learning.

Analysis, synthesis, and evaluation are higher-order thinking skills. Analysis indicates that the learner can deconstruct or break apart the concept. Synthesis indicates that the learner can connect the concept with other concepts and apply it in new ways. Finally, evaluation indicates that the learner can make judgments about how well they understand the concept. Virtual laboratories, computer simulation models, and case studies assist in the development of higher-order thinking skills in learners. The design of multiple-choice test questions can teach higher-order thinking skills (Lord & Baviskar, 2007).

E-LEARNING BASICS

We can use the myriad educational resources that make up e-learning to supplement course content to substitute for one or more sessions of a class, or as an entire course. Web-based instruction has uses in all educational venues, including degree programs and CE. E-learning is multidimensional. One has to consider the e-learning purpose, type or method of instruction, quality of instruction, role of the instructor, accessibility of learning, and the pros and cons.

Examples of E-Learning Purposes

Healthcare agencies that find it difficult to release employees at given times for classroom sessions use e-learning. Although there are upfront costs for the technology and software, there are also savings. The appropriate learning management software can greatly reduce the costs of faculty and materials, the difficulty in releasing employees at set times, and the clerical costs of keeping necessary records.

Many vendors offer e-learning tools that meet the criteria for the mandatory educational programs, such as cardiopulmonary resuscitation (CPR) required by accreditation agencies. For example, Family and Friends CPR Anytime Personal Learning Program produced for the American Heart Association includes a DVD, small resuscitation manikin, and a reminder card to assist with teaching cardiovascular life support CPR skills. The minimum competency, basic life support CPR skills, is a standard required competency for nurses and other healthcare providers. In 2009, the Los Angeles Unified School District nurses trained 2,027 students on how to perform

Learning Assessment Techniques	Bloom	Anderson & Krathwohl
Virtual labs, computer simulation models, case studies, multiple-choice questions Higher-order thinking skills	Evaluation Synthesis Analysis	Creating Evaluating Analyzing
Interactive tutorials, simulations, instructional games, case studies	Application	Applying
Simulations, animations, tutorials	Comprehension	Understanding
Flash cards, games, quizzes	Knowledge	Remembering

Figure 22-2. Learning assessment techniques in relation to learning taxonomies.

CPR and how to use an AED (American Heart Association, 2015). The students took their CPR kits home and trained 14,901 members of their communities. Advanced cardiac life support and pediatric advanced life support training is also available as e-learning. Users complete an online module and then attend a 2-hour class to demonstrate practice skills.

E-learning is useful for patient education. Office and clinic waiting rooms are excellent locations for the use of e-learning. Computer-aided instruction in a waiting room can provide patient education as part of a one-on-one session or group teaching. McMullen et al. (2011) reported equipping eight free medical clinics with computers and MedlinePlus Interactive tutorials for patient education. The University of South Caroline School of Medicine Library staff trained over 2,000 staff and volunteers about how to use the computers and tutorials. The clinics served over 12,800 patients. Smartphones apps can deliver patient education and serve as reminders for appointments and medications times. One example is the use of smartphones to deliver patient education to spinal cord–injured patients (Shepherd et al., 2012). Researchers found the smartphone use to be effective mechanism for patient education.

Types and Methods of Instruction
Multimedia

Multimedia describes any combination of hardware and software that displays images or plays sound. Today's computers often include multimedia software and are equipped with CD-ROM and DVD players. Smartphones and tablet devices usually include camera apps that allow users to record and edit video. Media apps allow faculty and students to view or create video and audio podcasts, audio files, and streaming video related to learning content. **Streaming video** is a technique where a sequence of compressed moving images, sent over the Internet, plays by a media viewer as they arrive. Streaming media is a combination of streaming video and audio.

Many nursing textbooks provide access to video learning materials so that students can hear and see essential concepts related to patient care. Broadband Internet access provides a way to use online multimedia learning resources. The Dalhousie University Common Currency Project (http://currency.medicine.dal.ca/video.htm) has links to videos on nursing procedures and gross anatomy. Martindale's Reference Desk (http://www.martindalecenter.com/) has links to many online multimedia resources for nurses. YouTube (http://www.youtube.com/) and Vimeo (https://vimeo.com/) include links to a variety of videos related to nursing and patient education. iTunes U, available for desktop and mobile devices, has free audio and video educational resources, including entire courses, which the user can view.

Distance Learning and Hybrid Courses

Distance learning is a phenomenon that has been with us since Roman times whenever and wherever a reliable postal service was available. In the United States and Europe, correspondence courses have been available since the 18th century. Although correspondence courses exist in many parts of the world, online courses continue to grow in popularity.

Distance learning means education in which the learners and students are in different locations. Distance education formats differ in the timeframes that they use; some are asynchronous, and others are synchronous. In the **asynchronous learning** format, learners use the learning resources at a time and place that is convenient for them. The asynchronous format is a common use of LMSs. In **synchronous learning**, class is held at set times and all participants are "present," either online or in the classroom. Web conferencing and webinars, often used to provide an educational session, are examples of synchronous learning.

There are many uses for distance learning in healthcare. One of the most widespread uses is for CE. This type of learning is available in different formats; some CE modules are free, and others are available for a small fee. The American Nursing Association provides a comprehensive listing of online CE learning resources at http://nursingworld.org/ce/cehome.cfm. Some of the CE resources are free for members. Most nursing journals that have an online presence provide access to journal articles and an associated quiz for CE credit. Staff educators may use many of these offerings as a part of an education for career ladder programs or other necessary learning.

There are full degree programs offered online. The major college-accrediting bodies offer accreditation of distance learning just as if the programs were all in a regular classroom. In addition, many higher education institutions offer certificate programs online. The programs vary in their requirements for a presence on campus during the program; some require none, and others may require a weekend presence during each course or a given on-campus presence sometime during the program.

The literature supports the potential value of online education. Du et al. (2013) conducted a systematic review to examine Web-based distance education for nursing education and identified encouraging results supporting acquisition of knowledge, skill performance, and self-efficacy when using Web-based distance education. One example of using distance education to improve access to nursing education is a project developed by the University of Notre Dame Australia to deliver Web-based nursing courses to remote areas of Australia (Clark & Piercy, 2012).

Learning Management Systems

Learning management is a concept that involves computer use in education. The term **learning management system (LMS)** describes software that facilitates delivering course content electronically. Examples of commercial LMSs include Blackboard, Canvas, ANGEL, ECollege, and Desire2Learn. Open-source solutions include Canvas, Moodle, Sakai, and ATutor.

LMS features can be as simple as delivering learning content, scoring computer learning activities, and providing printable certificates of course completion. Other LMS features include email, discussion forums, virtual student work areas, chat, wikis, and blogs. Sophisticated enterprise solutions synchronize with student registration database systems so that when students register for courses, they are automatically enrolled in the course's LMS. Courses using LMS systems offer primarily asynchronous access to learning resources.

LMSs can supplement or replace face-to-face classes. LMSs provide a means for faculty/student interaction, collaborative learning, and prompt feedback on learning progress. Many faculty use the concept of the **flipped classroom** in which students complete learning activities (videos, interactive learning modules, etc.) in advance, which allow learners to spend class time using engaged learning activities. The use of technology serves as a foundation for the design of a variety of interactive instructional methods. Different combinations of the methods serve as building blocks to provide learning content. When using the flipped classroom approach, it is important for the faculty to prepare the students with the rationale for use and student expectations (Hawks, 2014).

Today, the more sophisticated e-learning products are often a combination of LMS and **learning content management system (LCMS)** functions. The purpose of LCMSs is to store and manage learning resources authored by faculty and content experts so for reuse by a variety of educators. The LCMS learning resources such as course content modules, slides, video clips, illustrations, and quiz questions can be assembled into course learning content by using infinitely changeable combinations according to the instructor's needs. LCMS can provide a single portal for students to access etextbook learning resources or other types of LMSs.

Quality of Instruction in E-Learning

Chickering and Ehrmann (1996) identified seven principles of quality undergraduate education long before e-learning gained popularity. These classic principles apply to today's e-learning environment. The principles address the following:

1. The importance of faculty–student contact in and out of class
2. Collaborative learning among students and faculty
3. Active learning techniques, which allow students to discuss, write reflectively, and incorporate learning into their lives
4. Opportunities for students to practice learning and receive just-in-time feedback
5. Learning strategies that help students to learn efficiently
6. High faculty expectations for student learning
7. Respect for various learning styles and individual student talents

LMSs can supplement or replace face-to-face classes. LMSs provide a means for faculty/student interaction, collaborative learning, and prompt feedback on learning progress. The use of technology serves as a foundation for the design of a variety of interactive instructional methods. The different combinations of methods form building blocks to provide learning content.

Evaluating e-learning and determining what computer technology to use depend on the learning module objectives and expected learning outcomes. Instructors should use Bloom's Taxonomy determine appropriate learning methods. Identifying learning outcomes helps to determine the selection of learning resources that develop psychomotor skills, critical thinking, memorization, or just knowledge assimilation. The instructor must also consider the learner's prerequisite knowledge.

One characteristic that sets e-learning above all other teaching mediums, with the exception of a human teacher or live experience, is interactivity. The effectiveness of interaction depends on the mental processing required and the nature of the learner's interaction with the content. Several tools are available to assess the quality of e-learning resources. Examples of assessment tools include MERLOT peer review at http://info.merlot.org/merlothelp/merlot_peer_review_information.htm and Sharable Content Object Repositories for Education at http://publications.sreb.org/2007/07T01_SREB_Score.pdf. Quality Matters (QM) Program (https://www.qualitymatters.org/) provides national benchmarking for online and blended courses. Some resources, such as the rubric to assess courses, are available at no charge. Other resources require a subscription. QM concept "aligns" eight standards into the QM rubric (Quality Matters, 2014):

- Course overview and introduction
- Learning objectives (competencies)
- Assessment and measurement
- Instructional materials
- Course activities and learner interaction
- Course technology
- Learner support
- Accessibility and usability

Because QM is quite complex and fee based, some colleges and universities are creating their own e-learning quality assessment tools.

Role of Instructor in E-Learning

The role of an instructor who uses e-learning varies. Although the instructor is an important part of the process, the learners play a key role too. The instructor designs the learning content and facilitates the learning process. Although instructors take more of a "guide-on-the-side" role in the electronic classroom, their focus is still on teaching. The electronic world with narrated slides, podcasts, audio clips, and/or streaming video might replace the traditional classroom lecture where the voice can convey emphasis. The challenge for faculty is in not being able to see the faces of students. As a result, the learners must take on the responsibility of providing feedback on the instruction electronically. Effective faculty–student collaboration often makes the difference between whether learners find success or experience frustration.

Accessibility of E-Learning

The need to make websites available to those with physical disabilities is important for all education programs. There are special considerations for the design of e-learning for persons with disabilities. The American Disabilities Act (ADA), Section 508, W3C, requires federal agencies to make information technology accessible to qualified persons with disabilities (United States Access Boards, n.d.). Section 508 refers to the Rehabilitation Act of 1973. The act was amended in 1998 to include electronic and information technology.

As an example of the problem, persons with vision problems use Braille readers to access online information. The design of websites must be compliant with Braille readers. When graphics are used, websites should have alternative text descriptors of the graphic. Additional information on ADA standards for e-learning is available at http://www.access-board.gov/508.htm and http://www.gatech.edu/accessibility.php.

The Universal Design for Learning (UDL) provides a set of principles for curricular design. The basis for UDL principles is the way that the brain works. The principles address the recognition networks or the "what" of learning, the strategic networks or the "how" of learning, and the affective networks or the "why" of learning. The National Center on Universal Design for Learning

---

BOX 22-1 Advantages and Disadvantages of Distance Learning

Advantages of Distance Learning

1. Depending on the structure, students can participate in their schedule.
2. Students without easy access to a college can participate.
3. Students may view distance learning as a perk that increases retention.
4. An expanded audience allows filling classes in a limited specialty.
5. Access to class is available 24 hours a day, 7 days a week.

6. Learners must think before they express their ideas rather than speaking impulsively. Organizing one's ideas increases learning.
7. All learners must participate.

Disadvantages of Distance Learning

1. Instructors and students require the assistance of additional resources.
2. Lack of face-to-face contact.
3. May not be suitable to all contents.
4. The technology may contribute to frustration.

---

has comprehensive resources that instructors can use to improve academic achievement and learning outcomes at http://www.udlcenter.org/.

Pros and Cons of E-Learning

E-learning is neither a panacea nor something that will replace teachers. Like all innovations, there are advantages and disadvantages (Box 22-1).

One advantage is accessibility. Online learning allows students to access course content anywhere in the world from a computer with Internet access. Online learning accommodates shift work, family obligations, and military duty deployment. Before signing up for a course that uses e-learning, students should make sure that they have the qualities leading to success (Box 22-2).

BOX 22-2 Qualities of Successful Online Learners

Learning Technology and Environment

The learner:

- Must be very committed and focused on learning. Work and home obligations can be very distracting and can interrupt the learning environment.
- Must give online learning a priority in daily activities.
- Must have access to a working computer with virus, malware, and spam protection, an Internet connection, required e-learning software, and a printer. The computer becomes an essential tool for online learning. To maintain a functioning computer, the learner should
  - Restrict the use of the personal computer from any other user who may inadvertently download a virus or corrupt the operating system
  - Have a "backup strategy" in case of computer problems, for example, using

the college or community library and college or hospital computer laboratory

Learner Qualities

The learner should

- Be self-motivated and exercise self-discipline; own responsibility for learning
- Be able to communicate effectively in writing
- Be open-minded about sharing experiences and willing to learn from others
- Be willing to ask for help
- Be respectful of others in the learning environment
- Participate in the virtual classroom 4 to 7 days/week
- Be willing to apply learning to everyday life
- Have the ability to commit the required number of hours per week for completing assignments and class participation

Students can access the learning resources when they are best able to learn. Online learning allows learners to participate in educational experiences that otherwise are not available outside of real life. It also permits the learners to set their own pace. Another advantage is that, unlike a traditional lecture, learners never have to miss a class; the learning content and class discussion are online. ADA-compliant courses make learning accessible to students who are physically unable to attend class. The design of courses can accommodate vision- and hearing-impaired students.

Online learning also has disadvantages. Learners need the required software and hardware. They also need to have a backup plan in case of a computer problem. They need to have sufficient technology skills to allow them to access online courses and to troubleshoot technology glitches. Online learning is a disadvantage to the learner who is not motivated to learn and who does not exercise self-discipline.

TYPES OF E-LEARNING

There are many types of e-learning discussed here as separate entities. As the power of computers increases with the development of new uses of technology for e-learning, the technologies meld together seamlessly, enhancing the learning environment. For example, LMSs contain presentation software, chat functions, email, discussion boards, survey/quizzing features, and links to Web resources. When enrolled in a course using an LMS, students experience these different technologies functioning as a whole.

There are numerous types of e-learning ranging from instructional games, tutorials, and **drill and practice** to simulations and virtual and augmented reality. The next section includes a brief overview of some of the e-learning types.

Drill and Practice

Drill and practice software was among the first educational software introduced. It was relatively simple to produce, and it freed teachers from the mundane chores and repetitive teaching. Flash cards and questions with answers are examples of drill and practice learning methods. Flashcard Friends at http://www.flashcardfriends.com/ is a free website that allows users to create and share flash cards. The users could be teachers and students. Users can also create questions with fill in the blanks, multiple-choice, matching, and true and false. Students can collaborate and share the learning resources with others.

Proprietary software such as StudyMate Author allows faculty to create flash cards for online use with an LMS, computer, or downloaded to a small-screen mobile device (Respondus, 2014). Learners can purchase electronic flash cards online from Skyscape at http://www.skyscape.com and Amazon at http://www.amazon.com. Printed textbooks often include video resources, flash cards, and other interactive learning activities.

Drill and practice can assist the learner to develop the cognitive structure necessary for the kind of reflective thinking that produces critical thinking. The best use of the drill and practice method is as an aid for memorization. Pure memorization provides learning at Bloom's Taxonomy knowledge level, which is essential in many areas to provide a foundation for higher-level learning. For example, it is essential to memorize information such as medical terminology along with rules for combining the terms to create other words to understand the nursing information in texts and articles.

Tutorials

Tutorials are step-by-step programs designed to guide learners to understand information. Well-designed tutorials are interactive, present the learning content, and then provide the learner with self-assessment multiple-choice questions. Most tutorials use programmed learning models. The quality of a tutorial is evident with the use of branching techniques. At the low end of the continuum are programs that just inform the learner whether the answer is correct. Those at the high end offer more than one explanation for the same phenomenon and provide feedback on incorrect answers.

Tutorials do not have to "tell" the learners what they need to know. Instead, tutorials can present learners with a situation and the tools necessary to discover the answer. Learners can proceed through the tutorials at their own pace. Examples of interactive tutorials are online at MedlinePlus (http://www.nlm.nih.gov/medlineplus/tutorials/). The interactive tutorials provide an opportunity for the learners to review the different modules and test their learning.

Simulations

In the campus environment, combinations of computers with **simulation** equipment provide high-fidelity interactive experiences. Many nursing programs use intravenous (IV) simulations, electronic medication administration systems, and simulation manikins to enhance learning.

Simulations imitate actual experiences. Simulations have many uses, such as part of an orientation or in-service program, a face-to-face classroom or clinical laboratory setting, or as part of a homework assignment. Effective simulations match the learner's knowledge background, or are, at least, only slightly above it, and the point of view addresses the learning needs.

Online Simulations

The Internet provides simultaneous use by a large number of learners. An online flash simulation, Care of a Client with Schizophrenia (http://www.wisc-online.com/objects/ViewObject.aspx?ID=NUR3704), allows the learner to apply knowledge about schizophrenia. Assessing blood pressure is also a complex skill for the novice healthcare provider student. The simulation Assessing Blood Pressure at http://www.csuchico.edu/atep/bp/bp.html provides essential knowledge about how to take blood pressure and interpret the sounds. The student uses a computer mouse to "pump" the virtual blood pressure bulb and then releases the valve to hear the sounds. An interactive quiz provides feedback on the learning.

Patient Simulators

Patient simulators allow the learner to practice a patient encounter by providing care to a computerized manikin. This problem-based learning approach provides opportunities for the learner to develop higher-order thinking skills. The primary objective for the use of patient simulators is to allow the learner to be an actual participant in a patient care situation that would be too difficult,

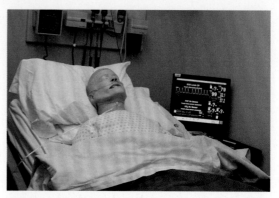

Figure 22-3. Patient simulator.

dangerous, or time consuming to provide in a real clinical. Manikins can be low or high fidelity. **Low fidelity** refers simulations that are not true to life. **High fidelity** refers to realistic simulated patients or situations (Figure 22-3). For example, instructors can program high-fidelity manikins to have heart and breath sounds, breathe, and perform physical acts associated with illness, such as coughing or bleeding. Many programs use high-fidelity patient simulators, such as those noted in Table 22-1. Research conducted by Hayden et al. (2014) indicated that it is possible to substitute patient clinical experiences with up to 50% simulation. The qualifiers for the substituting simulation for clinical experience were that

- The simulation experiences must be comparable to the ten sites described in the study.
- The faculty have formal training for use of simulation.
- The faculty-to-student ratio is sufficient for learning.
- Theory-based debriefing is done by subject matter experts.
- The simulation environment is realistic (Hayden et al., 2014, p. S38).

Research studies support the effective use of patient simulators. Johnson and Johnson (2014) compared the use of human patient simulators to the use of a CD-ROM training program, examining critical thinking and performance of nurse anesthesia participants. The researchers found that performance was better using the human patient simulator versus using the CD-ROM. Research reports on the use of patient simulators indicate

TABLE 22-1 Patient Simulation Resources

Manufacturer	High-Fidelity Patient Simulators	Website Address
CAE Healthcare	METIman, PediaSIM, BabySIM, HPS, iStan, Caesar, Emergency Care Simulator (ECS), Fidelis Lucina	http://www.caefidelis.com/
Laerdal	SimMan 3G, SimMan Essential, SimMan 3G Trauma, SimMan 3G Mystic, SimJunior, SimMom, SimBaby, SimNewB, ALS Simulator, Resusci Anne, MamaNatalie Birthing Simulator, Harvey The Cardiopulmonary Patient Simulator	http://www.laerdal.com/nav/207/Patient-Simulators
Wolters Kluwer Health and Laerdal	vSim for Nursing	http://thepoint.lww.com/vsim
Laerdal	Infant Virtual IV	http://laerdalcdn.blob.core.windows.net/downloads/f2387/13-13363_Infant_Virtual_IV_SS_v.6.pdf
Laerdal	Virtual IV	http://www.laerdal.com/doc/245/Virtual-I-V-Simulator

that students consistently value the learning experiences (Cardoza & Hood, 2012; Howard et al., 2010; Kaplan & Ura, 2010; Roh, 2014). There are, however, downfalls to the use of more complex simulators. Purchase costs for manikins, hardware, and software and training costs can be prohibitive. Moreover, time is an issue; time is required for faculty training and learning content development.

Electronic Health Record Simulation

Due to the complexity of the healthcare setting, simulations are becoming increasingly important. Nursing students should have basic proficiencies prior to providing care to patients/clients in the healthcare setting. The use of electronic health records (EHRs) is changing the teaching methods used by nursing programs. It was easy to simulate paper and pencil documentation, but its use is waning quickly. Nursing programs are adopting the use of a simulated EHR in nursing practice laboratories.

Figure 22-4 is an example of a simulated EHR. The simulated EHR allows the nursing student to practice entering patient documentation, accessing the laboratory, and other testing data, similar to the hospital or clinic work setting. Examples of EHR simulations are DocuCare (http://thepoint. lww.com/lwwdocucare), NurseSquared (http://www.nursesquared.com/), SIMchart (https://evolve. elsevier.com/studentlife/media/SimChart/story. html), iCare (http://www.icareacademic.com/), and Neehr Perfect (http://www.neehrperfect.com/). The University of Kansas School of Nursing is using a Simulated E-hEalth Delivery System (SEEDS) that incorporates the use of the EHR along with independent learning activities, case studies, simulation support for medication administration, and interprofessional collaboration simulation (Manos, 2014).

Animations

Animations provide visual representations of difficult concepts, processes, and models. You can create animations in a number of file formats. One common format used is Flash. You can use Flash player, a free download from http://www.macromedia. com/software/flash/about/, to view the files.

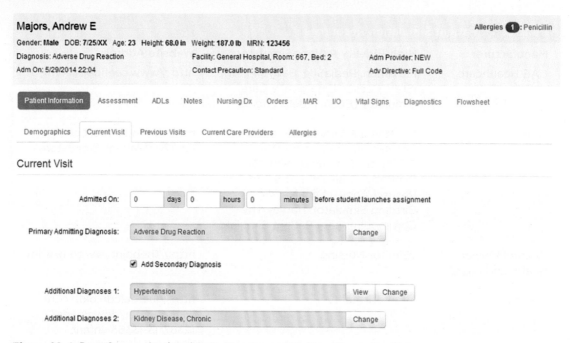

Figure 22-4. DocuCare, a simulated EHR. (Courtesy of Wolters Kluwer Health.)

The best use of animations is to supplement to written information. The KidneyPatientGuide (http://www.kidneypatientguide.org.uk/site/treatment.php) uses several animations to demonstrate concepts related to dialysis, transplants, and diet. The design of the animation is for patients, but it is useful for nursing students.

Virtual Reality (VR)

The use of **virtual reality (VR)** technology is to allow the participant to exist in another reality using allusions, where the participant experiences an event that appears real but does not physically exist. The objective is to create a scene in which the participant is free to concentrate on the tasks, problems, and ideas that he or she would face in the real situation. The primary criterion is that the participant be surrounded by an environment and be "inside" the information.

There are two main components of VR. One is the model or visualization that resembles reality and allows manipulation of the environment. Manipulation can be by virtual keyboard enabled with Bluetooth technology that can display on any surface for computer data entry. The second

VR component is an interface that resembles the three-dimensional world. During the VR experience, the "environment" reacts just as it would in the real world.

Nurses learning how to use surgical endoscopic equipment use VR as a training mechanism. Nyswaner (2007), a surgery research coordinator, described the learning challenges associated with video endoscope simulation use: "You need to realize that looking to the right translates into steering to the left. Don't be surprised if it takes a while to get the hang of 'driving' [the endoscope]—or that the OR is a high-stress place to learn this skill." Research results verify that nurses can perform virtual colonoscopy safely and accurately (Kruglikova et al., 2010).

The IV simulator for adults and pediatrics, discussed with human simulators, uses virtual reality to simulate IV insertion in various settings. Jenson and Forsyth (2012) conducted a small study with eight faculty members about the benefit of using an IV simulator and virtual reality for nursing students. All study participants agreed or strongly agreed that the simulator would assist students' knowledge about IV insertion.

Virtual Worlds

Students can use VR to enhance learning by using online sites such as OpenSimulator, or Second Life. OpenSimulator and Second Life are online three-dimensional VR environments. Open Simulator (http://opensimulator.org/wiki/Main_Page) is an open-source software application. Second Life (http://www.secondlife.com/) is proprietary. All virtual world participants must first register on the site to obtain a login ID and password and then download virtual world software applications. Participants interact by using **avatars**. An avatar is a fictionalized computer representation of oneself (Figure 22-5). Avatars can be custom designed with different looks. Because avatars can fly, they can "teleport" to different locations.

There are strengths and limitations for using virtual worlds as a part of instruction. Because avatars fictionalize representations of the users, any user disabilities are invisible. Everyone can walk and fly. The sites provide many opportunities

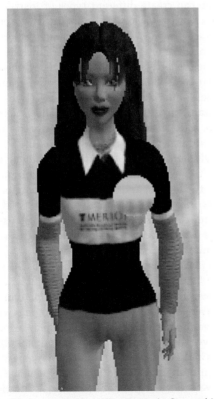

Figure 22-5. Jeanne Sewell's avatar in Second Life.

for experimentation and research while enhancing learning in safe environments (Miller & Jensen, 2014). A potential limitation is that virtual world learning has technical requirements and computer skills that not all learners may have. Navigating in a virtual world is a learned skill; fortunately, tutorials and videos are available for use. Learners should have specific learning goals prior to engaging with the learning content. Learners must also be very self-directed; otherwise, they could become lost in VR and end up very frustrated. The process to create a virtual world can be time intensive and challenging.

Virtual Communities

In order to simulate the experience of caring for a community with diverse members throughout a curriculum, many nursing programs have adopted virtual communities, such as the community of Mirror Lake developed by Ohio Lake University's College of Nursing (Curran et al., 2009). Virtual communities contain fictional characters complete with families, organizations, neighborhoods, and health centers. These virtual communities support student learning by situating learning within a cohesive, realistic environment. For example, in fundamentals, the student may meet the Scott family and learn about the hypertension experienced by the father and the diabetes of the mother. Later in the program, students may interact with this same family as the plan community health fairs and provide childbirth care in the local hospital. Engaged learning results when students interact with familiar virtual communities. Giddens et al. (2012) found that the use of virtual learning environments increased learning engagement and communication exchanges.

Augmented Reality

Augmented reality provides a representation of real life with digital images. The concept has fascinating implications for the teaching/learning process. Imagine holding a piece of paper with a block-like stamp (similar in function to a bar code) on it in front of a computer camera and watching images come to life, allowing you to interact with the images. You probably have encountered the concept, perhaps without realizing it. If you watch television, you probably have viewed some commercial advertisements with augmented reality.

The number of augmented reality apps continues to increase. An example of augmented reality for nursing is Anatomy 4D, a free app in the Apple App and Google Play stores. The user first prints a "target" for the app and then points the camera on the mobile device over the target to view the image. Anatomy 4D allows the user to change the gender for the image. You can learn more about augmented reality at http://www.howstuffworks.com/augmented-reality.htm.

Gesture-Based Computing

Gesture-based computing allows users to provide computer input with body motions (ELI, 2014). Gesturing can range from swiping a computer screen with fingers to playing virtual golf or tennis with a Nintendo Wii. Nintendo introduced gesture-based computing in 2006, and Xbox Kinect introduced it in 2010. Gesture-based computing is still in its infancy. As developers recognize the possibilities for nursing education, the possibilities are endless. Since gesture-based computing using body motions, including facial expressions, and multiple users, users might use the associated apps to learn effective communication techniques and create imaginative learning environments to improve population-based care outcomes.

Resources Supporting Affective Component of Learning

In addition to programs developed for knowledge, comprehension, and application, extensive resources are available on the Web to support the affective component of learning. Blogs are an online tool many people use as an online diary. Students can examine experiences of patients with various disorders to understand what it is like to have these disorders. YouTube is another resource for short videos where patients often share their experiences. Students can use the Internet to explore global health, or just about anything. Faculty can create activities to guide student tours of the Internet to enhance learning.

Some programs have incorporated the use of social networking sites such as Facebook to enhance learning through relationship building.

For example, by creating Facebook identifiers for lab manikins, the instructor can enhance the student connection to the learning experience. Similarly, some faculty have used social networking presence as a way of connecting with students, recognizing the importance of social media to the current generation (Skiba, 2010).

Instructional Games

Online **instructional games** can add a competitive contest aspect to learning. The purpose for the use of games is to motivate students to learn the needed information. Games can foster collaboration, problem solving, and analytical thinking. Learners must be clear about the purpose when using games. They should also be sure that they have the technology hardware and software necessary to play the game. Games that are successful must meet instructional requirements and be enjoyable for players. Games should be appropriate and not trivialize learning content or encourage guessing (Benner et al., 2010).

You can create different types of instructional games with a variety of software. Hot Potatoes software provides a variety of game formats; it is freeware. Some examples of games include those that select letters to identify words or phrases—similar to a popular television show—crossword puzzles, and fill in the blanks (Half-Baked Software Inc., 2014). Quandary allows users to create action mazes, which are interactive online case studies (Half-Baked Software Inc., 2009). StudyMate Author, a commercial product, allows users to create games such as crossword puzzles, fill in the blanks, and pick a letter and upload the games into LMSs (Respondus, 2014). SoftChalk, another commercial product, also allows users to create interactive learning resources with a variety of games (SoftChalk LLC, 2014).

Games are also available on the Web. The online game Outbreak at Water's Edge: A Public Health Discovery Game at http://www.mclph.umn.edu/watersedge/ uses a Java applet, a program written in Java programming language, to play a game to discover the source of contamination making residents in the local community sick. The game is available in both English and Spanish. The Nobelprize.org website at http://nobelprize.org/educational_games/medicine/ offers fun interactive games on topics that are difficult for learners to understand, such as blood typing, malaria, and the immune system.

Educational games are also available for mobile devices. Play to Cure: Genes in Space, a free gaming app available for Apple and Android devices, allows players to analyze actual genetic data using a fictional spaceship in space (Cancer Research UK, 2014). Cancer researchers are using the gaming results to assist with the development of cancer lifesaving treatments. Solve the Outbreak (Centers for Disease Control and Prevention, 2014) allows players to become disease detectives and earn badges for solving the source of a disease outbreak. The epidemiology game is available for Apple and Android mobile devices as well as on the Web.

Online Assessments and Surveys

Computers allow for many testing functions. Quizzes and surveys provide a means for assessing learning and are therefore termed **learning assessment**. LMSs and numerous companies include tools to create quizzes and anonymous surveys. You can create quizzes using the forms function of word processing software or sophisticated proprietary software. Quizzes found on the Web are often self-tests associated with tutorials. Self-tests are categorized as formative assessments because they provide information about ongoing learning. Quizzes associated with course grades are summative assessments because they sum up learning. Instructors often administer summative tests in a proctored testing environment.

Quiz Software

Quiz software is specially designed database software with a variety of uses. It allows faculty to create online quizzes either administered on the Web or integrated for use as a testing function within an LMS. Quiz software can also be useful in creating paper tests. Sophisticated testing software allows for feedback for right and wrong answers, the ability to categorize questions, test item analysis, and scoring student performance. Quiz software may allow the teacher to create a test bank of questions for reuse in various classes. You can import data from most testing software into a spreadsheet or database as part of an electronic grading book.

Question Writer from http://www.question-writer.com/free-quiz-software.html is a free (for noncommercial use) program that allows the creation of multiple-choice quizzes that can be posted to the Internet. Question Writer is also available for use with mobile devices. Users are able to print out a results report and view question feedback for correct/incorrect responses.

Surveys

Surveys provide a way to aggregate information anonymously from learners. You can use surveys in LMSs for learning assessment, such as "the muddiest point" technique and course evaluations. The "muddiest point" assessment is one where the student describes a topic that is least clearly understood. Surveys are a tool that provides evaluation information.

Several survey services are available on the Web. For example, SurveyMonkey (http://www.surveymonkey.com/) and Zoomerang (http://www.zoomerang.com/) provide free and for-purchase survey tools. Qualtrics (http://www.qualtrics.com/) is a robust online survey tool used by many higher education institutions. Students and faculty often use online surveys for research. When using online survey tools for research involving people, users much assure that the online survey has certification for HIPAA and FERPA (Family Education and Rights Policy Act).

SCORM Tools

Sharable Content Object Reference Model (SCORM) refers to a learning module that can be imported into any SCORM-compliant LMS; think of it as one design fits all (Advanced Distributed Learning, 2014). Typically, the SCORM module is designed to include a self-test associated with one or more learning tools such as flash cards, games, and tutorials. The learner has an opportunity to interact with the learning tools and then take the associated self-test. The self-test resides within the SCORM module, as opposed to the assessment/quiz section of the LMS, but a record of the self-test grade is in the LMS grade book.

Department of Defense in 2002 designed SCORM tools to save design costs associated with multiple systems. You can export course designer tools compliant with SCORM standards and specifications to all the popular LMSs. Examples of software to create SCORM tools are Hot Potatoes, Adobe Captivate, TechSmith Camtasia, Articulate, SoftChalk, and StudyMate Author.

Computer-Adaptive Testing

Computer-adaptive testing is a type of online testing that is familiar to most licensed registered nurses because since 1994, it has been the type of testing done to assess knowledge for licensure. The design of computer-adaptive testing makes the testing process more efficient because it adapts the questions to the candidate's responses. The basis of the nursing licensure exam—the NCLEX exam—is on the licensure test plan. The basis for the difficulty of the question presented on the computer screen is on the candidate's previous right or wrong response. Candidates who pass can answer 50% or more of the more difficult questions (NCSBN, 2014). A simulation of the exam is available at http://www.pearsonvue.com/nclex/#tutorial.

Web-Based Polling Technology

Web-based polling technology is available for use with online courses to provide assessment-centered instruction. Web-based polling simulates the use of clicker technology. Many of the polling resources are free (Table 22-2). To use a Web-based poll in an LMS, the faculty would first create the poll on the polling website. After creating the poll, the user copies and pastes the code to a course Web page and invites participants to vote. The poll provides a link so that participants can view the polling results. Anonymous polling can provide valuable feedback to faculty and students with regard to issues such as personal values, ethics, and beliefs.

Audience Response Systems (Clickers)

The term *audience response systems* refers to clicker-type devices used to provide assessment-centered instruction. The response system may use a separate wireless device or an app on a mobile device, such as the smartphone. The wireless response devices, which look similar to remote control devices used to control television sets and other media devices, are useful in both small and large classrooms. The two basic requirements for response system technology are that faculty must have response software on the instructor's computer used in the classroom and the students must have a device that communicates with the response system software used by the instructor.

Response system software is also available for use with smartphones, laptops, and tablet computers. An example is eClicker (http://eclicker.com/). The eClicker app is free for students and available for a nominal fee (under $15) for the instructor. Poll Everywhere is a free app that presenters can use in a classroom with PowerPoint or online with an LMS or website. Poll Everywhere will install an associated polling menu in PowerPoint. The presenter creates the poll on the Poll Everywhere website and then chooses the poll from the PowerPoint menu. The polling participants can respond using a text message, using a website provided by the presenter, using Twitter, or using a private link, whichever the presenter chooses to use.

TABLE 22-2 Free Web-Based Polling/Survey Solutions	
Polling Solution	**Website Address**
Bravenet Web Poll	http://www.bravenet.com/webtools/minipoll/
EasyPolls	https://www.easypolls.net/
MicroPoll	http://www.micropoll.com/
PollDaddy	http://polldaddy.com/
SurveyMonkey	https://www.easypolls.net/

Web-based response technology is available for use with online courses to provide assessment-centered instruction. Web-based polling simulates the use of clicker technology. To use a Web-based poll in an LMS, the faculty member creates the poll on the polling website, copies and pastes the code to his or her course Web page, and then invites participants to vote. The poll provides a link so that participants can view the polling results. Anonymous polling can provide valuable feedback to faculty and students with regard to issues such as personal values, ethics, and beliefs.

Faculty can assess students' understanding of key concepts by asking students to answer multiple-choice questions projected on a screen in front of the classroom. In this sense, clickers provide assessment feedback on "muddiest points" of learning. The assessment feedback creates the "teachable/learning moment" in the classroom. Because clicker responses can be anonymous, the students can use the technology to respond to sensitive issues such as ethics and personal beliefs. Reports in the literature support the use of clickers to create an interactive and meaningful learning environment (Sternberger, 2012; Vana et al., 2011).

Web-based polling technology is available for use with online courses to provide assessment-centered instruction. Web-based polling simulates the use of clicker technology. To use a Web-based poll in an LMS, the faculty would first create the poll on the polling website. After creating the poll, the user copies and pastes the code to their course Web page and invites participants to vote. The poll provides a link so that participants can view the polling results. Anonymous polling can provide valuable feedback to faculty and students with regard to issues such as personal values, ethics, and beliefs.

> ### QSEN Scenario
> Your nursing program uses a simulation lab to teach barcode medication administration, electronic documentation, hand-offs for care transition, and cultural-sensitive care concepts. What are some examples of scenarios that are appropriate for simulation experiences?

MERLOT: WEB-BASED LEARNING RESOURCES

Many e-learning resources are available on the Web, but discovering excellent resources can be like finding a needle in a haystack. Multimedia Education Resource for Online Learning and Teaching (MERLOT) at http://www.merlot.org is the first place that faculty and students should search (Figure 22-6). MERLOT is an online repository of peer-reviewed learning resources. Faculty members or students who want to share what they perceived as valuable teaching–learning resources contribute the learning resources you find in MERLOT. The learning resources actually reside in the computer of the author or sponsor. MERLOT simply provides a hyperlink to the resource along with a peer-reviewed rating and comments, user comments, and user-suggested learning assignments. In addition to searching MERLOT, users have the option of searching other digital libraries (federated search). The MERLOT vision is to become the "premiere online community where faculty, staff, and students from around the world share their learning materials and pedagogy" (MERLOT, 2014).

To take advantage of the community aspects of MERLOT, register for membership, which is free. MERLOT membership has many benefits. Members can do the following:

- Contribute new learning resources
- Provide users with comments about learning resources
- Publish a user profile to facilitate networking with others who have similar interests
- Save personal collections of favorite teaching and learning resources
- Build interactive learning Web pages by using MERLOT Content Builder
- Use MERLOT Voices to participate in a collaborative community with others interested in teaching and learning with technology

MERLOT membership offers faculty members the opportunity to become a peer reviewer in their discipline. MERLOT offers free "GRAPE (Getting Reviewers Accustomed to the Process of Evaluation) Camp," peer-reviewed how-to courses for faculty who have an interest in learning the peer-reviewed process.

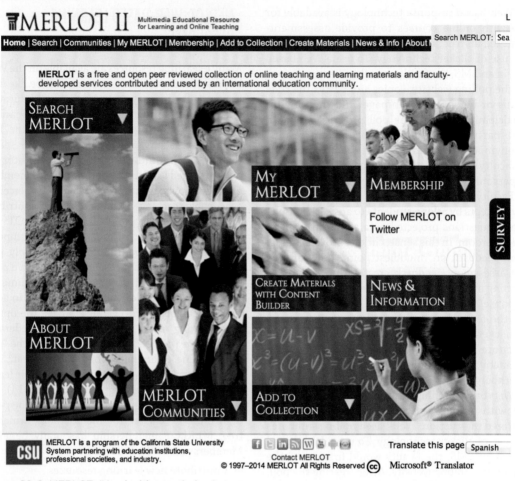

Figure 22-6. MERLOT. (Used with permission.)

FUTURE TRENDS

Ward once said, "If you can imagine it, you can achieve it; if you can dream it, you can become it" (ThinkExist.com, 2010). In 1993, futurist Marc Smith described cyberspace and virtual communities (Smith, 1993). In 1996, Chris Dede portrayed the social aspect of e-learning based on Smith's work: "Social network capital (an instant Web of contacts with useful skills), knowledge capital (a personal, distributed 'brain trust' with just-in-time answers to immediate questions), and communion (psychological/spiritual support from people who share common joys and trials) are three types of 'collective goods' that bind together

virtual communities enabled by computer-mediated communication" (Dede, 1996, p. 11). The imaginations of Smith and Dede helped to set the stage for the interactive Web e-learning environment. Technologic advances will continue to impact e-learning and the design of the learning environment.

Learners who grew up using technology are changing learning experiences to "connected learning" environments (Ito et al., 2013). Connected learning takes into consideration the learners' experiences, personal goals, motivation, and long-term memories. Connected learners are goal driven and learn without a formal education program using social networking.

Each year, EDCAUSE (http://educause. edu/) publishes the Horizon Report. The 2014 EDUCAUSE Horizon Report described six developments in technologies likely to impact teaching and learning between 2014 and 2019. The technologies were (1) the flipped classroom, (2) learning analytics, (3) 3D printing, (4) games and gamification, (5) quantified self, and (6) virtual assistants (Johnson et al., 2014). Technologic advances and free Web-enabled creative resources are empowering the learners to custom design their personal learning environment.

SUMMARY

In the information age, it is imperative that higher education prepare learners to be active, independent learners and problem solvers. E-learning, when used appropriately, facilitates this process and provides a venue for lifelong learning. E-learning can be classified by the learning method or the technology. There are numerous learning methods including drill and practice, tutorials, simulations, gaming, and testing. Effective learning methods, whether used online or face-to-face, must provide interactivity and prompt feedback to learners. The various technologies meet different learning needs.

Using e-learning successfully depends on how it is integrated into the total learning program. The level of interactivity also needs to be considered and matched with program goals. Like all teaching methods, e-learning has advantages and disadvantages. Advantages include interactivity and the flexibility of the medium. Disadvantages can include lack of familiarity with the technology, technology glitches, lack of access, and cost.

With the advent of the Internet, distance learning continues to gain in popularity for educational offerings. Programs offered via distance learning vary from correspondence courses and magazine articles to full degree programs. Distance learning requires the development of skills not always needed in traditional education including the ability to discipline oneself to set aside time for the program and the ability to communicate effectively in writing.

APPLICATIONS AND COMPETENCIES

1. Differentiate between the characteristics of the learning methods drill and practice, tutorial, and game, providing an example related to nursing for each one. Explain the connection of each learning method to Bloom's Taxonomy of Learning.

2. Compare the different modes of computerized testing and give examples for appropriate use. If you have used computerized testing, identify the strengths and limitations form the learner's perspective.

3. Research at least two types of simulations used in nursing education. What are the strengths and limitations of each type for both instructors and students? What instruction methods best enhance student learning?

4. Join MERLOT. Search for two online learning resources of value to nursing and then add them to the MERLOT collection.

5. Research emerging trends for e-learning using the Internet and online library. Create a bullet listing of "talking points" for at least three emerging trends.

REFERENCES

Advanced Distributed Learning. (2014, April). *Advanced distributed learning*. Retrieved from http://www.adlnet.org/

American Heart Association. (2015). *Los Angeles ISC case study*. Retrieved from http://commerce.workflowoneaccess.com/Themes/Custom/dabab82a-1302-4cc0-b5e6-55d349494117/cpr/events_programs.html

Anderson, L. W., Krathwohl, D. R., & Bloom, B. S. (2001). *A taxonomy for learning, teaching, and assessing: A revision of Bloom's taxonomy of educational objectives* (complete edition). New York, NY: Longman.

Atherton, J. S. (2013). *Learning and teaching; misrepresentation, myths and misleading ideas [On-line: UK]*. Retrieved from http://www.learningandteaching.info/learning/myths.htm

Benner, P. E., Sutphen, M., Leonard, V., et al. (2010). *Educating nurses: A call for radical transformation* (1st ed.). San Francisco, CA: Jossey-Bass.

Bloom, B. S. (1956). *Taxonomy of educational objectives, handbook 1: Cognitive domain*. New York, NY: Addison-Wesley.

Cancer Research UK. (2014). *Play to cure: Genes in space*. Retrieved from http://www.cancerresearchuk.org/support-us/play-to-cure-genes-in-space

Cardoza, M. P., & Hood, P. A. (2012). Comparative study of baccalaureate nursing student self-efficacy before and after simulation. *Computers, Informatics, Nursing: CIN*, *30*(3), 142–147. doi:10.1097/NCN.0b013e3182388936.

Centers for Disease Control and Prevention. (2014, August 18). *Solve the Outbreak app*. Retrieved from http://www.cdc.gov/mobile/applications/sto/

Chickering, A. W., & Ehrmann, S. C. (1996). *Implementing the seven principles: Technology as lever*. Retrieved from http://www.tltgroup.org/programs/seven.html

Clark, S. and Piercy, C. (2012). E-learning provides nursing education in remote areas. *Australian Nursing Journal*, *20*(4), 49. Retrieved from http://trove.nla.gov.au/work/35538060

Curran, C. R., Elfrink, V., Mays, B., et al. (2009). Building a virtual community for nursing education: the town of Mirror Lake. *Journal of Nursing Education*, *48*(1), 30–35. Retrieved from http://www.healio.com/nursing/journals/jne

Dede, C. (1996). The evolution of distance education: Emerging technologies and distributed learning. *American Journal of Distance Education*, *10*(2), 4. Retrieved from http://www.msmc.la.edu/include/learning_resources/emerging_technologies/ajde.pdf

Du, S. S., Liu, Z. Z., Liu, S. S., et al. (2013). Web-based distance learning for nurse education: A systematic review. *International Nursing Review*, *60*(2), 167–177. doi:10.1111/inr.12015.

ELI. (2014, January). *7 things you should know about gesture-based computing*. Retrieved from http://www.educause.edu/library/resources/7-things-you-should-know-about-gesture-based-computing

Giddens, J., Hrabe, D., Carlson-Sabelli, L., et al. (2012). The impact of a virtual community on student engagement and academic performance among baccalaureate nursing students. *Journal of Professional Nursing*, *28*(5), 284–290. doi:10.1016/j.profnurs.2012.04.011.

Half-Baked Software Inc. (2009). *What is quandary?* Retrieved from http://www.halfbakedsoftware.com/quandary.php

Half-Baked Software Inc. (2014). *Hot Potatoes*. Retrieved from http://hotpot.uvic.ca/

Hawks, S. J. (2014). The flipped classroom: Now or never? *AANA Journal*, *82*(4), 264–269. Retrieved from http://www.aana.com/newsandjournal/pages/aanajournalonline.aspx

Hayden, J. K., Smiley, R. A., Alexander, M., et al. (2014). The NCSBN national simulation study: A longitudinal, randomized, controlled study replacing clinical hours with simulation in prelicensure nursing education. *Journal of Nursing Regulation*, *5*(2), S3–S64. Retrieved from http://jnr.metapress.com/home/main.mpx

Howard, V. M., Ross, C., Mitchell, A. M., et al. (2010). Human patient simulators and interactive case studies: A comparative analysis of learning outcomes and student perceptions. *Computers, Informatics, Nursing: CIN*, *28*(1), 42–48. doi:10.1097/NCN.0b013e3181c04939.

Ito, M., Gutiérrez, K., Livingstone, S., et al. (2013). *Connected learning: an agenda for research and design*. Irvine, CA: Digital Media and Learning Research Hub. Retrieved from http://eprints.lse.ac.uk/48114/

Jenson, C. E., & Forsyth, D. M. (2012). Virtual reality simulation: Using three-dimensional technology to teach nursing students. *Computers, Informatics, Nursing: CIN*, *30*(6), 312–318; quiz 319–320. doi:10.1097/NXN.0b013e31824af6ae.

Johnson, L., Adams Becker, S., Estrada, V., et al. (2014). *The 2014 Horizon Report*. Austin, TX: The New Media Consortium. Retrieved from http://www.nmc.org/pdf/2014-nmc-horizon-report-he-EN.pdf

Johnson, D., & Johnson, S. (2014). The effects of using a human patient simulator compared to a CD-ROM in teaching critical thinking and performance. *U.S. Army Medical Department Journal*, 59–64. Retrieved from http://www.cs.amedd.army.mil/amedd_journal.aspx

Kaplan, B., & Ura, D. (2010). Use of multiple patient simulators to enhance prioritizing and delegating skills for senior nursing students. *Journal of Nursing Education*, *49*(7), 371–377. doi:10.3928/01484834-20100331-07.

Kruglikova, I., Grantcharov, T. P., Drewes, A. M., et al. (2010). Assessment of early learning curves among nurses and physicians using a high-fidelity virtual-reality colonoscopy simulator. *Surgical Endoscopy*, *24*(2), 366–370. doi:10.1007/s00464-009-0555-7.

Lord, T., & Baviskar, S. (2007). Moving students from information recitation to information understanding: Exploiting Bloom's taxonomy in creating science questions. *Journal of College Science Teaching*, *36*(5), 40–44. Retrieved from http://www.nsta.org/college/

Manos, L. (2014). *Academic electronic health record*. Retrieved from http://www.kumc.edu/documents/seeds/091511-lmanos.pdf

McMullen, K. D., McConnaughy, R. P., & Riley, R. A. (2011). Outreach to improve patient education at South Carolina free medical clinics. *Journal of Consumer Health on the Internet*, *15*(2), 117–131. doi:10.1080/15398285.2011.572779.

MERLOT. (2014). *MERLOT: About us*. Retrieved from http://taste.merlot.org/

Miller, M., & Jensen, R. (2014). Avatars in nursing: An integrative review. *Nurse Educator*, *39*(1), 38–41. doi:10.1097/01.NNE.0000437367.03842.63.

NCSBN. (2014). *NCLEX using CAT*. Retrieved from https://www.ncsbn.org/3761.htm

Nyswaner, A. (2007). "Driver's ed" for the OR nurse. *RN*, *70*(3), 45–48. Retrieved from http://rnjournal.com/

Quality Matters. (2014). *Quality Matters™ rubric standards, fifth edition, 2014, with assigned points*. Retrieved from http://www.qualitymatters.org

Respondus. (2014). *StudyMate learning activities and games*. Retrieved from http://www.respondus.com/products/studymate.shtml

Roh, Y. S. (2014). Effects of high-fidelity patient simulation on nursing students' resuscitation-specific self-efficacy. *Computers, Informatics, Nursing: CIN*, *32*(2), 84–89. doi:10.1097/CIN.0000000000000034.

Shepherd, J. D., Badger-Brown, K. M., Legassic, M. S., et al. (2012). SCI-U: e-learning for patient education in spinal cord injury rehabilitation. *Journal of Spinal Cord Medicine*, *35*(5), 319–329. doi:10.1179/2045772312Y.0000000044.

Skiba, J. (2010). Nursing education 2.0: Social networking and the WOTY... "word of the year". *Nursing Education Perspectives*, *31*(1), 44–46. Retrieved from http://www.nln.org/nlnjournal/

Smith, M. (1993). *Voices from the WELL: The logic of the virtual commons*. Los Angeles, CA: University of California, Los Angeles.

SoftChalk LLC. (2014). *SoftChalk*. Retrieved from http://www.softchalk.com/

Sternberger, C. S. (2012). Interactive learning environment: Engaging students using clickers. *Nursing Education Perspectives*, *33*(2), 121–124.

Thalheimer, W. (2006, May 1). *People remember 10%, 20%... Oh really?* Retrieved from http://www.willatworklearning.com/2006/05/people_remember.html

ThinkExist.com, Q. (2010). *William Arthur Ward quotes*. Retrieved from http://thinkexist.com/quotation/if_you_can_imagine_it-you_can_achieve_it-if_you/15190.html

United States Access Boards. (n.d.). *E-learning: Conforming to section 508*. Retrieved from http://www.access-board.gov/guidelines-and-standards/communications-and-it/25-508-standards/719-e-learning-conforming-to-section-508?highlight=WzUwOF0=

Vana, K. D., Silva, G. E., Muzyka, D., et al. (2011). Effectiveness of an audience response system in teaching pharmacology to baccalaureate nursing students. *Computers, Informatics, Nursing: CIN*, *29*(6), TC105–TC113. Retrieved from doi:10.1097/NCN.0b013e3181f9dd9c.

CHAPTER 23

Informatics in Management and Quality Improvement

OBJECTIVES

After studying this chapter, you will be able to:

1. Identify the tools necessary to manage business processes in nursing services.

2. Demonstrate basic competencies in spreadsheets and flowcharting in nursing administration.

3. Discuss data management to improve outcomes using quality improvement and benchmarking in patient care.

4. Explore the use of specialized applications in nursing administration, including scheduling systems and patient classification systems.

KEY TERMS

Benchmarking

Big data

Business intelligence

Cause-and-effect chart

Clinical information systems

Consumer Assessment of Health Providers and Systems

Core Measures

Dashboards

Data analytics

Demand forecasting

Employee scheduling system

Financial management

Flowcharting

Forecasting

Gantt chart

Human resource management system

National Database of Nursing Quality Indicators (NDNQI)

Patient classification systems

Patient throughput

Process improvement

Quality improvement

Value-based purchasing

There is little doubt that nurse administrators and managers must have competency in a wide range of technology skills to be effective in their roles. According to the American Organization of Nurse Executives (American Organization of Nurse Executives, 2005), one of the five leadership domains is business skills, which includes information management and technology. Competencies in email, word processing, spreadsheets, and the Internet are basic skills. Beyond these, nurse administrators use management information systems for the purposes of

---

BOX 23-1   AONE Nurse Executive Competencies. Business Skills: Information Management and Technology Competencies

AONE believes that managers at all levels must be competent to

• Demonstrate use of email, word processing, spreadsheets, and Internet programs
• Recognize the relevance of nursing data for improving practice
• Use telecommunication devices
• Utilize hospital database management, decision support, and expert system programs to access information and analyze data from disparate sources for use in planning for patient care processes and systems
• Participate in system change processes and utility analysis
• Participate in the evaluation of information systems in practice settings
• Evaluate and revise patient care processes and systems
• Use computerized management systems to record administrative data (billing data, quality assurance data, workload data, etc.)
• Use applications for structure data entry (classification systems, acuity level, etc.)
• Recognize the utility of nursing involvement in the planning design and choice and implementation of information systems in the practice environment
• Demonstrate awareness of societal and technologic trend issues and new developments as they apply to nursing
• Demonstrate proficient awareness of legal and ethical issues related to client data, information, and confidentiality
• Read and interpret benchmarking, financial, and occupancy data

---

financial management, **process improvement**, human resource management, **quality improvement**, **benchmarking**, and **business intelligence**. Because of the nurse administrator's unique role as a leader of nursing services, knowledge of **clinical information systems** is important as well. Box 23-1 specifies the competencies needed by nurse managers and nurse executives (American Organization of Nurse Executives, 2005). This chapter focuses on unique uses for applications in the work of an administrator.

TOOLS

Nurse managers use various desktop computer applications to increase their efficiency. Earlier chapters of this textbook include a description of the basic skills.

Financial Management: Spreadsheets

Chapter 7 provides an overview of how to create spreadsheets, insert formulas to perform calculations, and display data in charts. These skills are useful to any nurse manager for following monthly budgets or creating a variance report if the accounting department does not provide one. However, a nurse manager might want to take data available from different sources and create a new spreadsheet to determine if relationships exist between two groups of information.

For example, Table 23-1 shows sample nursing hours per patient day for registered nurses (RNs) and nursing assistants (NAs). Taken alone, the manager can see that nursing hours go up and down depending on the quarter. Table 23-2 shows the patients' average length of stay (LOS) on the unit

TABLE 23-1 Staffing Report: Hours per Patient Day	Quarter 1	Quarter 2	Quarter 3	Quarter 4
Registered nurses	9	15	10	12
Nursing assistants	2	3	1	3

for the same time periods. There are variations in LOS between quarters. The manager should consider hours per patient day and LOS simultaneously to see if a relationship exists.

Creating a chart that shows relationships starts with entry of staffing and LOS data into the cells of the same spreadsheet. You can create a column and line chart (Figure 23-1) that reveals a pattern: as the number of RN hours goes up (nursing hours are plotted on the left-hand axis), the patient LOS goes down (LOS is plotted on the right-hand axis). You might miss this important trend if you view the data independently.

The nurse manager must use data to show a need for staffing. Certainly, a chart showing that better staffing reduces the number of patient days in the hospital creates a positive financial impact and a substantial argument for appropriate staffing levels. You can make other similar comparisons with nurse-sensitive outcomes including falls, pressure ulcers, and infections.

Another way to use a spreadsheet is to trend historical data to forecast for future needs. Unfortunately, in nursing and healthcare, there is no perfect way to predict the demand for services. However, nurse leaders can use knowledge of their facilities, historical data, graphing techniques, assessment of trends or seasonal patterns, and formulas to make reasonable estimates (Finkler et al., 2012). Data collection is the first step in **forecasting** future events. The nurse leader needs to determine what data are most helpful and what length of time would be most appropriate. Finkler et al. suggest using 1 to 5 years of data for

forecasting. False conclusions might result if the time period is too short. For example, Figure 23-2 shows only 4 months of data, so an office manager in a primary care practice viewing it might misinterpret the a trend in number of visits for respiratory illnesses. More data are needed to ascertain the real pattern.

When viewed within a 5-year period, the office manager can clearly see a seasonal pattern: respiratory infections increase during the months of October to January and return to a lower level during the spring and summer months (Figure 23-3). However, the office manager might note that the number of respiratory infections appears to be on the increase overall in the last year. The office manager applies a linear forecast line to the chart and sees that respiratory infections could be expected to increase in coming winter months. With this knowledge, the office manager might suggest reassignment of a nurse practitioner to see "walk-in" patients with infections.

Process Improvement

Process improvement is the application of actions taken to identify, analyze, and improve existing processes within an organization to meet requirements for quality, customer satisfaction, and financial goals. Administrators can use a particular strategy such as total quality management, six sigma, lean, or a general process improvement framework called plan-do-study act (Gillam & Siriwardena, 2013; Simon & Canacari, 2012). Whatever the strategy used for improvement, an

TABLE 23-2 Patient Length of Stay	Quarter 1	Quarter 2	Quarter 3	Quarter 4
Length of stay	5	3.75	5.25	4.5

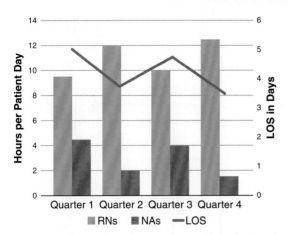

Figure 23-1. Nursing hours per patient day and average patient length of stay. (Used with permission from Microsoft.)

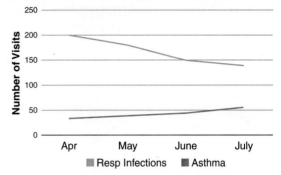

Figure 23-2. Line chart showing number of respiratory visits in 4 months. (Used with permission from Microsoft.)

organized approach is necessary to understand the current state of the process and plan for changes to improve outcomes. Process improvement should be an analytical process where you use tools such as flowcharts, cause-and-effect charts, and other control methods to make changes to targeted processes.

Analysis of Processes with Flowcharting

Flowcharting software applications can be useful because nurse administrators can map processes in patient care. There are many instances in healthcare where care processes need to be examined to make them more efficient or to reduce unwanted variation in care. For example, the movement of patients from the emergency department into a hospital inpatient room for admission is a complicated process. Delays in starting care are unnecessary and costly; analysis through flowcharting may reveal opportunities for improvement in the admission process. In Figure 23-4, it is possible to avoid unnecessary delays if the path from decision to admit and the transfer of the patient is a straight line (Figure 23-4A). When multiple decisions need to be made or multiple people are involved (Figure 23-4B), the process becomes more complicated and delays occur. The use of flowcharting is

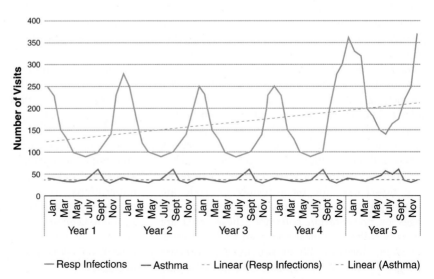

Figure 23-3. Line chart showing number of respiratory visits in 5 years. (Used with permission from Microsoft.)

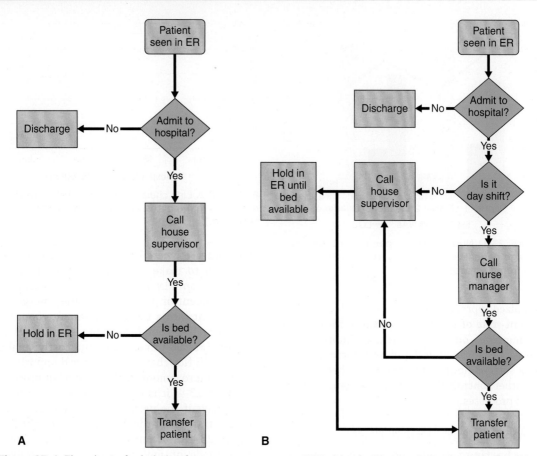

Figure 23-4. Flowchart of admission from emergency room (ER). (Used with permission from Microsoft.)

a powerful way to identify reorganization of steps in a process for better flow.

When examining relationships among complex processes, a **cause-and-effect chart** is another useful diagram for nurse administrators to use. The cause-and-effect chart places the effect at one end of the chart with the many suspected causes branching out from it. The resulting chart resembles a fish; thus, it is commonly referred to as a fishbone chart. Figure 23-5 depicts a simple cause-and-effect chart; charts that are more complex show multiple related causes under each branch.

There are many software options for developing flowcharts. The most readily available are drawing tools included in word processing packages or presentation software. These tools are usually sufficient unless you need to depict complicated processes. When you need a software program with more sophisticated flowcharting

abilities, the nurse administrator should analyze the products on cost and capabilities. The Microsoft product is called Visio, and other similar products are WizFlow (from Pacestar software), FlowBreeze Software, SmartDraw, EdrawSoft, and ConceptDraw (from Computer Systems Odessa Corp.) to name a few. Most of the products are $50 to $200 for a single-user license.

Project Management

Nurse administrators often oversee planning and implementation of complex projects with numerous stakeholders, resources, and financial implications. In many cases, the use of project management software can provide needed organization to keep projects on time and within budget. This type of software is not one nursing administration offices typically use—a purchase may be necessary.

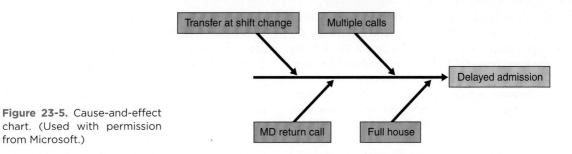

Figure 23-5. Cause-and-effect chart. (Used with permission from Microsoft.)

The benefit of using project management software is the ability to track the project's progress using tools such as a **Gantt chart**, which can show start to end dates and associated costs with tasks (Figure 23-6). Milestones can be marked on the chart to highlight important parts of a task. Links between tasks depict when tasks need to be completed before others start. Linking tasks is a good practice to use because when a date changes in one task, all other dates to linked tasks update. Some project management software can be set to send email reminders to individuals responsible for milestones or tasks within the project. This automation frees the administrator to focus on the big picture and leaves the details to the software.

You can generate reports of tasks and costs. These reports provide a snapshot of the progress, resources, and finances for the project. Depending on the level of integration, you can export these reports to a spreadsheet application for sharing with others in the organization.

Many vendors make project management software for personal computers including Microsoft Project; Standard Register, which produces SmartWorks; Intuit QuickBase; and Experience In Software, Inc., which develops Project Kickstart. Other options include purchasing a Web-based service if the nurse administrator needs to collaborate with others in a multihospital network. You should consider several factors when making a decision about purchasing project management software. The first is the degree of integration with other administrative tools such as spreadsheets, email, and calendars. The second is the number of users who would access the information contained in the project management software. The third is the security of Web-based systems compared with other deployment methods. Finally, consider the cost of the software: single-user licenses are relatively inexpensive but do not encourage collaboration. If a nurse administrator needs collaboration and has a secure Web solution, the cost of a multiuser license may be well worth the investment.

Human Resource Management

Personnel management is one of the most important parts of the job of a nurse manager. The use of a **human resource management system (HRMS)** is essential for planning and staffing nursing services appropriately. You can use HRMS, which generally contains four categories: personnel profiles including demographic data; daily work schedules and time-off requests; payroll data; and education, skill qualifications, and licensure information.

Not only can an HRMS serve as a scheduling system and repository of personnel data, but you can purchase a productivity module, which can pull nursing data (hours of care and skill mix) together with patient data (patient days, average LOS, and patient acuity). This productivity information is critical for nurse managers and nurse administrators to track,

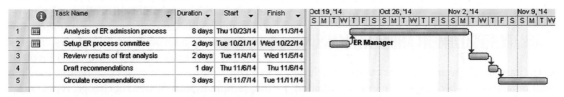

		Task Name	Duration	Start	Finish	Oct 19, '14	Oct 26, '14	Nov 2, '14	Nov 9, '14
1		Analysis of ER admission process	8 days	Thu 10/23/14	Mon 11/3/14				
2		Setup ER process committee	2 days	Tue 10/21/14	Wed 10/22/14				
3		Review results of first analysis	2 days	Tue 11/4/14	Wed 11/5/14				
4		Draft recommendations	1 day	Thu 11/6/14	Thu 11/6/14				
5		Circulate recommendations	3 days	Fri 11/7/14	Tue 11/11/14				

Figure 23-6. Gantt chart. (Used with permission from Microsoft.)

trend, and analyze productivity for meaning within their organizations and benchmark against similar organizations across the United States. This is likely the most powerful information produced for managers and administrators in healthcare today.

Because regulators and accreditation agencies require information about employees such as competencies, certifications, and evaluations, HRMS may provide a solution for managing these data too. Many HRMSs will contain employee appraisals; orientation checklists; employee competency checklists; development plans; compensation adjustments based on the achievement of personal, unit, or organization goals; and possibly succession plans. The HRMS may also generate reports for The Joint Commission (TJC).

Nurse administrators who might be involved in the decision to purchase an HRMS should be certain to view demonstrations from vendors whose products are specialized to healthcare. Because the work of nursing services is so different from manufacturing or other service-related industries, it is important to have systems that meet many specifications. The HRMS needs to meet the following minimum requirements:

1. Handle scheduling for 24 hours per day, 7 days per week
2. Accommodate different scheduling rules for units across an entire organization or network
3. Allow for staff self-scheduling
4. Determine the right number and mix of nursing staff for patient needs
5. Provide an analysis of nursing staff usage to manage productivity and support quality patient outcomes
6. Track time and attendance
7. Provide real-time analysis of overtime
8. Connect to the payroll system
9. Retain certification and licensure information
10. Serve as a repository for competency assessments and annual employee appraisals

USING DATA TO IMPROVE OUTCOMES: QUALITY IMPROVEMENT AND BENCHMARKING

In the past, nurses were viewed as overhead to hospital organizations because revenue was generated by admissions to the hospital, not by the quality of patient care that was provided. This view changed with **value-based purchasing** initiatives. Nurses are in pivotal positions to improve quality, prevent errors, and improve patient satisfaction in hospitals. For example, if nurses prevent nosocomial infections in postoperative patients, the hospital will receive full reimbursement allowed under the Centers for Medicare & Medicaid (CMS.gov, 2014a, 2014b). However, if a patient develops a catheter-associated urinary tract infection after hospital admission, CMS will not reimburse for additional treatment or days of hospitalization associated with the nosocomial infection. In order for excellence in patient care to be the norm for hospitals, nurse administrators must follow the progress of improvements in care and keep nursing staff informed about how their performance affects the hospital's reimbursement.

Not only do nurse administrators engage in quality improvement projects specific to their hospitals, but they must also provide leadership for the required hospital participation in improvement initiatives mandated by the CMS. These mandated programs include **Core Measures** and **Consumer Assessment of Health Providers and Systems**, Hospital Survey (HCAHPS) (CMS.gov, 2013; HCAHPS, 2015). In addition, nurse administrators may choose to join the **National Database of Nursing Quality Indicators (NDNQI)**. These quality improvement initiatives require the nurse administrator to designate staff and resources to the collection of data, aggregation of data for submission to databases, and response to reports.

Quality Safety Education for Nurses (QSEN)

Because of the roles nurses have in improving quality and safeguarding patients, education at the bachelor's and master's levels includes competencies in six critical areas: patient-centered care, teamwork and collaboration, evidence-based practice, quality improvement, safety, and informatics (Cronenwett et al., 2007). Informatics is at the core of modern quality improvement and safety practices; the ability to collect, aggregate, store, and access data appropriately is a prerequisite to quality improvement techniques. Nurses and other healthcare providers are often involved in quality improvement cycles that require baseline measurement, introduction of change, repeat measurement, and comparison of outcomes over time

(U.S. Department of Health and Human Services [HHS], n.d.). Likewise, safety practices require a culture of safety across the entire healthcare organization (Agency for Healthcare Research and Quality [AHRQ], 2014). Nurses and other healthcare providers must have a preoccupation with preventing errors by reporting and investigating near misses and errors without fear or blaming. Each near miss or error is viewed as an opportunity to find the underlying problems that put safety at risk and develop solutions to those system problems. Workflow analysis, root cause analysis, and cause-and-effect charts can be used to investigate the circumstances around a near miss or error (Agency for Healthcare Research and Quality [AHRQ], 2014).

Core Measures

In the late 1990s, TJC in cooperation with the CMS and the Hospital Quality Alliance (HQA) established standardized core measurements required for all accredited healthcare organizations (The Joint Commission, 2014). A few standardized core measurements were required in the first year. In subsequent years, more core measures were added in areas including myocardial infarction, congestive heart failure, pneumonia, pregnancy, treatment of asthma in children, surgical care improvement project, venous thromboembolism, immunizations, smoking treatment, and stroke. Each of these core measures required extensive data collection, aggregation, and reporting to stay in compliance. Once reported, the core measures are available for the public at http://www.hospitalcompare.hhs.gov.

Consumer Assessment of Health Providers and Systems: Hospital Survey

Beginning in 2008, the CMS in collaboration with the HQA required hospitals to survey patients and families to gather information about their experiences with healthcare (CMS.gov, 2013). The AHRQ developed the tool, known as HCAHPS, as a standardized survey tool designed for administration to a sample of discharged patients. Hospitals are required to submit data to the CMS website so that patients' experiences can be trended over time in one hospital and benchmarked to other hospitals. These data are available to the public

to provide accountability in healthcare at http://www.hospitalcompare.hhs.gov.

Hospitals may use a vendor to survey patients or elect to conduct surveys with its employees. Regardless of this choice, surveyors must use a standardized method of collecting data and reporting data. The HCAHPS survey includes six composite measures, two individual items, and two overall items (CMS.gov, 2013). Hospitals can add other questions to customize the survey to meet their own needs for data on the patient experience. Initially, the federal government only required inpatient hospitals to participate in HCAHPS; failure to participate resulted in 2% reduced payments by Medicare. However in 2012, a hospital's performance on HCAHPS was linked to its Medicare reimbursement using a formula (CMS.gov, 2013).

National Database of Nursing Quality Indicators

The quality of nursing care has an influence on a hospital's performance in some of the areas of core measures and patients' experiences in healthcare as measured by HCAHPS. A more direct measurement of the quality of nursing care is possible when nurse administrators choose to participate in the NDNQI. The American Nurses Association (ANA) in partnership with the University of Kansas, School of Nursing began the development of its safety and quality initiative, which resulted in NDNQI. After a development period of approximately four years, the NDNQI began accepting data for comparison from hospitals in 1998. The service was free until 2001 when a fee was established for joining the database. As of 2014, over 2000 hospitals participated in the service (American Nurses Association, 2014). In 2014, Press Ganey, an organization that focuses on improving healthcare, acquired NDNQI.

The NDNQI is a national database to which hospitals submit nursing-sensitive data about structure, process, and outcomes of nursing care. The NDNQI aggregates the data quarterly and returns reports to participating hospitals. Nurse administrators and managers receive unit-level information that is compared across time periods and benchmarked to similar units from other hospitals. The NDNQI data include nursing hours per patient day, staff mix, falls, nursing turnover, pressure ulcers, infections, restraint use, intravenous infiltration, and nosocomial infection, to name a few (American Nurses Association, 2014). You can find more information at http://www.nursingquality.org.

BIG DATA

Business Intelligence in Healthcare Systems

Nursing services collect hundreds of thousands of data elements every day in the delivery of patient care and in management processes such as utilization review, case management, and infection control. The creation of tremendously large amounts of data, both structured and unstructured that is created, collected, and accessed at different times, is called **big data** (Roski et al., 2014). There is no need for additional measurements; the critical part to making big data work in healthcare is an infrastructure to handle big data. Nurse administrators need to focus on measurements that are the key drivers of effective, quality care (Frith et al., 2010). There needs to be alignment of decisions about quality measurements throughout the healthcare organization to provide information about the outcomes of patient care, patient satisfaction, costs, and revenue. This alignment and linking of data to transform them into information for decision making is called business intelligence (Elliot, 2004). Another related term is **data analytics**, which is "a process of reviewing large amounts of raw and unorganized data to identify patterns or trends that will help organizations better understand behavior and outcomes" (Murphy et al., 2013).

Developing a plan for business intelligence is a strategic process with engagement of executives, including the nurse administrator. Other key positions in a healthcare organization include information management specialists, informatics nurse specialists, and statisticians who have domain knowledge required to develop or select data warehousing software, data integration software, querying software, and **dashboard** software to present performance indicators. Nurse administrators have domain knowledge of the questions that need the data contained in the warehouse to answer. All must work together to have a robust business intelligence that can be used to collect, store, and analyze data to answer relevant clinical and management questions and to track outcomes.

Data analytics and business intelligence go through a maturity process; early phases of business intelligence result in descriptive outputs to executives (Murphy et al., 2013). As a healthcare organization's business intelligence matures, the outputs become predictions of healthcare outcomes and prescriptive suggestions for optimizing healthcare outcomes (Roski et al., 2014).

The delivery of business intelligence and data analytics must be user-friendly for viewers. Most often, these are in the form of dashboards to deliver real-time information on key performance indicators to drive decision making in healthcare (Table 23-3). Malik (2005) makes an analogy

TABLE 23-3	Effective Dashboards
Synergetic	Dashboard components must work together to relay information on a single screen.
Monitor	Dashboards must display key performance indicators for the user's decision-making needs.
Accurate	Data on the dashboard must be valid and reliable.
Responsive	When key performance indicators are below established targets, a flag or alarm must alert the user.
Timely	Dashboards must display data in real time.

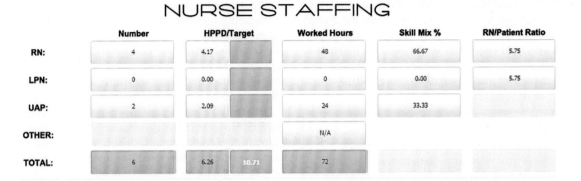

Figure 23-7. Example nurse staffing dashboard.

between a pilot's uses of a dashboard of instruments to fly a jet and an administrator's need for a dashboard of key performance indicators to make operational decisions in healthcare. This analogy makes sense if we believe that administrators of complex healthcare organizations need information to make critical decisions just as pilots need information when making decisions while flying. Malik further states that for dashboards to be effective and useful for decision making, they must be SMART (see Table 23-3).

The use of dashboards in healthcare is playing an important role at senior administrative levels. Dashboards are not just for executives; anyone who has decision-making responsibility should have access to information in the timeliest manner possible (Figure 23-7). Nurse managers need access to real-time data about staffing, productivity, costs, and quality through the use of dashboards to guide operations effectively (Anderson et al., 2011).

Patient Care Management

Forward-thinking leaders can use big data too by integrating publically available datasets with communication technologies to improve patient care management in primary or specialty practices. For example, in the care of patients with asthma or chronic obstructive pulmonary disease (COPD), environmental conditions can trigger exacerbations resulting in an office or emergency room visit (Moineddin et al., 2008). A common trigger for people with asthma and COPD is poor air quality, which is a particular problem in large cities in the summer months (Figure 23-8). With knowledge of air quality problems and a free mobile warning system from the U.S. Environmental Protection Agency, a primary care provider could encourage patients with asthma and COPD to download the AirNow app to receive air quality warning, sign up for free email or twitter messages from EnviroFlash,

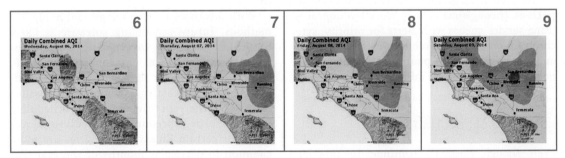

Figure 23-8. AirNow from the U.S. Environmental Protection Agency (http:\\www.airnow.gov). Note: The EPA defines the color coding according to an air quality index, where green is good, yellow is moderate, orange is unhealthy for sensitive groups, and red is unhealthy for everyone.

or give permission for the office to send text messages to them on days with poor air quality (AirNow, n.d.). During office visits, healthcare providers could emphasize to the need for patients to use their individualized asthma action plan on days with poor air quality warnings (Booth, 2012).

QSEN Scenario

You learned that the healthcare agency where you work uses data analytics from data stored in a data warehouse. What are some potential benefits for improving the quality and safety of nursing practice from data analytics?

WORKFLOW

One of the challenges in complex, acute care hospitals is the workflow, also known as throughput. Delays in patient care because of miscommunication, unavailable transport services, overdue room cleaning, and poor patient scheduling decrease patient satisfaction and decrease the profitability of a hospital. Systems are emerging on the market, which have the potential to innovate hospital operations. One such system, Horizon Enterprise Visibility, is available from McKesson Corporation. The system provides a visual presentation of all patients on whiteboards with updates on patients' locations, the status of test results, and updates on discharges; the system communicates this information through existing enterprise software. Another software package developed by CareLogistics for hospital management delivers innovation in **patient throughput** as well. Workflow improves using service queues with alerts for priority; synchronization of patient rooms, tasks, equipment, and services; and hospital performance dashboards to keep managers informed in real time.

EMPLOYEE SCHEDULING

Even though hospitals continue to function by scheduling nursing staff using a paper system, there are many reasons to change to a computerized **employee scheduling system**. Scheduling nurses' work is a repetitive task, and nurse managers spend hours developing biweekly or monthly schedules. Computerized scheduling systems can handle scheduling rules such as master schedules and shift rotations, repeating patterns to make a quick first draft of a schedule. It is easier to make modifications when the availability of nurses shows in the system. Scheduling systems can often prevent errors such as scheduling nurses for a double shift, for overtime, during overlapping shifts, or during requested time off. Often, scheduling systems are capable of generating reports to show the number of productive hours, education, vacation, and family medical leave hours in a period. Some scheduling systems allow managers to share the schedule with nurses by Intranets, Internet, email, or printing schedules. With an Intranet or Internet interface, nurses can interact with scheduling systems to make requests, view schedules, or fill open shifts.

Some hospitals are successful with centralized, self-scheduling software to fill open shifts (Ellerbe, 2007; Russell et al., 2012). Most of these programs provide a Web-based system for hospitals to use to fill their open shifts. The software matches the qualifications of the RN with the job requirements of the shift and offers an incentive for the RN to bid for the open shift. Hospitals have reported a reduction of $1 to 4 million per year in costs for contract labor using this system of competitive bidding for open shifts. Nurses report satisfaction because they see open shifts across the entire hospital, bid for the ones that most interest them, and receive fewer calls at home requesting them to work on their off days (AORN).

With advances in technology and analytical methods, future scheduling software is likely to include **demand forecasting** capabilities, which takes historical data on patient acuity and census to predict the needs for nurse staffing. Demand forecasting in healthcare is possible because of the repetitive nature of scheduling for surgery or procedures and because admissions for certain illnesses or injuries are more common in particular months of the year. For example, admissions for respiratory infections (pneumonia and influenza) are more common in the winter months, so demand forecasting can take information from previous winter months to predict the need for nurses on medical units in a particular hospital.

PATIENT CLASSIFICATION SYSTEMS (ACUITY APPLICATIONS)

Staffing is one of the most difficult decision-making roles a nurse manager fulfills. The purpose of **patient classification systems** is to estimate the care needs of inpatients for prudent staffing decisions. Most patient acuity systems generate data to calculate the number of full-time equivalents needed for a nursing unit (Finkler et al., 2012). Some look at self-care deficits such as those related to activities of daily living, treatments, medications, and patient teaching. Another approach assigns time to each task based on hospital-specific, predetermined measures. Another method is the use of specific nursing diagnoses based on patient dependency. This approach uses decisions made by the primary nursing care provider.

All patient classification systems depend on accurate and timely data input. Some patient classification systems use computer-based data entry and require the nurse to enter characteristics or tasks for use in the scoring of the patient's acuity. Other systems draw data from nurses' documentation in the computerized patient record, which relieves nurses of the additional step of data entry for patient classification. If nurses delay documentation (regardless of the reason), the patient's acuity is downgraded because the documentation of vital signs, education, dressing changes, and other nursing activities are not present in the record to reflect the patient's true acuity.

CLINICAL INFORMATION SYSTEMS

The CMS created regulations for Stage 1 and Stage 2 meaningful use of electronic health records (EHRs) and exchange of health information to improve the quality of healthcare in Medicare-eligible hospitals and healthcare providers (CMS.gov. 2014a). The CMS and the Office of the National Coordinator of Health Information Technology outlined a phased-in approach for the implementation of EHRs, and the failure of eligible hospitals or professionals to meet meaningful use requirements of EHRs by deadlines set by the CMS results in reductions in Medicare reimbursement (Recovery.gov, n.d.).

Many of the elements of meaningful use impact the work of nurses and nurse practitioners (Fuchs, 2014). The required core objectives, in particular, depend on the accurate collection and recording of data in an EHR, including patient demographics, vital signs, and smoking status (CMS.gov, 2014a). Other core objectives begin to focus nurses and other healthcare providers on patient safety with requirements for medication reconciliation, summaries of care for transitions, and provision of patient-specific health education (CMS.gov, 2014a). Nurses and other healthcare providers must use secure reminder systems to communicate with patients about their preventive care services and follow-up on medical information (CMS.gov, 2014a).

Only 3.4% of hospitals and 4.3% of providers in the United States have implemented complete electronic medical records (EMRs), defined by the Healthcare Information and Management Systems Society (HIMSS) as Stage 7 (Healthcare Information and Management Systems Society, HIMSS Analytics, 2013). This means that nurse administrators should be involved in the evaluation and purchase decision of many different parts of information systems including nursing and clinical documentation, clinical decision support systems for error checking and for clinical protocols, computerized provider order entry, closed-loop medication administration systems, data warehousing, and information exchanges. Meaningful involvement requires nurse administrators to understand the workflow in their own hospitals and the capability and limitations of clinical information systems so that purchased systems support clinical practice patterns. Although the nurse administrator may not have knowledge of the technical aspects, the administrator must be the voice of nursing when purchases are considered. The nurse administrator is in the best position to advocate for all nursing services and place nurses on purchase committees to make product selections that streamline work processes and put information in the hands of nurses.

The AONE released the guiding principles for the role of the nurse administrator in the selection and implementation of information systems (American Organization of Nurse Executives, 2007). This document clearly states that although the nurse administrator may delegate operational aspects of the acquisition and implementation of an information system, the administrator retains accountability for the process. Some key points include the following:

1. Describe the strategic nursing plan so that the chief information officer and members of the task force understand the information needs of nurses now and in the future.
2. Know about the planned technology purchases that will occur during the information system acquisition and consider the implications on nursing services.
3. Develop an understanding of contracts and legal issues surrounding data ownership.
4. Make site visits to hospitals where proposed information systems have been implemented and talk to the chief nurse executives at those facilities.
5. Get a clear understanding of the responsibility for training (when, where, how long, who provides, and who pays).
6. Develop metrics for implementation and monitor the implementation process using them.
7. Include deans from schools of nursing, pharmacy, and others to lessen the impact on their programs.
8. Be prepared for system downtimes.

In addition to the guiding principles for selection and implementation of information systems, the American Organization of Nurse Executives (2010) released a toolkit for the acquisition and implementation of information systems, which provides nurse administrators with three broad suggestions to deal with the meaningful use legislation: (1) Strategize about the implementation of information systems with careful attention to workflow implications, (2) understand the phased-in regulations and use project management to optimize incentives and avoid reductions in reimbursement, and (3) work closely with vendors to ensure that information systems meet certification requirements.

SUMMARY

Nurse administrators, like all other healthcare professionals, use computer applications in their daily work to communicate by email, find resources on the Internet, and develop documents with word processors and spreadsheets. Use of these tools, in addition to applications that can assist in the analysis of processes and in the planning for change, is an essential competency for today's nurse administrator. Moreover, nurse administrators are routinely involved in monitoring data from quality improvement studies (core measures, HCAHPS, NDNQI, and other measures) to implement change in nursing practice and patient care.

The nurse administrator's need for tools and information to support decisions on financial matters, to develop strategies for improvement in patient care, and to meet regulatory requirements has never been greater. Systems that support administrative work include human resource management systems, scheduling systems, patient management systems, and acuity systems. Information from these systems assists the nurse administrator to use nursing services wisely and to assess the effectiveness of decisions over time.

The nurse administrator should always have a strong voice in the decision to purchase an information system, whether it is a management system or clinical system. This involvement begins well before selection of an information system and continues after implementation to evaluate the performance metrics, costs, and vendor responsibility. The nurse administrator must ensure that decisions about systems that affect nursing services remain within the authority of the nurse administrator. Examples of the systems include clinical information systems, expert systems to support clinical decision making, medical technology, databases, and data warehousing systems. The reason is that the nurse administrator retains responsibility and accountability for providing the resources to accomplish patient care in a safe and efficient manner.

APPLICATIONS AND COMPETENCIES

1. Copy the data from the table below into a spreadsheet. Develop a chart (custom type) with a line column on two axes. Place the patient outcomes (falls and pressure ulcers) in the columns and the percentage of RNs on the line.

	Quarter 1	Quarter 2	Quarter 3	Quarter 4
Number of falls	5	8	9	4
Number of pressure ulcers	4	6	7	5
Percentage of registered nurses	0.80	0.75	0.76	0.81

2. Using drawing tools in a word processing software or presentation software, diagram the process for hiring an RN in your organization.
   a. Analyze the process.
      i. Are there ways that the hiring process can stagnate?
      ii. Are there steps that can be streamlined?
   b. Draw the ideal process.
   c. Consider ways to implement change in your organization.

3. Search the Internet and find five software vendors for project management.
   a. List the strengths and weaknesses of each.
   b. Download a trial version of at least two project management software packages.
   c. Develop a Gantt chart for a simple project in your organization to learn to use the software.

4. Go to http://www.hospitalcompare.hhs.gov and compare your hospital's outcome on core measures with three others in your area and two from different areas that have services similar to your own.

   a. Review the following outcomes:
      i. Surgical care improvement/surgical infection prevention
      ii. HCAHPS
      iii. Pneumonia
   b. Develop a plan for improvement in areas where the hospital is below the state and national average.

5. Investigate the use of dashboards in your organization. If dashboards are in use, clarify your understanding of the metrics included on the dashboard. If dashboards are not currently used, develop necessary knowledge of dashboards.
   a. Read more about dashboards from publications in nursing and business.
   b. Look for vendors offering healthcare dashboard services on the Internet.
   c. Discuss options with the chief information officer.

REFERENCES

Agency for Healthcare Research and Quality [AHRQ]. (2014). *Patient Safety Network. Patient Safety Primers*. Retrieved from http://psnet.ahrq.gov/primerHome.aspx

AirNow. (n.d.). *AirNow EnviroFlash: Air Quality Notifications*. Retrieved from http://www.airnow.gov/

American Nurses Association. (2014). *NDNQI Quality Improvement Solutions from ANA*. Retrieved from http://www.nursingquality.org/About-NDNQI

American Organization of Nurse Executives. (2005). AONE nurse executive competencies. *Nurse Leader, 3*(1), 15–22. Retrieved from http://www.aone.org/aone/certification/docs%20and%20pdfs/NurseExecCompetencies.pdf

American Organization of Nurse Executives. (2007). *AONE guiding principles for defining the role of the nurse executive in technology acquisition, implementation, and evaluation of information technology*. Retrieved from http://www.aone.org/aone/resource/PDF/AONE_GP_Technology_and_Acquisition_and_Implementation.pdf

American Organization of Nurse Executives. (2010). *AONE Toolkit for the nurse executive in the acquisition and implementation of information systems*. Retrieved from http://www.aone.org/aone/member/ResourceCenter/Toolkits/AONE_Toolkit_Nurse_Executive_Acquisition.pdf

Anderson, E. F., Frith, K.H., & Caspers, B. A. (2011). Linking economics and quality: Developing an evidence-based nurse staffing tool. *Nursing Administration Quarterly, 35*(1), 53–60. doi:10.1097/NAQ.0b013e3182047dff.

Booth, A. (2012). Benefits of an individual asthma action plan. *Practice Nursing*, 23(12), 594–602. Retrieved from http://www.practicenursing.com/

CMS.gov. (2013). *HCAHPS Fact Sheet*. Retrieved from http://www.hcahpsonline.org/files/August%202013%20HCAHPS%20Fact%20Sheet2.pdf

CMS.gov. (2014a). *EHR Incentive Programs: Stage 2*. Retrieved from http://www.cms.gov/Regulations-and-Guidance/Legislation/EHRIncentivePrograms/Stage_2.html

CMS.gov. (2014b, September). *Hospital-Acquired Conditions and present on admission indicator reporting system*. Retrieved from http://www.cms.gov/Outreach-and-Education/Medicare-Learning-Network-MLN/MLNProducts/Downloads/wPOAFactSheet.pdf

Cronenwett, L., Sherwood, G., Barnsteiner, J., et al. (2007). Quality and safety education for nurses. *Nursing Outlook*, 55(3), 122–131. doi:10.1016/j.outlook.2007.02.006.

Ellerbe, S., (2007). Practice matters. Staffing through web-based open-shift bidding. *American Nurse Today*, 2(4), 32–34. Retrieved from http://www.americannursetoday.com

Elliot, T. (2004). *Choosing a business intelligence standard*. Retrieved from http://www.businessobjects.com/pdf/solutions/evaluate/evaluating_bi.pdf

Finkler, S., Kovner, C., & Jones, C. (2012). *Financial management for nurse managers and executives* (4th ed.). St. Louis, MO: Saunders Elsevier.

Frith, K., Anderson, F., & Sewell, J. (2010). Assessing and selecting data for a nursing services dashboard. *Journal of Nursing Administration*, 40(1), 10–15. doi:10.1097/NNA.0b013e3181c47d45.

Fuchs, J. (2014). Stage 2 Meaningful Use—Implications for Ambulatory Care Nursing. *AAACN Viewpoint*, 36(4), 1–11. Retrieved from https://www.aaacn.org/viewpoint

Gillam, S., & Siriwardena, A. N. (2013). Frameworks for improvement: clinical audit, the plan-do-study-act cycle and significant event audit. *Quality in Primary Care*, 21(2), 123–130. Retrieved from http://www.radcliffehealth.com/shop/quality-primary-care

Hospital Consumer Assessment of Healthcare Providers & Systems [HCAHPS]. (2015). *CAHPS hospital survey*. Retrieved from http://www.hcahpsonline.org/

Healthcare Information and Management Systems Society (HIMSS) Analytics. (2013). *Electronic Medical Record Adoption Model (EMRAM)^SM*. Retrieved from http://www.himssanalytics.org/emram/emram.aspx

Malik, S. (2005). *Enterprise dashboards, design and best practices for IT*. New York, NY: John Wiley & Sons.

Moineddin, R., Nie, J., Domb, G., et al. (2008). Seasonality of primary care utilization for respiratory diseases in Ontario: A time-series analysis. *BMC Health Services Research*, 28(8), 160. doi:10.1186/1472-6963-8-160.

Murphy, S. L, Wilson, M. L., & Newhouse, R. P. (2013). Data analytics: Making the most of input with strategic output. *The Journal of Nursing Administration*, 43(7/8), 367–370. doi:10.1097/NNA.0b013e31829d60c7.

Recovery.gov. (n.d.). *The Recovery Act*. Retrieved from http://www.recovery.gov/

Roski, J., Bo-Linn, G. W., & Andrews, T. A. (2014). Creating value in health care through big data: Opportunities and policy implications. *Health Affairs*, 33(7), 1115–1122. doi:10.1377/hlthaff.2014.0147.

Russell, E., Hawkins, J., & Arnold, K. A. (2012). Guidelines for successful self-scheduling on nursing units. *Journal of Nursing Administration*, 42(9), 408–409. doi:10.1097/NNA.0b013e3182664dd8.

Simon, R. W., & Canacari, E. G. (2012). A practical guide to applying lean tools and management principles to health care improvement projects. *AORN Journal*, 95(1), 85–103. doi:10.1016/j.aorn.2011.05.021.

The Joint Commission. (2014). *Core Measurement Sets*. Retrieved from http://www.jointcommission.org/core_measure_sets.aspx

U.S. Department of Health and Human Services (HHS), (n.d.). *Quality improvement*. Retrieved from http://www.hrsa.gov/quality/toolbox/methodology/qualityimprovement/

CHAPTER 24

Informatics and Research

OBJECTIVES

After studying this chapter, you will be able to:

1. Demonstrate basic competencies using statistical analysis software.
2. Identify sources of data for research.
3. Discuss the use of data to conduct research in nursing service, education, and administration.
4. Synthesize research findings in informatics in selected topics.

KEY TERMS

Business intelligence

Codebook

DataFerrett

Descriptive data analysis

Evidence-based practice

Healthcare data analytics

Meta-analysis

Microdata

Output

Statistical analysis

In this data-rich healthcare environment, the need to turn data into useable information is imperative. There is a movement to develop **business intelligence** (also known as **healthcare data analytics**), which can integrate financial data, patient data, and quality data to produce predictive and prescriptive analytics for decision makers in healthcare (Anderson et al., 2011). Nurse informatics specialists need to understand this next wave of innovation. Moreover, nurses in all roles need skills and tools to summarize sets of numbers into understandable pieces of information and to interpret the meaning of evidence produced through research. The purpose of this chapter is to develop basic competencies in data analysis and research to form a foundation for decision making in nursing and healthcare.

DATA ANALYSIS AND RESEARCH IN MEDICINE AND NURSING

History

The use of data analysis and research in medicine has an interesting history, which began in France and England (Chen, 2003). During the early 19th century, one of the first uses of statistical procedures to influence medical decision making was to demonstrate the harm of performing bloodletting to treat infection. Physicians debated the appropriateness of using mathematics to understand the individual responses of humans to treatments. They argued that medicine was an art that could not be subjected to methods used in science such as astronomy. Even in 1870, when Joseph Lister published his findings on the effect of antiseptic methods in surgery on the mortality rate of patients, physicians rejected the use of statistical methods in medicine. As a professor at the University College in London, Dr. Karl Pearson developed the first inferential statistical methods in the 1880s. At the turn of the century, Major Greenwood furthered the work of Lister and Pearson at the Lister Institute for Preventive Medicine, the first establishment of a statistics department (Chen, 2003).

Unfortunately, medicine did not accept the use of **statistical analysis** until the 1920s, nearly 100 years after the first use of statistics in medicine (Chen, 2003). By that time, others believed that premedical students should learn statistics. Later in the 1940s, the British Medical Research Council conducted the first clinical trial to test the effectiveness of streptomycin compared with the usual treatment of bed rest for tuberculosis. Patients' clinical conditions and radiological findings improved when treated with an antibiotic. Following this study, the acceptance of statistics in medicine was secured (Chen, 2003).

The use of statistics and research in nursing has a similar history. The pioneer of statistical thinking was Florence Nightingale, whose work in the 1850s to 1860s showed that clean conditions in field hospitals in the Crimean War reduced the mortality rate for soldiers (Brown, 1993). Despite Miss Nightingale's groundbreaking work, the use of statistical analysis and research did not develop until the 1920s when case studies were used to describe the effectiveness of nursing interventions (Gortner, 2000). Between 1930 and 1960, nursing research in the United States was generally concentrated on nurses, nursing education, and the practice of professional nursing. The first publication of *Nursing Research* was in 1952; however, the emergence of nursing as a clinical science did not develop until nearly a quarter century later. The National Institute of Nursing Research (NINR), established in the mid-1980s, provided federal funding to nursing studies aimed at prevention of illness, promotion of healthy lifestyles, and support of quality of life (Gortner, 2000). Since that time, nurse scientists have been providing research evidence to change traditional ways of caring for patients. This emphasis on evidence-based practice is an important step in the development of nursing science and the improvement in patient care.

Use of Technology Today

Today, statistical analysis and research in nursing are increasing in complexity, in large part, because of the availability of personal computers and statistical analysis programs. Nurse researchers can collect data, manage them in databases, and analyze them with specialized programs. With attention to the principles of data analysis, other nurses (e.g., informatics nurse specialists, managers, educators, clinical nurses, and advanced practice nurses) can benefit from the use of statistical analysis to improve decision making and outcomes.

Personal computers are capable of performing many complex statistical analyses. There are a number of alternatives for statistical analysis including purchasing commercial statistical analysis programs, using spreadsheet programs, or downloading free programs from the Internet. Most commercial programs are comparable. Cost and user preference are likely to be the deciding factors. The most popular commercial programs are Statistical Package for Social Sciences (SPSS provided by IBM), Statistical Analysis Software (SAS provided by SAS Institute Inc.), and Minitab (provided by Minitab Inc.). Microsoft Excel (included with Microsoft Office) is useful because many nurses have the spreadsheet software readily available. Free statistical analysis programs are available on the Internet. A comparison of analysis capabilities of free programs is available at http://freestatistics.altervista.org/en/comp.php. Most of these programs are not as user-friendly as commercial software because they do not have a graphical user interface (GUI). Instead, they require the use of command lines to input data and run analyses. BrightStat overcomes this problem, does not require the download of a program because it is an Internet-based program, and provides commonly used statistical procedures (Stricker, 2008).

STATISTICS BASICS

Because data are readily available in healthcare settings today, nurses have an obligation to use them responsibly. Nurses must collect, aggregate, analyze, and interpret data correctly. Nurses who wish to analyze data should refresh their knowledge of statistics either through an academic course or by using reliable sources such as printed textbooks or online textbooks.

Online Resources for Statistics Basics

Several online sites are excellent sources of information about the basics of statistics and correct application of statistical procedures to data. Readers are encouraged to review one of the following online sources to understand statistical concepts before undertaking an analysis:

- StatSoft: http://www.statsoft.com/textbook/stathome.html
- Online statistics: An interactive multimedia course of study: http://onlinestatbook.com/
- Rice virtual lab in statistics: http://onlinestatbook.com/rvls.html
- Research methods knowledgebase: http:// http://www.socialresearchmethods.net/kb/
- National Library of Medicine: National Information Center on Health Services Research and Health Care Technology: http://www.nlm.nih.gov/nichsr/outreach.html

Software for Statistical Analysis
Spreadsheet Software

You can use a spreadsheet to complete simple **descriptive data analysis**. The first step in any data analysis is to put data in the correct format. Enter data on the row, with variable labels in the columns. Code categorical data with numbers. For example, gender is male or female, but statistical programs understand numbers. Change the word "female" into the number "0" and "male" into "1." Make a **codebook** to remember what the numbers represent.

The next step is to create or insert formulas into the spreadsheet. Fortunately, spreadsheets have built-in formulas for many statistical procedures such as mean, median, standard deviation, variance, and correlation. You can select a cell on the spreadsheet and insert a formula using the "Formulas" menu. Add a formula selecting the "more functions" option on the ribbon and then selecting "statistical" to display a list of statistical formulas. You can scroll down until the formula you want to use appears. Finally, define the numbers used in the statistical formula by adding them to the "argument." You can accomplish this by clicking the icon inside the number field. After the window minimizes, you can select the numbers you need to use for the formula. Once you have inserted the formula and defined the arguments, the result is the display of the statistical procedure.

Spreadsheets also provide graphical presentation of data. As described in Chapter 7, you can easily create charts using the chart wizard. Besides pie, bar, and line charts, you can use scatter charts to show relationships between two pieces of data.

BrightStat Software

Even though you can use spreadsheets to calculate many descriptive statistics, your data analysis will be more efficient when using a program designed for that purpose. BrightStat, an Internet-based statistical analysis program, can be used for descriptive, nonparametric, and parametric tests. The GUI of BrightStat operates in a manner similar to those in SPSS, making its use practical for any person with a basic understanding of statistics. BrightStat is located at http://www.brightstat.com, and users can simply register with the site to use it. Users should set their browser options to allow pop-up windows and make sure they have the Adobe Flash Player plug-in. Although there is no users' manual, there are context-specific help screens inside the program and video tutorials on YouTube.

To use BrightStat, upload data from a spreadsheet into the program. Format the spreadsheet in the manner described earlier in the chapter. Once the data are available, there are several steps to uploading, browsing, and importing data files (Figures 24-1 and 24-2).

Summarizing data with descriptive statistics using BrightStat is quite easy. Select the variables for analysis, and choose the statistical procedures (Figures 24-3 and 24-4). You can run more sophisticated statistical analyses, such as *t*-test, variance, correlations, and linear regression using BrightStat too. You can create graphs including line, bar, scatterplot, histograms, and boxplots. The capability of this free software makes running statistical analyses available to any nurse who

Data File	Edit	Data	Analyze	Charts
Download from Server	Find	Data Description	Descriptives	Line
Upload to Server	Find Next	Filter Data	Frequencies	Bar
Load from Local Storage	Find and Replace	Weight Cases	Chi-Squared	Area
Save to Local Storage	Define Value Labels	Split Data	Binomial Test	Error bars
Upload Datafile	Add New Variable	Compute Variable	NP. Central Tendencies	Scatter
Preferences	Delete Variable	Recode Variable	Kolmogorov-Smirnov	Histogram
	Add Data Row	Automatic Recode	Compare Means	Boxplot
	Delete Data Row		ANOVA	Pie
			ANOVA Rep. Measurements	Spider
			Compare Variances	Heat map
			Bivariate Correlations	
			Linear Regression	
			Logistic Regression	
			Reliability	
			Kaplan Meier	

▲ DATA MENU ▲

| Data | Variables | Output | | weight cases | filter cases | split file |

Figure 24-1. Upload data file.

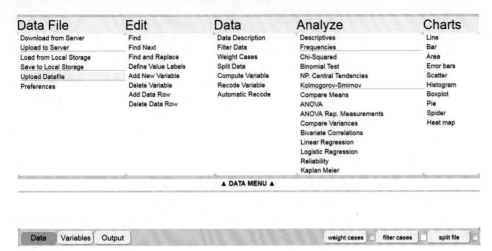

Your data files:

please select your file ▼

please select your file
BodyFat
Patient Outcomes

cancel

Data description:

load

| Data | Variables | Output | | weight cases | filter cases | split file |

Figure 24-2. Select data file.

▼ DATA MENU ▼

BS brightstat.com   Logout

Patient Outcomes

ID	Name	Label	Type	Scale
0	Time	Click to edit	NUMBER	SCALE
1	RR_intervals	Click to edit	NUMBER	SCALE
2	Abs_Differences_of_RR_Intervals	Click to edit	NUMBER	SCALE
3	Breathing_Rate	Click to edit	NUMBER	SCALE

Showing 1 to 4 of 4 entries

| Data | Variables | Output | | weight cases | filter cases | split file |

Figure 24-3. Select variables and statistics.

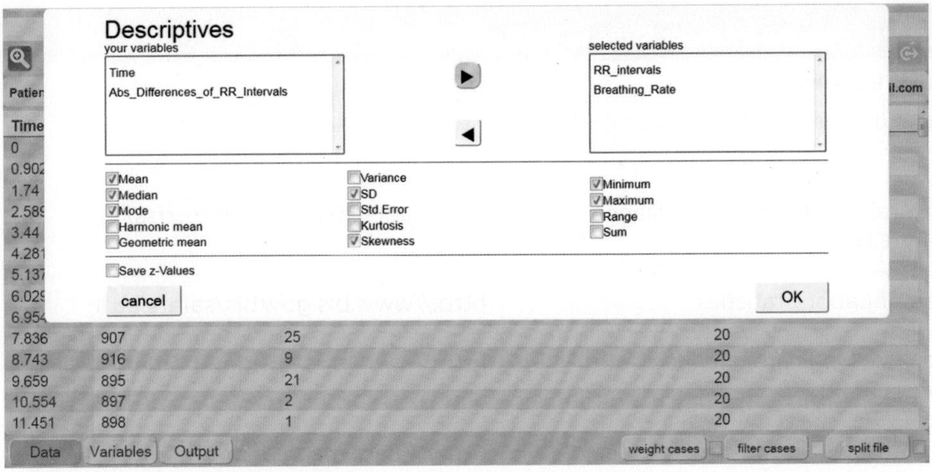

Figure 24-4. Select Descriptive Statistics

needs to find specific answers to questions about patient outcomes, nursing practice, or processes in a healthcare facility. The **output** window displays graphs and statistical analyses, which you can save inside BrightStat, export, or print.

OBTAINING DATA SETS FROM THE INTERNET

Occasionally, nurses need data from sources other than their own facilities to make comparisons. For example, a nurse manager of an emergency department might like to compare wait times for certain diagnoses across all hospitals in the United States. **DataFerrett**, a browser provided by the U.S. Census Bureau (http://dataferrett.census.gov/), provides access to publicly available data. There is a video and tutorial on the website to guide users. You must download and install DataFerrett on a local computer. Once installed, you can access public **microdata** (individual responses—not aggregated) from various federal agencies. You can use DataFerrett to export data from approximately 20 national surveys including the National Health and Nutrition Examination Survey (NHANES), National Health Interview Survey (NHIS), and the National Center for Health Statistics, to name a few.

Another useful site for health information on the Internet is the Agency for Healthcare Research and Quality (AHRQ) at http://www.ahrq.gov/research/data/dataresources.html. The AHRQ also provides tools (software downloads), evaluation toolkits, and databases for conducting research.

Nurses can use tools such as the following to mine for data in several national initiatives:

- Medical Expenditure Panel Survey (MEPS)
- Healthcare Cost and Utilization Project (HCUP)
- HIV and AIDS Costs and Use
- Safety Net Monitoring Initiative

In addition, nurses can find research on quality, access, cost, and information technology at the AHRQ website. Research findings are synthesized or provided in fact sheets for easy reading.

The Centers for Medicare and Medicaid Services (CMS) provide access to research, statistics, data, and systems at its website http://www.cms.hhs.gov/home/rsds.asp. Nurses can locate information on patient satisfaction, outcomes of care, and cost. Findings from the required Hospitals Consumer Assessment of Health Providers and Systems are available for review and comparison. You can download data from https://data.medicare.gov/ into a comma separated values file or into Microsoft Access Database. You can import the data into a software program to run statistical analyses once you locate the file on your local computer.

No discussion of research on the Internet would be complete without looking at the NINR located at http://www.ninr.nih.gov/. Publications from the NINR provide the latest scientific evidence on clinical topics. The NINR makes monthly summaries of research available at http://www.ninr.nih.gov/newsandinformation/newsnotesarchive#.Ur3R__RDvEw. Table 24-1 lists other Internet sites with useful health statistics.

TABLE 24-1 Helpful Internet Sites to Find Health Statistics

Name of Internet Source	URL
Agency for Healthcare Research and Quality	http://www.ahrq.gov/data/
Behavioral Risk Factor Surveillance System (CDC)	http://apps.nccd.cdc.gov/brfss/
Bureau of Labor Statistics	http://www.bls.gov/bls/safety.htm
Centers for Medicare and Medicaid Services (CMS)	http://www.cms.hhs.gov/home/rsds.asp
CMS Data Download	https://data.medicare.gov/
Department of Health and Human Services, the HHS Data Council	http://aspe.hhs.gov/datacncl/
FedStats	http://www.fedstats.gov/
FirstGov	http://www.usa.gov/
Health Insurance Information from the Census Bureau	http://www.census.gov/hhes/www/hlthins/hlthins.html
Health Resources and Services Administration, Geospatial Data Warehouse	http://datawarehouse.hrsa.gov/
Healthy People 2020	http://www.healthypeople.gov/Data/
Morbidity and Mortality Weekly Report	http://www.cdc.gov/mmwr/weekcvol.html
National Cancer Institute	http://www.cancer.gov/statistics/finding
National Center for Health Statistics	http://www.cdc.gov/nchs/express.htm
National Program of Cancer Registries	http://www.cdc.gov/cancer/npcr/
National Vital Statistics Survey	http://www.cdc.gov/nchs/nvss.htm
Substance Abuse and Mental Health Services Administration: National Outcome Measures	http://www.nationaloutcomemeasures.samhsa.gov/outcome/sa_pre.asp
Web-Based Injury Statistics Query and Reporting System	http://www.cdc.gov/ncipc/wisqars/

RESEARCH EVIDENCE IN NURSING

Single research studies produce evidence that can be useful in nursing practice. However, the use of evidence-based practice can bring about scientifically sound changes in nursing practice. Evidence-based practice is the scholarly process of synthesizing evidence from multiple studies and combining it with the expertise of nurses and the preferences of patients (Melnyk & Fineout-Overholt, 2014). It is the responsibility of every nurse to keep current in practice by using research evidence. There are several ways to stay current: read research literature in the specialty area, subscribe to clinical practice journals, attend professional meetings, review clinical practice guidelines, and participate in quality improvement or clinical practice committees.

Even though evidence-based practice is taught in baccalaureate programs, there are barriers to applying research findings to change clinical practice. First, nurses might not subscribe to journals that publish research, and nurses may be in work settings where evidence-based practice is not used. Second, there may be little or replication of studies with important findings on a particular topic. Single studies are not usually the basis for changing practice. Third, even when there are multiple research studies on a topic, the methods may be so disparate that combining findings into an integrative review or **meta-analysis** may not be possible. The replication and synthesis of findings to change practice builds stronger evidence for practice change.

The skills needed to find research reports, read, and critique them for use in practice begin in a nurse's basic educational program. Students need practice and positive reinforcement to improve their health information literacy skills to prepare for the workplace (Chang & Levin, 2014). Students who practice should be able to overcome the challenges of finding and using research in clinical practice. Table 24-2 provides some learning strategies to overcome challenges associated with nursing research.

TABLE 24-2	Learning Strategies to Overcome Challenges Associated with Nursing Research
Challenge	**Learning Strategy**
Research is intimidating	Attend class and listen to explanations about the research. Synthesize literature reviews and discuss the results with faculty. Ask faculty for feedback to validate knowledge. Practice reviewing research studies, looking for similarities and differences.
Difficulty in identifying research articles	Ask a librarian for assistance in locating journals specializing in nursing research. Search digital library databases that index nursing journals. Specify research in digital library database queries. Ask faculty for feedback on search techniques and quality of search results. Practice search skills.
Difficulty in analyzing research results	Learn to identify the sections of a research article in which the results, limitations, and conclusions are summarized. Consult research and statistics textbooks to review qualitative or quantitative analysis information. Ask faculty for feedback to validate knowledge. Practice data analysis skills.

The passage of The Patient Protection and Affordable Care Act of 2010 has brought urgency to using data analytics to bear on health information contained in EMRs (Meek, 2012). For example, readmission to acute care hospitals within 30 days of discharge is costly to hospitals. Teams composed of nurses, other healthcare providers, informaticists, case managers, and quality improvement specialists can examine current process, mine data from EMRs, and conduct statistical analyses to identify at-risk patients. A redesign process for discharge planning could be based on the results from data analyses. Once the most common factors are known and built into new processes and screening tools, nurses and case managers can more easily determine what resources patients need to avoid readmission (Meek, 2012).

RESEARCH FINDINGS IN INFORMATICS

Research in informatics focuses on the use of technology to connect interdisciplinary researchers across a continuum of laboratory-based studies to practice-based implementation and back again (Bakken et al., 2012). This broad conceptualization can be boiled down to a simple but powerful focus: Informatics must harness the power of new technologies to handle massive amounts of data to support or redesign nursing practice, empower patients and families, and support new research or evaluation methodologies (Bakken et al., 2012).

The following sections describe the current state of research in three major areas: health information technology (health IT), electronic medical records (EMRs), and clinical decision support systems (CDSSs). Although the presentation of research findings is not exhaustive, it does provide readers with a snapshot of topics and methods under investigation in informatics.

Internet Access and Health Information–Seeking Behaviors

Adoption of technology to access the Internet has been rapid and widespread. The Pew Research Center reported that in 2000, only 46% of American households used the Internet, and 25% of Americans reported using it to obtain health information (Zickuhr & Smith, 2013). Nearly

15 years later, the Pew Research Center reported that 70% of households have broadband Internet access, and only 3% have dial-up service (Zickuhr & Smith, 2013). Ninety-one percent of Americans own cell phones, and 63% of them use their smartphones to access information on the Internet and via smartphone apps (Duggan & Smith, 2013). Among households without broadband Internet access, 10% report having smartphones with 3G or 4G service, providing adequate access to online information (Zickuhr & Smith, 2013).

Seeking health information online is prevalent; nearly 60% of Americans report looking for health information on the Internet (Fox & Duggan, 2013). Thirty-five percent of Americans used the Internet for medical information to diagnose themselves or others. Of these "diagnosers," half of them talked with a clinician about the information, and 40% of them had their diagnosis confirmed (Fox & Duggan, 2013). Americans also report using the Internet for peer-to-peer support, although this type of health information seeking behavior occurs at a lower percent, typically 16% to 26%. However, when asked about a serious illness, most Americans still seek health information from physicians and other healthcare providers in their offices (Fox & Duggan, 2013).

Meaningful Use Stage 2 ushers in the requirement for patient portals or other communication technologies to connect patients to their healthcare provider (CMS, 2014). To date, studies show that patients have positive perceptions about portals (Goldzweig et al., 2013; Lam et al., 2013). There is limited evidence that portals can decrease the number of office visits and lower the number of telephone calls because patients use them to ask health questions, request appointments, request medications, and get laboratory results (Ammenwerth et al., 2012). However, more research is needed to quantify health outcomes based on use of patient portals.

Use of Electronic Health Record Systems

The adoption of EMRs has escalated due to mandated use of EMRs and meaningful use regulations. The Health Information and Management Systems Society (HIMSS) Analytics documented that only 5.8% of hospitals in the United States have not implemented any part of an EMR by the fourth quarter of 2013 (Health Information and Management Systems Society Analytics, 2013). Nearly 32% of hospitals have nursing documentation fully implemented, leaving the majority of US hospitals with much work to implement EMRs.

Using an EMR or electronic health record (EHR) does not guarantee good patient outcomes. It is important to prepare nurses and other healthcare providers for change. Nurses need to have computer and informatics competencies and receive support during implementation of an EHR or EMR to avoid patient safety threats (Poe, 2011). The most failure prone time for EMRs is the "go-live" period (Gruber et al., 2009). In addition to technical support personnel being present during the go-live period, the healthcare organization may need to schedule more nursing staff to ensure that patients' needs do not suffer while nurses learn to use the system (Gruber et al., 2009).

Once the initial go-live period is over, nurses and other healthcare providers can often experience major changes in workflow. Investigating this phenomenon, Lee and McElmurry (2010) conducted an extensive review of literature on workflow after implementation of EMRs. The authors found that the implementation of EMRs created new work including time-consuming data entry because of structure issues in the EMRs, awkward navigation that was not intuitive to healthcare providers, and decreased clinical reasoning ability of healthcare providers because of massive amounts of data. There were reports of errors in entering physician orders due to confusing order options and inappropriate order templates. Physicians reported a variety of workflow issues created by EMRs—all stemming from system inflexibility and inappropriate customization. For nurses, there was no improvement in documentation completeness with EMRs, particularly when documentation occurred at the end of shifts rather than in real time. Lee and McElmurry found mixed results regarding nurse attitudes and acceptance of EMRs.

Nurses' and other healthcare providers' perceptions of EMRs depend on the usability of the system. In a study by Rantz and colleagues (2011), nurses reported that evaluation of patients' clinical trends and communication with other healthcare providers was easier after the implementation of the EMR than previous paper systems had

been. However, nurses also expressed concerns citing inconsistent use of the system, difficulty for some nursing staff to find documentation once entered into the system, and late documentation. While nursing staff perceived implementation at 24 months as successful, most reported the need for additional staffing during the first 12 months due to increased time for documentation, pulling them away from patient care.

Adoption of EMRs or EHRs does not automatically improve patient outcomes (Crosson et al., 2012), but some studies show promising results. Kern et al. (2014) investigated the effect of an EMR on 10 outcomes in a patient-centered medical home. They found that four outcome measures (eye examinations, hemoglobin A1c, chlamydia screening, and colorectal cancer screening) improved after the implementation of EMR as compared to a paper-based system. Dowding and colleagues (2012) studied the incidence of nurse-sensitive outcomes after EMR implementation and found that pressure ulcer assessment increased and incidence decreased. The researchers did not find significant changes in fall rates. In another study, Longhurst and colleagues (2010) studied the mortality rates post implementation of EMRs. They found 36 fewer deaths (20% decrease in adjusted mortality) in the 18 months after implementation of an EMR (Longhurst et al., 2010).

Researchers who plan to study the impact of using EMRs or EHRs need to build on the research base already in place. Assessments of user satisfaction, clinical outcomes, and financial impact are the most widely studied aspects, but there is little consistency in methods or measures. The heterogeneous methods severely limit the ability to synthesize findings to determine the best practices in EHR planning, implementation, and evaluation. Nurse informatics specialists should use published instruments (if validity and reliability are acceptable) and employ standardized evaluation techniques whenever possible to address the identified shortcomings in the informatics literature.

Use of Clinical Decision Support Systems

Clinical Decision Support Systems (CDSS) are information systems deployed to improve clinical decision-making and patient outcomes. Reminders

TABLE 24-3 **Research Studies that Show Positive Changes Resulting from the Use of CDSS**

Authors	Function of CDSS	Outcome	Improvement
Alvey et al. (2012)	Support assessment and documentation of pressure ulcer stage by nurses	Accuracy of pressure ulcer staging based on depth, color, and characteristics	Nurses who used the CDSS were significantly more accurate in pressure ulcer staging than nurses who overrode the CDSS staging.
Cho et al. (2010)	Diagnostic computer-based decision support	Amounts of information preferred by expert and novice nurses	Experts preferred a moderate amount of information and novices preferred high amounts of information.
Fossum et al. (2011)	Support for pressure ulcer assessment and guidance for nursing and nutritional interventions Prevent pressure ulcers, manage pressure ulcers, and support nutrition in elders residing in nursing homes.	Number of residents in long-term care with pressure ulcers Number of residents in long-term care with malnutrition	The number of residents in long-term care with malnutrition was significantly decreased.
Harrison et al. (2013)	Adherence to hypoglycemia protocols to keep blood glucose levels within normal range	Percent of nurse compliance with hypoglycemia protocol and blood glucose levels	The level of compliance significantly increased; however, only 25% of nurses used the protocol by the end of the research study.
Lyerla et al. (2010)	Reminder to nurses to measure head of bed (HOB) for ventilator patients	Degree of elevation of HOB and percentage of patients with HOB >30 degrees	Use of CDSS improved adherence to guidelines for HOB settings.

for preventive care, order sets, evidence-based suggestions for disease management, and alerts for drug prescribing are the primary support functions provided in CDSS (Bright et al., 2012). Most often, use of CDSS is to improve care for patients with chronic illness or with care processes that are prone to errors, such as medication prescription or administration. Researchers initially conducted descriptive research on CDSS, but there are randomized controlled trials and quasiexperimental studies in the literature.

Bright and colleagues (2012) conducted a systematic review of 148 controlled trials; they analyzed findings in six primary outcomes: healthcare processes, clinical outcomes, user workload and efficiency outcomes, relationship-centered outcomes, economic outcomes, and use and implementation outcomes. Studies of the effect of CDSS on healthcare processes predominated research literature they reviewed, and the evidence strength was the highest in healthcare processes. In other words, when CDSS provide automatic recommendations at the point of care, appropriate ordering of preventive care procedures, diagnostic studies, and treatment significantly improved. The strength of evidence was low to moderate regarding clinical outcomes (length of inpatient stay, mortality, health-related quality of life, and adverse events). The strength of evidence about the effect of CDSS on user workload and efficiency and on relationship-based outcomes was low or insufficient. Bright and colleagues found moderate strength of evidence about the effect of CDSS on cost; with use of CDSS, there was a "trend toward lower treatment costs, total costs, and greater cost savings" (p. 32). Finally, use and implementation outcomes had mixed strength of evidence with insufficient, low, and moderate levels, as assessed by Bright and colleagues. The strongest evidence of provider satisfaction with CDSS was found in studies where there was integration of CDSS into computerized provider order entry or EHRs and when CDSS alerts were automatically delivered at the point of care without a mandatory response by the provider.

Research about the effect of CDSS on nursing processes and outcomes are more difficult to find. However, a few examples show positive changes resulting from the use of CDSS (Table 24-3).

QSEN Scenario

The healthcare facility where you work has adopted a sepsis alert program to reduce morbidity, mortality, and length of stay for patients. How could use of a clinical decision support system (CDSS) be effective as a component of the sepsis prevention program?

SUMMARY

Research in medicine and nursing has a short history. Most scholars point to the beginning of clinical trials in the 1940s as a significant marker. Since that time, healthcare professionals have engaged in research to find the best way to produce good patient outcomes. Personal computers are now capable of performing complex statistical analyses that were not possible before the 1990s. Data are available in healthcare settings through EHRs, administrative databases, and the Internet. We have the ability to provide meaningful information from discrete data, and we must use it. Decision makers at the bedside, in boardrooms, and in educational settings need to examine the effects of practice on outcomes.

Evidence to guide the practice of nursing informatics is beginning to emerge, and informatics specialists need to keep their knowledge current. Yet, the research methodology used in existing studies is mostly descriptive. We need designs that are more rigorous to test the effectiveness of technology to improve patient care and outcomes. Nurse informatics researchers are in a good position to lead change by using evidence produced in research.

APPLICATIONS AND COMPETENCIES

1. Copy the data from the table below into a spreadsheet. Perform a statistical analysis to obtain descriptive statistics that summarize the data (complete using spreadsheet or BrightStat). Remember to split the data by hospital first.

   a. Obtain the mean, median, minimum, maximum, and standard deviation for length of stay (LOS) and age.

   b. Find the frequency count of male and female patients and for type of hospital.

   c. Write a paragraph to summarize the LOS of patients at the rural and city hospitals.

   d. Write a paragraph to describe the age of the patients at both hospitals.

LOS	Age	Gender	Hospital
3	50	Male	City
4	65	Male	Rural
7	72	Female	City
5	72	Male	Rural
2	45	Male	City
2	68	Male	Rural
8	82	Female	City
7	70	Male	Rural
5	72	Female	City
4	50	Male	Rural
7	85	Male	City
6	62	Male	Rural
3	67	Male	City
5	65	Male	Rural
7	66	Male	City
8	80	Female	Rural
5	62	Female	City
8	71	Female	Rural
10	78	Female	City
5	55	Male	Rural
7	77	Male	City
5	47	Male	Rural
8	81	Male	City
10	77	Female	Rural

LOS	Age	Gender	Hospital
6	70	Male	City
10	82	Female	Rural
4	63	Female	City
9	85	Female	Rural
8	90	Male	City
8	76	Female	Rural
8	77	Male	City
7	77	Female	Rural
6	79	Female	City
10	81	Female	Rural
7	82	Female	City
8	67	Female	Rural
3	55	Male	City
7	73	Male	Rural
9	57	Male	City
6	66	Male	Rural
4	60	Male	City
10	63	Female	Rural
5	62	Male	City
9	74	Female	Rural
6	78	Male	City
10	80	Female	Rural
6	73	Female	City
6	72	Female	Rural

LOS	Age	Gender	Hospital
7	69	Male	City
6	72	Female	Rural
7	70	Female	City
7	67	Female	Rural
9	77	Female	City
3	73	Male	Rural
2	57	Male	City
4	76	Male	Rural
6	59	Male	City
7	72	Male	Rural
7	52	Male	City
10	88	Female	Rural
6	83	Female	City
3	67	Male	Rural

2. Using the same data set, determine the relationship of age and LOS in each hospital.

   a. Make a scatter chart for both hospitals.

   b. Calculate the correlation of age and LOS at both hospitals.

   c. Write a paragraph to describe the findings.

3. Using the same data set, compare the LOS for males and females at both hospitals.

   a. Run a *t*-test to determine if there is a significant difference in mean LOS.

   b. Write a paragraph to describe the findings.

4. Search for research findings at the AHRQ located at http://www.ahrq.gov/research/.

   a. Find a fact sheet regarding the health of minority women in the United States and summarize the findings.

   b. Look for research synthesis on hospital nurse staffing and quality of care. Summarize the main findings.

5. Search for current nursing informatics research in databases at your local hospital, college, or university. Find at least three research reports in your area of interest. Think about how the research could be used in your work setting.

REFERENCES

Alvey, B., Hennen, N., & Heard, H. (2012). Improving accuracy of pressure ulcer staging and documentation using a computerized clinical decision support system. *Journal of Wound, Ostomy and Continence Nursing*, 39(6), 607–612. doi:10.1097/WON.0b013e31826a4b5c.

Ammenwerth, E., Schnell-Inderst, P., & Hoerbst, A. (2012). The impact of electronic patient portals on patient care: A systematic review of controlled trials. *Journal of Medical Internet Research*, 14(6), e162–e162. doi:10.2196/jmir.2238.

Anderson, E. F., Frith, K. H., & Caspers, B. A. (2011). Linking economics and quality: Developing an evidence-based nurse staffing tool. *Nursing Administrative Quarterly*, 35(1), 53–60. doi:10.1097/NAQ.0b013e3182047dff.

Bakken, S., Stone, P. W., & Larson, E. L. (2012). A nursing informatics research agenda for 2008–18: Contextual influences and key components. *Nursing Outlook*, 60(5), 280–288.e3. doi:10.1016/j.outlook.2012.06.001.

Bright, T. J., Wong, A., Dhurjati, R., et al. (2012). Effect of clinical decision-support systems: A systematic review. *Annals of Internal Medicine*, 157(1), 29–43. doi:10.7326/0003-4819-157-1-201207030-00450.

Brown, P. (1993). *Florence Nightingale: The tough British campaigner who was the founder of modern nursing*. Watford, England: Exley Publications.

Chang, A., & Levin, R. F. (2014). Tactics for teaching evidence-based practice: Improving self-efficacy in finding and appraising evidence in a Master's evidence-based practice unit. *Worldviews on Evidence-Based Nursing*, 11(4), 266–269. doi:10.1111/wvn.12050.

Chen, T. (2003). The history of statistical thinking in medicine. In Y. Lu, & J.-Q. Fang (Eds.), *Advanced medical statistics*. Singapore: World Scientific Publishing Company. Retrieved from http://www.worldscibooks.com/lifesci/etextbook/4854/4854_chap1.pdf

Cho, I., Staffers, N., & Park, I. (2010). Nurses responses to differing amounts and information content in a diagnostic computer-based decision support application. *CIN: Computers, Informatics, Nursing*, 28(2), 95–102. doi:10.1097/NCN.0b013e3181cd8240.

CMS.gov. (2014). *EHR incentive programs: Stage 2*. Retrieved from http://www.cms.gov/Regulations-and-Guidance/Legislation/EHRIncentivePrograms/Stage_2.html

Crosson, J. C., Ohman-Strickland, P. A., Cohen, D. J., et al. (2012). Typical electronic health record use in primary care practices and the quality of diabetes care. *Annals of Family Medicine*, *10*(3), 221–227. doi:10.1370/afm.1370.

Dowding, D. W., Turley, M., & Garrido, T. (2012). The impact of an electronic health record on nurse sensitive patient outcomes: An interrupted time series analysis. *Journal of the American Medical Informatics Association*, *19*(4), 615–620. doi:10.1136/amiajnl-2011-000504.

Duggan, M. & Smith, A. (2013). *Cell Internet use 2013. Pew Research Center's Internet & American Life Project*. Washington, DC: Pew Research Center. Retrieved from http://www.pewinternet.org/2013/09/16/cell-internet-use-2013/

Fossum, M., Alexander, G. L., Ehnfors, M., et al. (2011). Effects of a computerized decision support system on pressure ulcers and malnutrition in nursing homes for the elderly. *International Journal of Medical Informatics*, *80*(9), 607–617. doi:10.1016/j.ijmedinf.2011.06.009.

Fox, S. & Duggan, M. (2013). *Health Online 2013. Pew Research Center's Internet & American Life Project*. Washington, DC: Pew Research Center. Retrieved from http://www.pewinternet.org/2013/01/15/health-online-2013/

Goldzweig, C. L., Orshansky, G., Paige, N. M., et al. (2013). Electronic patient portals: Evidence on health outcomes, satisfaction, efficiency, and attitudes: A systematic review. *Annals of Internal Medicine*, *159*(10): 677–687. doi:10.7326/0003-4819-159-10-201311190-00006.

Gortner, S. (2000). Knowledge development in nursing: Our historical roots and future opportunities. *Nursing Outlook*, *48*(2), 60–67. Retrieved from http://www.nursingoutlook.org/

Gruber, D., Cummings, G., Leblanc, L., et al. (2009). Factors influencing outcomes of clinical information systems implementation: A systematic review. *CIN: Computers, Informatics, Nursing*, *27*(3), 151–163. doi:10.1097/NCN.0b013e31819f7c07.

Harrison, R. L., Stalker, S. L., Henderson, R., et al. (2013). Use of a clinical decision support system to improve hypoglycemia management. *Medsurg Nursing*, *22*(4), 250–263. Retrieved from http://www.medsurgnursing.net/

Health Information and Management Systems Society Analytics. (2013). *United States EMR adoption model*. Retrieved from http://www.himssanalytics.org/home/index.aspx

Kern, L. M., Edwards, A., & Kaushal, R. (2014). The patient-centered medical home, electronic health records, and quality of care. *Annals of Internal Medicine*, *160*(11), 741–749. doi:10.7326/M13-1798.

Lam, R., Lin, V. S., Senelick, W. S., et al. (2013). Older adult consumers' attitudes and preferences on electronic patient-physician messaging. *American Journal of Managed Care*, *9*(10 Spec. No.), eSP7–eSP11. Retrieved from http://www.ajmc.com/publications/issue

Lee, S., & McElmurry, B. (2010). Capturing nursing workflow disruptions: Comparison between nursing and physician workflows. *CIN: Computers, Informatics, Nursing*, *28*(3), 151–159. doi:10.1097/NCN.0b013e3181d77d3e.

Longhurst, C. A., Parast, L., Sandborg, C. I., et al. (2010). Decrease in hospital-wide mortality rate after implementation of a commercially sold physician order entry system. *Pediatrics*, *126*(1), 14–21. doi:10.1542/peds.2009-3271.

Lyerla, F., LeRouge, C., Cooke, D. A., et al. (2010). A nursing clinical decision support system and potential predictors of head-of-bed position for patients receiving mechanical ventilation. *American Journal of Critical Care*, *19*(1), 39–47. doi:10.4037/ajcc2010836.

Meek, J. (2012). Affordable care act: Predictive modeling challenges and opportunities for case management. *Professional Case Management*, *17*(1), 15–23. doi:10.1097/NCM.0b013e318234e7dd.

Melnyk, B., & Fineout-Overholt, E. (2014). *Evidence-based practice in nursing & healthcare: A guide to best practice* (3rd ed.). Philadelphia, PA: Lippincott Williams & Wilkins.

Poe, S. S. (2011). Building nursing intellectual capital for safe use of information technology: A systematic review. *Journal of Nursing Care Quality*, *26*(1), 4–12. doi:10.1097/NCQ.0b013e3181e15c88.

Rantz, M. J., Alexander, G., Galambos, C., et al. (2011). The use of bedside electronic medical record to improve quality of care in nursing facilities: A qualitative analysis. *CIN: Computers, Informatics, Nursing*, *28*(2), 1–8. doi:10.1097/NCN.0b013e3181f9db79.

Stricker, D. (2008). BrightStat.com: Free statistics online. *Computer Methods and Programs in Biomedicine*, *92*(1), 135–143. doi:10.1016/j.cmpb.2008.06.010.

Zickuhr, K., & Smith, A. (2013). *Home Broadband 2013. Pew Research Center's Internet & American Life Project*. Washington, DC: Pew Research Center. Retrieved from http://www.pewinternet.org/2013/08/26/home-broadband-2013-2/

CHAPTER 25

Legal and Ethical Issues

OBJECTIVES

After studying this chapter, you will be able to:

1. Discuss the similarities and differences between professional nursing codes of ethics and professional informatics associations' codes.

2. Identify at least three ways that privacy of information can be breached.

3. Identify the strengths and weaknesses of the Health Insurance Portability and Accountability Act (HIPAA).

4. Discuss current telehealth issues associated with practicing nursing across state lines.

5. Discuss the pros and cons of the implantable patient chip using radiofrequency identification (RFID) microchip technology.

6. Give examples of appropriate and inappropriate professional nurse use of interactive Web applications.

7. Apply the use of copyright law to activities associated with the scholarship of professional publications by nurses.

KEY TERMS

Code of ethics

Code of ethics for nurses

Coordinated Licensure Information System

Copyright

Fair use

Fixed tangible medium

Health Insurance Portability and Accountability Act (HIPAA)

Nurse Licensure Compact (NLC)

Privacy Rights Clearinghouse

Restricted license

TEACH Act

Informatics applications and competencies are essential skills for all nurses. The rapid change in technology development behooves us to stay abreast of new knowledge. We need to have factual knowledge of technology changes and the potential implications for making our patients safe. Healthcare personnel and those involved with informatics with access to confidential information have a special obligation to abide by the professional ethical standards and legal statutes in the handling of information. This chapter addresses the ethical and legal responsibilities of the nurse as they relate to informatics. Topics that are discussed include the pertinent professional codes of ethics, **Health Insurance Portability and Accountability Act (HIPAA)**, the interactive Web, telehealth, the implantable patient microchipping using RFIC, nanotechnology, wearable computing, and copyright issues.

ETHICS

Professionals are bound by their pertinent **code of ethics**. A code of ethics is made up of statements of the professionals' values and beliefs, which are based on ethical principles (Table 25-1). According to Curtin (2005), ethical choices have three characteristics. First, choices always involve conflict of values that are extremely important. Second, scientific inquiry can influence the choice made in a value conflict, but it cannot provide an answer. Finally, the process involves deciding which value is most important. Curtin suggests that any decision made about conflicts of fundamental values will have lasting and unexpected consequences on human concern areas. For the public good and protection, professionals who are involved with the use of healthcare informatics "must be bound by

TABLE 25-1 Ethical Principles

Principle	Description
Autonomy	Self-rule/determination
Beneficence	Doing what is best for the individual
Nonmaleficence	Doing no harm
Veracity	Truth telling
Fidelity	Honesty
Paternalism	Making decisions on behalf of others
Justice	Being fair
Respect for others	Appreciation for human dignity

ethical, moral, and legal responsibilities" (Curtin, 2005, p. 352).

The concept of conflicting values is central to informatics. As an example, the ethical principles of autonomy and beneficence are often in conflict when discussing the use of radiofrequency identification (RFID) to track the whereabouts of nursing staff or patients and for telehomecare monitoring to assess symptoms changes of patients. Relationships between two or more people are subject to conflict of ethical principles, depending on the situation. Nurses must be knowledgeable about ethical principles, the professional **code of ethics for nurses**, pertinent laws, and conflict resolution skills. Even without a universal structured curriculum in ethics, nurses abide by ethical principles while caring for patients and families. In fact, according to the Gallup Poll, nurses have been named the number 1 ethical professionals since 1999, with the exception of 2001—the year of the World Trade Center terrorist attacks (firefighters were number 1 that year) (Gallup Inc., 2014).

Code of Ethics for Nurses

Professional nursing associations worldwide have established codes of ethics. Not surprisingly, there are marked similarities between all of them. They all address principles and values of ethical practice, although the exact wording may vary slightly. Professional nurses must adhere to their code of ethics in their personal lives, not just in the workplaces. Informatics competencies and applications pertain to the personal use of the computer as well as the use of health information technology (HIT) in the workplace.

The American Nurses Association (ANA) Code of Ethics for Nurses (2015) is available online at http://nursingworld.org/MainMenuCategories/EthicsStandards/CodeofEthicsforNurses.aspx. The code addresses issues that concern acting on behalf of the patient's interests, privacy, and confidentiality. It provides general statements that could be useful when addressing conflicts or dilemmas in interactions with others (within and outside the agency) resulting from the creation of, access to, and/or disposition of electronic health information data.

Simpson (2006) asserts that the ANA Code of Ethics Provisions 3, 5, 7, and 8 are particularly applicable for electronic health information. Provision 3, confidentiality and patient safety, addresses the nurse's ethical responsibility to safeguard the patient's right to privacy and confidentiality. Provision 5, competence and continuing education, addresses the nurse's ethical responsibility to maintain competence and ongoing learning. Provision 7, contribution to advancement of the profession, addresses the nurse's ethical responsibility to contribute to the nursing research, scholarly inquiry, and the development of nursing and health policies. Lastly, Provision 8, collaborating with health professionals and the public, addresses the nurse's ethical responsibility to protect the public from misinformation and misinterpretation.

The International Council of Nurses Code of Ethics for nurses is available online at http://www.icn.ch/about-icn/code-of-ethics-for-nurses/. Most countries with professional nurses have codes of ethics. The International Council of Nurses website has links to codes of ethics for nurses in other countries, including France, Italy, Germany, Japan, Sweden, and Brazil.

Code of Ethics for Informatics Professional Organization Members

Informatics specialists may belong to one or more informatics professional organizations. Each organization has formulated a code of ethics for its members. Although the principles identified for the various health informatics organizations are implied in the nursing codes of ethics, in this time of worldwide adoption of HIT, it may be pertinent to update the nursing codes so that the ethics associated with information technology become more explicit.

LAWS, RULES, AND REGULATIONS

Laws state exactly what is expected, unlike codes of ethics, which are open to interpretation. A person or an organization caught breaking a law can expect to be penalized. If the offender breaks a criminal law, the penalty could involve a jail or prison sentence; if it is a civil law, the offender can be fined.

Regulatory agencies, such as the State Board of Nursing, Centers for Medicare & Medicaid

(CMS), and The Joint Commission provide rules for persons or organizations to follow. A person or an agency not following a rule and caught doing so may be penalized as when breaking a law. The penalty for breaking a rule might be temporary or permanent loss of privileges.

Data Security Breaches

A data security breach is unlawful and can result in fines, imprisonment, or both. When discussing informatics, you might think that security breaches are always done using a computer, but that is not true. These can happen when a truck carrying paper records is involved in an auto accident and overturns, spilling records; tampering of postal mail; stolen patient paper files; stolen or lost computers or computer drives; as well as theft of computer data using electronic transmission. The criminal hacker receives lots of media attention because it is possible to steal thousands of records containing private information relatively invisibly and quickly.

Prevalence of Breaches

According to the Identity Theft Resource Center (2014), in terms of the percentage of security breaches in 2013, medical/healthcare ranked first (43.8%) followed by business (34.4%) and education (9%) (Figure 25-1), and medical/healthcare ranked second (8,811,051) for the *number* of known breaches (Figure 25-2). The ramifications

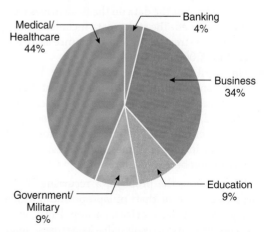

Figure 25-1. Percentage of records breached by type of service—2013. (Data from ITRC, 2014.)

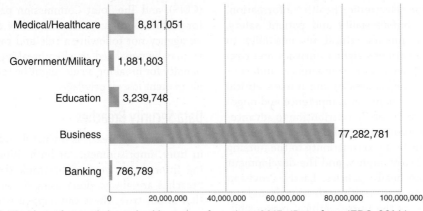

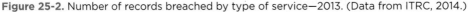

Figure 25-2. Number of records breached by type of service—2013. (Data from ITRC, 2014.)

for those who were affected are potentially devastating if the persons in possession of that private information use it maliciously for personal gain. These statistics give credence to concerns that we must do more to protect the private and confidential information of healthcare consumers.

The **Privacy Rights Clearinghouse** (2013) maintains an online record of all types of security breaches at http://www.privacyrights.org/. According to the website, there have been a staggering number of security breaches in recent years. A few examples of the enormous problem are as follows:

■ On March 28, 2014, a laptop and two flash drives were stolen from an employee's vehicle. The employee worked for Palomar Health in Escondido, California. The laptop data were encrypted, but the data on the flash drives were not encrypted. The stolen data included names, diagnoses, treatment, and insurance information for 5,000 patients.

■ On April 2, 2014, server security barriers were compromised due to malware at Kaiser Permanente Northern Division of Research in Oakland, California. As a result, hackers were able to obtain patient information for 5,100 patients including names, addresses, medical record numbers, and lab results.

In reviewing the problem, a recurring theme involves the loss or theft of laptops and portable storage devices (flash drives, backup drives, etc.). Breaches were also a result of hacks, viruses, unauthorized access to digital records, and loss of paper records, although loss of paper records information breaches were much less common. In some cases, data on the devices were not encrypted.

Cost of Breaches

Data breaches are expensive. The average per-incident cost in 2009 was $6.75 million (Ponemon Institute & Intel, 2010). In 2009, the average cost of a lost laptop used in healthcare was $49,246. The replacement costs of laptops are just one component of the loss; others include the cost of an employee's time while attempting to recover the loss and reporting the incident, the data breach cost, the forensics and investigation cost, the lost productivity cost, and the legal and regulatory cost. According to one study, the average cost for *each* breached *record* was $188 in 2012 (Ponemon Institute & Symantec, 2013). Because the public is made aware of data breaches as well as each individual who is affected, loss of reputation is yet another cost of breaches (and maintaining a good reputation is a stimulus to prevent breaches).

Laws Enacted

The Health Information Technology for Economic and Clinical Health (HITECH) Act that went into effect in 2009 includes rules to ensure the privacy and security of health information. The HITECH Act defined unsecured protected health information as well as security breach (HHS.gov, n.d.). The HITECH Act required agencies to assure that private health information is secure and to prevent a breach or unauthorized access or disclosure of the information.

In January 2013, the law was strengthened. The updated rule made business associates of healthcare agencies liable for information breaches. It also gave patients the right to obtain electronic copies of their health records and to restrict disclosures of their health information. As a result of the law, healthcare agencies are taking additional steps to ensure health information privacy and security.

Risk Assessment and Prevention of Breaches

The prevention of data security breaches is paramount. The actions must be proactive and must involve all employees who have access to protected health information, not just the information technology staff.

Risk Assessment

Healthcare organizations are using risk assessment to mitigate data breaches. The HealthIT website has a comprehensive Security Assessment Tool that users can download. The tool addresses administrative, technical, and physical safeguards. Components of risk assessment include (HealthIT. gov, 2014):

- Reviewing policies and procedures
- Analyzing system vulnerabilities
- Taking inventory of personally identifiable information (PII) and personal health information (PHI)
- Reviewing pertinent regulations
- Monitoring employee compliance
- Tracking external threats

Prevention Measures

In addition to performing risk assessment, healthcare agencies are taking measures to prevent data breaches. Several methods are currently in use to prevent breaches. They include the following:

- Performing employee privacy and security training
- Using data encryption software
- Performing an inventory of PII and PHI
- Using data loss prevention software
- Purchasing cyber liability insurance

Privacy and security training must include more than understanding the HIPAA. Employees must understand the differences between a system login, secure access, and data encryption. They must also have the ability and know-how to encrypt files and drives. They must also have plans to prevent the loss of portable computers and drives.

The differences between operating system login, secure access, and data encryption may not be taught in a nursing program or in orientation to a healthcare organization. A system login provides basic protection of personal data and files. To access email accounts and other secure websites, additional logins may be required. A common misconception is that data sent from a secure email server are protected. If you need to send a secure message, check with your agency or school information security officer for guidance. If you need to send a secure personal message, search for online resources. For example the How-to-Geek has an article "The Best Free Ways to Send Encrypted Email and Secure Messages" at http://www.how-togeek.com/135638/the-best-free-ways-to-send-encrypted-email-and-secure-messages/.

Encryption software is available without a fee. Users can encrypt the entire computer hard drive or individual folders and files. Encryption software should be a requirement for all portable healthcare agency computers and associated portable devices.

Data loss prevention software can be used to track and locate lost/stolen portable computers. The loss prevention software is proprietary and may require a subscription fee for use. The software is very sophisticated. After the computer is determined as lost or stolen, the owner would contact the software company and the police. When the lost/stolen computer connects to the Internet, the locator software sends a message to the recovery team. The recovery team works with the local police to find the missing computer. If the computer locator software includes data security features, all computer data can be deleted remotely from the missing computer. If the located software package includes geolocation software, the physical location of the computer can be identified using Wi-Fi or global positioning system technology. As an example, the Apple iPad and iPhone include geolocation software and the ability to conduct a remote wipeout of data. However, the user must activate the geolocation feature and the device must be turned on at the remote location in order to locate it.

The healthcare agency's information security officer and information technology personnel should be able to provide information on data encryption and data loss prevention software. All users of mobile devices must take a proactive stance to protect electronic health information. Inattention to data security can cause devastating results for healthcare consumers whose personal information has been confiscated maliciously by a cybercriminal.

The Limitations of HIPAA Protection

The general public and healthcare professionals have heard so much about the HIPAA that some have come to believe mistakenly that all health records are private and confidential. Consider the following example. In the case of *Beard v. City of Chicago*, a paramedic was terminated from the city's fire department (*Beard v. City of Chicago*, 2004). The plaintiff pleaded that she was discriminated against and cited that others too had taken medical leaves of absence. The fire department happened to keep copies of medical records for all their employees. The fire department staff physician provided the medical records. These were patient records from physicians outside the fire department, with the patient's consent. The fire department resisted providing the records of other employees, citing HIPAA regulations. The court ruled that HIPAA was not applicable because the fire department did not fall into any one of the three categories that HIPAA covered: It was not a fee-for-service healthcare provider, a health plan, or a healthcare clearinghouse that electronically billed the CMS.

The HIPAA ruling has been criticized for not protecting all private health information. The HITECH Act serves to bridge the limitations of HIPAA. However, if the health information does not fall under HIPAA or the HITECH Act, the information is not protected. Examples include patients' health records in a filing cabinet at home, on their personal computers, or filed at their health club.

LEGAL AND ETHICAL ISSUES ASSOCIATED WITH TELEHEALTH

The Tenth Amendment to the U.S. Constitution guarantees states those powers neither delegated nor prohibited by the Constitution. Under this amendment, individual states have assumed the power to regulate healthcare practitioners for the protection of their citizens. No state, however, has authority over practice in another state. Transport nursing and telehealth both create problems with these assumptions. If a nurse practicing and licensed in state A provides nursing care to a client in state B in which she or he is not licensed, which state has the responsibility and authority to regulate the practice? Malpractice issues associated with telehealth are slowly being addressed. Perhaps, the lack of urgency to address this issue relates to the quality of care rendered and lack of need.

The various state boards involved in regulating healthcare practitioners have been wrestling with the various questions this issue involves. Is the care provided at the location of the provider or the patient? Should the healthcare provider be licensed in both the state where the patient resides and the state where the provider is located? Licensure for physicians and nurses is at the state level. The HealthIT.gov (2013) has links to the most current information regarding licensure for telehealth. The Federation of State Medical Boards developed a framework for regulating interstate practice in 1996 (ATAwiki, 2014; Federation of State Medical Boards, 2013). The framework created a "**restricted license**" for practicing telemedicine across state lines; however, the decision to adopt the license was left to the individual state boards.

In 1998, the National Council of State Boards of Nursing (NCSBN) endorsed the **Nurse Licensure Compact (NLC)** as a framework for regulating the interstate practice of nursing for RNs and LPNs/VNs (NCSBN, 2014). Under this concept, nurses holding a valid license in one state could practice (both physically in person and electronically by using the telephone or telemedicine connectivity to assess and provide care) in other states, according to the rules and regulations of the states. This is similar to a driving license in which a person is licensed in one's state of residence but may drive in another state as long as, while driving in that state, the person follows its laws. The NCSBN maintains up-to-date information for current licensure, as well as pending legislation on the NLC website. The NLC stipulates that certain data about personal licensure be stored in a **Coordinated Licensure Information System** (Box 25-1). In 2002, the NCSBN adopted a framework similar to the NLC for advance practice registered nurses

---

BOX 25-1 Data Required by the Nurse Licensure Compact Coordinated Licensure Information System

- Name of the nurse
- Licensure jurisdiction(s)
- License expiration date(s)
- Licensure classification(s) and status(es)
- Public emergency and final disciplinary actions (defined by contributing state authority)
- Multistate licensure privileges status

(APRNs); however, it stipulated that the APRN compact could only be implemented in states that had endorsed the RN and LPN/VN compact.

IMPLICATIONS OF IMPLANTABLE MICROCHIP DEVICES

Use of the implantable RFID microchip, originally produced by the VeriChip Corporation, serves to polarize individuals' beliefs. When the patient microchip is scanned using an RFID handheld device, the chip information transmits to a computer application, which displays the patient chip information.

The implantable device was originally marketed for use to display identification information for patients with chronic diseases who may require emergency treatment, such as diabetes mellitus and stroke, cognitive impairment such as Alzheimer disease, and those who have some type of implantable devices such as pacemakers and joint replacements. Proponents envisioned a chip containing a unique patient identifier that would allow healthcare providers access to the electronic health record. Supporters stated that the use of the implantable chip is voluntary.

The Electronic Privacy Information Center (n.d.), the American Civil Liberties Union, and certain religious conservatives had issues with the implantable RFID VeriChip (Lewan, 2007). Concerns voiced were about the loss of individual civil liberties and the possibility of mandatory chipping of humans. Opponents saw chipping as just another way the government is stripping the privacy rights of citizens. The opponents won. The implantable device for humans is no longer marketed and the VeriChip merged to form a company, PositiveID. One can only surmise that ethical concerns about human chipping are the reason that the chip is no longer marketed.

However, PositiveID has not given up on using an implantable chip. The company continues to develop innovative products for healthcare. The Breath Glucose Detector and an implantable glucose chip are examples (PositiveID, 2014). The Breath Glucose Detector is designed to measure exhaled acetone for diabetes management. The implantable glucose chip is designed to measure blood glucose levels for management of diabetes.

LEGAL AND ETHICAL ISSUES FOR THE USE OF INTERACTIVE WEB APPLICATIONS

Although interactive Web applications such as Facebook, blogs, podcasts, video, and picture sharing open up a world of opportunities for sharing thoughts, opinions, and experiences, the use must be approached with measured caution. All shared media are open to the world, including attorneys, nursing colleagues, patients and families, charities, and advocacy associations.

As noted in Chapter 4, nurse authors who share information on any type of social media must adhere to a set of ethical and legal guidelines. Nurses should use the online resources at the National Council of State Boards of Nursing at https://www.ncsbn.org/2930.htm and the American Nurses Association at http://www.nursingworld.org/FunctionalMenuCategories/AboutANA/Social-Media/Social-Networking-Principles-Toolkit.aspx to guide their use of the interactive Web. The owner of the blog is responsible for blog content. Nurses should be familiar with employer policies and procedures for social media use by staff members and must avoid all negative references to healthcare agencies or other employers. Shared social media must never contain names or identifiers of patients, families, or other staff members. Moreover, it should not contain any type of information that might *indirectly* identify persons in the clinical setting.

All postings should be respectful of others. Dark humor used by some nurses as a coping mechanism in stressful situations is not appropriate within the privacy of the break room and never appropriate in the public blog arena. The ethical principle, respect for others, must always be used by healthcare professionals who use interactive Web applications.

LEGAL AND ETHICAL ISSUES FOR THE USE OF NANOTECHNOLOGY

The ethical use of nanotechnology in healthcare is an emerging topic. Nanotechnology is work done at the nanoscale, which is 1 to 100 nm in diameter (Nano.gov, n.d. a). To provide a comparison, hemoglobin is 5.5 nm, and a strand of DNA is 2 nm in diameter. It is a relatively recent scientific breakthrough made possible with development of special microscopes that allow scientists to view an atom.

Scientists envision many benefits from use of nanotechnology in medicine (Nano.gov, n.d. b), for example, using a nanosilver-coated bandage to treat an infection from a bug bite, instead of administering antibiotics, and using nanoballoons and laser technology to deliver chemotherapy directly to cancer cells. Another example is using nanobubbles to detect low levels of malaria through the skin.

The legal and ethical concerns surpass the protection of individuals participating in research projects. Resnik (2012) asserts that because the work is done at the atomic level, there are risks to others—for example, family members, research investigators, workers in manufacturing companies developing nanotechnology, as well as others who may come into contact with the nanomaterials. The long-term effects for use of nanotechnology in medicine are unknown, and analysis of literature published about nanotechnology reveals that the risks and benefits are not well understood. Therefore, there is no consensus on how to "protect against occupational and environmental safety concerns" (Fleege & Lawrenz, 2012, p. 761). Nanotechnology may sound like science fiction, but in reality, it is under development in medicine and has the possibility of changing the ways we detect and treat disease.

LEGAL AND ETHICAL ISSUES FOR THE USE OF WEARABLE COMPUTING

There are legal and ethical issues associated with wearable computing—specifically, Google Glass. Google Glass has a wearable computer and video camera built into optical glass frames (Google, n.d. a). The computing capabilities include the ability to take videos and photos, listen to music, send text messages, and provide turn-by-turn directions using GPS. In the operating room, Google Glass could guide a surgeon using visuals of the technique or allow a surgeon to view radiology images during surgery. In the patient care setting, Google Glass could allow care providers to view health records while caring for patients.

The legal and ethical concerns relate to persons who misuse Google Glass to spy, steal, or invade the privacy of others. Unscrupulous people who wear Google Glass could take videos in healthcare settings that violate the privacy of others or take photos of patient records to steal a person's identity. Only time will reveal whether the benefits of using Google Glass will outweigh the detriments.

COPYRIGHT LAW

The U.S. Copyright Office defines **copyright** as a law, Title 17, which provides protection to authorships that are original, thereby protecting intellectual property rights. The keyword in that definition is "original"; examples include books, music, movies, and software. Just about every imaginable **fixed tangible medium** is copyrighted whether or not the individual has applied for copyright protection. Users should assume that all written or recorded mediums are copyrighted even if there is no © symbol. The copyright protection allows registered copyright owners the right to sue over infringements (Copyright Clearance Center, 2005). The law is available online at https://www.copyright.com/Services/copyrightoncampus/basics/law.html.

Fair Use

The copyright law does allow for limited use of copyrighted material under the doctrine of **fair use** (U.S. Copyright Office, 2012). Unfortunately, copyright law provides little direction in determining what amount is fair to use; however, the consideration of the following four factors of fair use should be used as a guide:

1. The purpose and character of the use, for example, nonprofit, educational, news reporting, or commercial
2. The nature of the work, for example, fact, published, unpublished, and imaginative
3. The amount of the work used, for example, small amount or a more substantial amount
4. The effect on the author or for permissions with widespread use, for example, little effect or competes with the owner's sales or royalties

Many colleges and universities have learning resources for copyright online. As an example, the University of Minnesota Libraries has a comprehensive, easy-to-use website about copyright at http://www.lib.umn.edu/copyright/. The website includes tools to assess fair use and information on how copyright applies to education.

Not Protected by Copyright

According to the U.S. Copyright Office, there are four exceptions to the copyright law.

- Work that is intangible, meaning that it is not well defined. Examples include unrecorded music or speeches put together without preparation that have never been recorded or written.
- Composites of information with no original author(s). Examples include calendars, height and weight charts, tape measures, and information in a telephone book.
- "Titles, names, short phrases, and slogans; familiar symbols or designs; mere variations of typographic ornamentation, lettering, or coloring; mere listings of ingredients or contents" (U.S. Copyright Office, 2012, p. 3).
- "Ideas, procedure, methods, systems, processes, concepts, principles, discoveries, or devices, as distinguished from a description, explanation, or illustration" (U.S. Copyright Office, 2012, p. 3).

How long is a copyright in effect? It depends on when the copyright went into effect and what the status of the law was at that particular time.

History of Copyright

The history of copyright development continues to unfold (Table 25-2). In early history, there really was no need for copyright law, as books were handwritten and very expensive to produce. The invention of the printing press by Johann Gutenberg in 1440 changed things. Authors lost ownership of their creations when the number of printing presses proliferated. In 1710, the Statute of Anne was passed in England to stop bookstores from reprinting books and reaping the associated profits. The Statute of Anne restored rightful ownership back to the authors when it made it illegal to reprint without the consent of the "author or proprietors" of the writings (Library of Congress, n.d.). Eighty years later, in 1790, the U.S. Congress passed the first copyright law protecting the ownership of charts, maps, and books for citizens of the United States for 14 years. If the authors were still living after that time, they could reapply for an extension of their copyright for another 14 years. In 1895, the law was amended to prohibit the copyright of government documents.

Copyright law continued to evolve, protecting poetry, drama, motion pictures, architecture, and music. In 1978, copyright protection was extended to the life of the author plus 50 years. In the meantime, computer technology was developing. The copyright law was amended in 1980 to address computer programs and again in 1998, extending copyright protection to the life of the author plus 70 years. A final significant milestone in the timeline was when the Technology, Education, and Copyright Harmonization (TEACH) Act was passed in 2002. The act allowed for the use of copyrighted material in distance education courses that are provided by accredited nonprofit educational institutions (Library of Congress, n.d.). The TEACH Act provides specific stipulations, including that the copyrighted material be used under instructor supervision and that the content is an integral component of the course.

TABLE 25-2 Timeline for the Development of the Copyright Law

1440	1710	1790	1895	1978	1980	1998	2002
Gutenberg invented the printing press.	Statute of Anne established copyright for owners.	U.S. Congress passed 11th copyright law.	Printing Act prohibited copyrighting government documents.	Copyright protection extended to life of the author plus 50 yr.	Copyright amended for computer programs.	Copyright protection extended to life of the author plus 70 yr. Digital Millennium Copyright Act of 1998	TEACH Act allowed for use of copyrighted works for distance learning[a]

[a]Applies only to nonprofit educational institutions.

From Taking the Mystery out of Copyright (n.d.) (http://www.loc.gov/teachers/copyrightmystery/text/files/).

CONFU and the TEACH Act

The U.S. National Information Infrastructure invited representatives from libraries, academic institutions, and industry to define fair use (Lehman, 1997). Although a consensus was never reached, an initiative undertaken from 1994 to 1996, the Conference on Fair Use (CONFU), proposed the following guideline suggestions for fair use: Text was 1,000 words or 10% of the work; images were 15 graphics or 10% of the total collection; music was 30 seconds or 10% of the total composition; and video was 3 minutes or 10% of the total video. These recommendations are taken into consideration for web-based courses (Dobbins et al., 2005). Although the **TEACH Act**, passed in 2002, relaxed the copyright law as it applies to distance learning and nonprofit educational institutions, what constitutes fair use is still blurred.

Faculty and students should follow their institutional guidelines for the interpretation of copyright fair use. There may be differences of opinion about requirements for the use of copyrighted media in password-protected course management systems and general use on the Web.

Plagiarism

Quoting a sentence, a few words, or paraphrasing an idea of another's work and giving credit to the author is considered fair use under copyright law; however, not giving the author credit is considered plagiarism (American Psychological Association, 2009, pp. 15–16). Plagiarism is the same as stealing another's intellectual property and is unethical. The origin for the word "plagiarism" is Latin, and it means kidnapper (The University of Melbourne, 2014). If there is a question about the need to obtain permission for the use of a more substantial amount of the material, the author or owner, such as the publisher, should be contacted for permission.

Use of word processors and the Internet makes it easy to avail the copy and paste functions when writing. Some writers may be tempted to steal the written words and use them as their own. What they may not realize is the Internet also provides a means for others to detect the plagiarism using tools like search engines or plagiarism detection software. Writers should take care when paraphrasing and quoting and use appropriate citation.

A periodic review of good tutorials on the topic is one way of becoming more conscientious about appropriate citation and referencing. The San Jose' public library at http://www.sjlibrary.org/services/literacy/info_comp/plagiarism.htm has good information on the topic and includes an animated tutorial. The Virtual Academic Integrity Laboratory is an award-winning interactive tutorial on plagiarism available through the University of Maryland University College (2003) at http://www-apps.umuc.edu/vailtutor/. Although the resource was developed more than a decade ago, it remains valid today. Most public, school, and college libraries have pertinent online resources on avoiding plagiarism.

Copyright Issues Associated with Google Books

In 2004, Google made the news when it launched the "Google Print" Library Project to scan books and make them searchable on the Web (Google, n.d. b). Google renamed the project "Google Books" in 2005. The inception of the project began in 1996 with a research project at Stanford University by two computer science students, Sergey Brin and Larry Page. The research entailed creating a search engine for book information. The Google search engine was the consequence of their research.

Google Books at http://books.google.com/ provides a way to search, browse, purchase, or borrow a book from an online library (Google, n.d. a). Google has collaborated with a number of large libraries internationally, including Columbia University Library, Harvard University, and Oxford University, for the liberty to scan their book collections and make that information available online. Proponents of Google Books Search state that Google is actually helping publishers and authors by making the books available to the public and that the project is assisting in the sale of books. It allows access to rare books that are otherwise unavailable and too fragile to be viewed by the public. The Google Books project moves the access of books residing in a digital library to the user.

Those opposed to the project state that the Google Books Project is copyright infringement and violates fair use practice. The problem is that Google did not ask for the permission of authors of copyrighted books. As a result, several lawsuits, including those by the Authors Guild, were filed against Google (*District Court Rules in Perfect 10 v. Google*, 2006). On November 14, 2013, the court system dismissed the case involving the Authors Guild. The Authors Guild planned to appeal the ruling (Stempel, 2013).

The Google Books Help Center notes that Google does respect the copyright law by the way the books are displayed (Google, n.d. c). If Google does not have permission from authors or publishers' participants, the only book information displayed is that similar to a card catalog citation. Google suggests that the use of Google Books is analogous to visiting a bookstore and thumbing through the books. The Google Books project challenged copyright law while at the same time changed to cohabitate with the intention of copyright law.

> **QSEN Scenario**
>
> You are preparing a patient education project for a group of newly diagnosed patients with insulin-dependent diabetes. You want to include pictures on a brochure for the patients. What copyright issues should you consider?

SUMMARY

Informatics is associated with multiple legal and ethical issues. This chapter has focused on a few issues in detail that were not addressed in previous chapters. Ethical issues in informatics have been addressed by professional organizations' codes of ethics. As technology matures and evolves, professional codes of ethics must be updated to ensure that patient information issues are clearly addressed. Professionals are constantly being asked to balance the risks associated with patient autonomy and the greater good. The use of RFID technology using the implantable chip with patients and employee tracking is an ethical example that was explored. Telehomecare monitoring is another ethical example that was provided. Does telehomecare monitoring invade the patient's privacy and/or does it provide unnecessary opportunities for security breaches? The legal and ethical issues associated with emerging technologies, such as nanotechnology and Google Glass wearable computing, were discussed.

The HIPAA law has strengths and weaknesses. The law was crafted with the introduction of the electronic transmission of patient record information for CMS billing. Because nurses and the general public have heard so much about the law, we have begun to develop misconceptions that HIPAA protects all patient information. There are concerns about the lack of adequate protection for electronic health records and personal health records. The HITECH Act was passed to provide additional security for health information.

Because boards for professional nursing practice rules vary from state to state, there is no uniform way to license practice that crosses state lines. The NCSBN did develop the compact licensure agreement, but the decision to have a licensure agreement is still at the state level. The implication for nursing is that the telehealth nurse may have to obtain a license to practice in each state practice area, if those states do not have an agreement. Nurses who practice across state lines must also be aware of the differences in state board rules and regulations for all states in which they are licensed.

Finally, there are legal and ethical issues associated with copyright. Copyright law has evolved so that it now covers all fixed tangible media whether or not the owner has paid a fee and registered their copyright with the government office. Copyright registration provides a mechanism for the owner to sue for infringements on unauthorized use. There is still no agreement on what constitutes fair use; the answers lie in "it depends" on when, where, why, and how the information is used. We are cautioned to notify the copyright owner to clarify any question about fair use. Even if the medium is not copyrighted, as is the case with government documents, we must always provide credit to the source to avoid plagiarism. Plagiarism is ethically wrong because it entails stealing the creation of others.

The legal and ethical aspects associated with informatics are very complex and constantly changing. Ignorance of the law has never provided any protection. What it means is that in addition to changes in practice, nurses must also stay abreast of the associated legal and ethical issues. It also means that to protect patient information, we must advocate for the necessary technology and policy changes.

APPLICATIONS AND COMPETENCIES

1. After reviewing the different codes of ethics discussed, select one for nursing and one other. Discuss the similarities and differences. Is nursing management of patient health information explicit enough? If not, make at least one recommendation for a change in the code.

2. Explore the Privacy Rights Clearinghouse website http://www.privacyrights.org/ on the subject of data breaches. Discuss at least three recent health information breaches and identify strategies to prevent those breaches.

3. Discuss the strengths and weaknesses of the HIPAA and the HITECH Act.

4. Identify one strategy that could be used to protect the privacy of the electronic health record and the personal health record. Explain how the strategy could be applied.

5. Discuss the pros and cons of an implantable patient chip that uses RFID microchip technology.

6. Conduct a search for nurse-authored features that use interactive Web applications. Were you able to identify any legal or ethical issues for the content that was displayed? Discuss your findings.

7. Compare and contrast the use of copyright law when writing a journal article versus the design of a personal blog space or social networking site posting.

REFERENCES

American Nurses Association. (2015). *Code of ethics for nurses* (2nd ed.). Silver Spring, MD: Author. Retrieved from http://nursingworld.org/MainMenuCategories/EthicsStandards/CodeofEthicsforNurses.aspx

American Psychological Association. (2009). *Publication manual of the American Psychological Association* (6th ed.). Washington, DC: Author.

ATAwiki. (2014, April 3). *Licensure*. Retrieved from http://atawiki.org.s161633.gridserver.com/wiki/index.php?title=Licensure

Beard v. City of Chicago, 299 F. Supp. 2d 872 C.F.R. (N.D. Ill, 2004).

Center for Intellectual Property at University of Maryland University College Staff. (2003). *Virtual Academic Integrity Laboratory (VAIL)*. Retrieved from http://www-apps.umuc.edu/vailtutor

Copyright Clearance Center. (2005). *Copyright basics: What is copyright law?* Retrieved from https://www.copyright.com/Services/copyrightoncampus/basics/law.html

Curtin, L. L. (2005). Ethics in informatics: The intersection of nursing, ethics, and information technology. *Nursing Administration Quarterly, 29*(4), 349–352.

Dobbins, W. N., Souder, E., & Smith, R. M. (2005). Living with fair use and TEACH: A quest for compliance. *Computers, Informatics, Nursing, 23*(3), 120–124.

Electronic Privacy Information Center. (n.d.). *Verichip*. Retrieved from http://epic.org/privacy/rfid/verichip.html

Federation of State Medical Boards. (2013, June). *Telemedicine overview: Board-by-board approach*. Retrieved from http://www.fsmb.org/pdf/GRPOL_Telemedicine_Licensure.pdf

Fleege, L., & Lawrenz, F. (2012). An empirical examination of the current state of publically available nanotechnology guidance materials. *Journal of Law, Medicine and Ethics, 40*(4):751–62. doi:10.1111/j.1748-720X.2012.00704.x

Gallup Inc. (2014). *Honest/ethics in professions*. Retrieved from http://www.gallup.com/poll/1654/honesty-ethics-professions.aspx

Google. (n.d. a). *Glass*. Retrieved from https://www.google.com/glass/start/

Google. (n.d. b). *About Google books*. Retrieved from http://books.google.com/googlebooks/about/index.html

Google. (n.d. c). *Does scanning comply with copyright law?* Retrieved from https://support.google.com/books/answer/43749?hl=en&ref_topic=9259

HealthIT.gov. (2013, January 15). *Are there state licensing issues related to telehealth?* Retrieved from http://www.healthit.gov/providers-professionals/faqs/are-there-state-licensing-issues-related-telehealth

HealthIT.gov. (2014, May 2). *Security Risk Assessment Tool*. Retrieved from http://www.healthit.gov/providers-professionals/security-risk-assessment-tool

HHS.gov. (n.d.). *Guidance to render unsecured protected health information unstable, unreadable, or indecipherable to unauthorized individuals*. Retrieved from http://www.hhs.gov/ocr/privacy/hipaa/administrative/breachnotificationrule/brguidance.html

Identity Theft Resource Center (ITRC). (2014, April 23). *2014 data breach stats*. Retrieved from http://www.idtheftcenter.org/images/breach/ITRC_Breach_Stats_Report_2014.pdf

Lehman, B. A. (1997, September). *The Conference on Fair Use: Report to the Commissioner on the conclusion of the first phase of the Conference on Fair Use*. Retrieved from http://www.uspto.gov/web/offices/dcom/olia/confu/conclu1.html

Lewan, T. (2007, July 2). *Microchips in humans spark privacy debate*. Retrieved from http://usatoday30.usatoday.com/tech/news/surveillance/2007-07-21-chips_N.htm?csp=34

Library of Congress. (n.d.). *Timeline of copyright milestones*. Retrieved from http://www.loc.gov/teachers/copyrightmystery/text/files/

NCSBN. (2014). *Nursing licensure compact*. Retrieved from https://www.ncsbn.org/nlc.htm

Nano.gov. (n.d. a). *What is nanotechnology?* Retrieved from http://www.nano.gov/nanotech-101/what/definition

Nano.gov. (n.d. b). *Nanotechnology highlights*. Retrieved from http://www.nano.gov/nanotech-101/what

Ponemon Institute & Intel. (2010, September 30). *The billion dollar lost laptop problem*. Retrieved from http://www.intel.com/content/www/us/en/enterprise-security/enterprise-security-the-billion-dollar-lost-laptop-problem-paper.html

Ponemon Institute & Symantec. (2013, May). *2013 cost of a data breach* Retrieved from http://www.symantec.com/about/news/resources/press_kits/detail.jsp?pkid=ponemon-2013 HealthID. (n.d.). *HealthID*. Retrieved from https://www.healthid.com/

PositiveID. (2014). *PositiveID Corporation*. Retrieved from http://www.positiveidcorp.com/

Privacy Rights Clearinghouse. (2013, December 31). *Chronology of data breaches*. Retrieved from https://www.privacyrights.org/data-breach

Resnik, D. B. (2012). Responsible conduct in nanomedicine research: Environmental concerns beyond the common rule. *Journal of Law, Medicine and Ethics, 40*(4), 848–855. doi:10.1111/j.1748-720X.2012.00713x.

Simpson, R. L. (2006). Ethics and information technology: How nurses balance when integrity and trust are at stake. *Nursing Administration Quarterly, 30*(1), 82–87.

Stempel, J. (2013, November 14). *Google beats authors in U.S. book-scanning lawsuit*. Retrieved from http://www.reuters.com/article/2013/11/14/us-google-books-idUSBRE9AD0TT20131114

The University of Melbourne. (2014, March 10). *Academic honesty & plagiarism*. Retrieved from https://academichonesty.unimelb.edu.au/plagiarism.html

U.S. Copyright Office. (2012, May). *Copyright basics*. Retrieved from http://www.copyright.gov/circs/circ01.pdf

Computer Hardware Overview

KEY TERMS

Bus

Central processing unit (CPU)

Cold boot

Compatibility

Driver

Ergonomics

FireWire

Hard disk drive (HDD)

Lithium-ion battery

Logical structure

Motherboard

Nickel–cadmium battery

Nickel–metal hydride battery

Nonvolatile memory

Object

Permanent memory

Physical structure

Random access memory (RAM)

Read-only memory (ROM)

Reboot

Solid-state drive (SSD)

Surge protector

Temporary memory

Thin client

Thunderbolt

Uninterruptible power supply

Universal serial bus (USB)

Volatile memory

Warm boot

In healthcare education, the purpose and parts of a stethoscope are explained before how to use it to listen to heart and lung sounds. To be effective in using the stethoscope, a clinician needs to know when to use the bell and when to use the diaphragm. In the same way, it is imperative to have some understanding of how and when to use the tool of informatics: the computer.

THE COMPUTER

A complete computer system is the integration of human input and information resources using hardware and software. In computer terms, hardware refers to objects such as disks, disk drives, monitors, keyboards, speakers, printers, mice, boards, chips, and the computer itself. Software includes programs that give instructions to the computer that make the machine useful. Information resources are data that the computer manipulates. Human input refers to the entire spectrum of human involvement, including deciding what is to be input and how it is to be processed as well as evaluating output and deciding how it should be used. This appendix focuses on the computer and the associated hardware components.

Computer Misconceptions

When computers were new, there were many fears and misconceptions about using them. Some of these were computers can think, computers require mathematical genius to be used, and computers make mistakes (Perry, 1982). Today, there are other misconceptions, perhaps born of familiarity, which can be dangerous to users. It is important to understand that computers cannot think, and they are not smart. Incidents like the one in which Deep Blue (the nickname given to an IBM computer specially designed to play chess) won a chess game against world champion Garry Kasparov led to such misperceptions (Computer History Museum, n.d.). Consider the game of chess. Although there are many possible combinations, there are a given set of moves, rules, and goals that make it a perfect stage to display the potential of computers. Deep Blue is a very powerful computer, capable of quickly analyzing hundreds of millions of possible moves and responding according to rules (known as algorithms) that were part of the software that beat Kasparov. It made use of these qualities to beat Kasparov. It did not use thinking in the human sense. To read more about the history of computer chess, go to http://www.computerhistory.org/chess/index.php.

The thought that only mathematical geniuses can use computers, although just as false, continues to flourish. This belief is linked to the development of the first computers as a means to "crunch numbers" or process mathematical equations. Hence, in colleges and universities, many computer departments are still housed in, or closely related to, the departments of mathematics. It did not take experts long to translate the mathematical concepts into everyday language, an accomplishment that made the computer available to everyone, regardless of level of proficiency in math.

The last myth that computers make mistakes makes it a wonderful excuse for human error. This was well illustrated by a cartoon in the early 1990s that showed a man saying, "It's wonderful to be able to blame my mistakes at the office on the computer, I think I'll get a personal computer." Computers act on the information they are given. As one humorist said, "Computers are designed to DWIS, or Do What I Say." As many a user will tell you, computers resist with great determination any inclination to DWIM, or "Do What I Mean!" Unlike a colleague to whom you only need to give partial instructions because the person is able to fill in the rest, a computer requires complete, definitive, black-and-white directions. Unlike humans, computers cannot perceive that a colon and semicolon are closely related, and in many cases, a computer believes that an uppercase letter and a lower case letter are as different as the letter A from the letter X. This is known as case sensitivity. There are no "almosts" with a computer.

Computer Characteristics

A computer accomplishes many things that are otherwise impossible. When programmed properly, it is superb in remembering and processing details, calculating accurately, printing reports, facilitating editing documents, and sparing users many repetitive, tedious tasks, which frees time for more productive endeavors. Remember, however, that computers are not infallible. Being electronic, they are subject to electrical problems. Humans build computers, program them, and enter data into them. For these reasons, many situations can cause error and frustration. Two of the most common challenges with computers are "glitches" and the "garbage in, garbage out" (GIGO) principle. That is, if data input has errors, then the output will be erroneous.

Anyone who was using a computer when it crashed or "went down" may have experienced a guilty feeling that she or he did something wrong. Unless the user was purposely engaged in something destructive, that person did not cause the crash; rather just found a flaw in the system that was inadvertently created by the programmer(s). There are times, however, when crashes occur for seemingly no reason. Computers, regardless of their manufacturer, will sometimes, for unknown reasons, perform in a totally unexpected manner. This is as true today as when computers were first introduced. The good news is that this is much less apt to happen despite the intricacy of today's computers.

Given the complexity of programming, it is not unusual to find "bugs" or glitches in a new system. You may have experienced a problem when a new information system was installed at your place of work. If you should be the unfortunate one who discovers a bug, you can help the programmers to correct it by carefully communicating the actions you took that preceded the problem (as far as you can remember) and the exact result. If an error number was presented on the screen, be sure to include this in your communication. Finding the problem is usually harder than fixing it. The hardest mistakes to fix are those that cannot be recreated.

Digital Native or Digital Immigrant?

Are you a digital native or digital immigrant? In a seminal essay, Marc Prensky (2001) stated that digital natives grew up with computers. They are comfortable with computers, surfing the Internet, emailing, gaming, and social networking. Prensky asserts that digital natives are "native speakers" of the digital computer language. Digital natives are very comfortable with using the Internet as a primary source of information.

However, digital natives do not necessarily have the technology literacy skills for use in higher education. In 2014, the Educause Center for Analysis and Research (ECAR) surveyed 5,473 college and university students about their use of technology (C. Bowen and E. Dahlstrom, *personal communication*, April 17, 2014). Forty-three of the survey participants agreed or strongly agreed they needed to be better prepared to use institution-specific technology and 32% agreed or strongly agreed that they needed to be better prepared to use basic software (C. Bowen and J. Reeves, *personal communication*, May 19, 2014).

Prensky (2001) said that digital immigrants who were born before computers were popular have a "digital language accent," for example, printing out email or turning to the Internet as a secondary source of information. If you have not grown up using computers, your attitude about their use may range from curiosity and excitement to complete dislike, frustration, and fear.

Addressing fears takes time for both a trainer and the individual experiencing the fears. One-on-one sessions for the person affected may be necessary and save time in the long run by preventing frantic calls to the help center. Studies show that the learning patterns of those afraid of computers can be improved by treating the bodily symptoms of anxiety and providing distracting thought patterns (Bloom, 1985). Techniques such as teaching relaxation methods before starting any hands-on training often helps, as does giving the anxious trainee something to repeat internally, such as "You're in control, not the computer." If you can reframe your negative feelings to positive feelings of excitement about discovery and new opportunities, it will be possible for you to overcome your anxieties.

Other helpful techniques include recognizing and accepting fear. One method is to have trainees check off from a list of possible feelings (e.g., panicky, lost, curious) those that they are feeling, a practice that can help them face their fears. Inherent in all these terrors is the fear of failure and of looking incompetent in front of their peers. This may be especially evident in people who see themselves as having a high degree of competence in their profession and to whom people look for answers. Therefore, placing themselves in a learning situation can be very threatening to their self-image.

If you are calling your information services (IS) department for help, it is sometimes difficult to understand what you are being told. One remedy for this is to say, "I just don't get it. Could you please explain it like you were talking to your non–computer-using friend?" We all tend to downgrade the knowledge that we possess, believing that others also possess this knowledge, which causes us to provide explanations that are unclear. IS department personnel are just as susceptible to this condition as nurses are when we talk with our patients.

Types of Computers

The progress in computers is measured by generations, each of which grew out of a new innovation (Table A-1). Computer sizes vary from supercomputers intended to process large amounts of data for one user at a time to small handheld computers. Each type has its niche in healthcare. However, it is becoming increasingly difficult to classify the different types of computers, because smaller ones are taking on the characteristics of their bigger brothers as the amount of space needed for processing lessens.

Supercomputers

Technically, supercomputers are the most powerful type of computers, if power is judged by the ability to do numerical calculations. Supercomputers can process hundreds of millions of instructions per second. They are used in applications that require extensive mathematical calculations, such as weather forecasts, fluid dynamic calculations, and nuclear energy research. Supercomputers are designed to execute only one task at a time; hence, they devote all their resources to this one situation. This gives them the speed they need for their tasks.

Mainframes

The first computers were large, often taking up an entire room. They were known as mainframes and were designed to serve many users and run many

TABLE A-1 The Five Generations of Computers

Generation	Dates	Innovation
1	1940–1956	Vacuum tubes
2	1956–1963	Transistors
3	1964–1971	Integrated circuits
4	1971–present	Microprocessors
5	Present and beyond	Artificial intelligence, voice recognition, quantum computation, molecular and nanotechnology. Includes devices that respond to natural language.

Source: Webopedia Staff. (2014, March 9). The five generations of computers. Retrieved from http://www.webopedia.com/DidYouKnow/Hardware_Software/2002/FiveGenerations.asp.

programs at the same time. These computers continue to be the backbone of many hospital information systems.

Servers

A server can be a mainframe or personal computer (PC) that is connected with other computers or terminals for the purpose of sharing databases, programs, and files. Server software allows these computers to perform functions like email exchange or offsite storage of files.

Thin Clients

Thin clients are computers without a hard drive and with limited, if any, processing power. Besides costing much less, thin clients do not need to be upgraded when new software is made available because they do not contain any applications. Because they do no processing, older PCs can function in this capacity instead of being retired. An example of a thin client is a computer terminal that allows access to only the electronic medical record for viewing and entering data.

Personal or Single-User Computers

PCs are designed for one individual to use at a time. PCs are based on microprocessor technology that enables manufacturers to put an entire processing (controlling) unit on one chip, thus

permitting the small size. When PCs were adopted in business, they freed users from the resource limitations of the mainframe computer and allowed data processing staff to concentrate on tasks that needed a large system. Today, although capable of functioning without being connected to a network, in businesses including healthcare, PCs are usually connected or networked to other PCs or servers. They still process information, but when networked, they can also share data.

In information systems, PCs often handle the tasks of entering and retrieving information from the central computer or server, although thin clients may be used for this purpose instead. When a full PC is available on the unit, personnel can use application programs such as word processing. PCs are available in many different formats such as a desktop or tower model and mobile computers.

Desktop and Towers

The original PC was a desktop model. You are probably familiar with these. The traditional desktop computer has a computer processor, monitor, and mouse. The computer processor component may be placed vertically on the desktop, inside a desk cabinet, or built into the monitor. Some desktop computers classified as "all-in-ones" have the processor built into the monitor and use a wireless keyboard and mouse for data input. A touch screen monitor may be used for data input instead of a mouse.

Mobile Computers

Handheld computers are mobile Internet devices. As computer usage became popular, people found that they needed the files and software on their computer to accomplish tasks away from their desks. The first mobile computer that made this practical was really more transportable than portable. Developed in the 1980s, it was about the size of a desktop and had a built-in monitor. Toward the end of the 1980s, the transportables were replaced by true portables: laptops, or computers small enough to fit on one's lap. As technology continued to place more information on a chip, mobile computers became smaller. Mobile computers are commonly classified as laptops, tablet PCs, tablets (includes e-book readers), netbooks, smartphones, and wearables, such as the smartwatch.

Laptops have some drawbacks. The screen is usually smaller than the one in a desktop, and the resolution may not be as crisp. Keyboards are also smaller. The mouse, or pointing and selecting device, can be a button the size of a pencil eraser in the middle of the keyboard, or a small square on the user end of the keyboard, or a small ball embedded in the keyboard. Many of the new lightweight laptops do not have an optical drive with CD/DVD capabilities. Some users purchase docking stations for their laptops. The laptop can be placed in the docking station (may be called a port replicator, or notebook extender), which is connected to hardware such as a larger monitor, keyboard, separate mouse, and printer. A port replicator enables the user to have access to these devices when at their desk but makes it easy to remove the laptop and enjoy its portability, albeit, without the hardware connected to the docking station. Some healthcare organizations use laptops for point-of-care data entry at the bedside or any place where care is delivered.

The tablet PC is a variation of the laptop. The tablet PC has a screen that swivels or folds so that it looks like a book. A tablet PC also has a touch screen and includes a special stylus for pen writing capabilities. The pen writing capability has handwriting recognition that converts it to text.

A tablet is a computer with only a flat touch screen. Instead of a keyboard or mouse, data is input using a fingertip or stylus. The most recent tablets are variations of the laptop where the user can attach a keyboard or a docking station. Many smartphones, e-book readers, and media players are classified as tablets. A tablet often has a much longer battery life than a laptop or tablet PC.

The netbook, a scaled down version of a laptop, was introduced in 2007. The netbook is lighter and less expensive than a laptop. They lack an optical drive, have less power, and smaller monitors and keyboards than a laptop PC. The screen sizes vary from 5 to 10 inches and the weight ranges from 2 to 3 pounds. The netbook lost popularity after the release of newer versions of tablets with faster processors and features similar to smartphones.

BATTERIES

One thing that all portable electronic devices share is a need for a rechargeable battery. Keeping batteries charged in healthcare agencies can be a difficult process. A multitude of devices we use in healthcare are battery powered, for example, intravenous (IV) controllers, pumps, Dopplers, otoscopes, cardiac defibrillators, laptop PCs, and medication carts. Selecting equipment with the right battery and caring for it properly will increase the battery life and length of time it will power a device. This time is related not only to the care a battery receives but also to the type, size, and age of the battery. As batteries age, they lose the ability to retain a full charge (Wikipedia Contributors, 2014a). There are several types of batteries: nickel–cadmium, nickel–metal hydride, lead–acid, and lithium-ion. With the exception of the lead–acid battery, any of these can be found in mobile computing devices (Buchmann, 2014).

Nurses often find themselves having to make decisions about the purchase of equipment that is battery powered. To that end, we need to be knowledgeable about the various types of batteries. Two resources that extend the information included in this textbook are How Stuff Works (http://www.howstuffworks.com/battery.htm) and Wikipedia (http://en.wikipedia.org/wiki/Battery_(electricity)).

Nickel-Based Batteries

The **nickel–cadmium batteries** were the first batteries used in laptops. They are relatively heavy and need to be fully discharged occasionally to avoid decreasing the usage time. This need is a result of crystalline formation on their cells, which decreases the length of time the battery can be used. Their life can be extended if they are fully discharged once every 3 months. They are useful where there is extended temperature range and the need for a long life. Smartphones, laptops, and tablets often use the **nickel–metal hydride battery**, which is replacing use of the nickel–cadmium battery. Nickel-metal hydride batteries suffer from the same memory problem as the nickel–cadmium battery, although to a lesser degree.

Lithium-Ion Batteries

The trend today is toward **lithium-ion batteries**. These batteries have a typical life span of 2 to 3 years whether or not they are used because of loss of capacity through cell oxidation, although they are continually being improved (Buchmann, 2014; Woodford, 2013). These batteries respond better if they are only partially discharged, and frequent full discharges are avoided. To maintain the battery life, charge the battery more often or use a larger battery. A lithium-ion battery must have a protection circuit to shut off the power source when it is fully charged. Overheating may result if this is not present and can cause batteries to explode. Since about 2003, the search for cheap batteries produced a flood of counterfeit batteries that have no protection against overheating. This is why manufacturers advise customers to buy only approved batteries.

Battery life is documented with watt hours. Mobile computers often use lithium-ion. The actual battery life will probably be less than noted in the manufacturer's information. Batteries are tested in ideal conditions, with a minimal processor speed, the screen dimmed, and wireless turned off. In reality, users that use devices with lithium-ion batteries prefer features that diminish the battery life.

Battery Self-Discharging

If you have ever used a laptop, you may have noticed that after it has been unplugged for a while, the battery charging light comes on when you plug the computer into an electrical outlet. This is a result of self-discharge, a characteristic common to all batteries (Buchmann, 2014). Interestingly, it is highest right after charge. The nickel-based batteries lose 10% to 15% of capacity in the first 24 hours after charge, which levels off to 10% to 15% a month. Lithium-ion batteries self-discharge only about 5% in the first 24 hours and then 1% to 2% in a month. Higher temperatures will increase the self-discharge rate, which doubles roughly with every 18°F (10°C) rise in temperature. Leaving the battery in a hot car will create a noticeable energy loss.

Solar-Powered Batteries

There are areas in the United States and other countries around the world where people live "off the grid," meaning that they have limited or no access to electricity or use solar or wind power to supply their own sources. Even if people are located in areas on the power grid, electricity may not be readily available to charge devices—for example, smartphones in airport terminal waiting areas. Solar-powered batteries are increasing in popularity. You can purchase a solar-powered battery to charge a smartphone for less than $50 in the United States.

PC SYSTEMS

Desktop and laptop computers consist of at least three components: a display screen, a keyboard for entering data, and the system components generally housed in a rectangular box often referred to as the CPU (**central processing unit**). These parts provide the input, processing, and output functions needed by a computer.

Surge Protectors and Uninterruptable Power Supplies

Computers, whether mobile or stationary, need a continuous nonvariable supply of power. Their operation can be affected by a power surge. Although the power surge may be generated by the electrical company, in some homes, this can occur when a large electrical device, such as an air conditioner, comes on. To protect against this, all computers come with some degree of built-in surge protection. When this protection is inadequate, the motherboard, or heart of the computer, may be damaged. For this reason, it is a good idea to use a separate, high-quality **surge protector**. If you use a broadband router, digital subscriber line (DSL), or a modem to connect to the Internet, use a surge protector that allows you to connect the telephone line since the phone line can also conduct high voltages.

Some surge protectors include a battery backup, or an **uninterruptible power supply** (UPS) (Figure A-1), which allows you time to power down the computer in the case of a power outage. No surge protector, however, will protect from a lightning strike. Some users elect to unplug their computer and monitor altogether during thunderstorms. Some situations require use of a UPS that runs until backup generators start, if the generators are available.

How a Computer Works

Did you ever wonder how a computer works? It requires a combination of components that are connected together with communication and power cables. The processing part of a computer consists of a motherboard, a central processing unit (CPU), bus, and cards. Consider watching a video, Computer Tour, which provides a tour of the inside of a PC at http://computer.howstuffworks.com/ultimate-computer-hardware-videos-playlist.htm.

Motherboard

The **motherboard** (Figure A-2) is the main circuit board with connecting points that determines the type of computer and power supply that the computer can support. The motherboard typically contains the CPU, the basic input–output system (BIOS), memory, and connections to all ports, expansion slots, disks, and all input–output devices. It contains the chip that is the microprocessor or CPU. A chip is a small box with prongs that enables it to be attached to the motherboard.

CPU/Microprocessor

The CPU is the heart or brains of the computer; it controls what the computer does. Some computer types such as supercomputers or mainframes may have many CPUs. PCs, however, have a single CPU that consists of a single chip called a microprocessor. The CPU consists of an arithmetic logic unit (ALU), a control unit, and some memory registers. The ALU performs all arithmetic and logical operations such as calculating a formula or comparing two items. The control unit directs the flow of information in the computer. It can be thought of as a combination traffic officer and switchboard. It gets instructions from memory, interprets them, directs them, and makes certain they are properly executed. It performs these operations in nanoseconds (one

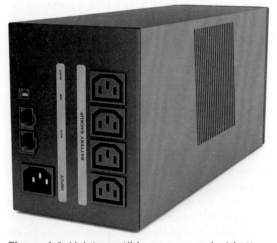

Figure A-1. Uninterruptible power supply (shutterstock.com/MileAtanasov).

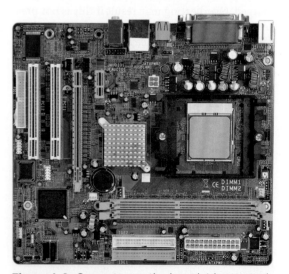

Figure A-2. Computer motherboard (shutterstock.com/HellenSergeyeva).

billionth of a second) so that to a user the results appear instantaneous.

These chips, smaller and thinner than a baby's fingernail, come in different varieties. They may be referred to by manufacturer and number or name. Intel and AMD are the largest processor manufacturers (Godbole, 2014). Intel produces three core series—the Core i7, Core i5, and Core i3—where the Core i7 has the most processing speed (Parkinson, 2012). Intel also produces the Xeon, Pentium, Celeron, and Atom chips. AMD produces FX Series, A Series, Phenom II, Athlon II, and Sempron chips. All chips with the same number or name are not the same, however. Differences may include power management modifications for battery-run computers or the speed at which the chip accomplishes its tasks.

The processing speed is referred to as the clock speed of the computer. The clock speed determines how often a pulse of electricity "cycles" or circulates through the circuits and, hence, how fast information is processed. The more cycles per given time period, the greater the processing speed will be. Clock speed is measured in hertz, which is one cycle per second. Computers today are capable of speeds in the gigahertz (GHz) range (one billion hertz).

The speed of processing is also affected by the type of system processor. If a CPU processes 32 bits of information at a time, it is a 32-bit computer. A 32-bit computer could manage 4 gigabytes (Gb) of RAM (random access memory) for a task. A computer that processes 64 bits of information at one time is a 64-bit computer. The 64-bit computer, of course, is faster and handles four times the RAM than that of the 32-bit system processor (Gizmo, 2014).

The Bus

The speed with which the computer returns results is affected not only by the speed of the CPU but also by the speed and width of a device called a **bus**. Like a bus one sees on a highway, a computer bus is a mode of transportation for data. Physically, a bus is a collection of wires that transmits data from one part of a computer to another, such as from the CPU to the main memory. It also transmits information about where the data should go. Like a CPU, the bus is measured by the number of bits it transfers at one time and the speed of this transfer.

Cards

Many of the functions that a computer performs are regulated by cards that are inserted into slots on the motherboard. These cards, which like the motherboard are printed circuit boards, are used for things such as the video display, RAM, sound, telephone modem, network connections, and expansion.

Bluetooth

Bluetooth, discussed in Chapter 11, allows us connection of multiple devices within a personal area network. Bluetooth was named after a Danish King Blåtand (Bluetooth in English), who in the 10th century settled countries at war with each other (Bluetooth SIG, 2014). Bluetooth symbolizes the connectivity and collaboration of the Danish king. Today, Bluetooth is used with computers to connect mice, printers, and headsets, and it is a common feature for vehicles that allows users to make phone calls and send text messages. It is used in healthcare with monitoring devices for glucometers and inhalers.

HOW A COMPUTER WORKS WITH DATA

A computer does all its work on the basis of whether electronic circuits are on or off. In giving information to the computer, these conditions are represented by a one (1) if the circuit is on and a zero (0) if it is off. Because only 1s and 0s are used, the data are termed binary system data (Roberts, 2009). The decimal system with which we are familiar is base 10, that is, we start expressing our numbers by reusing the last numbers in multiples of 10, for example, the number 11 reuses the 1 from the 10 and adds the 1, 20 reuses the 2 and adds numbers zero to nine, etc. In a binary system, which is base 2, numbers are reused starting with 3. Besides the binary system, two other numbering systems may be seen in computers: octal or base 8, and hexadecimal, which is base 16. To learn more about the binary system, go to a tutorial, Computer Tutorial How Binary Code Works, at http://www.youtube.com/watch?v=ETsfylK7kzM.

Bits and Bytes

The amount of data that can be represented by one circuit is formally called a binary digit and is usually referred to as a bit. Bits hold only one of two values: 0 or 1. They are the smallest unit of information that a machine can hold. When eight of these bits are combined, there is enough memory, or on–off switches, to represent a letter, number, or other character. This amount of memory is called a byte.

ASCII

Standards were set very early in the evolution of the computer for how the on–off switches in a byte would be used for each character to allow computers to exchange data. The standard for PCs is the American Standard Code for Information Interchange (ASCII). Under this system, each character on the keyboard is represented by a number.

Memory

To work with data, to store it, and report it to users, computers need two types of memory: temporary and permanent. **Volatile memory** is what the computer uses to hold program instructions and data that are being created, edited, or used by a user. Anything temporary that the memory contains is deleted when the computer is turned off, unless it is a permanent resident on the computer such as software, or saved by the user when it is something the user created. **Permanent memory** or **nonvolatile memory** is a form of storage. Permanent memory saves any changes in the software or files created by the user when the power is turned off.

Memory is available for the software you use and the files you create. A file is anything that you create on a computer, including a word-processed document or a presentation slideshow. There are two types of memory. One is the memory that you, the user, have access to for the software you are using and the files that you create and is called **random access memory (RAM)**. The second type is pre-programmed, unchangeable by the user, permanent and is known as **read-only memory (ROM)**.

Random Access Memory

RAM is the working or primary memory of the computer. It is temporary, or what is termed "volatile," and everything in it is lost when the computer is turned off unless it has been stored or saved. RAM is the memory area, where temporary files are stored before you save the files to the hard drive. When you close the program, it is erased from memory, but not from its storage place. To preserve the files that you create using a program, you must save the file before closing it or the program or shutting down the computer.

When you open a program or a file, you are not removing it from its storage place but asking that a copy of the program or file be placed in RAM for your use. The original, however, remains on the storage device unless you give a command to delete it. What is not in storage, however, is any change you make to a file after it has been saved. That is, if you retrieve a file from storage and make changes to it, what is in storage is the file that was there when you retrieved it or last saved it. Thus, you must resave a file for it to reflect what is currently in RAM. What does not need to be resaved is the application program because you have generally not changed it, but just used it. In the rare instance that you have made any changes to the program itself, such as changed what it contained on the top of the screen, you will be asked if you want to save these changes. If you like your changes, click Yes.

The amount of RAM that is needed depends on how the computer is used. If using a computer for accessing the Web and perhaps a little word processing, it needs only enough RAM to accommodate the operating system's requirements and the applications. Users who routinely keep several programs open at once will want more than the minimum amount of RAM. When the RAM is inadequate to perform the tasks, the computer slows down. This is caused when the computer has to exchange parts of the application that are in RAM with the parts needed in the drive. Because this exchange is slower than the amount of available RAM, the program slows down. Graphical programs, such as picture-editing programs and many games, require a lot of RAM, hence using more than the average amount of RAM. Because the amount of RAM that a computer can support depends on the processor, you need to know the information before purchasing a computer. A good rule of thumb is to buy double as much RAM that the operating system lists as required.

For example, if Windows 7 requires 2 Gb of RAM for 64-bit computers, purchase the computer with 4 Gb. Avoid purchasing a computer with the minimum amount of RAM.

Read-Only Memory

The second type of memory, ROM, can only be read by the computer; no information can be written to it and no information can be erased or deleted from it. The users' only awareness of ROM may be when they see information flashing on the screen when the computer is turned on. The information in ROM is written to a chip before installation at the factory. It has no relationship to programs installed by a user or any data that a user creates on the computer. The set of instructions it contains are part of the processor of the computer. ROM is used to store critical programs that all computers need, such as the program that boots (starts) the computer. The BIOS, built-in software that determines what the computer can do without accessing any additional software, is usually found on a ROM chip. The last instruction that the BIOS executes is to look for an operating system and install it.

Cache

Cache, which is pronounced "cash," is a special high-speed storage mechanism that permits rapid access to frequently used data. It may be an independent storage device or a reserved section of main memory. Cache is often used by hard drives, CPUs, and Web browsers. You may have heard the term "cache" in connection to your Web browser's memory or history of recently viewed pages. Two types of caching are commonly used in PCs: memory caching and disk caching. In memory caching, a special high-speed static RAM known as SRAM contains the data. In disk caching, the hard drive's hardware disk buffer stores the most recently accessed data from the disk. When there is a need to access data from the disk, the computer first checks the disk cache, because retrieving data from there is faster than from the disk.

Measurement of Memory

The measurement of memory of any type is based on the byte, or the amount of memory required to store one character, such as the letter "L." It is

TABLE A-2   Terms that End with "Byte"

Name	Number of Bytes
Kilobyte	1024
Megabyte	1024^2
Gigabyte	1024^3
Terabyte	1024^4
Petabyte	1024^5
Exabyte	1024^6
Zettabyte	1024^7
Yottabyte	1024^8

expressed by placing prefixes in front of the word byte that denote increments of approximately 1,000. A kilobyte is 1,024 bytes, whereas a megabyte is more than 1 million bytes. Although the prefixes in Table A-2 are from the decimal system, the words they create do not represent numbers divisible by 10 because the amounts are translations from the binary numbering system. The same prefixes are used to describe the number of hertz or the measurement of the computer's clock speed. Thus, a GHz would be 1,073,741,824 Hz or cycles per second.

Secondary or "Permanent" Memory

Secondary memory provides a form of permanent storage for a computer. This type of storage is permanent only in that the user determines whether or not this data will be retained. Except for files in ROM, a user can delete any data in secondary memory. For many programs and users, this type of storage is on the computer's hard disk, (a large storage device internal to PCs). For those who might be concerned that they would accidentally delete an application program from the hard disk, be assured that this action requires a great deal of effort and is very unlikely to be done accidentally. Additionally, a copy of any application programs on the computer should be either on another storage mechanism that is not attached to the computer or available from the Internet. Many devices are used to provide storage. They employ either magnetic or optical methods of storing data.

Magnetic Storage

Some computer hard drives are types of magnetic storage devices still currently in use (Wikipedia Contributors, 2014b). Audio and videotape examples of earlier magnetic storage devices have since been replaced. The drive has a magnetic coated surface used to store the information.

Storage Devices

The type of "permanent" storage available is constantly changing. A good rule of thumb is to update the storage media used every time you buy a new computer. The most versatile storage method today is a flash drive that attaches to a **universal serial bus (USB)** port. Continue reading for more information about this storage device and others.

Internal Hard Drive

A hard drive is a large capacity storage disk. Hard drive storage capacity in today's PCs is measured in gigabytes (Gb) and terabytes (Tb) storage. Home PCs and many found in agencies have an internal hard drive. Users often install the software that they have purchased on this hard drive. Hard drives must be formatted for use with the operating system. On computer with the Windows OS, the drive is usually named "C:" this drive contains the operating system. There is no similar designation on Mac computers.

Internal Hard Drive Storage Types

There are two main types of hard drive storage, the **hard disk drive (HDD)** and the **solid-state drive (SDD)** (Santa Domingo, 2014). The HDD is a magnetic storage device, the traditional spinning hard drive. It requires power to store and display information. If you boot a computer that uses an HDD, it may take several minutes (5 to 10 minutes) to display the start-up window.

In contrast, the SDD uses interconnected flash memory chips that retain data without power. Therefore, when you turn a computer on that uses a SDD, the boot is instantaneous, taking only seconds. The SDD is durable and not subject to data disruption

with jarring, such as being dropped. Furthermore and the SDD is very fast, has no physical size limitation, therefore, amenable small computers, such as very thin laptops and tablets. Because there are no moving parts, the SDD makes no noise when it works. The limitation of the SDD over the HDD relates to cost and capacity. The SDD is more expensive than the HDD. Although it will change, the SDD has a storage capacity limit of 1 terabyte.

External hard drives or storage devices that can be connected to the computer when desired are also available. The portable drives are often used for backing up information on the computer and storing pictures and video. External hard drives usually come preformatted for use with Windows and/or Mac operating systems. When selecting an external hard drive, look for storage space, backup/synchronization software, and transfer speeds. The latest drives use USB 3.0 technology (discussed later in this appendix). Information stored on internal hard drives uses the same method as on smaller removable disks.

Flash Drive

A flash drive is a flash memory storage device that plugs into a USB port (Figure A-3). One can think of it as both the drive and the disk in one, although the similarity ends there. Flash memory is memory that can be erased and reprogrammed in units termed "blocks." It differs from the more common type of erasable memory by erasing and rewriting these blocks in a "flash" from which its name is derived (Wikipedia Contributors, 2014c). Disks write and rewrite using individual bytes. Flash

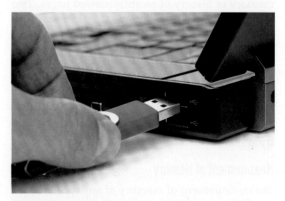

Figure A-3. USB flash drive being connected to a computer (shutterstock.com/rian A Jackson).

drives are popular because they are rewritable, can hold up to several gigabytes of information, and are small, fast, reliable, relatively inexpensive per byte, and portable. They are also easily lost!

One caution with flash drives, including card readers for cameras, is that unlike other nontemporary memory, a flash drive is the drive and disk in one small piece of hardware. Consequently, the flash drive is powered by the computer. Although you can insert the flash drive into a USB port with the computer on, you should remove it with more thought and never in the middle of being written to or reading from them. Wait a few seconds after saving a file to remove the drive.

Optical Disks

The computer writes and reads data to an optical disk by light (Smith, 2014). A laser burns microscopic pits onto the surface to record data. Another laser beam reads the data. Changes in the reflection pattern detect the pits. When a reflection is detected, the bit is on; when there is no reflection, the bit is off. Optical disks replaced diskettes for storage. However, flash drives and the availability of cloud storage are beginning to make optical disks obsolete.

The three kinds of optical storage used in computers today are the compact disk (CD), the digital versatile disk (DVD) and the Blu-ray Disc. CD storage originated on the same disks used with audio disks. A CD can store about 650 to 700 megabytes of data. CDs can contain audio, video, or both on the same disk. DVDs replaced in CDs in many cases. The amount of data that a DVD can store varies from 4.7 to almost 10 Gb depending on the disk. Software is often sold today on a CD or DVD. Blu-ray Discs (BD) are used for file storage, high-definition video, and PlayStation 3 video games. Blu-ray gets its name from the violet colored laser used to read the data. BDs hold 25 to 50 Gb of data. The BD players are backward compatible and can play CDs and DVDs (Blue-ray Disc Association, n.d.).

Whether you can write to an optical disk is dependent not only on the drive but also on the type of disk you are using and the available software. Information about the type of disk, whether a CD-ROM (read only), a CD-RW (read/write), a DVD that is read only, or a DVD with read/write

capabilities and whether it supports a double layer, will be available on the label of the container in which you purchase the disk. Software affects not only if the computer can write to a disk but is also a component of the speed with which the drive writes data to the disk. The amount of available disk space and the RAM in your computer also affect the speed that the drive writes data. If you burn video DVDs or BDs for patient education or other uses, investigate the many options available for making a video, including the aspect ratio and video format that are available in the help feature for the computer operating system. Optical disks have several advantages, including size and not being subject to corruption from magnetic fields or to "head" crashes. They are, however, not immune to damage from scratches or high temperatures.

Permanently Destroying Data on Disks

Today, many computers in healthcare agencies have data that would violate the Health Insurance Portability and Accountability Act (HIPAA) or other privacy acts if it were released. Although your personal computer is not protected by HIPAA, you probably have files with private information such as your social security number and/or banking account numbers. You must remove all confidential information prior to discarding an old computer or the associated drives.

Reformatting a hard drive erases only the filing, or address of the files on the disk, but leaves the files intact (Fisher, 2014). In Windows OS prior to NT and 2000, the file system was called File Allocation Table (FAT or FAT32). Windows NT, 2000, and later use New Technology File System (NTFS) to provide an improved method for securing files (Santa Domingo, 2013). Unless the disk is wiped clean, it is possible to retrieve old files using any number of products easily obtainable on the Web.

A more permanent form of disk cleansing is called disk wiping (Fisher, 2014). There are three ways to make data on a hard drive impossible to retrieve. The first is to use free data destruction software, which you can find with a Web search. The second is to physically destroy the drive, for example, using a drill or hammer to create several holes in the drive. If the drive is an HDD, you could use a degausser to dislocate the magnetic fields on the drive. The drawback to degaussing is that the specialized equipment costs several hundred dollars. It is easier and less expensive to destroy the drive and replace it with a new one if you want to sell or give away a used computer.

PERIPHERALS

Types of Peripherals

A peripheral is any device, such as a keyboard, monitor, mouse, digital camera, scanner, or printer, which is not an essential component of the computer. In general, peripherals are the devices that allow inputting of data to a computer and outputting of information from a computer. A keyboard, monitor, mouse, and camera are standard features in today's computers.

Printers

Printers allow users to print information from a computer, a flash drive, and from storage cards. With current technology, printers can be shared by multiple users. Modern-day printers are multifunctional. For example, they allow remote connecting for printing using Wi-Fi. Some printers have computer capabilities that allow users to email print jobs to the computer via the Internet. All-in-one printers have paper copier, scanning, and fax capabilities. Inkjet printers are popular with home users because they are relatively inexpensive and can print in color and black and white. Some inkjet computers use special ink for printing photographs. Print from inkjet printers will smear when wet.

Laser printers use a dry powder ink and special technology to apply the ink to the paper. Print from laser printers does not smear when wet. Laser printers are more expensive than inkjet printers; for example, laser printers that print in color are often four to five times as expensive as inkjet printers. However, the long-term cost of printing with inkjet printers is higher due to the cost of the ink (Rouse, 2010). Because printer technology continues to improve, nurses making printer purchase decisions, for either home or work, should consider researching online reviews to make informed decisions relating to performance and costs.

Digital Cameras

Healthcare providers might use a digital camera for purposes such as recording the healing progress of wounds. Text descriptions cannot compare with a picture in letting clinicians and patients see healing progress. However, nurses must follow the agency's policies and procedures before using a camera in the clinical setting to assure that there are no HIPAA violations. Cameras are also used for video teleconferencing. The built-in camera on today's computer or smartphone allows the user to take forward and backward facing video and images.

Scanners

Scanners take a picture of a document and then allow users to save this as a file. Unless there is character recognition software available, any text that is scanned will be in a picture format and uneditable. Additionally, some healthcare agencies input clinical records into electronic health records by scanning free text. Even when you use character recognition software to translate the words in the "picture" to text, you need to check the results for accuracy.

Clinical Monitors

Clinical monitors can be part of a network and monitored at a central location. They can also be programmed to provide alarms, either at the central station or to individual pagers, when the monitor shows something beyond the norm. A clinical monitor whether attached to a network, or not, can input patient data, such as vital signs, cardiac, or fetal monitoring tracing, directly to a computer. The advantage of computerized clinical monitoring is that it allows one person to monitor many patients at once as well as provide notification of problems. It should never be allowed to reduce nurse–patient interaction.

Connecting Peripherals

A peripheral connects to a computer through a port. Although today, the USB port is the de facto standard for PCs; in the past, there were other types of ports such as serial and parallel. Computers manufactured in recent years do not have serial or parallel ports.

USB Port

A USB port or universal serial bus is a standard originally created in 1995 (AllUSB, 2014; Intel, 2014). These ports are thin slots found on the sides of laptops and on the front of desktops or towers. USB ports are standard ports on computers using the Windows OS and Mac computers. There are micro versions of some of the USB connections. A graphic depicting the various types of USB ports is available at http://www.flickr.com/photos/dullhunk/7277528920/in/photostream/.

The original, USB 1.0, port transmitted data at only 12 megabits per second (AllUSB, 2014; Intel, 2014) (remember, it takes 8 bits to form a byte, which is required to transfer one letter), making it useful for only mice and keyboards. This easy connection method, however, created a revolution resulting in devices, such as flash drives, external hard drives, and webcams, which needed faster transmission speeds. USB 2.0 technology released in 2000, transmitted data at 480 megabits per second. USB 3.0 technology, released in 2010, transmits data at 5 gigabits per second (Gb/s), which is ten times faster than USB 2.0. USB 3.0 technology (Figure A-4) allows for two-way data transfer, one to send and one to receive (Diffen.com, n.d.; Gailbraith, 2013). USB 3.1 technology, released in 2014, transmits data at 10 Gb/s, twice as fast as USB 3.0 (Shah, 2014). USB 3.1 ports are slimmed down versions of older USB technology, making them amenable for slimmer laptops, tablets, and smartphones. Furthermore, unlike USB 1.0, 2.0, or 3.0 devices, there is no plug orientation for the device insertion.

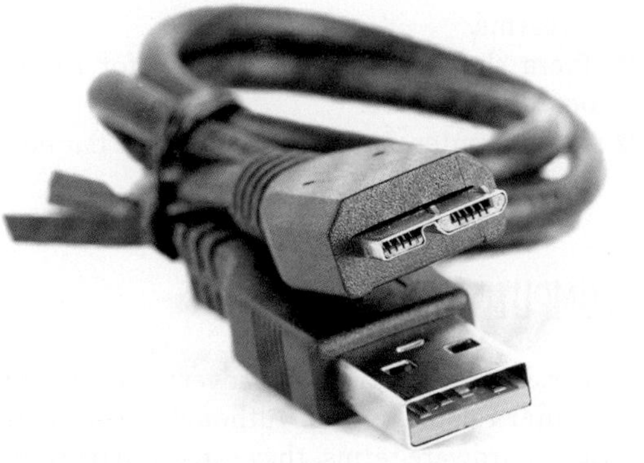

FireWire and Thunderbolt

FireWire originated in the mid-1980s as a high-speed data transfer method for Macintosh external hard drives (Wikipedia Contributors, 2014d; F. Lowney [personal communication, June 7, 2014]). Apple presented this technology to the Institute of Electrical and Electronics Engineers (IEEE), who in December 1995, released IEEE 1394, which is an official FireWire standard. It was often referred to as FireWire 400 and had transfer speeds of 100 to 400 megabits per second. In April 2002, the IEEE released a new standard for FireWire 800, which transferred data at 786 megabits per second. FireWire 3200, released in 2010, transferred data at 3.2 gigabits per second (Wikipedia Contributors, 2014d).

In 2011, Apple replaced FireWire with the faster **Thunderbolt** technology (Figure A-5). Similar to USB 3.0, Thunderbolt supports two-way data transfer, however much faster (Wikipedia Contributors, 2014e). Thunderbolt provides a transfer speed of 10 Gb/s each way, for a total of 20 Gb/s. Thunderbolt 2 was released in 2013 and was a standard on the new Mac Pro and MacBook Pro with Retina display computers (Apple, 2014).

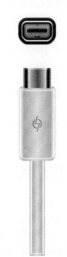

Figure A-4. USB 3.0 cable connectors (shutterstock.com/AnakeSeenadee).

Figure A-5. Thunderbolt cable and socket (shutterstock.com/TheVectorminator).

Thunderbolt 2 technology allows the user to connect UltraHD (very high-definition) monitors and use other peripherals.

Infrared Port

An infrared (IR) port is a connection on a computer that uses IR signals to wirelessly transmit information between devices such as a PDA and a computer. It has a range of about 5 to 10 feet. Most handheld devices have the capability to communicate via IR ports that allow the device to directly interface with another device to exchange data.

Infection Control

Computers, particularly keyboards, are commonplace in healthcare settings and are easily contaminated with potentially pathogenic microorganisms. Reports from studies demonstrate the presence of pathogens, not only in healthcare agencies but also on nurses' home computers (Anderson & Palombo, 2009; Po et al., 2009). These studies also demonstrated that these organisms can be spread to patients.

Although hand washing before touching a keyboard or any other computer part can help, all computer peripherals in a room should be routinely cleaned with a solution recommended by infection control personnel. Research conducted by D'Antonio et al. (2013) identified that plastic keyboard covers impregnated with an antimicrobial polymer can reduce bacterial survival. Some healthcare facilities are using tablet devices, which can be cleaned between patients for improved infection control. If possible, engineering the physical environment to prevent contamination should also be done. For example, hand gesturing may replace use of hardware and the associated infection control problems in certain settings, such as the operating room (Jacob et al., 2013).

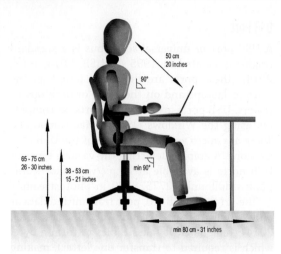

Figure A-6. How to sit and use a computer to avoid musculoskeletal disorders (shutterstock.com/Maluson).

agency as well as the home computer work setting. Figure A-6 depicts the design of a safe work setting. A summary of the key design elements is noted below (Occupational Safety and Health Administration, OSHA, n.d.b).

■ The top of the computer monitor should be at or just below eye level.
■ Computer monitor should be about 20 inches from the user's eyes.
■ The head and neck should be balanced and in-line with the torso.
■ The elbows should be close to the body and supported.
■ There should be support for the lower back.
■ The wrists and hands should be in-line with the forearms.
■ There should be adequate room for the keyboard and mouse.
■ The computer user's feet should rest flat on the floor.

ERGONOMICS WITH COMPUTER USE

The U.S. Occupational Safety and Health Administration (OSHA) (n.d.a) defines **ergonomics** as fitting the job to the person. The OSHA provides resources to analyze a computer workstation and also provides a purchasing guide checklist. The resources are beneficial to the healthcare

COMPUTERESE

Discussion, instruction, and advertising use many computer-related terms. Although they are not strictly hardware terms, they can often be confusing. Booting refers to loading the software that starts the computer. The term **"reboot"** means to restart the computer. A **warm boot** is restarting the computer without turning it off. A **cold boot** is starting the computer when the power is completely off.

Compatibility refers to whether programs designed for one chip will work with an older or newer chip or whether files created with one version of a program will work with another version of the same program. Most computer chips and software are backward compatible, that is, they will work with older versions of a program or files created with an older version of a program. Some are not, however, forward compatible, or the situation in which an older program does not recognize files created by a newer version of the same program. This is particularly true of spreadsheets, databases, and presentation programs.

A **driver** is a software program that allows data to be transmitted between the computer and a device that is connected to the computer. Drivers are generally specific to the brand and model of the device. They may come with a new peripheral or can often be downloaded from the vendor's website.

When used with a computer, the terms "logical" and "physical" refer to where data are located in the computer. The **physical structure** is the actual location, whereas a logical structure is how users see the data. For example, when a user requests information about laboratory tests, he or she may see the indications for the test, the normal values, the cost of a test, and the patient's test results. Although this information may be presented as one screen, which is a **logical structure**, different pieces will have been retrieved from different files in different locations, which is the physical structure of the information.

Another potentially confusing computer term is object. Although the more common use of the term "**object**" is for a physical entity, or at least a picture on the screen, to a computer, an object is anything the computer can manipulate. That is, an object can be a letter, word, sentence, paragraph, piece of a document, or an entire document. Objects can be nested, that is, a word is an object nested within a sentence object. A paragraph is an object that is contained in a document. When an object is selected, clicking the right mouse button presents a menu of properties of that object that can be changed.

GLOBAL PERSPECTIVES ON COMPUTERS AND USE OF THE INTERNET

The use of computer devices to access the Internet continues to grow at a rapid pace. A 2014 report from Cisco (2014), a major provider of networking equipment, predicted that Internet traffic will increase five-fold between 2013 and 2018. By 2018, most Internet traffic will be devices other than PCs. Internet traffic is growing most quickly in the Middle East, Africa, and Asia Pacific. The global growth in Internet use serves to improve communication in healthcare and among healthcare consumers worldwide.

SUMMARY

Understanding how computers function forms the background for a beginning understanding of informatics. Computers are devices, which, although we may anthropomorphize them, are still inanimate objects. Computers do not think; they need explicit instructions and are incapable of interpreting gray areas. This is not to say that gifted programmers cannot make one think a computer is behaving in a seemingly human manner.

Like informatics, computers have many different types and parts. When all these parts function together along with human interventions, the results benefit healthcare. Regardless of size, all computers possess some given parts, a CPU, memory, storage devices, and ways to both enter and retrieve data. How many and how much of each of these parts a computer needs depends on the function the computer is intended to serve and often the depth of the owner's pocketbook. Understanding the function of each of these parts allows nurses to creatively and effectively use a computer both professionally and personally.

Computers, however, are not without their hazards in healthcare. Their parts, particularly mice and keyboards, are capable of harboring pathogenic microorganisms, which have been known to create infections in patients. Data that they can contain could create harm if it became known; hence, computers that will need to be discarded must have their internal storage devices thoroughly wiped before being released.

REFERENCES

AllUSB. (2014). USB history. Retrieved from http://www.allusb.com/usb-history

Anderson, G., & Palombo, E. A. (2009). Microbial contamination of computer keyboards in a university setting. *American Journal of Infection Control*, 37(6), 507–509.

Apple. (2014). Thunderbolt: Next generation high speed I/O technology. Retrieved from http://www.apple.com/thunderbolt/

Bloom, A. J. (1985). An anxiety management approach to computer phobia. *Training and Development Journal*, 19(1), 90–94.

Blue-ray Disc Association. (n.d.). History of Blu-Ray disc. Retrieved from http://www.blu-raydisc.com/en/AboutBluray/WhatisBlu-rayDisc/HistoryofBlu-rayDisc.aspx

Bluetooth SIG. (2014). Fast facts: Bluetooth technology. Retrieved from http://www.bluetooth.com/Pages/FastFacts.aspx

Buchmann, I. (2014). Battery University table of contents: Basic to advanced. Retrieved from http://batteryuniversity.com/learn

Cisco. (2014, June 10). Cisco visual networking index: Forecast and methodology, 2013-2018. Retrieved from http://www.cisco.com/c/en/us/solutions/collateral/service-provider/ip-ngn-ip-next-generation-network/white_paper_c11-481360.html

Computer History Museum. (n.d.). Mastering the game: A history of computer chess. Retrieved from http://www.computerhistory.org/chess/index.php

D'Antonio, N. N., Rihs, J. D., Stout, J. E., et al. (2013). Computer keyboard covers impregnated with a novel antimicrobial polymer significantly reduce microbial contamination. *American Journal of Infection Control*, 41(4), 337–339. doi: 10.1016/j.ajic.2012.03.030.

Diffen.com. (n.d.). USB 2.0 vs USB 3.0. Retrieved from http://www.diffen.com/difference/USB_2.0_vs_USB_3.0

Fisher, T. (2014). How to completely erase a hard disk drive: Several ways to completely erase a hard drive of all data. Retrieved from http://pcsupport.about.com/od/toolsofthetrade/tp/erase-hard-drive.htm

Gailbraith, J. (2013, May 24). How fast is USB 3.0 really? Retrieved from http://www.macworld.com/article/2039427/how-fast-is-usb-3-0-really-.html

Gizmo. (2014, July 13). 32-bit and 64-bit explained. Retrieved from http://www.techsupportalert.com/content/32-bit-and-64-bit-explained.htm

Godbole, M. (2014, April 30). AMD vs. Intel processors. Retrieved from http://www.buzzle.com/articles/amd-vs-intel-processors.html

Intel. (2014). Universal serial bus overview. Retrieved from http://www.intel.com/content/www/us/en/io/universal-serial-bus/universal-serial-bus.html

Jacob, M. G., Wachs, J. P., Packer, R. A. (2013). Hand-gesture-based sterile interface for the operating room using contextual cues for the navigation of radiological images, *Journal of the American Medical Informatics Association*, 20(e1), e183–e186. doi: 10.1136/amiajnl-2012-001212.

Occupational Safety & Health Administration (OSHA). (n.d.a). Prevention of musculoskeletal disorders in the workplace. Retrieved from https://www.osha.gov/SLTC/ergonomics/

Occupational Safety & Health Administration (OSHA). (n.d.b). OSHA solutions: ergonomics workstations etool. Retrieved from https://www.osha.gov/SLTC/etools/computerworkstations/index.html

Parkinson, D. (2012, December 26). What's the difference between an Intel Core i3, i5 and i7? Retrieved from http://www.pcadvisor.co.uk/buying-advice/pc-components/3417091/whats-difference-between-intel-core-i3-i5-i7/

Perry, W. E. (1982). *Survival guide to computer systems*. Boston, MA: CBI Publishing Company.

Po, J. L., Burke, R., Sulis, C., et al. (2009). Dangerous cows: an analysis of disinfection cleaning of computer keyboards on wheels. *American Journal of Infection Control*, 37(9), 778–780.

Prensky, M. (2001). Digital natives, digital immigrants: Do they really think differently? *On the Horizon*, 9(6), 15–24. Retrieved from http://www.marcprensky.com/writing/Prensky%20-%20Digital%20Natives,%20Digital%20Immigrants%20-%20Part2.pdf

Roberts, B. (2009, February 21). Computer tutorial how binary code works. Retrieved from http://www.youtube.com/watch?v=ETsfylK7kzM

Rouse, M. (2010). Laser printer. Retrieved from http://whatis.techtarget.com/definition/laser-printer

Santa Domingo, J. (2014, February 20). SSD vs. HDD: What's the difference? *PC Magazine*. Retrieved from http://www.pcmag.com/article2/0,2817,2404258,00.asp

Santa Domingo, J. (2013, July 16). FAT32 vs. NTFS: Choose your own format. *PC Magazine*. Retrieved from http://www.pcmag.com/article2/0,2817,2421454,00.asp

Shah, A. (2014, April 2). Fumble-free USB 3.1 connector will be in products by year end. *PC World*. Retrieved from http://www.pcworld.com/article/2139041/fumblefree-usb-31-connector-will-be-in-products-by-year-end.html

Smith, J. (2014). Computer basics: Storage optical disks. Retrieved from http://www.jegsworks.com/lessons/lesson6/lesson6-7.htm

Wikipedia Contributors. (2014a, May 2). Battery (electricity). Retrieved from http://en.wikipedia.org/wiki/Battery_%28electricity%29

Wikipedia Contributors. (2014b, May 27). Computer data storage. Retrieved from http://en.wikipedia.org/wiki/Computer_data_storage

Wikipedia Contributors. (2014c, May 26). Flash memory. Retrieved from http://en.wikipedia.org/wiki/Flash_memory

Wikipedia Contributors. (2014d, May 31). IEEE. Retrieved from http://en.wikipedia.org/wiki/Firewire

Wikipedia Contributors. (2014e, May 5). Thunderbolt (interface). Retrieved from http://en.wikipedia.org/wiki/Thunderbolt_%28interface%29

Woodford, C. (2013, September 8). How lithium-ion batteries work. Retrieved from http://www.explainthatstuff.com/how-lithium-ion-batteries-work.html

Glossary

abstract: summarizes the information presented in an academic paper; one of four sections of an APA paper

academic papers: papers written for an instructor or professor in an educational setting

accessibility: the design of a resource, such as a website, that allows individuals with disabilities the ability to access the resource; the resource design should allow for use of screen readers for persons with limited eyesight as well as for those who are hearing disabled

accuracy of data: the quality of data can be improved with methods that check the data during input; for example, when a user chooses phrases for input from a predefined list

active cell: the location where you enter data in a spreadsheet; analogous to the insertion point in other programs

active RFID: a radio frequency identification (RFID) tag that is battery powered and constantly transmitting signals and used to track and identify objects

advanced encryption standard (AES): an encryption standard found in Wi-Fi used to protect electronic data

advanced search: a search method that allows users to enter multiple search terms as well as define fields to narrow the search; often used in database searches, such as with a digital library search

adware: software that includes pop-up advertisements; paying to register the software installation may remove these ads

aggregated data: data from more than one source and grouped for comparison

Alliance for Nursing Informatics (ANI): a professional informatics nursing organization which is composed of many member organizations; the organization is sponsored by the American Medical Informatics Association

(AMIA) and the Healthcare Information Management Systems Society (HIMSS)

alt tag: a text alternative for a graphic because screen readers cannot "read" a graphic; the tag should provide either textual information used by a screen reader in place of the illustration or a link to a site that explains the illustration in text

American Health Information Management Association (AHIMA): a professional organization formed by the American College of Surgeons in 1928 to improve clinical records; the name reflects today's situation in which clinical data have expanded beyond either a single hospital or a provider

American Medical Informatics Association (AMIA): a professional organization made up of informatics professionals and students, with a goal to advance informatics, promote education, and assure effective informatics use

American Nursing Informatics Association (ANIA): the largest nursing informatics professional association; has annual educational conferences, provides continuing education forums, and disseminates informatics updates with an organization newsletter

animations: static images displayed in a sequence that provide an illusion of a motion picture; often used to display difficult concepts, processes, and models; the best use of animations is to supplement written information

APA (American Psychological Association) 6th Style: a style for authoring scholarly papers in many nursing education programs, journals, and textbooks

Apple iCloud: a cloud sharing program accessible on the web that includes syncs apps, mail, contacts, etc.; allows for file sharing

application (app): various types of software, such as office software and web browsers

area charts: communicates the proportion of various items in relation to the whole (pie charts are an example); they are "part-to-whole" charts designed to show numbers or percentages

asynchronous learning: learners use the distance learning resources at a time and place that is convenient for them

augmented reality: provides a representation of real life with digital images

atomic level: data in a cell that cannot be reduced; when designing a database, each field must contain atomic level data

authentication: verifying the identification of the person logging into the system; it can be accomplished by using passwords, smartcards, biometrics, or a combination of these

attribute: instructs the database about the type of datum in each field name; may be a date, time, currency, number, or text

axes: divisions that include a list of terms with agreed upon definitions that can be used to create combinational vocabulary

avatar: a fictionalized graphical computer representation of oneself that can be custom designed with different looks

background layer: sometimes called the master layer in slide presentation software that holds the design of the slides, or the theme; is important because it keeps all the slides in the presentation consistent in looks

backup: a duplicate copy of a digital file

bandwidth: the rate of digital communication for data transmission

bar chart: generally associated with comparisons of amounts; data in bar charts can be displayed either vertically or horizontally, and varieties include simple, clustered, and stacked

beaming: allows for wireless, very short-ranged (4 inches to 3 feet), transmission of information to other beam-enabled devices with the same operating system using infrared, Bluetooth, or near field communication (on Android devices); AirDrop emulates beaming with Mac devices for file sharing

benchmarking: a process for comparing performance using metrics; nurses are in pivotal positions to improve quality, prevent errors, and improve patient satisfaction in hospitals that will improve benchmarking ratings

best of breed: a computer system that best meet the needs of particular services or departments; it requires building an integrated interface at the institutional level to communicate with other computer systems

best research evidence: clinically relevant research, which includes outcomes and effectiveness patient care

big-bang conversion: used when switching from one computer system to another; the entire institution implements the system at the same time

big data: creation of tremendously large amounts of data, both structured and unstructured that is created, collected, and accessed at different times

biometric garment: emerging wearable technology that allows for a proactive approach for early identification of symptoms before problems develop; has the potential for maintaining the patient's quality of life, reducing acute exacerbations of disease processes, and avoiding unnecessary medical costs

biometrics: a secure method of authentication, it is the use of physiological characteristics such as iris scan, fingerprint, or a voiceprint that is presumably unique to the particular person

blended course: a combination of the traditional face-to-face classroom and online formats for learning

blog: an online web log or discussion about thoughts or topics of interest

Bloom's Taxonomy of Learning: delineates progressively complex domains of learning to include knowledge, comprehension, application, analysis, synthesis, and evaluation; was later modified to make "creating" rather than "evaluating" the highest level of learning

Bluetooth: allows for a wireless, short-ranged (32 feet), low-powered radio frequency connection to other Bluetooth-enabled devices

body of the paper: a section of a written paper supporting an argument or thesis; begins with an introduction and ends with a conclusion or summary; one of four sections of a paper written using APA style

Boolean logic: a form of algebra in which matches are either true or false, named after the 19th century mathematician George Boole; three concepts make up Boolean logic: "AND," "OR," and "NOT"

botnet: a malware threat comprised a group of computers connected to the Internet that, unbeknownst to their owners, have software installed on their computers to forward items such as spam or viruses to other computers; also known as a zombie army

Braille reader: a screen reader that can send information to a Braille reader placed near or under the keyboard; users then use their fingers to "read" the information

British Computer Society (BCS): a professional organization group supporting the use of information technology in the United Kingdom and internationally

broadband: high speed or wide data transmission via computers

bugs: computer system errors and issues

business continuity plan: the term used by information technology (IT) for disaster recovery; some resources differentiate the two terms, indicating that "business continuity" refers to how to continue IT services in the case of a disruption and "disaster recovery" refers to the recovery of IT services after a disaster

business intelligence: a movement to integrate financial data, patient data, and quality data to produce predictive and prescriptive analytics for decision makers; also known as healthcare data analytics

campus area network (CAN): a network that encompasses a defined geographic area, such as a college campus

cause-and-effect chart: a chart that places the effect at one end with the many suspected causes branching out from it; the resulting chart resembles a fish, thus it is commonly referred to as a fishbone chart

cell: the rectangles contained in a grid of a spreadsheet that are arranged in columns and rows; each cell can be formatted to display numbers, text data, and formulas

cell address: the name given to a cell in a spreadsheet; uses the letter of the column and the row number where it is located

cell range: a group of contiguous cells in a spreadsheet (e.g., B11:D13); users can name ranges of cells and use this name in commands instead of the cell location to create formulas

cell phone: a shortwave wireless communication phone that has a connection to a transmitter to receive calls over a wide geographic area; requires a paid subscription to the transmission service provider

Certification Commission for Healthcare Information Technology (CCHIT): pioneered the electronic health record (EHR) certification process for the U.S. government; in 2014, CCHIT took a strategic direction to provide assistance to healthcare providers and vendors attempting to meet the HIT regulations

chaos theory: a theory that deals with the differences in outcomes depending on conditions at the starting point; first encountered by a meteorologist, Edward Lorenz, in 1963

chat: interactive e-mail that involves two or more individuals; users type their conversation and tap the Enter key to send the message and then others respond

chart: a graphical presentation of a set of numbers; provide a means to interpret the relationships of quantitative and categorical data in a table

classify: to group terms so that they can be analyzed beyond the individual term

clinical decision support system (CDSS): a computer application that uses a complex system of rules to analyze data and presents information to support the decision-making process of the knowledge worker

Clinical Document Architecture (CDA): used in the electronic health records, these data standards devised by Health Level 7 (HL7) provide a common structure for clinical documents; the structure has three levels that provide the ability to send documents that have sufficient "code" in them to be machine-readable and yet are easily interpretable as a document by a human

clinical expertise: the ability to use clinical skills and past experience to rapidly identify each patient's unique health state and diagnosis, individual risks and benefits of potential interventions, and personal values and expectations

clinical information systems: computer systems designed for use in healthcare delivery

clinical reasoning: decision making that uses critical thinking skills and considers all factors influencing patient preferences by nurse care provider; the nurse uses clinical reasoning to determine pertinent factors to assist the patient to maintain or attain health

clipboard: software where cut or copied data are stored for transfer between documents

closed-loop safe medication administration: the term "closed loop" means that the right patient received the right medication and right dose at the right time; it is an essential component of patient safety improvements

cloud computing: use of remote computers for applications and file storage

code of ethics: statements of the professionals' values and beliefs, which are based on ethical principles

codebook: a document with records of codes assigned for numbers used for statistical categorical data in descriptive data analysis

cognitive load theory: the brain has limited short-term memory and unlimited long-term memory; therefore, it is difficult for the brain to process reading words on a slide while listening to a presenter unless the two are congruent

cognitive science: the study of the human mind and intelligence and how information can be applied; it is interdisciplinary, includes philosophy, psychology, artificial intelligence, neuroscience, linguistics, and anthropology, and is a part of social informatics

collective intelligence: intelligence that emerges from group collaboration

column: a vertical group of cells in a spreadsheet or table

combinational vocabulary: a term is created by combining terms from lists in different axes or categories

combo box: a list to validate data that appear from a drop-down menu, created in spreadsheet or database software

computer fluency: understanding how to use computers and the related computer concepts

computer literacy: the ability to perform various tasks with a computer

computer virus: a malware program from the Internet designed to execute and replicate itself without the user's knowledge

confidentiality: authorized care providers maintaining all personal health information as secret, except to other care providers who need access to that information and to others that the patient has consented to allow access

Consumer Assessment of Health Providers and Systems: a standardized survey tool designed for administration to a sample of discharged patients; hospitals are required to submit data to the Centers for Medicare & Medicaid website so that patients' experiences can be trended over time in one hospital and benchmarked to other hospitals

consumer informatics: a field of study related to healthcare information that is accessible to consumers in a useful, understandable manner

content layer: the slide presentation layer use to enter text or other objects, such as images, tables, and charts

context-sensitive help: help that is modified based on where in the computer system help was accessed

contingency plan: a computer plan for unexpected outcomes that is detailed and addresses risks of significant implementation problems

Continuity of Care Document (CCD): the clinical document architecture for shared data that provides a "snapshot" of a patient's health information, including insurance information, medical diagnoses and problems, medications, and allergies

controlling: the fourth phase of the systems life cycle, which includes the ongoing process of systems maintenance, such as having trained staff work on the help desk

Coordinated Licensure Information System: the Nurse Licensure Compact stipulates that certain data about personal licensure be stored in this system, which includes the name of the nurse, the licensure of jurisdiction, the license expiration date, the licensure classification and status, public emergency and final disciplinary actions, and multistate licensure privileges status

copyright: the U.S. Copyright Office defines copyright as a law, Title 17, which provides protection to authorships that are original, thereby protecting intellectual property rights; the keyword in that definition is "original"—examples include books, music, movies, and software

core measures: national scientifically based standards used to compare quality of healthcare

cost-benefit: an examination of the difference between the projected revenues and expenses

crashes: computer programs that close without notice; work that has not been saved will be lost

crop: allows the designer to trim the vertical or horizontal edges of a graphic

dashboards: a user-friendly way to deliver business intelligence and data analytics; deliver real-time information on key performance indicators to drive decision making in healthcare

data: individual facts

data analytics: examination of large amounts of raw and unorganized data to identify patterns or trends in order to make business decisions

data mining: a process that extracts from data potentially useful information that was previously unknown

data security: the responsibility of the computer user; has three aspects: ensuring the accuracy of the data, protecting the data from unauthorized eyes, and dealing with internal or external damage to the data

data warehouse: a comprehensive collection of clinical and demographic data on large populations

database: software that is a collection of related objects, such as tables, forms, queries, and reports

database model: the way data are organized in a database; several models exist, including flat, hierarchical, network, relational, and object oriented

Database Management System (DBMS): a software application that provides tools for creating a database, entering data, retrieving, manipulating, and reporting information contained within the data

DataFerrett: a browser provided by the U.S. Census Bureau that provides access to publicly available data

debugging: process of correcting computer system errors

default settings: the software presets, such as line spacing, margins, default font, and paragraph headings

deidentified data: data stripped of subject identifiers

demand forecasting: predictive decision making that takes historical data on patient acuity and census to predict the needs for nurse staffing

digital subscriber line (DSL): a home network that connects a router to the Internet; uses a regular phone line

disaster recovery: referred to as a business continuity plan in information technology (IT) referring to the recovery of services after a disaster

disjunctive: a taxonomy where each term can belong to only one overall concept or have only one parent

distributed denial of service (DDoS): when a botnet owner (or herder) directs all the computers in its botnet to send requests to the same site at the same time, overwhelming the website and preventing legitimate access

drill and practice: repeated practice that provides feedback to reinforce learning; examples are flash cards and questions with answers

dynamic IP address: the Internet protocol (IP) address that changes each time a user connects to the Internet

eBook: an electronic book

e-learning: learning using computer technology; the term places the emphasis on student learning and pedagogy

electronic health record (EHR): an electronic record of a patient's health history, established by President George W. Bush in 2004; one's health information is available from any location where there is Internet access and a health information exchange

electronic medical record (EMR): the focus of most healthcare providers today, the institution or provider that creates EMRs owns and manages them, and they are accessible to consumers; not a true electronic health record because outside agencies cannot interface with them

electronic medication administration record (eMAR): a multidisciplinary electronic record that communicates the complex process of medication use; provides a mechanism for efficient nurse time utilization as well as facilitates the delivery of safe care

Electronic Numerical Integrator and Computer (ENIAC): the first computer by today's perception, built in 1946 at the Moore School of Engineering at the University of Pennsylvania in partnership with the U.S. government

e-intensive care: a form of telemedicine designed to enhance the delivery of intensive patient care

e-mail: electronic mail

e-mail virus: a malicious file attached to an e-mail message

employee scheduling system: an electronic system with scheduling rules such as master schedules and shift rotations, repeating patterns for creating a work schedule; used to prevent errors, generate reports, and share data with employees

encryption: a method of protecting vulnerable data from cyber thieves; requires a password to decode and read the files

endnotes: notes displayed at the end of the document

entity: a discrete unit

European Federation for Medical Informatics (EFMI): a professional informatics group representing Europe; has a nursing working group to support European nurses and nursing informatics as well as to build informatics contact networks

Evidence–assertion order (assertion–evidence order): a slide presentation style with visual evidence precedes a slide with the assertion or statement of meaning; termed assertion–evidence order when the assertion slide appears before the evidence slide

evidence-based care: a method of care based on the scientifically proven research

evidence-based nursing: nursing care based upon scientifically proven nursing research

evidence-based practice (EBP): a cyclical process of moving knowledge from original research into patient care

executing: the third stage of the systems life cycle; this phase involves customizing the system to meet the needs of the organization

export: a way to share computer files between programs

external reference: references (links) a cell or a cell range in a spreadsheet located in another workbook; values changed in a linked cell change the referenced cell in another workbook

extraneous cognitive load: unnecessary information delivered in the design of instruction

extranet: an extension of an intranet with added security features, providing accessibility to the intranet to a specific group of outsiders

Facebook: a social media website that provides the ability for users to create personal pages, groups, and includes e-mail messaging and chat features

FaceTime: an app created by Apple that allows iPhone and iPad users to have video calls over Wi-Fi with others who have a Mac computer, iPhone, or iPad

FaceTime Audio: an app created by Apple that allows Apple Mac computers, iPhone, and iPad users to call others using Wi-Fi

factual database: a database that replaces reference books with searchable and updatable online information—for example, drug and laboratory manuals

federated search: a type of computer search that allows you to search several databases simultaneously

fair use: limited use of copyrighted material under the doctrine of fair use; though there is little direction in determining what is fair to use, there are four factors that should be used as a guide: the purpose and character of the use, the nature of the work, the amount of the work used, and the effect on the author or for permissions with widespread use

field: a column in a database table; the smallest structure in a database

figures: graphs, charts, maps, drawings, and photographs

financial management: management of money for decision making; often accomplished using specialized software programs

firewall: a computer network system that blocks incoming and outgoing data using a set of rules

fixed tangible medium: just about every imaginable fixed tangible medium is copyrighted whether or not the individual has applied for copyright protection; users should assume that all written or recorded mediums are copyrighted even if there is no © symbol

flash drive: a data storage device that connects to a computer using a universal serial bus (USB)

flash memory: computer memory that it is nonvolatile, meaning that the applications and data will not disappear after the loss of battery power

flat database: all of the data are located in one table, such as a spreadsheet, worksheet, or an address book, in a word processor; very simple to construct and use but have limitations when it comes to tracking items that belong in a record when there are more than one of the same item

Flesch Reading Ease: measures how easy it is to read text from a formula using the average sentence length and the average number of syllables per word; the recommended score is between 60 and 70

Flesch-Kincaid Grade Level: calculates a U.S. school grade level with a formula that uses the average number of words per sentence and the average number of syllables per word; the recommended Flesch-Kincaid Grade Level for patient education resources is 6

flipped classroom: students complete learning activities (videos, interactive learning modules, etc.) in advance, allowing learners to spend class time using engaged learning activities that reinforce learning

folksonomy: word descriptor tags used for content and often achieved by group consensus

flowcharting: a diagram that uses symbols and arrows to a map process

footnotes: notes located at the bottom of a page

forecasting: determining future needs by reviewing historical trends; data collection is the first step in the process, and 1 to 5 years of data are ideal for forecasting to avoid false conclusions

foreign key: database field located in the detail (child) table that contains data identical to that in the master table, which relates the two tables

form: used to add, edit, and view data from a database table or query; shows all the fields related to that record for which data must be entered, regardless of the base table in which the data are stored

foundational interoperability: the transmission and reception of information so that it is useful, but with no need for interpretation; these systems are able to send and receive usable data from different systems

freeware: an application the programmer has decided to make freely available to anyone who wishes to use it, but it is protected by copyright

freeze: a method to keep one part of a spreadsheet (rows, columns, or both) visible while scrolling to another area on the spreadsheet; important for accurate data entry when the data refer to a heading in a column or row

Gantt chart: tracks a project's progress by showing start to end dates and associated costs with tasks

general systems theory: a method of thinking about complex structures such as an information system or an organization; von Bertalanffy (1973), a biologist, introduced the original theory

genomics: a discipline of genetics related to the study of DNA

germane cognitive load: thought processes or schemas that organize categories of information for storage in long-term memory; slide design should have minimal text, appropriate visual images, and facilitate learners to process information

go-live: the implementation of a new computer system (also known as rollout)

Google Drive: a cloud sharing app that includes software including a word processor, presentation program, spreadsheet, a drawing program, form creator; files can be shared and edited with others

gradient background: a presentation slide that is gradually shaded from a lighter to a darker shade of the same color

grammar check: a proofreading feature that alerts the user of errors, such as subject/verb disagreement, run-one sentences, and split infinitives; a squiggly blue underline is the universal alert for grammatical errors

granularity: the most specific terms, which are on the lowest level of a taxonomy of a database

graphical user interface (GUI): the point and click interface used on computers today

hacked: unauthorized use of an account

handheld computer: handheld mobile devices

hardwired: computers wired together or wired to something that physically exists

harmonization: all the degrees of making standardized terminologies partially interoperable

hashtag: the # sign that identifies the keyword or topic of a social media post

health literacy: the ability to obtain and understand health information for decision making; it includes the capacity to understand instructions on prescription drug bottles, appointment slips, medical education brochures, doctor's directions, consent forms, and the ability to negotiate complex healthcare systems

health numeracy: the ability of a consumer to interpret and act on numerical information to make effective health decisions

health information exchange (HIE): exchange of health information facilitated by the Office of the National Coordinator for Health Information Technology (ONC); includes three types of exchanges: directed, query-based, and consumer mediated

health information technology (HIT): a workforce that can innovate and implement information technology specifically for healthcare

Health Information Technology for Economic and Clinical Health (HITECH) Act: part of the American Recovery and Reinvestment Act and signed into law in 2009, it outlined four purposes: to define meaningful use, to use incentives and grant programs to foster the adoption of EHRs, to gain the trust of the public regarding the privacy and security of electronic healthcare data, and to promote IT innovation

Health Insurance Portability and Accountability Act (HIPAA): a law passed in 1996 that protects the privacy and security of health information and provides patients the right to see their own healthcare records

healthcare data analytics: a movement to integrate financial data, patient data, and quality data to produce predictive and prescriptive analytics for decision makers; also known as business intelligence

healthcare informatics: a discipline specializing in the management of healthcare information with computer technology

healthcare information system (HIS): is a composite made up of all the information management systems that serve an organization's needs. The complexity of HIS is largely independent of the size of the organization because healthcare provides a common core of patient care services

Healthcare Information and Management Systems Society (HIMSS): a not-for-profit professional organization dedicated to promoting a better understanding of healthcare information and management systems; in 2003, HIMSS formed a Nursing Informatics Community to provide support to the nursing role in informatics

hibernate: a deeper sleep than sleep mode for some computers and other devices

hierarchical database: an early database model, it has tables that are organized in the shape of an inverted tree, like an organizational chart; often called a tree structure, records are linked to a base, or root, but through successive layers

high-fidelity manikins: realistic simulated patients or situations; for example, instructors can program high-fidelity manikins to have heart and breath sounds, breathe, and perform physical acts associated with illness, such as coughing or bleeding

HONcode: This icon signifies certification of the website certifies the quality of website health information by the Health on the Net Foundation, an international nonprofit

hotspot: a term used to identify a Wi-Fi–enabled area that allows Wi-Fi–enabled mobile device to connect to the Internet; many hotspots use encryption for security reasons and require the user to enter an access code or pay a fee for use

hoax: a sensational message claiming to contain a virus, though it does not contain one; damaging hoaxes can direct a user to delete a file that is necessary for a computer to function properly

human resource management system (HRMS): a business database system for managing personnel; generally contains four categories: personnel profiles including demographic data; daily work schedules and time-off requests; payroll data; and education, skill qualifications, and licensure information

image map: clickable spots on a graphic, which have hyperlinks to other websites

implementation: a significant milestone in transitioning to a new computer system that needs to be carefully planned

index: a system used to file or catalog references and provides the mechanism for database searches

informatics: computer information systems science

informatics nurse: one who enters the nursing informatics field because of an interest or experience

informatics nurse specialist: a nurse with either a graduate education degree in nursing informatics or a field relating to informatics who has successfully passed an American Nurses Credentialing Center (ANCC) specialty certification exam

informatics theory: a branch of applied probability theory that builds on information theory and uses concepts from change theories, systems theory, chaos theory, cognitive theory, and sociotechnical theory

information literacy: the ability to know when one needs information and how to locate, evaluate, and effectively use it

information technology: the use of informatics, with a focus on information management, not computers

information technology skills: the ability to use computers, computer software, and peripherals to access electronic information efficiently

initiating: every computer system begins with an idea; in the critical initiating phase, project planners identify and analyze the project goals and needs

instructional games: educational games that add a competitive contest aspect to learning by motivating students to learn the needed information, foster collaboration, problem solving, and analytical thinking

intangibles: those values that are not easily calculated or in which the results cannot be directly attributed to the investment; examples include improved decision-making, communication, and user satisfaction

integrated: uniting separate entities into a whole

integrated enterprise system: information system designed to meet the needs of the organization at large, which may include multiple geographically separated hospitals and clinics

integrated interface: the selection of a collection of health information systems that are already interfaced; however, the systems may not all be best of breed

interdisciplinary terminology: terminology that can be used across disciplines in healthcare; the ANA recognizes three interdisciplinary terminologies: the Systematized Nomenclature of Medicine Clinical Terminology (SNOMED CT); Logical Observations: Identifiers, Names, Codes (LOINC); and the Alternative Billing Codes (ABC)

interface terminology: terminology that allows the exchange of computer clinical information with the user

International Medical Informatics Association (IMIA): an international scientific organization established in 1967 as TC4, a Technical Committee within the International Federation for Information Processing; the goals include promoting informatics in healthcare, promoting biomedical research, advancing international cooperation, stimulating informatics research and education, and exchanging information

Internet protocol (IP): a computer communication technology created by the U.S. Defense Advanced Research Projects Agency

Internet radio: a social media form for streaming audio using the Internet

Internet telephone: computer software and hardware that can perform functions usually associated with a telephone

interoperable: data can be shared electronically, such as in an electronic health record

interoperability: is the ability of two or more systems to pass information between them and to use the exchanged information; in healthcare, it means that healthcare information systems can transmit and receive information within and across organizational boundaries to provide the delivery of optimum healthcare to individuals and communities

intrinsic cognitive load: the difficulty of problem solving or making sense of the learning material

invisible/deep web: sites not reachable by traditional search tools

IP address: an identifier of four sets of numbers separated by periods or dots, making it possible for each computer on the Internet to be electronically located

Internet service provider (ISP): a company that provides Internet access; uses a modem and router to connect devices to the Internet

intranet: a private network within an organization, which allows users of an organization to share information, including features similar to the Internet, such as e-mail, mailing lists, and user groups

journal manuscripts: a paper written for journal readers

keylogger: a software program that tracks all keystrokes made by a user; can be used to trace and steal passwords and bank account numbers

keywords: tags used to identify the topics discussed in a paper, which serve as search terms

knowledge-based database: indexes published literature; focuses on areas such as health sciences, business, history, government, law, and ethics

layout layer: builds on the background layer in the number and types of placeholders it has for different layouts in a presentation file

learning assessment: quizzes and surveys provide a means for assessing learning, which can be administered via a computer

learning content management system (LCMS): a database system that stores and manages learning resources authored by faculty and content experts; LCMS learning resources such as course content modules, slides, video clips, illustrations, and quiz questions can be assembled into course learning content by using infinitely changeable combinations according to the instructor's needs

learning management system (LMS): database software that facilitates delivering course content electronically; can be as simple as delivering learning content, scoring computer-learning activities, and providing printable certificates of course completion, but other features include e-mail, discussion forums, virtual student work areas, chat, wikis, and blogs

learning style: the way a person perceives, remembers, expresses, and solves problems

learning theories: conceptual frameworks that support how people learn

lecture replacement model: a slide presentation style that requires text or narration to guide the audience viewer; because the tutorial replaces a lecture, the learning objectives must be explicit to the viewer and very detailed

lecture support model: also known as the slide presentation supplement model, can guide audiences to follow the oral presentation; the slides should help an audience keep track of ideas and illustrate points but not include the entire talk

Lessig style: a fast-paced slide presentation style used when the content is not detailed; slides use text visuals of a few words or quotes to engage the viewers

lexical: a word-for-word match when mapping terminology

line chart: a chart that uses lines to connect data: one type communicates changes in elapsed time period data and one type shows data trends; the category data are displayed on the horizontal axis and the data values displayed on the vertical axis

line spacing: the amount of space between lines of text; the default setting in word processors is single space

linear list: an alphabetical list such as a dictionary

linked: one term is related, or often used, with another; terms may be presented together for documentation purposes

LinkedIn: a professional social networking site that provides a way to connect with other business professionals, share information, or look for new career opportunities

Listserv: an e-mail discussion list that has participants who discuss various aspects of a topic

local area network (LAN): a network confined to a small area such as a building or groups of buildings

lookup table: a database table that provides a list of allowable entries for a field that is linked to that field

low-fidelity manikin: a human simulation that is not true to life; often used for learning skills such as nasogastric insertion

mail merge: a word processing feature that takes a set of data and places the different pieces into the desired place in a document; it can be used for labels, letters, and e-mail

malware: all forms of computer software designed by criminals, often for a profit, to damage or disrupt a computer system

mapping: a form of matching concepts from one standardized terminology with those having similar meaning from another

margins: the amount of white space between the edge of the document and the text

meaningful use: the use of aggregated data from electronic health records for decision making to improve healthcare delivery

medical subject headings (MeSH): the controlled vocabulary of terms used to index materials in PubMed and MEDLINE databases; MeSH differs from many other subject heading lists because the basis is a hierarchal structure

meta-analysis: research on previous research—systematic reviews

Metathesaurus: developed by UMLS, it is a list of concepts and terms from health-related standardized vocabularies and is used by the UMLS to index literature

metropolitan area network (MAN): a network that encompasses a city or town

microblogging: very brief web journaling; text-based communication tools include Twitter, text messaging, and chat

microdata: nonaggregated, individual responses

minimum data set: a list of categories of data, each of which has an agreed definition as to what it includes; they specify the type of data that will meet the essential needs of data users for a specific purpose, such as billing

mission critical: the services are vital to the existence of the organization

modem: a device that transmits digital information

multiaxial taxonomies: a classification system with two or more axes, used for standardizing nursing language in computer documentation

multimedia: any combination of hardware and software that displays images or plays sound

National Database of Nursing Quality Indicators (NDNQI): a national database to which hospitals submit nursing-sensitive data about structure, process, and outcomes of nursing care; the NDNQI aggregates the data quarterly and returns reports to participating hospitals

Nationwide Health Information Network (NwHIN): a foundation for secure information exchange of healthcare data over the Internet using a "a set of standards, services, and policies," according to HealthIT.gov

natural language: one's everyday speaking tongue, which is very expressive and requires no change in how you think when using it in documentation

navigation bars: graphical bars across the top of a page that provide multiple choices and need alternative methods of access

needs assessment: an initial step of the systems life cycle that comparable to a brainstorming session to identify the requirements of a computer system

network: a connection of two or more computers, which allows the computers to communicate

network authentication: a standard for work and home computer networks that requires a user to enter an authentication code to use a secure Wi-Fi network

network model: similar to the hierarchical database model, but the trees can share branches; because of the data structure, the network model is complex and inflexible

nodes: tiny routers with a few wireless cards and antennas that pick up signals sent by a user and transmit them to the central server or rebroadcast them to another node

normal view: the default creation mode in a slide presentation file

normalization rules: used in relational databases to organize, aggregate, and display data; each table represents a category of data, and each field should be unique to the database

nursing informatics: subspecialty of nursing that focuses on managing information pertaining to nursing

Nursing Informatics Working Group (NIWG): responsible for promoting the integration of nursing informatics into the broader context of healthcare; also works to influence U.S. policy makers regarding the use of nursing information

nursing knowledge: information known to nursing practice, which defines the profession

Nurse Licensure Compact (NLC): endorsed by the National Council of State Boards of Nursing (NCSBN) as a framework for regulating the interstate practice of nursing for RNs and LPNs/VNs; under this concept, nurses holding a valid license in one state could practice (both physically in person and electronically by using the telephone or telemedicine connectivity to assess and provide care) in other states, according to the rules and regulations of the states

Office of the National Coordinator for Health Information Technology (ONC): created by President George W. Bush in 2004 to move toward electronic health records, creates and implements strategic plans to improve health and healthcare for all Americans through information and technology

one-to-many relationship: a database concept that describes the relationship of records in tables where one record in a table can have many records in a related table; for example, one patient can have many medications or hospitalizations

OneDrive: a Microsoft cloud storage app that allows a user to access and sync files from a computer, tablet, or smartphone

ontology: the highest level of organization of a terminology; complex and powerful, it provides the ability for concepts to be represented and linked to more than one concept

open access journals: journals that publish peer-reviewed articles with no user fees; many have limited copyright/licensing restrictions and allow anyone with an Internet connection to download, copy, and distribute the articles

open source: software that has copyright protection, but the source code is available to anyone who wants it

operating system: the most important program on a computer; coordinates input from the keyboard with output on the screen, responds to mouse and touchpad clicks, heeds commands to save a file, retrieves files, transmits commands to printers and other peripheral devices, and provides access to applications

out-of-office reply: a feature that will automatically send an out-of-office e-mail to each person who sent an e-mail

outline view: a viewing mode in a presentation file that provides a user the ability to enter and edit information

output: the end result of input, whether it is from a computer or a process

page break (hard page return or forced page break): begins the next section of text on a new page; the four main sections of an APA paper (title page, abstract, body of the paper, and reference list) must be separated with a page break

page header: a separate section located at the top of a page that can be used for a running head and page number

page ruler: assists with formatting functions, such as modifying/setting tabs and creating a hanging indent used for the reference list

paragraph headings: name the sections of a paper and assist the reader to understand what to anticipate in the section that follows a heading

parallel conversion: information system transition that requires the operation and support of the new and the old computer system for a period of time

parameter query: queries that require the user to enter a constraint to define data output; only records that match that "parameter" are returned

parent–child relationship: a database term that describes the master table and the associated related tables

passive RFID: requires the use of a barcode or radio frequency identifier (RFID) scanner that is either handheld or built into a laptop or tab-

let computer; often used in closed loop medication administration in healthcare settings

patient classification systems: database systems that estimate the care needs of inpatients for prudent staffing decisions

patient portal: a secure website that provides patients access to their EHR data

patient throughput: also known as workflow, it is one of the challenges in complex, acute-care hospitals, which improves using service queues with alerts for priority; synchronization of patient rooms, tasks, equipment, and services; and hospital performance dashboards to keep managers informed in real time

patient values: according to the Institute of Medicine, "refers to the unique preferences, concerns, and expectations that each patient brings to a clinical encounter" that are used when making clinical decisions (Institute of Medicine (U.S.). Committee on Quality of Health Care in America. (2001; p. 47, para 2). *Crossing the quality chasm: A new health system for the 21st century.* Washington, DC: National Academy Press. Retrieved from http://www.nap.edu/openbook. php?isbn=0309072808)

peer-reviewed article: a journal article that was blind reviewed by two or more nurse experts for a blind review to assure the validity, quality, and reliability of information

personal health record (PHR): a record of health information owned by the individual; may be maintained using computer document or a paper record

personal identification number (PIN): an identifier used to gain computer access

personal information management: most mobile devices include this software, such as contact information, a calendar, and a clock

personal reference manager: a user can export search findings into this software; other common features include the ability to store digital copies of full-text articles and the ability to cite sources and automatically generate a formatted reference list while writing with word processing software

pharming: a web scam that tries to get personal information from an individual, resulting from when an attacker infiltrates a domain name server and changes the routing for addresses

phased conversion: a computer system implementation strategy used to bring up a new system gradually in a controlled environment; done incrementally with several alternative approaches

phishing: a web scam that tries to get personal information from an individual, resulting from an individual receiving an e-mail message with a web address hyperlink, clicking on it, and confirming an account or entering personal information

photo sharing: a popular social media form that provides the ability to share photos with others as well as the ability to upload files

Physician Quality Report Initiative (PQRI): an innovative reimbursement incentive effort to reward quality care by the Centers for Medicare & Medicaid Services (CMS).

PICO (PICOT, PICOTT): a standard used today to investigate evidence-based care in medicine and nursing; the abbreviation stands for patient, problem, or population; intervention; comparison; outcome; and in some cases represents time, type of question, and/or type of study (if added to the end of the abbreviation)

piconet: a personal area connection created when a user has Bluetooth enabled on a mobile device and pairs it with another Bluetooth device

pie charts: communicate the proportion of various items in relation to the whole (classified as area charts); they are "part-to-whole" charts designed to show percentages, not amounts, and use only one data series

pilot conversion: a computer system implementation strategy done to "test the waters" to see what issues might occur when making a transition to a new computer information system; this approach enables the testing of a system on a smaller scale

plain old telephone service (POTS): an Internet connection using a dial-up modem through a regular telephone line, often used in rural areas

plagiarism: using another's work as your own; two common types include copying the exact text written by others without citing the source and reordering the words of a source text without citing the source

Plaxo: a social networking online address book that syncs the cloud address book with other devices, such as smartphones and tablets

podcasting: sharing audio and video content on the web; some developers publish podcasts as a theme series on a specific subject and make the podcasts available as RSS feeds

podcatching: software that allows users to aggregate podcast feeds and play podcasts on their computers, smartphones, and tablet devices

portable monitoring devices: include an input device and various types of peripheral monitoring equipment; many of the input devices use a touch screen with text and audio to ask assessment questions about the patient's health

positive patient identifier (PPID): uses a bracelet with a barcode to verify the patient's identification

post-coordinated terms: taxonomy terms used in documentation that follow the axes and categories determined for combinational vocabulary

pre-coordinated terms: taxonomy terms prepared by experts in a field by combining the terms from the various axes

Prezi: presentation software that uses zooming to navigate to images on a single canvas

primary key: the unique identifier of a record in a table of a database

privacy: the right of patients to control what happens to their personal health information

Privacy Rights Clearinghouse: maintains an online record of all types of security breaches at http://www.privacyrights.org/; according to the website, there have been a staggering number of security breaches in recent years

process improvement: the application of actions taken to identify, analyze, and improve existing processes within an organization to meet requirements for quality, customer satisfaction, and financial goals

professional networking: a subset of social media, where interactions focus on business themes

progressive disclosure: a slide presentation technique in which items are revealed one at a time until all the items on a slide display

project goal: a succinct statement that describes the project in the systems life cycle

project requirements: involves using a needs assessment to identify the expectations or requirements of the computer system in the systems life cycle; data and information pertinent to the project goal and scope are put together and translated to the needs for the system

project scope: all the elements that are entailed in the project in the systems life cycle

proprietary: commercial software that has copyright protection and must be purchased; users must accept the terms of use prior to installation

protocols: a system of rules required for data transfer

public domain software: software with no copyright restrictions that can be used in any way the user desires, including making changes

quality improvement: a process to improve outcomes by the introduction of change, repeat measurement, and comparison of outcomes over time

Quality and Safety Education for Nurses (QSEN): an initiative initially funded by the Robert Wood Johnson Foundation that is now hosted by Case Western Reserve University, which focuses on six competencies of nursing, including patient-centered care, teamwork and collaboration, evidence-based practice, quality improvement, safety, and informatics

query: the search function for a relational database; one of the characteristics that make databases powerful

QWERTY keyboard: a keyboard layout common to the PC and typewriter that comprises the first six letters on the top row of letters; data using a QWERTY keyboard is available on all smartphones and tablets

radio frequency identifier (RFID): data stored on a small microchip, which a specialized reader can interpret; used on bracelets as a positive patient identifier (PPID) to verify the patient's identification and also used to track medical equipment

random-access memory (RAM): one of three types of built-in memory for mobile devices, it stores all of the add-on applications and data files and requires a small amount of continuous battery power; this memory is volatile; hence, all of the data stored in RAM are lost with the depletion of the battery life

randomized controlled trials (RCTs): highest priority or evidence is derived from meta-analysis of these trials and evidence-based clinical guidelines based on systematic reviews of them

readability: the difficulty of reading text

read-only memory (ROM): one of three types of built-in memory for mobile devices, it stores the operating and standard applications such as contacts, calendar, and notes

real simple syndication (RSS): a feed for websites such as news and blogs to notify a user when there is new information on the site; also called rich site summary

real-time telehealth: involves the patient and the provider interacting at the same time by using interactive video/television; requires the use of telecommunications devices that permit two-way communication

record: a row in a database table; all the information about a single "member" of a table

reference terminology: works behind the scenes, taking a documentation term and giving it a code related to concepts at a higher level to allow a broader analysis

reference terminology model: refers to a set of terms based upon evidence-based research; some of the potential uses for this model include facilitating the documentation of nursing problems (diagnosis) and actions (interventions) in electronic information systems

references: a list of sources used in a paper; the fourth section of an APA paper

Regional Extension Centers (RECs): a component of the Health Information Technology Extension Program; trained staff members assist healthcare providers to understand and implement the electronic health record adoption, and educational components include vendor selection, workflow analysis necessary to decide on a vendor, and how to meet meaningful use requirements.

regression testing: refers to application functionality in computer systems

relational database: a flexible database model which uses two or more tables connected by identical information in key fields in each table, which allows the data in a record from one table to be matched to any piece or pieces of data in records in another table

repeat header row: a word processing table feature, when selected, the header row will appear on the subsequent page(s); use with tables that span across multiple pages

report: often used for printing information from data in a table(s) or query, it provides data organized to fulfill user need

request for information (RFI): a document sent with a summary of information to vendors, and the information from the return of the RFI is used to determine which vendors should be considered in the development of a new computer system

request for proposal (RFP): a detailed document sent to potential vendors asking for information on how their product will meet the users' needs

Research Information Systems (RIS): this format consists of a standardized tag that allows for data exchange between digital library databases and reference citation managers

research practice gap: emerges when there are differences between clinical practice and the research on effective clinical practice; nurses must expedite closing the research practice gap in order to make dramatic, needed improvements to our healthcare delivery system

ResearchGate: a professional networking site for researchers and scientists that allows members to share research, post published papers, and collaborate with others

restricted license: the result of a framework for regulating interstate practice developed by the Federation of State Medical Boards in 1996; allowed for the ability to practice telemedicine across state lines, though the decision to adopt the license was left to the individual state boards

return on investment (ROI): the cost savings that are realized as a result of an investment

rich site summary (RSS): a feed for websites such as news and blogs to notify a user when there is new information on the site; also called real simple syndication

robotics: the use of robots; used in a variety of healthcare settings

Rogers' Diffusion of Innovations Theory: first published in a 1962 book of the same name; the theory examines the pattern of acceptance that innovations follow as they spread across the population and the process of decision making that occurs in individuals when deciding whether to adopt an innovation

rollback: backing out of the implementation of a computer system; the cancellation of the system implementation

rollout: once there is agreement that the computer system meets the user requirements, the staff members are trained and the system is implemented (also known as go-live)

router: a device that connects multiple devices to the same network; has one or two antennas (which may be internal) to transmit the Wi-Fi signal

save as: in many software programs, a way to save a file in a different format

scholarly nursing journal: written by only qualified nurses with expertise in the subject area; articles are rigorously peer reviewed prior to publication

scholarly writing: includes a variety of venues, including online discussion postings, master's theses, doctoral dissertations, and journal manuscripts

scope creep: describes unanticipated growth of the project that can result in cost overruns; it can develop because of "we don't miss what we never had" situations

screen reader: computer accessibility feature with speech recognition for those with limited eyesight; can translate text to speech, and some readers can send information to a Braille reader

secondary data: data analyzed for purposes other than the purpose of the original collection

security: the measures implemented to prevent unauthorized users access to the personal health information of patients

self-plagiarism: it occurs when authors take work they previously published and present it as new

semantic: a match on the same meaning or a synonym when mapping terminology

semantic interoperability: information transmitted is understandable, and at its highest level, the interpretation and action on messages exchanged by two computers occurs without human intervention; the effectiveness of it depends on the interaction between algorithms (rules), the data used in the message, and the terminology used to designate that data

seminal work: work frequently cited by others or that influences the opinions of others

Sharable Content Object Reference Model (SCORM): technical standard that allows sharing of learning content with SCORM compliant learning management systems (LMSs)

shareware: developers encourage users to give copies of the software to friends and colleagues to try out for a trial period; the software is protected by copyright

Skype: a Voice over Internet Protocol program that allows free Skype-to-Skype voice and video calls, instant messaging, and file sharing

simulation: imitates actual experiences and has many uses, such as part of an orientation or in-service program, a face-to-face classroom or clinical laboratory setting, or as part of a homework assignment; effective simulations match the learner's knowledge background, or are, at least, only slightly above it, and the point of view addresses the learning needs

single sign-on: allows the user to access multiple clinical applications with only one login/password for authentication; an issue for the use of clinical information systems

sleep mode: occurs after a given period of inactivity on all computers, including tablets and smartphones; saves energy but allows a user quick access to files after taking a break

slideshow view: the view that audiences see in a slide presentation; only for viewing, not editing

slide sorter view: a slide presentation view that shows many slides on one screen and is used for viewing and rearranging all the slides

smart card: looks like a plastic credit card and, like a credit card, has embedded information that a smart card reader can read; requires the appropriate computer system and access code to read and write, encrypts the data on the card

smartphone: cell phones with Internet connectivity

social bookmarking: saves bookmarks to the cloud where they are available on an individual's computers and devices with an Internet connection

social engineering: tricks victims into downloading and installing malware

social informatics: holds that a good design is based on an understanding of how people work and the context of the work, not just technologic considerations

social media: allows people to share their stories, pictures, videos, and thoughts with others online using the Internet; there are four main classifications of social media: networking sites, blogging, microblogging, and content sharing

social networking: websites that serve to connect millions of users worldwide

sociotechnical theory: originated in the middle of the last century when it became evident that not all implementations of technology were increasing productivity; the overall focus of this

theory is the impact of technology's implementation on an organization

software piracy: using a copyrighted program without following the rules for use

speaker notes: a feature in slide presentation software that can help a speaker remember information for a given slide; when the slideshow is projected, only the slide is visible to the audience, but the speaker can print notes associated with the slides

spear phishing: a tactic used to steal patient information, criminal hackers use it to lure the care provider into revealing private information; in this case, hackers send what appears to be legitimate business e-mail from a person well known to the e-mail recipient, which lures an employee into revealing private login information

speech recognition: the ability to translate the spoken work into text

spelling check: a tool in word processors to avoid misspelled words; a squiggly red underline is a universal alert for a misspelled word

spreadsheet: an electronic version of a table consisting of a grid of rectangles (cells) arranged in columns and rows; can be uniquely formatted to display numbers, text data, and formulas

spyware: tracks web surfing to tailor advertisements to the user, often appearing like legitimate adware; can monitor keystrokes and transmit it to a third party as well as scan hard drives, read cookies, and change default home pages on web browsers

stacked chart: a bar chart that is a part-to-whole chart that measures in percentage; each data set uses as its baseline the previous data set, and stacked bar charts compare differences in groups of clustered data

standards: an agreement to use a given protocol, term, or other criterion formally approved by a nationally or internationally recognized professional trade association or governmental body

Stark Rules: the name for the Physician Self-Referral Law, which is an effort to prevent Medicare fraud; however, it has been criticized for interfering with collaborative innovations and limiting the ability of healthcare agencies and providers to design seamless solutions for sharing healthcare information using technology, so the law was relaxed in August 2006 to provide an incentive for physicians to adopt a certified electronic health record

statistical analysis: nurse researchers can collect data, manage them in databases, and analyze them with specialized programs; with attention to the principles of data analysis, other nurses can benefit from the use of statistical analysis to improve decision making and outcomes

static IP address: an Internet protocol (IP) address that remains the same each time a computer connects to the Internet

stop words: words, such as articles and prepositions, which a search engine generally does not search for unless they are a part of a phrase enclosed with quotes

store and forward (S&F): a telehealth technology where a digital camera, scanner, or technology (e.g., x-ray machine) that generates electronic images captures a still image electronically and then that image is sent to a specialist for interpretation later

storyboard: a plan for the visuals of a presentation that forces a presenter to organize thoughts and assemble them into a coherent presentation

strategic plan: a roadmap that guides the institution in meeting its mission, directs decision-making practices over a 3- or 5- to 10-year period, guides the acquisition of resources and budget priorities, and serves as a living and breathing document that allows for flexibility

streaming video: a technique where a sequence of compressed moving images, sent over the Internet, plays by a media viewer as they arrive

structural interoperability: a concept intended to coordinate work processes and refers to the uniform format or structure of the exchanged messages; data exchanged between information systems allows for interpretation at the data field level

Structured Query Language (SQL): the name of the coding that is used for querying in many databases; an ANSI (American National Standards Institute) standard computer language for retrieving and updating data in a database

subset: a smaller set of terms from a larger group of terms

subject heading: a standardized term used to index or catalog reference materials; each library chooses a standard subject authority or thesaurus for all of its cataloging

superuser: an individual identified to assist in the computer system building and testing; should be clinical nurses and staff who are recruited from each of the areas where the system will be deployed

support groups: use a variety of online forums, for example, patient portals, social networking websites, message boards, e-mail lists, chat rooms, or any combination of these

synchronize (sync): technology that allows users to share files between devices through a cloud sharing application where changes are copied back and forth

synchronistic learning: class is held at set times and all participants are "present," either online or in the classroom

systematic review: a research process designed to carefully review and analyze the results of multiple, similar research studies; reduces three types of bias inherent in individual research studies: selection, indexing, and publication

systems life cycle: the process that begins with the conception of a computer system until the system is implemented

table of contents: a table that includes the main headings used in a paper and the associated page numbers

table: a database collection of related information that consists of records, and each record is made up of a number of fields; database professionals refer to a table as an entity or file

tangibles: those values that can be clearly measured, calculated, and quantified with numerical data; examples include a decrease in length of stay, a decrease in anti-infective medication costs, a decrease in the number of unnecessary medications and tests, and a decrease in charges per admission

taxonomic vocabulary: grouping terms with conceptual similarities into groups that share a common concept, such as pain; examples of taxonomic vocabularies are the North American Nursing Diagnosis Association–International (NANDA-I) and the Nursing Interventions Classification (NIC)

TEACH Act: passed in 2002, it relaxed the copyright law as it applies to distance learning and nonprofit educational institutions, though what constitutes fair use is still blurred

Technology Informatics Guiding Educational Reform (TIGER): an initiative whose objective is to make nursing informatics competencies part of every nurse's skillset for the 21st century so nurses can deliver safer, high-quality, evidence-based care

TED (Technology-Entertainment Design) style: a slide presentation style that uses commanding images with or without a few words to convey meaning in a presentation; each slide conveys a message

telehealth: health services delivered using electronic technology to patients at a distance; extends beyond the delivery of clinical services

telehomecare: the monitoring and delivery of healthcare in the patient's home rather than the provider's work setting; the greatest use of telehomecare is that it allows the patient the comforts of his or her own home, improves quality of life, and avoids time-consuming costly visits to office appointments or hospital admissions

telemedicine: the electronic exchange of health information between two sites using telecommunication tools

telemental health: use of telehealth to deliver psychiatric healthcare

telenursing: using telehealth to provide home nursing care; defined by the International Council of Nursing as telecommunications technology in nursing to enhance patient care

telepresence: the use of technology to provide the appearance of a person's presence, although he or she is located at a remote site

teletrauma: used to obtain second opinions and advice from trauma care experts; used by rural hospitals and clinics and parts of the world torn by violence and war

test scripts: a set of situations devised to depict normal and abnormal events that could occur; also called scenarios and used to test computer systems

text speak: a new language system that uses letter, numbers, and symbols instead of spelling out words

theme: a predesigned combination of background colors, font style, size, and color in a slide presentation file

title page: contains the running head, page number, author name, and institutional affiliation; one of four sections of an APA paper

track changes: a review feature to use when collaborating with others; the tool will enable the author to see proposed changes while maintaining the ability to see the original document

transmission control protocol (TCP): a computer communication technology created by the U.S. Defense Advanced Research Projects Agency

Trojan horse: appears to be a program that performs a useful action or is fun, such as a game, but when the program runs, it places malicious software on a computer or creates a backdoor

Tumblr: is part microblog and part social networking that allows for posting text, customizing photos, links, quotes, videos, and e-mail from any location

tutorial: step-by-step program designed to guide learners to understand information; well-designed tutorials are interactive, present the learning content, and then provide the learner with self-assessment multiple-choice questions

Twitter: a mini-blogging platform where an individual can send messages of 140 characters or less, known as "tweets," to family, friends, or the general web community; photos and short videos can also be shared

two-factor authentication: requires personal information for account changes to prevent unauthorized users from hacking an account

Unified Medical Language System (UMLS): according to the National Library of Medicine, "the UMLS integrates and distributes key terminology, classification and coding standards, and associated resources to promote creation of more effective interoperable biomedical information services, including electronic health records" (National Library of Medicine. (2014, February 18). *UMLS®*. Retrieved from http://www.nlm.nih.gov/research/umls/

unintended consequences: outcomes, good or bad, that were not planned or deliberate

unique patient identifier (UPI): a single source that links each patient with his or her individual health record

universal resource locator (URL): assigned to all web documents and contain descriptors, a domain name (a unique name that identifies a website), and may include a folder name, a file name, or both

USB port: installed on a computer that allows a device with a universal serial bus (USB) connection to be plugged in and accessed on the computer

urban legends: stories thought to be factual by those who pass them on that are often sensationalist, distorted, or exaggerated; often sent through e-mail

usability: websites should meet certain criteria to make them useable for their audience, including considering location of drop-down menus, the amount of information on the screen, the font size, the amount of instructions for finding videos, and navigation issues; the site needs to be compliant with the American Disability Act usability principles

usability theory: represents a multidimensional concept and involves users' evaluation of several measures, each one representative of their effectiveness in performing a task; involves the ease of use, users' satisfaction that they have achieved their goals, and the aesthetics of the technology

user liaison: in this role, the informatics nurse is the communications link between nurses and others involved in computer-related matters

value-based purchasing: a Centers for Medicare & Medicaid initiative that reward hospitals with incentives to improve the quality of care, prevent errors, and improve patient satisfaction in hospitals

vanilla product: a standard product provided by a computer vendor without any enhancements; it is similar to the default formatting in a word processing program

vaporware: broken promises of computer system products made by the vendor

video sharing: a popular social media form that provides the ability to share videos with others as well as the ability to upload files; popular video sharing sites include YouTube and Vimeo

Vimeo: a video sharing website that includes the ability to search and find video, as well as post user-generated video

virtual private network (VPN): an intranet with an extra layer of security that operates as an extranet, which allows an organization to communicate confidentially by transmitting a file using an encrypted tunnel blocking view of the file by others

virtual reality (VR): allows the participant to exist in another reality using allusions, where the participant experiences an event that appears real but does not physically exist; the objective is to create a scene in which the participant is free to concentrate on the tasks, problems, and ideas that he or she would face in the real situation

visible/surface web: sites reachable by traditional search engines

visual literacy: a "set of abilities that enables an individual to effectively find, interpret, evaluate, use, and create images and visual media" (Association of Colleges and Research Libraries. (2011). ACRL Visual Literacy Competency Standards for Higher Education. Accessed from http://www.ala.org/acrl/standards/visualliteracy); the level of visual literacy must be considered when using visuals in a presentation

Voice over the Internet Protocol (VoIP): terminology for telephony products, which allow one to make a telephone call anywhere in the world with voice and video by using the Internet, thereby bypassing the phone company

voice recognition: another type of biometric used for security; creates voiceprints using a combination of two authentication factors: What is said and the way that it is said

warez: illegal and pirated software used by botnets

Web 2.0: a descriptor for what online companies/services that survived the dot.com bubble burst in 2000 had in common; includes the shift from only reading to reading, interacting, and writing on the Internet

Web browser (browser): a tool enabling users to retrieve and display files from the Internet

Web conferencing: similar to an open telephone call, but with the added element of video; provides participants with the ability to mark up documents or images, as well as "chat" by using a keyboard

Webcast: a one-way presentation, usually with video, to an audience who may be present either in a room or in a different geographical location

Webinar: a live seminar over the Internet where users must log in to a website address;

audience members can ask questions during the presentation and the speaker can ask for feedback

wide area network (WAN): a network that encompasses a large geographical area; might be two or more local area networks

Wi-Fi protected access (WPA): a Wi-Fi security measure

Wi-Fi protected access 2 (WPA2): a Wi-Fi security measure that is better than Wi-Fi protected access because it uses an advanced encryption standard

wiki: a piece of server software that allows users to freely create and edit content on a web page using any web browser; allows for collaborative knowledge sharing

wired equivalent privacy (WEP): a Wi-Fi security measure

wireless (Wi-Fi): a network connection where a device does not need to be hard wired to the Internet but connects to it using a modem and router, which emits a signal through an antenna

workbook: a spreadsheet file containing one or more spreadsheets; a user can change the order of the sheets, add, or delete sheets from a workbook

workflow analysis: analyzes and depicts how work is accomplished; a critical component of the computer system planning phase

workflow redesign: one of the many difficult issues that healthcare providers face when planning and designing the application of electronic systems; this includes the lack of experience or lack of knowledge about other ways to accomplish work, resistance to change, the tedious processes involved in identifying how work changes with a technology solution, which involves creating process flow diagrams that paint "before" and "after" pictures of workflow and the nuts-and-bolts questions about the presence of computers

worksheet: one spreadsheet in a workbook file; it is best to use a separate worksheet for each table in a workbook

worm: a small piece of malware that uses security holes and computer networks to replicate itself

writing bias: distortion of information that others might interpret as prejudice, such as terminology used for labels, gender, sexual orientation, racial and ethnic identity, disabilities, and age

YouTube: a video sharing website that includes the ability to search and find video, as well as post user-generated video

Index